How to access the supplemental online course, *Cardiorespiratory Fitness Assessment and Prescription, Version 1.2*

We are pleased to provide access to an online course that supplements your textbook *Advanced Fitness Assessment and Exercise Prescription, Fifth Edition*. This course is a great way for you to apply what you have learned in the text. The course has four main units that can be completed at your own pace over the course of a semester.

Accessing the online course is easy! Simply follow these steps:

1. Using your Web browser, go to the Academic Online Education Center Web site at: **http://academic.hkeducationcenter.com**.

2. Click on the MY COURSES button on the left navigation bar.

3. Click on the **Click Here To Register with HK Academic OEC** link. You will create your personal profile and password at this time.

4. Write your e-mail and password down for future reference. Keep it in a safe place.

5. Once you are registered, on the My Courses page of the site, click on the Enter Key Code button.

6. Enter your code exactly as it is printed at the right, including all hyphens. Click Verify

7. Once you have successfully registered, use the <u>click here to continue</u> link to advance to the My Courses page.

8. Click on » **Cardiorespiratory Fitness Assessment & Prescription, Version 1.2** to access the course and test. You will have 1 year from your first course entry to complete the course and test.

If you are taking the course as part of a university or academic course, you may be requested to register as part of your class. To do this, follow the steps above. When you have reached step 8:

- Click the <u>Join Class</u> link located under the course title.
- To join a class, you will be asked to enter your Student ID number (this is your university student ID) and your class code. You should obtain the class code from your instructor.

After you enter the key code the first time, you will not need to use it again to access the course or test. In the future, simply log in (after clicking on the My Courses link) using your e-mail and the password you created.

For technical support, send an e-mail to:
support@hkusa.com . . . . U.S. and international customers
info@hkcanada.com . . . . Canadian customers
academic@hkeurope.com . . . . European customers
keycodesupport@hkaustralia.com . . . . Australian customers

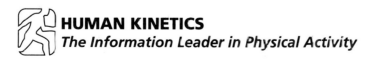

HUMAN KINETICS
The Information Leader in Physical Activity

Product: Cardiorespiratory Fitness Assessment and Prescription, Version 1.2

HFFT115V12-TS4V77J3-OEC

Key code:

This unique code allows you access to the online course

Access is provided if you have purchased a new book. Once submitted, the code may not be entered for any other user.

Fifth Edition

Advanced Fitness Assessment and Exercise Prescription

Vivian H. Heyward, PhD
University of New Mexico

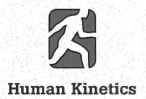

Human Kinetics

Library of Congress Cataloging-in-Publication Data

Heyward, Vivian H.
Advanced fitness assessment and exercise prescription / Vivian H. Heyward. -- 5th ed.
    p. cm.
Includes bibliographical references and index.
ISBN-13: 978-0-7360-5732-5 (hard cover)
ISBN-10: 0-7360-5732-3 (hard cover)
1. Physical fitness--Testing. 2. Exercise tests. 3. Health. I. Title.
GV436.H48 2006
613.7--dc22   2006011631

ISBN-10: 0-7360-5732-3
ISBN-13: 978-0-7360-5732-5

The Web addresses cited in this text were current as of June 14, 2006 unless otherwise noted.

Acquisitions Editor: Michael S. Bahrke, PhD; **Developmental Editor:** Amanda S. Ewing; **Assistant Editors:** Lee Alexander and Maureen Eckstein; **Copyeditor:** Jocelyn Engman; **Proofreader:** Erin Cler; **Indexer:** Betty Frizzéll; **Permission Manager:** Carly Breeding; **Graphic Designer:** Bob Reuther; **Graphic Artist:** Angela K. Snyder; **Photo Manager:** Sarah Ritz; **Cover Designer:** Keith Blomberg; **Photographer (interior):** Sarah Ritz, except where otherwise noted. Figures 8.1, 8.2, & 8.12a-b © Human Kinetics. **Art Manager:** Kelly Hendren; **Illustrator:** Craig Newsom; **Printer:** United Graphics

We thank the Exercise Physiology Laboratory at the University of New Mexico in Albuquerque, New Mexico, for assistance in providing the location for the photo shoot for this book.

Printed in the United States of America

10   9   8   7   6   5   4   3   2   1

Human Kinetics
Web site: www.HumanKinetics.com

United States: Human Kinetics
P.O. Box 5076
Champaign, IL 61825-5076
800-747-4457
e-mail: humank@hkusa.com

Canada: Human Kinetics
475 Devonshire Road Unit 100
Windsor, ON N8Y 2L5
800-465-7301 (in Canada only)
e-mail: orders@hkcanada.com

Europe: Human Kinetics
107 Bradford Road
Stanningley
Leeds LS28 6AT, United Kingdom
+44 (0) 113 255 5665
e-mail: hk@hkeurope.com

Australia: Human Kinetics
57A Price Avenue
Lower Mitcham, South Australia 5062
08 8277 1555
e-mail: liaw@hkaustralia.com

New Zealand: Human Kinetics
Division of Sports Distributors NZ Ltd.
P.O. Box 300 226 Albany
North Shore City
Auckland
0064 9 448 1207
e-mail: info@humankinetics.co.nz

In memory of Mom—for her gentle encouragement
and unwavering confidence in me.

Contents

Preface

Advanced Fitness Assessment and Exercise Prescription, Fifth Edition is written primarily for exercise science students in advanced professional courses dealing with physical fitness appraisal and exercise prescription. This book is also a resource for exercise physiologists or personal trainers working in the public or private sectors. Previous editions of this text have been adopted for course use by numerous universities and colleges and have been translated into Greek, Italian, Korean, Portuguese, and Spanish.

This book provides exercise scientists with the knowledge and skills needed to assess the physical fitness of apparently healthy individuals rather than individuals who have suspected or documented cardiovascular disease. Since this text is not clinically oriented, it provides limited information on the etiology and pathophysiology of chronic diseases, on clinical exercise testing, and on exercise prescriptions for clinical populations. Exercise scientists working with clinical populations are encouraged to consult clinically oriented books that provide detailed information for exercise testing and prescriptions for these populations.

In its well-balanced approach to the assessment of physical fitness, *Advanced Fitness Assessment and Exercise Prescription* addresses four components:

- Cardiorespiratory endurance
- Muscular fitness
- Body weight and composition
- Flexibility

This text is unique in its scope and in the depth of its content, organization, and approach to the subject matter. Introductory texts typically focus on field testing for evaluating physical fitness. Although this text includes some field tests, it emphasizes laboratory techniques for assessment. The scope and depth of information make this text an important resource for practitioners, especially those employed in health and fitness settings. This text is organized around the four physical fitness components, providing for each of them one chapter

on assessment followed by one chapter on exercise prescription. The multidisciplinary approach of this text synthesizes concepts, principles, and theories based on research in exercise physiology, kinesiology, measurement, psychology, and nutrition. The result is a direct and clear-cut approach to physical fitness assessment and exercise prescription.

The scope and organization of the fifth edition of *Advanced Fitness Assessment and Exercise Prescription* are not substantially different from previous editions. Pedagogical tools include *Key Questions* at the beginning of each chapter and *Key Points*, *Review Questions*, and *Key Terms* at the end of each chapter. Each of the key terms is defined in the *Glossary of Terms* at the back of this book. These tools will help you identify the key terms and concepts and test your knowledge and understanding of the material in each chapter.

Pertinent information from the latest edition (2006) of *ACSM's Guidelines for Exercise Testing and Prescription* is incorporated throughout the text. Updated addresses, phone numbers, and Web sites are included for equipment manufacturers and suppliers. The following list highlights some of the chapter changes in *Advanced Fitness Assessment and Exercise Prescription, Fifth Edition:*

Chapter 1

- Recent global and U.S. statistics on the prevalence of chronic diseases
- New research substantiating the link between physical activity and disease risk
- Risk factors for metabolic syndrome
- General guidelines for prescribing exercise for clients with hypertension
- Exercise prescription guidelines for improving bone health of adults, children, and adolescents

Chapter 2

- Modified criteria for evaluating risk factors for coronary heart disease

- Revised terminology for blood pressure classification
- Criteria used to judge the accuracy of blood pressure measuring devices
- ACSM's risk stratification criteria
- ACSM's guidelines for medical examination and exercise testing

Chapter 3

- Updated information about the certification and licensure of exercise professionals
- Comparison of selected professional certifications
- Evaluation criteria for judging the relative worth of physical fitness tests and prediction equations for groups and individuals

Chapter 4

- Updated norms for evaluating cardiorespiratory fitness of adults (20-79 yr)
- Latest (2006) ACSM guidelines for exercise testing
- New exercise test protocols including treadmill and cycle ergometer ramp protocols
- Field tests and norms for evaluating cardiorespiratory fitness of older adults (60-94 yr)

Chapter 5

- Latest (2006) ACSM guidelines for designing aerobic exercise programs
- Using the talk test for monitoring exercise intensity
- Treading, spinning, and water-based exercise as alternative modes of aerobic exercise

Chapter 6

- Updated norms for push-up and trunk-curl tests
- Guidelines for testing muscular fitness of children and older adults
- Field tests and norms for testing the functional strength of older adults

Chapter 7

- Guidelines for designing resistance training programs for children

- New guidelines for developing resistance training programs for novice, intermediate, and advanced weightlifters
- Updated guidelines for developing periodized resistance training programs
- Sample resistance training programs using linear and undulating periodization methods
- New information about functional training and exercise progressions
- Updated information about the effectiveness of supplements for increasing strength

Chapter 8

- Expanded information about air displacement plethysmography and dual-energy X-ray absorptiometry as reference methods for body composition assessment
- Updated population-specific conversion formulas for estimating body fat from body density
- Comparison of high-quality and plastic skinfold calipers
- Using anthropometric indices to classify disease risk

Chapter 9

- Updated statistics on the global prevalence of obesity in children and adults
- New 2005 *Dietary Guidelines for Americans* and healthy eating pyramids
- Methods and formulas for estimating total energy expenditure
- Updated information on weight-loss diets, including low-carbohydrate diets
- Physical activity and exercise recommendations for health benefit, healthy weight loss, and weight management

Chapter 10

- Field tests and norms for assessing the flexibility of older adults (60-94 yr)
- Updated norms for the standard sit-and-reach test
- Field tests and reference values for assessing lumbar stability of healthy adults

Chapter 11

- Updated guidelines for designing stretching programs
- Sample flexibility exercise program
- Updated information about stretching and injury prevention
- Expanded information about lumbar stability exercises for low back care programs

Appendixes

- Updated PAR-Q & YOU and PARmed-X forms
- Updated Web sites for professional organizations
- Asian, Latin American, Mediterranean, and Vegetarian healthy eating pyramids
- Photographs of selected isometric exercises and flexibility exercises.
- Descriptions and illustrations of additional exercises for low back care

These updates and additions provide a more comprehensive and advanced approach to physical fitness appraisal and exercise prescription. I hope you will use *Advanced Fitness Assessment and Exercise Prescription, Fifth Edition* to improve your knowledge, skill, and professional competence as an exercise scientist.

Acknowledgments

Many people have made unique and important contributions to the evolution of this text. In addition to all of the individuals I acknowledged in previous editions of this book, I would like to thank Dr. Len Kravitz for his helpful suggestions for this edition. Also, I would like to acknowledge Dr. Cristine Mermier, Dr. Virginia Wilmerding, and Matthew Gordon for their cooperation and assistance in securing models and equipment for the new photographs in this edition. I am indebted to each of you and truly appreciate your effort, cooperation, and support.

chapter 1

Physical Activity, Health, and Chronic Disease

Key Questions

- Are adults in the United States getting enough physical activity?
- What diseases are associated with a sedentary lifestyle, and what are the major risk factors for these diseases?
- What are the benefits of regular physical activity in terms of disease prevention, and how does physical activity improve health?
- How much physical activity is needed for improved health benefits?
- What kinds of physical activities are suitable for typical people, and how often should they exercise?

Although physical activity plays an important role in the prevention of chronic diseases, an alarming percentage of adults in the United States report no physical activity during leisure time. One of the national health objectives for the year 2010 is to increase to 30% the proportion of people aged 18 years and older who regularly (preferably daily) engage in moderate physical activity at least 30 min per day (U.S. Department of Health and Human Services 2000a). According to a recent U.S. national survey from the Centers for Disease Control (CDC) (2003b), we are achieving this objective. At present in the United States, 45% of adults get the recommended amount of physical activity, but 55% do not. Approximately 26% of the American population report no physical

activity (< 10 min/wk of moderate physical activity). Women 45 yr and older are less active than their male counterparts, and older adults are less active than younger adults.

Physical inactivity is not just a problem in the United States; it is a global issue. According to the World Health Organization (2002b), ~60% of the global population do not meet the daily minimum recommendation of 30 min of moderate-intensity physical activity. Thus, as an exercise specialist, you face the challenge of educating and motivating your clients to incorporate physical activity as a regular part of their lifestyles.

This chapter deals with physical activity trends, risk factors associated with chronic diseases, the role of regular physical activity in disease prevention and health, and physical activity recommendations for improved health. For definitions of terminology used in this chapter, see the glossary on page 379.

PHYSICAL ACTIVITY, HEALTH, AND DISEASE: AN OVERVIEW

Our increased reliance on technology has substantially lessened work-related physical activity, as well as the energy expenditure required for activities of daily living like cleaning the house, washing clothes and dishes, mowing the lawn, and traveling to work. What would have once required an hour of physical work now can be accomplished in just a few seconds by pushing a button or setting a dial. As a result, more time is available to pursue leisure activities. The unfortunate fact, however, is that many individuals do not engage in physical activity during their leisure time.

Although the human body is designed for movement and strenuous physical activity, exercise is not a part of the average lifestyle. One cannot expect the human body to function optimally and to remain healthy for extended periods if the body is abused or is not used as intended. Physical inactivity has led to a rise in chronic diseases. Individuals who do not exercise regularly are at greater risk than others of developing chronic diseases such as coronary heart disease, hypertension, hypercholesterolemia, cancer, obesity, and musculoskeletal disorders (see figure 1.1).

For years, exercise scientists and health/fitness professionals have maintained that regular physical activity is the best defense against the development of many diseases, disorders, and illnesses. The importance of regular physical activity in preventing disease and premature death and in maintaining a high quality of life received recognition as a national health objective in the first U.S. Surgeon General's report on physical activity and health (U.S. Department of Health and Human Services 1996). This report identifies physical inactivity as a serious nationwide health problem, provides clear-cut scientific evidence linking physical activity to numerous health benefits, presents demographic data describing physical activity patterns and trends in the U.S. population, and makes physical activity recommendations for improved health (see page 3).

But how much physical activity is enough? The answer depends on your clients' goals. In 1995 the CDC and the American College of Sports Medicine (ACSM) endorsed the following statement regarding physical activity for health benefits (Pate et al. 1995):

Every U.S. adult should accumulate 30 min or more of moderate-intensity physical activity on most, preferably all, days of the week.

This amount of physical activity equates to exercising 150 min/wk or to expending approximately 1000 kcal/wk. Participating in moderate-intensity physical activity on a daily basis reduces the risk of coronary heart disease by 50% and the risk of hypertension, diabetes, and colon cancer by 30% (U.S. Department of Health and Human Services 1996). Also, the risk of breast cancer decreases by 18% in women who walk briskly 1.25 to 2.5 hr/wk (McTiernan et al. 2003).

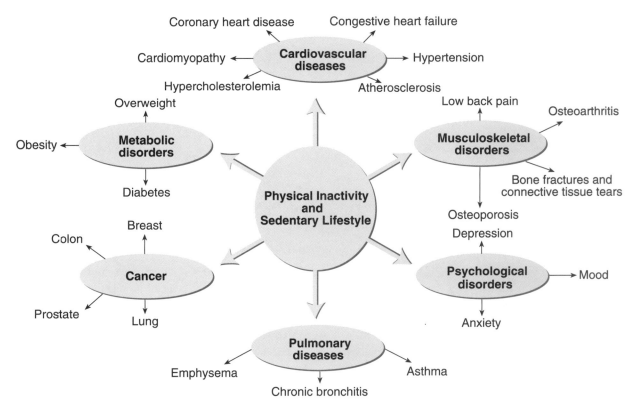

Figure 1.1   Role of physical activity and exercise in disease prevention and rehabilitation.

Improvements in health benefits depend on the volume (i.e., combination of frequency, intensity, and duration) of physical activity. This is known as the **dose-response relationship** (Bouchard 2001; Canadian Society of Exercise Physiology 2003;

Health Benefits of Physical Activity

Reduced risk of

- dying prematurely,
- dying prematurely from heart disease,
- developing diabetes,
- developing high blood pressure, and
- developing colon cancer.

Reduction of

- blood pressure in people who already have high blood pressure, and
- feelings of depression and anxiety.

Help in

- controlling body weight;
- building and maintaining healthy bones, muscles, and joints;
- developing strength and agility in older adults so they are better able to move about without falling; and
- creating a sense of psychological well-being.

Data from U.S. Department of Health and Human Services, 1996, *Physical Activity and Health: A Report of the Surgeon General–At a Glance* (Washington, DC: Author).

Kesaniemi, Danforth, Jensen, Kopelman, Lefebvre, and Reeder 2001). Figure 1.2 illustrates the general dose-response relationship between the volume of physical activity participation and selected health benefits that do not require a minimal threshold intensity for improvement like muscular strength and aerobic fitness. The volume of physical activity participation needed for the same degree of relative improvement (%) varies among health benefit indicators. For example, to improve triglycerides from 0 to 40% requires 250 kcal/wk of physical activity compared to 1800 kcal/wk for the same relative improvement (0 to 40%) in high density lipoprotein (see figure 1.2). Additionally, you should note that too much physical activity defined as engaging in 5 hr of structured high-intensity activity per week, may be associated with negative health consequences or overuse injuries. For extensive reviews of literature dealing with the dose-response relationship between physical activity and health, see *Medicine & Science in Sports & Exercise* (June 2001, Supplement).

Although following the CDC and ACSM recommendation (30 min/day of moderate-intensity physical activity) reduces disease risk, it may not be optimal for maintaining a healthy body weight. In 2002, the Institute of Medicine (IOM) recommended 60 min of daily moderate-intensity physical activity, twice the amount recommended by the CDC and ACSM. In the IOM report, the expert panel stated that 30 min of daily physical activity is insufficient to maintain a healthy body weight and to fully reap its associated health benefits. Initially, the IOM recommendation created

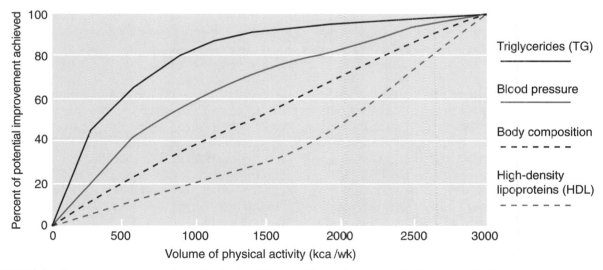

Figure 1.2 Dose-response relationship for health benefits and volume of physical activity.

Source: *The Canadian Physical Activity, Fitness and Lifestyle Approach: CSEP—Health and Fitness Program's Health-Related Appraisal and Counselling Strategy*, 3rd edition © 2003. Reprinted with permission from the Canadian Society for Exercise Physiology. Schematic developed by N. Gledhill and V. Jamnik of York University.

Examples of Moderate Amounts of Physical Activity

This list contains examples of moderate amounts of physical activity. (A moderate amount of physical activity is roughly that which uses approximately 150 kcal energy per day, or 1000 kcal per week. Some activities can be performed at various intensities; the suggested durations correspond to expected intensity of effort.) More vigorous activities, such as stair-climbing and running, require less time (15 min). On the other hand, less vigorous activities, like washing and waxing the car, require more time (45 to 60 min).

Less Vigorous, More Time

- Washing and waxing a car for 45-60 min
- Washing windows or floors for 45-60 min
- Playing volleyball for 45 min
- Playing touch football for 30-45 min
- Gardening for 30-45 min
- Wheeling self in wheelchair for 30-40 min
- Walking 1.75 miles (2.8 km) in 35 min (20 min/mile pace)
- Basketball (shooting baskets) for 30 min
- Bicycling 5 miles (8.0 km) for 30 min
- Dancing fast (social) for 30 min
- Pushing a stroller 1.5 miles (2.4 km) for 30 min
- Raking leaves for 30 min
- Walking 2 miles (3.2 km) in 30 min (15 min/mile pace)
- Water aerobics for 30 min

More Vigorous, Less Time

- Swimming laps for 20 min
- Playing wheelchair basketball for 20 min
- Playing basketball for 15-20 min
- Bicycling 4 miles (6.4 km) in 15 min
- Jumping rope for 15 min
- Running 1.5 miles (2.4 km) in 15 min (10 min/mile pace)
- Shoveling snow for 15 min
- Stair walking for 15 min

Data from U.S. Dept. of Health and Human Services, 1996, *Physical Activity and Health: A Report of the Surgeon General—At a Glance* (Washington, D.C.: Author), 2.

much confusion for fitness professionals and the general public about how much physical activity is enough. However, the apparent discrepancy can be reconciled by examining the goals of these two public health recommendations. The goal of the CDC and ACSM recommendation is to increase physical activity to reduce morbidity and mortality from chronic diseases, especially among sedentary individuals (Blair, LaMonte, and Nichaman 2004). The IOM recommendation addresses the amount of physical activity necessary to maintain a healthy body weight and to prevent unhealthful weight gain (Brooks, Butte, Rand, Flatt, and Caballero 2004). The IOM recommendation of 60 min of daily physical activity is consistent with recommendations for preventing weight gain made by other organizations (i.e., Health Canada, the International Association for the Study of Obesity, and the World Health Organization) (Brooks et al. 2004). The bottom line is that 30 min/day of moderate-intensity physical activity provides substantial health benefits but may be insufficient to prevent weight gain for many individuals. It is a good initial goal and a sufficient amount of activity to move individuals from a sedentary to low physical activity level (Brooks et al. 2004). As individuals adopt regular physical activity and improve their lifestyle and fitness, they should increase the duration of daily physical activity to a level (~60 min) that prevents weight gain and provides additional health benefits. This goal is especially important for individuals who have difficulty controlling their body weight (Blair et al. 2004; Lohman, Going, and Metcalfe 2004), and it is sufficient to move individuals from a sedentary to active physical activity level (Brooks et al. 2004).

The Exercise and Physical Activity Pyramid, developed by the Metropolitan Life Insurance Company (1995), illustrates a balanced plan of physical activity and exercise to promote a healthy lifestyle and improve physical fitness (see figure 1.3). You should encourage your clients to engage in physical activities around the home and work-

place on a daily basis to establish a foundation (base of pyramid) for an active lifestyle. They should perform aerobic activities and flexibility exercises at least 2 to 3 days/wk; they should do weight-resistance exercises and recreational, sport activities, 3 to 5 days/wk (middle levels of pyramid). High-intensity training and competitive sports (top of pyramid) require a solid fitness base to prevent injury, and they offer relatively few health benefits. Most people should engage in these activities only sparingly.

Canada's Physical Activity Guide to Healthy Active Living (Health Canada 2003) recommends accumulating 60 min of daily physical activity to stay healthy and improving health by participating in aerobic activities (4-7 days/wk), strength activities (2-4 days/wk), and flexibility activities (4-7

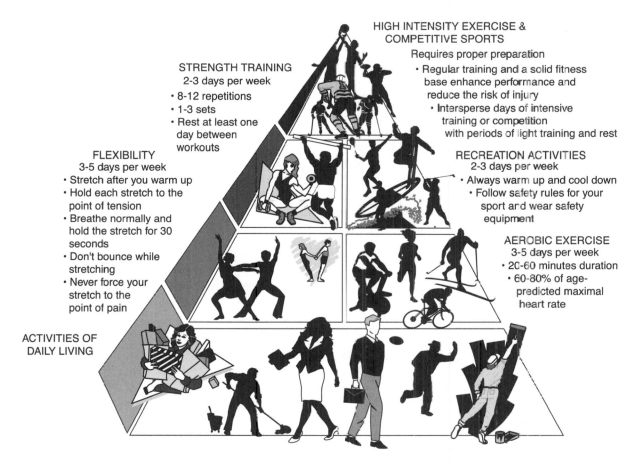

Figure 1.3 The Exercise and Physical Activity Pyramid.

Adapted from "Exercise and Activity Pyramid," Metropolitan Life Insurance Company, 1995.

days/wk). The duration of the activity depends on the intensity or effort: Perform light activities (e.g., walking or gardening) for 60 min, moderate activities (e.g., brisk walking or swimming) for 30 to 60 min, and vigorous activities (e.g., jogging or hockey) for 20 to 30 min. Later chapters of this text contain detailed information regarding aerobic, muscular fitness, and flexibility exercise prescriptions.

CARDIOVASCULAR DISEASE

Cardiovascular disease (CVD) causes 16.7 million deaths worldwide each year. According to the World Health Organization (2004a), approximately 85% of cardiovascular deaths occur in low- and middle-income countries. CVD is the principal cause of mortality in Europe, accounting for nearly half of all deaths (American Heart Association 2004). In developing countries in Africa, Western Asia, and Southeastern Asia, 15% to 20% of the annual deaths are due to CVDs (American Heart Association 2001). The proportion of deaths from CVD ranges from 25% for Latin American countries to 45% for eastern Mediterranean countries (American Heart Association 2001). In 1997, diseases of the heart and blood vessels claimed the lives of 931,108 people in the United States alone. CVD accounted for 38.5% of deaths (1 out of every 2.6) in the United States in 2001 (American Heart Association 2004). More than 64 million Americans have some form of CVD such as hypertension (50.0 million), coronary heart disease (13.2 million), congestive heart disease (5.0 million), and stroke (4.8 million) (American Heart Association 2004).

One myth about CVD is that it is more prevalent in men than in women. In terms of total deaths, since 1984 CVD has claimed the lives of more females than males (American Heart Association 2004). Nearly 500,000 females die from CVD each year in the United States. Another misconception about CVD is that it only afflicts the older population. Although it is true that older people are at greater risk, over 60% of the people in the United States with CVD are less than 65 yr, and CVD ranks as the third-leading cause of death for children under age 15 (American Heart Association 2004).

Coronary heart disease accounts for more deaths annually than any other disease, with more than 500,000 people dying each year from CHD (American Heart Association 2004). Among American adults 20 years of age or older, the estimated age-adjusted prevalence of CHD is higher for Black and Hispanic men and women compared to White men and women (American Heart Association 2004).

Coronary heart disease (CHD) is caused by a lack of blood supply to the heart muscle (**myocardial ischemia**), resulting from a progressive, degenerative disorder known as atherosclerosis. **Atherosclerosis** involves a buildup and deposition of fat and fibrous plaques in the intima, or inner lining, of the coronary arteries. These plaques restrict the blood flow to the myocardium and may produce **angina pectoris**, which is a temporary sensation of tightening and heavy pressure in the chest and shoulder region. A **myocardial infarction**, or heart attack, can occur if a blood clot, or thrombus, obstructs the coronary blood flow. In this case, blood flow through the coronary arteries is usually reduced by over 80%. The portion of the myocardium supplied by the obstructed artery dies and is replaced eventually with scar tissue.

Coronary Heart Disease Risk Factors

Epidemiological research indicates that many factors are associated with the risk of CHD. The greater the number and severity of risk factors, the greater the probability of CHD. The positive risk factors for CHD are

- family history,
- hypercholesterolemia,
- hypertension,
- current cigarette smoking,
- impaired fasting glucose (diabetes mellitus),
- obesity, and
- physical inactivity.

An increased level of high-density lipoprotein cholesterol or **HDL-cholesterol** (HDL-C >60 mg · dl^{-1}) in the blood decreases CHD risk. If the HDL-C is high, you should subtract one risk factor from the sum of the positive factors when assessing your client's CHD risk.

Physical Activity and Coronary Heart Disease

Nearly 22% of all cases of CHD worldwide can be attributed to a lack of physical activity and a sedentary lifestyle (World Health Organization 2004a). As an exercise scientist, you must educate your clients about the benefits of physical activity and regular exercise for preventing CHD. Physically active people have lower incidences of myocardial infarction and mortality from CHD and tend to develop CHD at a later age compared to their sedentary counterparts (Berlin and Colditz 1990). Individuals who exercise regularly reduce their relative risk of developing CHD by a factor of 1.5 to 2.4 (American Heart Association 1999; Powell, Thompson, Casperson, and Kendrick 1987). Physical activity exerts its effect independently of smoking, hypertension, hypercholesterolemia, obesity, diabetes, and family history of CHD (Bouchard, Shephard, and Stephens 1994). Also, in a meta-analysis of studies dealing with the dose-response effects of physical activity and cardiorespiratory fitness on CVD and CHD risk, Williams (2001) reported that cardiorespiratory fitness and physical activity have significantly different relationships to CVD and CHD risk. Although physical fitness and physical activity each lower the risk of developing CVD and CHD, the reduction in relative risk was almost twice as great for cardiorespiratory fitness as for physical activity. These findings suggest that in addition to physical activity level, cardiorespiratory fitness level should be considered a potential risk factor for CHD.

HYPERTENSION

Hypertension, or high blood pressure, is a chronic, persistent elevation of blood pressure that is clinically defined as a systolic pressure ≥ 140 mmHg or a diastolic pressure ≥ 90 mmHg or as taking antihypertensive medicine. **Prehypertension** is a new term to describe individuals with a systolic pressure of 120 to 139 mmHg, a diastolic pressure of 80 to 89 mmHg, or both (Chobanian et al. 2003). About 62% of strokes and 49% of heart attacks are caused by hypertension (World Health Organization 2004a).

About 15% to 40% of the global adult population have hypertension. Generally, the average blood pressure of adults from European countries (England, Finland, Germany, Italy, and Spain) is higher than that of American and Canadian adults (Wolf-Maier et al. 2003). In England, approximately 36% of adult women and men are

hypertensive (British Heart Foundation 2004). In comparison, the prevalence of hypertension is estimated to be 10% to 17% for adults in the eastern Mediterranean region, 4% to 12% for adults in India, 8% for people 15 yr and older in China, and 5% to 12% for adults in Africa (American Heart Association 2001).

In the United States, more than 1 out of 4 adults (29%) have high blood pressure, and 22% are prehypertensive (American Heart Association 2004). Up to age 55, the percentage of American men with hypertension is greater than that of women. The percentage of women with high blood pressure progressively increases from ages 55 to 74. After age 74, the percentage of women with hypertension is greater than that of men. Women with hypertension have a 3.5 times greater risk of developing CHD than do women with normal blood pressure. Also, the prevalence of high blood pressure for Blacks in the United States (43%) is among the highest in the world and is substantially greater than that of American Indians or Alaskan Natives, Asians or Pacific Islanders, Hispanics, and Whites in the United States (American Heart Association 2004). Table 1.1 summarizes the risk factors associated with developing hypertension.

Epidemiological studies indicate an inverse relationship between the resting blood pressure and the level of physical activity in women and men (Fagard 1999; Hagberg 1990; Paffenbarger, Jung, Leung, and Hyde 1991; Reaven, Barrett-Connor, and Edelstein 1991). Regular physical activity prevents hypertension and lowers blood pressure in younger and older adults who are normotensive, prehypertensive, or hypertensive. Compared to normotensive individuals, training-induced changes in resting systolic and diastolic blood pressures (5-7 mmHg) are greater for hypertensive individuals who participate in endurance exercise. However, even modest reductions in blood pressure (2-3 mmHg) by endurance or resistance exercise training decrease CHD risk by 5% to 9%, stroke risk by 8% to 14%, and all-cause mortality by 4% in the general population (Pescatello, Franklin, Fagard, Farquhar, Kelley, and Ray 2004). In a recent position paper on exercise and hypertension (Pescatello et al. 2004), the ACSM endorsed the following exercise prescription to lower blood pressure in adults with hypertension.

TABLE 1.1 Summary of Factors Associated With Disease Risk

Factor	CHD	Diabetes	Hypertension	Hypercholesterolemia	Low back pain	Obesity	Osteoporosis
Age	↑	↑	↑	↑	↑	↑	↑
Gender	M>F[a]	F>M	F>M[b]	F>M[b]	F=M	F>M	F>M[b]
Race	B, H>A, AI, W	AI, B, H>A, W	B>A, AI, H, W	B, H, W>A, AI		AI, B, H, W>A	A, W>AI, B
Family history	↑	↑	↑	↑		↑	↑
SES	↓	↓	↓	↓		↓	
Alcohol use			↑	↑			↑
Smoking	↑		↑	↑			
Nutrition							
Na intake			↑				
Ca intake			↓				↓
Fat/cholesterol intake	↑	↑		↑		↑	
CHO intake				↓			
Intake>expenditure		↑				↑	
Physical activity	↓	↓	↓		↓	↓	↓
Exercise amenorrhea							↑
Flexibility					↓		
Muscular strength					↓		↓
Skeletal frame size							↓
Other diseases							
Anorexia nervosa							↑
Diabetes	↑						
Hypertension	↑						
Hypercholesterolemia	↑						
Obesity and overweight	↑	↑	↑	↑	↑		↓

↑ = Direct relationship; as factor increases, risk increases.

↓ = Indirect relationship; as factor increases, risk decreases.

[a] Males (M) at higher risk than females (F) up to age 55 years.

[b] Menopausal females at higher risk than males.

CHD = coronary heart disease; CHO = carbohydrate; A = Asian; AI = American Indian; B = Black; H = Hispanic; W = White; Na = sodium; Ca = calcium; SES = socioeconomic status (reflects income and education levels).

<table>
<tr><td>

Exercise Prescription for Hypertension (Pescatello et al. 2004)

Mode: Primarily endurance activities supplemented by resistance exercises
Intensity: Moderate (40% to 60% $\dot{V}O_2R$)*
Duration: 30 min or more of continuous or accumulated physical activity per day
Frequency: Most, preferably all, days of the week

*$\dot{V}O_2R$ is the difference between the maximum and the resting rate of oxygen consumption. See "VO$_2$ reserve (MET) Method" on page 98 for more information.

</td></tr>
</table>

HYPERCHOLESTEROLEMIA AND DYSLIPIDEMIA

Hypercholesterolemia, an elevation of total cholesterol (TC) in the blood, is associated with increased risk for CVD. Hypercholesterolemia is also referred to as hyperlipidemia, which is an increase in blood lipid levels; dyslipidemia refers to an abnormal blood lipid profile. Approximately 18% of strokes and 56% of heart attacks are caused by high blood cholesterol (World Health Organization 2002b). Nearly 37 million Americans have TC levels that are classified as high risk ($\geq$240 mg · dl^{-1}); in Americans aged 50 and older, more women (19.1%) than men (17.2%) have TC levels equaling or exceeding 240 mg · dl^{-1} (American Heart Association 2004). Compared to those in Western countries, the average TC levels for adults in China, Japan, and Indonesia are uniformly lower (190-207 mg · dl^{-1}) (American Heart Association 2001). Risk factors for hypercholesterolemia are identified in table 1.1.

LDLs, HDLs, and TC

Cholesterol is a waxy, fatlike substance found in all animal products (meats, dairy products, and eggs). The body can make cholesterol in the liver and absorb cholesterol from the diet. Cholesterol is essential to the body and is used to build cell membranes, to produce sex hormones, and to form bile acids necessary for fat digestion. Lipoproteins are an essential part of the complex transport system that exchanges lipids among the liver, intestine, and peripheral tissues. Lipoproteins are classified by the thickness of the protein shell that surrounds the cholesterol. The four main classes of lipoproteins are chylomicron, derived from the intestinal absorption of triglycerides; very low-density lipoprotein (VLDL), made in the liver for the transport of triglycerides; low-density lipoprotein (LDL), a product of VLDL metabolism that serves as the primary transporter of cholesterol; and high-density lipoprotein (HDL), involved in the reverse transport of cholesterol to the liver. The molecules of LDL are larger than those of HDL and therefore precipitate in the plasma and are actively transported into the vascular walls. Excess LDL-cholesterol stimulates the formation of plaque on the intima of the coronary arteries. Plaque formation reduces the cross-sectional area and obstructs blood flow in these arteries, eventually producing a myocardial infarction. Therefore, LDL-cholesterol (LDL-C) values less than 100 mg · dl^{-1} are considered optimal for reducing CVD and CHD risk (National Cholesterol Education Program 2001).

The smaller HDL molecules are suspended in the plasma and protect the body by picking up excess cholesterol from the arterial walls and delivering it to the liver where it is metabolized. HDL-cholesterol (HDL-C) values exceeding 45 mg · dl^{-1} are desirable; women tend to have higher HDL-C compared to men.

Individuals with low HDL-C or high TC levels (dyslipidemia) have a greater risk of heart attack. Those with lower HDL-C ($\leq$37 mg · dl^{-1} for men or $\leq$47 mg · dl^{-1} for women) are at higher risk regardless of their TC level. This fact emphasizes the importance of screening for both TC and HDL-C in adults.

Physical Activity and Lipid Profiles

Regular physical activity, especially habitual aerobic exercise, positively affects lipid metabolism and lipid profiles (Durstine, Grandjean, Cox, and Thompson 2002). Cross-sectional comparisons of lipid profiles in physically active and sedentary women and men suggest that physical fitness is inversely related to TC and the TC/HDL-C ratio (Despres and Lamarche 1994; Shoenhair and Wells 1995).

Regular endurance exercise usually lowers plasma triglycerides but rarely reduces TC and LDL-C levels in individuals with initially high levels unless dietary fat intake is reduced and body weight is lost (Durstine et al. 2002). HDL-C increases in response to endurance training. This response appears to relate to the exercise training dose (interaction of the intensity, frequency, and duration of each exercise session and the length of the training period) and is less dramatic in women than in men (Kokkinos and Fernhall 1999; Lokey and Tran 1989). An analysis of longitudinal and cross-sectional exercise studies concluded that 15 to 20 mi/wk of brisk walking or jogging (equivalent to 1200-2200 kcal of energy expenditure) decreases blood triglyceride levels by 5 to 38 mg·dl[-1] and increases HDL-C by 2 to 8 mg·dl[-1] (Durstine et al. 2002). In comparison, resistance training has no effect on blood triglyceride levels, and TC and LDL-C are lowered only when the training increases lean body mass and decreases relative body fat (Durstine et al. 2002). Also, resistance training has little or no effect on the HDL-C levels of men at risk for CHD (Kokkinos et al. 1991).

CIGARETTE SMOKING

The World Health Organization (2002c) estimates that about one-third of the global adult population smokes. In the United States, the prevalence of adults (age 18 and older) who smoke has declined by 40% since 1965 (Centers for Disease Control 2003b). Approximately 21% of American women and 25% of American men are smokers. Globally, the prevalence of smoking is highest for men in Asian countries. About half of all men in Malaysia and Japan smoke, whereas in China, Cambodia, and Korea 67% of men smoke (World Health Organization 2002c). While the prevalence of smoking is falling in well-developed countries, tobacco consumption is rising in developing countries by 3.4% per year (World Health Organization 2002c). Worldwide, 1 in 5 teenagers (13-15 yr) is a smoker. Also, the risk of death from CHD increases by 30% in those exposed to environmental tobacco smoke at home or at work (American Heart Association 2004).

Smoking is the largest preventable cause of disease and premature death. Cigarette smoking is linked to CHD, stroke, and chronic lung disease. It causes cancer of the lungs, larynx, esophagus, mouth, and bladder and is also associated with cancer of the cervix, pancreas, and kidneys (World Health Organization 2002c). Compared to non-smokers, smokers have more than twice the risk of heart attack. The nicotine in cigarette smoke increases heart rate and blood pressure and inhibits the anticlotting mechanisms of the blood.

When individuals stop smoking, their risk of CHD declines rapidly, regardless of how long or how much they have smoked. One year after quitting, the risk of CHD decreases by 50%, and within 15 yr the relative risk of dying from CHD almost matches that of a longtime nonsmoker (American Heart Association 2004).

DIABETES MELLITUS

There is a global diabetes epidemic. Over a period of 10 yr (1985-1995), the number of people with diabetes increased by 78% worldwide. The World Health Organization (2002a) predicts that by 2025 the global prevalence of diabetes will have continued to escalate, with the number of individuals with diabetes increasing relatively more in developing countries than in developed countries. Since 1994, the age-adjusted prevalence of diabetes for adults in the United States increased by 54%, from 4.8% to 7.3% (American Heart Association 2004). Compared to White adults in the United States, the prevalence of diabetes and impaired blood glucose levels for Blacks, Hispanics, and American Indians is higher (Centers for Disease Control 2003a). In fact, the prevalence of diabetes for American Indians and Alaska Native adults (15.3%) is one of the highest in the world; 43.5% of American Indian men and 52.4% of American Indian women have diabetes (American Heart Association 2004).

Type 1, or **insulin-dependent diabetes mellitus (IDDM)**, usually occurs before age 30 but can develop at any age. Type 2, or **non-insulin-dependent diabetes mellitus (NIDDM)**, is more common; 90% to 95% of individuals with diabetes mellitus have type 2 diabetes (Kriska, Blair, and Pereira 1994). Risk factors for developing diabetes are presented in table 1.1. Healthy nutrition and increased physical activity can reduce the risk of diabetes by as much as 60% in high-risk individuals.

Research suggests that regular physical activity reduces one's risk of developing NIDDM through its association with weight loss and the effects of exercise on insulin sensitivity and glucose tolerance (Kelley and Goodpaster 1999; Kriska, Blair, and Pereira 1994; Wells 1996). Manson et al. (1991) reported that women who engaged in vigorous exercise at least once a week have a reduced risk of diabetes. The reduction in diabetes risk, however, appears to be associated with the frequency of exercise. The risk of diabetes decreased 23%, 38%, and 42%, respectively, in male physicians who exercised vigorously one time, two to four times, and five or more times a week (Manson, Nathan, Krolewski, Stampfer, Willett, and Hennekens 1992). Vigorous exercise was defined as physical activity of sufficient duration to produce sweating. Specific guidelines for prescribing exercise programs for people who have type 1 and type 2 diabetes are available elsewhere (ACSM and American Diabetes Association 1997; Campaigne 1998; Colberg 2001).

OBESITY AND OVERWEIGHT

In clinical guidelines established by the Obesity Education Initiative Task Force of the National Institutes of Health and National Heart, Lung, and Blood Institute (1998), overweight and obesity are classified using the body mass index (BMI = weight [kg]/height squared [m²]). Individuals with a BMI between 25 and 29.9 kg/m² are classified as overweight; those with a BMI of 30 kg/m² or more are classified as obese.

Using these definitions, the World Health Organization (2004b) reported that more than 1 billion people worldwide are overweight and that at least 300 million of overweight individuals are obese. The prevalence of obesity increases with the development of countries, as is seen in the data for undeveloped countries (1.8%), developing countries (4.8%), countries in transition (17.1%), and developed countries (20.4%) (World Health Organization 2001). In Indonesia, 12.5% of adults ages 25 to 64 are obese; in Beijing, China, a 1988-1989 survey indicated that 35.2% of men and 39.5% of women were overweight; and in Africa, 8.3% of men and 36% to 50% of women are obese (American Heart Association 2001). Since 1960, the prevalence of overweight and obesity in the United States has increased across all age, gender, and ethnic groups (Flegal, Carroll, Kuczmarski. and Johnson 1998). According to the most recent National Health and Nutrition Examination Survey (NHANES IV), almost 66% of American adults are overweight and over 30% are obese (Hedley, Ogden, Johnson, Carroll, Curtin, and Flegal 2004). Childhood obesity is also a global problem (see chapter 9, pp. 214-216). The prevalence of children at risk for overweight in Canada and the United States ranges from 29% to 35% (Hedley et al. 2004; Tremblay and Willms 2000). Since 1980, the number of overweight American children has doubled and the number of overweight American adolescents has tripled (World Health Organization 2004b). Table 1.1 summarizes factors associated with increased risk of obesity.

Excess body weight and fatness pose a threat to both the quality and quantity of one's life. Obese individuals have a shorter life expectancy and greater risks of CHD, hypercholesterolemia, hypertension, diabetes mellitus, certain cancers, and osteoarthritis (Grundy, Blackburn, Higgins, Lauer, Perri, and Ryan 1999; National Institutes of Health and National Heart, Lung, and Blood Institute 1998). Although obesity is strongly associated with CHD risk factors such as hypertension, glucose intolerance, and hyperlipidemia, the contribution of obesity to CHD appears to be independent of the influence of obesity on these risk factors (Grundy et al. 1999). For a comprehensive report and roundtable discussion of the role of physical activity in the prevention and treatment of obesity and its comorbidities, see the November 1999 supplement to *Medicine & Science in Sports & Exercise*.

Obesity may be caused by genetic and environmental factors. Although studies suggest that genetic factors contribute to some of the variation in body fatness, there has been no substantial change in the genotype of the American population over the past 30 years (Hill and Melanson 1999). Thus, the major cause of obesity in the United States may be linked to our environment. Over the past three decades, we have been exposed to an environment that strongly promotes not only the consumption of high-fat, energy-dense foods (increased energy intake), but also reliance on technology that discourages physical activity and reduces the amount of physical activity (decreased energy expenditure) needed for daily living (e.g., use of energy-saving devices and prepared foods) (Hill and Melanson 1999). As an exercise specialist, you play an important role in combating this major health problem by encouraging a physically active lifestyle and by planning exercise programs and scientifically sound diets for your clients, in consultation with trained nutrition professionals. Restricting caloric intake and increasing caloric expenditure through physical activity and exercise are effective ways of reducing body weight and fatness while normalizing blood pressure and blood lipid profiles.

METABOLIC SYNDROME

Metabolic syndrome describes a combination of CVD risk factors associated with hypertension, dyslipidemia, insulin resistance, and abdominal obesity. According to clinical criteria adopted by the National Cholesterol Education Program (2001), individuals with three or more CVD risk factors are classified as having metabolic syndrome (see table 1.2). Approximately 24% of adults in the United States have metabolic syndrome. Metabolic syndrome increases the risk of developing CHD (by fourfold), CVD (by twofold), and diabetes (by five- to ninefold).

Age and BMI directly relate to metabolic syndrome (National Cholesterol Education Program 2001). The prevalence of this syndrome is higher for older (>60 yr) adults (>40%) than for younger

TABLE 1.2   Risk Factors for Metabolic Syndrome*

Risk factor	Risk criteria
Waist circumference	>102 cm (>40 in.) for men
	>88 cm (>35 in.) for women
Blood pressure (BP)	≥130 mmHg (systolic BP) or
	≥85 mmHg (diastolic BP) or both
Fasting blood glucose	≥100 mg/dl or ≥6.1 mmol/L
Triglycerides	≥150 mg/dl or ≥1.6 mmol/L
HDL-C	<40 mg/dl or <1.04 mmol/L for men
	<50 mg/dl or <1.29 mmol/L for women

*Metabolic syndrome is defined as 3 or more risk factors.

National Cholesterol Education Program 2001

(20-29 yr) adults (7%). Also, the prevalence of metabolic syndrome is much higher for obese (BMI > 30 kg/m²) individuals (~50%) than for normal weight (BMI ≤ 25 kg/m²) individuals (6.2%). Lifestyle must be modified in order to manage metabolic syndrome. The combination of healthy nutrition and increased physical activity is an effective way to increase HDL-C and to reduce blood pressure, body weight, triglycerides, and blood glucose levels.

MUSCULOSKELETAL DISEASES AND DISORDERS

Diseases and disorders of the musculoskeletal system, such as osteoporosis, osteoarthritis, bone fractures, connective tissue tears, and low back syndrome, are also related to physical inactivity and a sedentary lifestyle. **Osteoporosis** is a disease characterized by the loss of bone mineral content and bone mineral density due to factors such as aging, amenorrhea, malnutrition, menopause, and physical inactivity (see table 1.1 for osteoporosis risk factors). Over 7.8 million women and 2.3 million men in the United States have osteoporosis. Individuals with osteoporosis have bone mineral density values that are more than 2.5 standard deviations below the young adult mean value. **Osteopenia,** or low bone mineral mass, is a precursor to osteoporosis. More than 1 of every 2 adults aged 50 or older has either osteoporosis or osteopenia (National Osteoporosis Foundation 2004). Adequate calcium intake and regular physical activity help counteract age-related bone loss.

Epidemiological studies show that the incidence of bone fracture is lower in women with higher levels of physical activity. Although no data have demonstrated that exercise alone can prevent the loss of bone mass during and after menopause, the ACSM suggests the following exercise prescription to help counteract bone loss due to aging and preserve bone health during adulthood (Kohrt, Bloomfield, Little, Nelson, and Yingling 2004).

Exercise Prescription for Bone Health (Kohrt et al. 2004)

Mode: Weight-bearing endurance activities (e.g., tennis, stair-climbing, jogging, and walking with intermittent jogging), activities that involve jumping (e.g., volleyball and basketball), and resistance training
Intensity: Moderate to high, in terms of bone-loading forces
Frequency: 3-5 times per week for weight-bearing endurance activities; 2-3 times per week for resistance exercise
Duration: 30-60 min/day of a combination of weight-bearing endurance activities, activities that involve jumping, and resistance training that targets all major muscle groups

Peak bone mass is developed during childhood and adolescence and is a major factor associated with the risk of osteoporosis. Bone mass is higher in physically active children compared to less active children. Given that exercise-induced gains in bone mass during childhood and adolescence are maintained into adulthood, the ACSM recommends the following exercise prescription for developing peak bone mass in children and adolescents (Kohrt et al. 2004).

Exercise Prescription for Peak Bone Mass in Children and Adolescents (Kohrt et al. 2004)

Mode: Impact activities (e.g., gymnastics, plyometrics, and jumping), moderate-intensity resistance training, sports that involve running and jumping (e.g., soccer and basketball)
Intensity: High in terms of bone-loading forces; for resistance training, <60% 1-RM.
Frequency: At least 3 days/wk
Duration: 10-20 min (twice a day may be more effective)

Low back pain afflicts millions of people each year. More than 80% of all low back problems are produced by muscular weakness or imbalance caused by a lack of physical activity (see table 1.1). If the muscles are not strong enough to support the vertebral column in proper alignment, poor posture results and low back pain develops. Excessive weight, poor flexibility, and improper lifting habits also contribute to low back problems. While gender and age are associated with low back pain and are not modifiable risks, lifestyle behaviors such as smoking, physical inactivity, flexibility, and muscular strength and endurance are all modifiable risk factors that are related to

low back pain (Albert, Bonneau, Stevenson, and Gledhill 2001).

Because the origin of low back problems is often functional rather than structural, in many cases the problem can be corrected through an exercise program designed to develop strength and flexibility in the appropriate muscle groups. Also, people who remain physically active throughout life retain more bone, ligament, and tendon strength and are, therefore, less prone to bone fractures and connective tissue tears (McGill 2002).

KEY POINTS

- More than 55% of all Americans do not get the recommended amount of physical activity needed for health benefits.

- Major chronic diseases associated with a lack of physical activity are CVDs, diabetes, obesity, and musculoskeletal disorders.

- Cardiovascular diseases are responsible for 38.5% of all deaths in the United States and more than 50% of all deaths in Europeans older than 65 years.

- The positive risk factors for CHD are the following: family history, hypercholesterolemia, hypertension, cigarette smoking, glucose intolerance, obesity, and physical inactivity.

- The prevalence of obesity is on the rise, especially in developed countries; in the United States, two of every three adults and more than one of every four adolescents and children are overweight or obese.

- Metabolic syndrome is a term used to describe individuals who have three or more cardiovascular disease risk factors.

- Osteoporosis and low back syndrome are musculoskeletal disorders afflicting millions of people each year.

- To benefit health and prevent disease, every adult should accumulate 30 min or more of moderate-intensity physical activity on most, preferably all, days of the week.

KEY TERMS

Learn the definition for each of the following key terms. Definitions of key terms can be found in the glossary on page 379.

angina pectoris
atherosclerosis
body mass index (BMI)
cardiovascular disease (CVD)
cholesterol
chylomicron
coronary heart disease (CHD)
dose-response relationship
dyslipidemia
HDL-cholesterol (HDL-C)
high-density lipoprotein
hypercholesterolemia
hyperlipidemia
hypertension
LDL-cholesterol (LDL-C)

lipoprotein
low back pain
low-density lipoprotein (LDL)
metabolic syndrome
myocardial infarction
myocardial ischemia
obesity
osteopenia
osteoporosis
overweight
prehypertension
total cholesterol (TC)
type 1 diabetes
type 2 diabetes
very low-density lipoprotein (VLDL)

REVIEW QUESTIONS

In addition to being able to define each of the key terms just listed, test your knowledge and understanding of the material by answering the following review questions.

1. What percentage of the American population does not get the recommended amount of physical activity for health benefits?

2. What is the recommended minimum amount of daily physical activity for health?

3. Give examples of moderate physical activity.

4. What percentage of Americans have some form of CVD?

5. Name four types of CVD. Which is most prevalent?

6. Explain the etiology of CHD.

7. Identify the positive and negative risk factors for CHD.

8. Explain how regular physical activity impacts each of the CHD risk factors, as well as overall CHD risk.

9. Define obesity and overweight relative to BMI.

10. What types of exercise are effective for counteracting bone loss due to aging?

11. Explain the relationship between physical inactivity and low back pain.

chapter 2

Preliminary Health Screening and Risk Classification

Key Questions

- What are the major components of the health evaluation, and how is this information used to screen clients for exercise testing and participation?

- What factors do I need to focus on when evaluating the client's medical history and lifestyle characteristics?

- How is the client's disease risk classified?

- Do all clients need a physical examination and medical clearance from their physician before taking an exercise test?

- What are the standards for classifying blood cholesterol levels?

- How is blood pressure measured and evaluated? Are automated blood pressure devices accurate?

- How is heart rate measured? Are heart rate monitors accurate?

- What is an ECG, and does every client need to have one before taking an exercise test?

- Is it safe to give a graded exercise test to all clients? When does a physician need to be present?

- What are the major components of the lifestyle evaluation, and how can this information be used?

- What are the purposes of informed consent?

Before assessing your client's physical fitness profile, it is important to classify the person's health status and lifestyle. You will use information from the initial health and lifestyle evaluations to screen clients for physical fitness testing. You also will use this information to identify individuals with medical contraindications to exercise, with disease symptoms and risk factors, and with special needs.

This chapter discusses the components of a comprehensive health evaluation, including a coronary risk factor profile, medical history questionnaire, lifestyle evaluation, and informed consent. It also presents guidelines and standards for classifying blood cholesterol levels, blood pressures, and disease risk, along with techniques and procedures for measuring heart rate and blood pressure at rest and during exercise and for conducting a resting 12-lead electrocardiogram (ECG).

PRELIMINARY HEALTH EVALUATION

The purpose of the health evaluation is to detect the presence of disease and to assess the initial disease risk classification of your clients. The components of a comprehensive health evaluation are listed in table 2.1. To evaluate the client's health status, information from questionnaires and data from clinical tests are analyzed. Minimally, for pretest health screening of clients for exercise testing and exercise program participation, you should:

- administer the Physical Activity Readiness Questionnaire (PAR-Q),
- identify signs and symptoms of diseases,
- analyze the coronary risk profile, and
- classify the disease risk of your clients.

Step-by-step procedures for conducting a comprehensive health evaluation are listed in "Procedures for Comprehensive Pretest Health Screening," on page 17.

Questionnaires and Screening Forms

Appendix A provides questionnaires and forms that may be used to obtain information for the preliminary health screening and evaluation of your clients. The client should complete the PAR-Q, medical history questionnaire, lifestyle evaluation, and the informed consent form. You will interview your client to gather information about signs/symptoms of disease, analyze your client's coronary heart disease (CHD) risk factors, and determine your client's disease risk classification. For some clients, it may be necessary to obtain a medical clearance from their physician.

Physical Activity Readiness Questionnaire

The PAR-Q has seven questions designed to identify individuals who need medical clearance from their physicians before taking any physical fitness tests or starting an exercise program (see appendix

---

TABLE 2.1 Components of a Comprehensive Health Evaluation

Component	Purpose
QUESTIONNAIRES/SCREENING FORMS	
PAR-Q	To determine client's readiness for physical activity
Signs and symptoms of disease and medical clearance	To identify individuals in need of medical referral and to obtain evidence of physician approval for exercise testing and participation
Coronary risk factor analysis	To determine the number of CHD risk factors for client
Disease risk classification	To categorize clients as low, moderate, or high risk
Medical history	To review client's past and present personal and family health history, focusing on conditions requiring medical referral and clearance
Lifestyle evaluation	To obtain information about the client's living habits
Informed consent	To explain the purpose, risks, and benefits of physical fitness tests and to obtain your client's consent for participation in these tests
CLINICAL TESTS	
Physical examination	To detect signs and symptoms of disease
Blood chemistry profile	To determine if client has normal values for selected blood values; values of blood cholesterol are used in the coronary risk factor analysis
Blood pressure assessment	To determine if client is hypertensive; these values are also used in the coronary risk factor analysis
12-lead ECG	To evaluate cardiac function and detect cardiac abnormalities that are contraindications to exercise
Graded exercise test	To assess functional aerobic capacity and to detect cardiac abnormalities due to exercise stress
Additional laboratory tests (e.g., angiograms, echocardiograms, pulmonary tests)	To provide a more in-depth assessment of clients' health status, particularly those with known disease

> ## Procedures for Comprehensive Pretest Health Screening
>
> Here are step-by-step procedures you should follow when conducting a comprehensive health evaluation:
>
> - Greet the client.
> - Explain the purpose of the health evaluation and lifestyle evaluation.
> - Obtain the client's informed consent for health screening.
> - Administer and evaluate the PAR-Q; refer client to physician if needed.
> - Administer and evaluate client's medical history, focusing on signs, symptoms, and diseases; refer client to physician if needed.
> - Evaluate client's lifestyle profile.
> - Evaluate and classify the client's cholesterol and lipoprotein levels if test results are available.
> - Measure and classify the client's resting blood pressure and heart rate.
> - Assess the client's coronary risk factors.
> - Classify the client's disease risk.
> - Evaluate the client's blood chemistry profile if test results are available.
>
> If so requested by the client's physician, you may do the following:
>
> - Explain the purpose of and answer any questions about the 12-lead resting ECG and graded exercise test (GXT).
> - Obtain the client's informed consent for these tests.
> - Prepare the client and administer the 12-lead resting ECG.
> - Have a physician interpret the results of the 12-lead resting ECG.
> - Use the client's disease risk classification to determine whether a maximal or submaximal GXT should be administered and whether a physician needs to be present during this test.
> - Assess the client's resting blood pressure and heart rate.
> - Administer the GXT.
> - Assess and classify the client's functional aerobic capacity.

A.1, "Physical Activity Readiness Questionnaire (Par-Q)," p. 278). If clients answer "yes" to any of these questions, they should be referred to their physicians to obtain medical clearance before engaging in physical activity. Also, older clients and those who are not used to regular physical activity should always check with their physicians before starting an exercise program.

Medical History Questionnaire

You should require your clients to complete a comprehensive medical history questionnaire that includes questions concerning personal and family health history (appendix A.2, "Medical History Questionnaire," p. 280). Use the questionnaire to

- examine the client's record of personal illnesses, surgeries, and hospitalizations (section A);

- assess previous medical diagnoses and signs and symptoms of disease that have occurred within the past year or are currently present (section B); and
- analyze your client's family history of diabetes, heart disease, stroke, and hypertension (section C).

Also, when reviewing the medical history, you should carefully focus on conditions that require medical referral (see "Absolute and Relative Contraindications to Exercise Testing" [Gibbons et al. 2002] on p. 18). If any of these conditions are noted, refer your client to a physician for a physical examination and medical clearance prior to exercise testing or starting an exercise program. It is also important to note the types of medication being used by the client. Drugs such as digitalis, beta-blockers, bronchodilators, vasodilators,

---

Absolute and Relative Contraindications to Exercise Testing[a]

Absolute Contraindications

1. Acute myocardial infarction (within 2 days)
2. Unstable angina
3. Uncontrolled cardiac arrhythmias causing symptoms or hemodynamic compromise
4. Uncontrolled symptomatic heart failure
5. Acute aortic dissection
6. Suspected or known dissecting aneurysm
7. Acute myocarditis or pericarditis
8. Acute pulmonary embolus or pulmonary infarction

Relative Contraindications

1. Left main coronary stenosis
2. Moderate stenotic valvular heart disease
3. Known electrolyte abnormalities (hypokalemia, hypomagnesemia)
4. Severe arterial hypertension; resting diastolic BP > 110 mmHg and/or resting systolic BP > 200 mmHg
5. Tachyarrhythmias or bradyarrhythmias
6. Hypertrophic cardiomyopathy and other forms of outflow tract obstruction
7. High-degree atrioventricular block
8. Mental or physical impairment leading to inability to exercise adequately

[a]For definitions of specific medical terms, refer to the glossary on page 379.

From Gibbons, R.J. et al. 2002. ACC/AHA 2002 Guideline update for exercise testing. A report of the American College of Cardiology/American Heart Association Task Force on Practice Guidelines (Committee on Exercise Testing). American College of Cardiology Web site. www.acc.org/clinical/guidelines/exercise/dirIndex.htm.

---

diuretics, and insulin may alter the individual's heart rate, blood pressure, ECG, and exercise capacity. If your client reports a medical condition or drug that is unfamiliar to you, be certain to consult medical references or a physician to obtain more information before conducting any exercise tests or allowing the client to participate in an exercise program.

Signs and Symptoms of Disease and Medical Clearance

As part of the pretest health screening, you should ask your clients if they have any of the conditions or symptoms listed in appendix A.3, "Checklist for Signs and Symptoms of Disease," page 282. Feel free to reproduce and use this checklist.

Clients with any of the signs or symptoms on the checklist should be referred to their physicians to obtain a signed medical clearance prior to any exercise testing or participation. The Physical Activity Readiness Medical Examination (PARmed-X) was designed for this purpose. The PARmed-X is a physical activity-specific checklist (see appendix A.4, page 284) that is used by the physician to assess and convey medical clearance for physical activity participation or to make a referral to a medically supervised exercise program for individuals who answered "yes" to one of the questions in the Physical Activity Readiness Questionnaire (PAR-Q). For definitions of specific medical terms used, refer to the glossary (p. 379).

Coronary Risk Factor Analysis

To assess your client's coronary risk profile, evaluate each item in table 2.2 carefully. Guidelines for classification of blood pressure and blood cholesterol levels in adults are presented in tables 2.3 and 2.4, respectively. If your client's high-density lipoprotein cholesterol (HDL-C) equals or exceeds 60 mg · dl^{-1}, subtract 1 from the total number of

TABLE 2.2　Coronary Heart Disease Risk Factors

Positive risk factors	Criteria
1. Family history	Myocardial infarction, coronary revascularization, or sudden death before 55 years of age for father or other first-degree male relative (brother or son); or before 65 years of age in mother or other first-degree female relative (sister or daughter)
2. Cigarette smoking	Current cigarette smoking, or smoking cessation within previous 6 months
3. Hypertension	Systolic BP ≥140 mmHg or diastolic BP ≥90 mmHg measured on two separate occasions, or individual taking antihypertensive medication
4. Dyslipidemia	TC ≥200 mg · dl^{-1}, or HDL-C <40 mg · dl^{-1}, or LDL-C ≥130 mg · dl^{-1} or on lipid-lowering medication
5. Impaired fasting glucose	Fasting blood glucose ≥110 mg · dl^{-1}, measured on two separate occasions
6. Obesity	Body mass index ≥30 kg/m^2 or waist circumference > 102 cm (40 in.) for men and >88 cm (35 in.) for women
7. Physical inactivity	Not participating in regular exercise program or not meeting the minimum physical activity recommendations from the U.S. Surgeon General's report (accumulating 30 min or more of moderate physical activity on most days of the week)

Negative risk factor[a]

High HDL-C	Serum HDL-C ≥60 mg·dl^{-1}

[a]If HDL-C is high, subtract one risk factor from the sum of the positive risk factors.

Data from National Cholesterol Education Program Committee, 2001, "Executive Summary of the Third Report of the National Cholesterol Education Program (NCEP) Expert Panel on Detection, Evaluation, and Treatment of High Blood Cholesterol in Adults (Adult Treatment Panel III)," *Journal of the American Medical Association* 285(19): 2486-2497.

TABLE 2.3　Classification of Blood Pressure for Adults, 18 Years or Older[a]

Systolic BP (mmHg)[b]	Category	Diastolic BP (mmHg)
<120	Normal	<80
120-139	Prehypertension	80-89
140-159	Stage 1 hypertension	90-99
≥160	Stage 2 hypertension	≥100

[a]For individuals not taking antihypertensive medication and not acutely ill. Based on average of two or more readings on two or more occasions.
[b]When systolic and diastolic pressures fall into different categories, use the higher category for classification.

Data from The Seventh Report of the Joint National Committee on Detection, Evaluation, and Treatment of High Blood Pressure, 2003, *Hypertension* 42: 1206-1252.

positive risk factors. This information is especially helpful in classifying the individual for exercise testing and in designing safe exercise programs.

Disease Risk Classification

On the basis of the results from the coronary risk factor analysis, you should classify individuals as low, moderate, or high risk. According to ACSM (2006), the **low CHD risk** category comprises younger men (< 45 years) and women (< 55 years) who are asymptomatic with no more than one major risk factor (see table 2.2). Older individuals (men ≥45 years and women ≥55 years) or those having two or more risk factors are classified as **moderate CHD risk.** The **high CHD risk** category includes individuals who have one or more signs or symptoms of cardiovascular, pulmonary, or metabolic disease or individuals with known cardiovascular, pulmonary, or metabolic disease (see p. 282).

TABLE 2.4	Classification of TC, LDL-C, Triglycerides, and HDL-C $(mg \cdot dl^{-1})$		

TOTAL CHOLESTEROL, LOW-DENSITY LIPOPROTEIN CHOLESTEROL, AND TRIGLYCERIDES

Classification	TC	LDL-C	Triglycerides
Optimal or desirable	<200	<100	<150
Near or above optimal	——	100-129	——
Borderline high	200-239	130-159	150-199
High	≥240	160-189	200-499
Very high	——	≥190	≥500

HIGH-DENSITY LIPOPROTEIN CHOLESTEROL

Classification	HDL-C
Low	<40
Normal	40-59
High	≥60

Data from National Cholesterol Education Program Committee, 2001, "Executive Summary of the Third Report of the National Cholesterol Education Program (NCEP) Expert Panel on Detection, Evaluation, and Treatment of High Blood Cholesterol in Adults (Adult Treatment Panel III)," *Journal of the American Medical Association* 285(19): 2487.

Lifestyle Evaluation

Planning a well-rounded physical fitness program for an individual requires that you obtain information concerning the client's living habits. The lifestyle assessment provides useful information regarding the individual's risk factor profile. Factors such as smoking, lack of physical activity, and diets high in saturated fats or cholesterol increase the risk of CHD, atherosclerosis, and hypertension. These factors can be used to pinpoint patterns and habits that need modification and to assess the likelihood of the client's adherence to the exercise program. You can obtain a lifestyle profile for your clients by using either the Lifestyle Evaluation form or the Fantastic Lifestyle Checklist provided in appendix A.5, page 288. The Fantastic Lifestyle Checklist is a self-administered tool designed to assess your client's present health-related behaviors.

Informed Consent

Before conducting any physical fitness tests or exercise programs, you should see that each participant signs the informed consent (see appendix A.6, "Informed Consent," p. 292). This form explains the purpose and nature of each physical fitness test, any inherent risks in the testing, and the expected benefits of these tests. The informed consent also assures your clients that test results will remain confidential and that their participation is strictly

voluntary. If your client is underage (< 18 years), a parent or guardian must also sign the informed consent. All consent forms should be approved by your institutional review board or legal counsel.

Clinical Tests

For a comprehensive health screening, you will need to evaluate information and data obtained from the physician's medical examination and clinical tests. Clinical tests provide data about your client's blood chemistry, blood pressure, cardiopulmonary function, and aerobic capacity.

Physical Examination

Your prospective exercise program participants should obtain a physical examination and a signed medical clearance from a physician (appendix A.4, "PARmed-X," p. 284), especially if they are

- men ≥45 years of age or women ≥55 years of age;
- individuals of any age with two or more major risk factors;
- individuals of any age with one or more signs/ symptoms of cardiovascular or pulmonary disease; or
- individuals of any age with known cardiovascular, pulmonary, or metabolic disease.

The physical examination should focus on signs and symptoms of CHD and should include an evaluation of body weight; orthopedic problems; edema; acute illness; pulse rate; cardiac regularity; blood pressure (supine, sitting, and standing); and auscultation of the heart, lungs, and major arteries. The physical examination and medical history may reveal signs or symptoms of CHD particularly if accompanied by shortness of breath, chest pains, leg cramps, or high blood pressure. Clients with these symptoms must obtain a signed medical clearance (p. 284) from their physician prior to exercise testing or exercise participation.

Blood Chemistry Profile

Information obtained from a complete blood analysis is used to assess your client's overall health status and readiness for exercise. Table 2.5 provides normal values for selected blood variables. If any of these values fall outside of the normal range, refer your clients to their physician. Pay special attention to your client's fasting blood glucose and blood lipid values.

The National Cholesterol Education Program (NCEP) (2001) established its guidelines for classifying lipoprotein levels and major risk factors that modify low-density lipoprotein cholesterol (LDL-C) treatment goals. For adults aged 20 years or older, NCEP (2001) recommends that a fasting lipoprotein profile (i.e., total cholesterol, LDL-C, HDL-C, and triglycerides) be obtained every five years. To classify your client's lipoprotein values, use the NCEP (2001) guidelines (see table 2.4). For nonfasting lipoprotein tests, only the total cholesterol (TC) and HDL-C values can be evaluated. If your client's TC is borderline high (200 to 239 mg · dl^{-1}) or high (≥240 mg · dl^{-1}), and the HDL-C level is less than 40 mg · dl^{-1}, a follow-up fasting lipoprotein test will be needed to assess LDL-C. Refer clients to their physicians for an extensive clinical evaluation and dietary therapy if they have high (160 to 189 mg · dl^{-1}) or very high (> 190 mg · dl^{-1}) LDL-C values. Treatment goals for lowering LDL-C depend on the number of major risk factors (exclusive of LDL-C) that the client has. To determine your client's risk category, focus on the following risk factors in table 2.2: cigarette smoking, hypertension, low HDL-C, family history of premature CHD, and age (men ≥45 years; women ≥55 years). Table 2.6 is NCEP's listing of three risk categories that modify LDL-C treatment goals. The NCEP (2001) dietary therapy guidelines for individuals with high LDL-C are included in table 9.4, page 223.

In addition to TC and lipoproteins, you can evaluate your client's triglyceride value and the ratio of TC to HDL-C. Clients with triglyceride levels of ≥150 mg · dl^{-1} or TC/HDL-C ratios >5.0 are at higher risk for CHD.

TABLE 2.5 Normal Values for Selected Blood Variables

Variable	Ideal or typical values
Triglycerides	<150 mg · dl^{-1}
Total cholesterol	<200 mg · dl^{-1}
LDL-cholesterol	<100 mg · dl^{-1}
HDL-cholesterol	≥40 mg · dl^{-1}
TC/HDL-cholesterol	<3.5
Blood glucose	60-109 mg · dl^{-1}
Hemoglobin	13.5-17.5 g · dl^{-1} (men) 11.5-15.5 g · dl^{-1} (women)
Hematocrit	40-52% (men) 36-48% (women)
Potassium	3.5-5.5 meq · dl^{-1}
Blood urea nitrogen	4-24 mg · dl^{-1}
Creatinine	0.3-1.4 mg · dl^{-1}
Iron	40-190 μg · dl^{-1} (men) 35-180 μg · dl^{-1} (women)
Calcium	8.5-10.5 mg · dl^{-1}

TABLE 2.6 Three Risk Categories That Modify LDL-C Goals (NCEP 2001)

Risk category	LDL-C goal (mg · dl^{-1})
CHD and CHD risk equivalents[a]	<100
Multiple (2+) risk factors[b]	<130
0-1 risk factor	<160

[a]CHD risk equivalents include diabetes and atherosclerotic disease (i.e., peripheral arterial disease, abdominal aortic aneurysm, and symptomatic carotid artery disease).
[b]Risk factors include cigarette smoking, hypertension, low high-density lipoprotein cholesterol, family history of premature CHD, and age.

Resting Blood Pressure

Blood pressure (BP) is a measure of the force or pressure exerted by the blood on the arteries. The highest pressure (**systolic blood pressure**) reflects the pressure in the arteries during systole of the heart when myocardial contraction forces a large volume of blood into the arteries. Following systole, the arteries recoil and the pressure drops during diastole, or the filling phase of the heart. **Diastolic blood pressure** is the lowest pressure in the artery during the cardiac cycle. The difference between the systolic and diastolic BPs is known as the **pulse pressure**. The pulse pressure creates a pulse wave that can be palpated at various sites in the body to determine pulse rate and to estimate BP.

Recently, the classifications of resting blood pressure were revised (see table 2.3) (Chobanian et al. 2003). Normal blood pressure (**normotensive**) is defined as values less than 120/80 mmHg. The **prehypertension** category (systolic BP = 120-139 mmHg; diastolic BP = 80-89 mmHg) is added to identify individuals at high risk of developing hypertension. **Hypertension** is defined as a resting blood pressure equaling or exceeding 140/90 mmHg on two or more occasions.

Although prehypertension is not considered a disease, prehypertensive individuals are encouraged to modify their lifestyle in order to reduce their risk of developing hypertension by

- losing body weight if overweight;
- adopting a healthy eating plan that includes a diet rich in fruits, vegetables, and low-fat dairy products but reduced in cholesterol, saturated fat, and total fat;
- restricting dietary sodium intake to no more than 2.4 g (100 mmol) per day;
- engaging in aerobic physical activities at least 30 min/day, most days of the week; and
- limiting alcohol consumption to no more than 1 oz (29.6 ml) per day for men and 0.5 oz (14.8 ml) per day for women.

When lifestyle modifications are ineffective, pharmacological therapy may be required to lower blood pressure. There are numerous drugs available to treat hypertension (see Chobanian et al. 2003), including

- diuretics to rid the body of excess salt and fluids;
- beta-blockers to reduce heart rate and cardiac output;

- sympathetic nerve inhibitors to prevent constriction of arterioles;
- vasodilators to induce relaxation in smooth muscles of arterial walls; and
- angiotensin-converting enzyme inhibitors to disrupt the body's production of angiotensin; which constricts arterioles.

Additional Clinical Tests

For individuals with known or suspected CHD, additional tests may be indicated. These may include a resting 12-lead ECG, angiogram, echocardiogram, and a physician-monitored graded exercise test. A chest X-ray, comprehensive blood chemistry, and complete blood count should also be obtained (ACSM 2006). For clients with known pulmonary disease, ACSM (2006) recommends a chest X-ray, pulmonary function tests, and specialized pulmonary tests (e.g., blood gas analysis).

Graded Exercise Test

Coronary heart disease often is not detectable from the resting ECG, and abnormalities may not appear until the individual engages in relatively strenuous exercise. The client's physician may recommend administration of a graded exercise test as part of the health evaluation to assess functional aerobic capacity of some individuals. Graded exercise tests should be administered only by trained, professionally certified personnel such as exercise scientists, physicians, and nurses.

Use the client's risk classification to determine whether the test should be a maximal or a submaximal exercise test and whether a physician needs to be present during the exercise testing (table 2.7). Also, you need to be familiar with medical conditions that are absolute and relative contraindications to exercise testing in an out-of-hospital setting (see "Absolute and Relative Contraindications to Exercise Testing" on p. 18). Individuals with absolute contraindications should not be given a graded exercise test unless their condition has been stabilized or medically treated. In cases in which the benefits outweigh the risks, individuals with relative contraindications may perform exercise tests. These tests, however, should use low-level end points and be administered with caution (ACSM 2006).

The ACSM (2006) recommends a maximal exercise test for older men (≥45 years) and women (≥55 years) before they begin a vigorous (>6 METs [metabolic equivalents] or >60% of functional aerobic capacity) exercise program

TABLE 2.7   ACSM Guidelines for Medical Examination and Exercise Testing Prior to Participation Based on Risk Classification (ACSM 2006)[a]

	Low risk	Moderate risk	High risk
MEDICAL EXAM AND EXERCISE TEST RECOMMENDED PRIOR TO PARTICIPATION IN:			
Moderate exercise (3-6 METs or 40-60% $\dot{V}O_2$max)	0[b]	0	+[c]
Vigorous exercise (>6 METs or >60% $\dot{V}O_2$max)	0	+	+
PHYSICIAN SUPERVISION RECOMMENDED DURING EXERCISE TEST[d]			
Submaximal test	0	0	+
Maximal test	0	+	+

[a]For definitions of low, moderate, or high risk, see page 19, "Disease Risk Classification."
[b]0 indicates that item is not necessary; however, it should not be viewed as inappropriate.
[c]+ indicates that item is recommended.
[d]For physician supervision—this suggests that a physician be in close proximity and readily available should there be an emergent need.

(see table 2.7). These maximal exercise tests should be administered with physician supervision. For low-risk individuals of any age, submaximal exercise testing can be done without physician supervision. However, the exercise tests should be conducted by exercise specialists, who are preferably ACSM certified and who are well trained and experienced in monitoring exercise tests and handling emergencies (ACSM 2006). The results from these tests provide a basis for prescription of exercise for healthy and coronary-prone individuals, as well as for cardiopulmonary patients.

TESTING PROCEDURES FOR BLOOD PRESSURE, HEART RATE, AND ELECTROCARDIOGRAM

One of your major responsibilities as an exercise scientist is to become proficient at measuring BP, heart rate, and ECGs during rest and exercise. During a graded exercise test, you will be expected to be able to obtain accurate and precise measurements of BP and heart rate while the client is exercising. Because of their importance and complexity, this section is devoted to a thorough discussion of these procedures.

Measuring Blood Pressure

Blood pressure can be measured directly or indirectly. The "gold standard" for assessing BPs is the direct measurement of intra-arterial BP. This method is invasive and requires catheterization. Therefore, in clinical or field settings, BP is typically measured indirectly by auscultation or oscillometry.

For auscultation, a stethoscope and a sphygmomanometer consisting of a blood pressure cuff (cloth cover and bladder) and either a mercury column or an aneroid manometer are used. Step-by-step instructions for the auscultatory method are presented in "Resting Blood Pressure Measurement" on page 24. Oscillometry uses an automated electronic manometer to measure oscillations in pressure (i.e., waveforms) when the cuff is deflated. Systolic and diastolic blood pressures are calculated with the use of proprietary algorithms provided by each manufacturer.

Blood Pressure Measurement Techniques

Measure resting BP in the supine and exercise (sitting or standing) positions prior to testing (ACSM 2006). The client should be wearing a short-sleeved or sleeveless garment and should be seated in a quiet room. Take BP measurements rapidly, and completely deflate the cuff for at least 30 sec between consecutive readings. For more accurate results, obtain two or three determinations of pressure from each arm.

It takes a great deal of practice to become proficient at measuring BPs. When you are first learning this method, it is highly recommended that you practice with a trained BP technician, using a dual- or multiple-head stethoscope so that you can listen simultaneously and compare BP readings for the same trial.

To measure resting BP (seated position), use the following recommended procedures (Reeves 1995):

1. Seat the client in a quiet room for at least 5 min. The client's bare arm should be resting on a table so that the middle of the arm is at the level of the heart.

2. Estimate the client's arm circumference or measure it at the midpoint between the acromion process of the shoulder and the olecranon process of the elbow (see appendix D.4, "Standardized Sites for Circumference Measurements," p. 337, for description of measuring arm circumference) using an anthropometric tape measure. The bladder of the cuff should encircle 80% of an adult's arm and 100% of a child's arm.

3. Palpate the brachial artery pulse on the anteromedial aspect of the arm below the belly of the biceps brachii and 2 to 3 cm (1 in.) above the antecubital fossa. Wrap the deflated cuff firmly around the upper arm so that the midline of the cuff is over the brachial artery pulse. The lower edge of the cuff should be approximately 2.5 cm (1 in.) above the antecubital fossa. If the cuff is too loose, BP will be overestimated. Avoid placing the cuff over clothing; and if the shirt sleeve is rolled up, make certain that it is not occluding the circulation.

4. Position the manometer so that the center of the mercury column or dial is at eye level and the cuff's tubing is not overlapping or obstructed.

5. Locate and palpate the radial pulse (see p. 29 for anatomical description of this site), close the valve of the BP unit completely by screwing it away from you, and rapidly inflate the cuff to 70 mmHg. Then slowly increase the pressure in 10-mmHg increments while palpating the radial pulse, and note when the pulse disappears (estimate of systolic BP). Partially open the valve by unscrewing it toward you to slowly release the pressure at a rate of 2 to 3 mmHg/sec and note when the pulse reappears (estimate of diastolic BP). Fully open the valve to completely release the pressure in the cuff. The estimate of systolic BP from the palpatory method is then used to determine how much the cuff needs to be inflated for measuring BP by means of the auscultatory technique. In this way, you can avoid over- or underinflating the cuff for clients with low or high BPs, respectively.

6. Position the earpieces of the stethoscope so that they are aligned with the auditory canals (i.e., angled anteriorly).

7. Place the head (bell) of the stethoscope over the brachial pulse (about 1 cm superior and medial to the antecubital fossa). Make certain that the entire head of the stethoscope is contacting the skin. To avoid extraneous noise, do not place any part of the head of the stethoscope underneath the cuff.

8. Close the valve, and quickly and steadily inflate the cuff pressure to about 20 to 30 mmHg above the estimated systolic pressure previously determined by palpation.

9. Partially open the valve to slowly release the pressure at a rate of 2 to 3 mmHg/sec. Note when you hear the first sharp thud caused by the sudden rush of blood as the artery opens. This is known as the first Korotkoff sound and corresponds to the systolic pressure (Phase I).

10. Continue reducing the pressure slowly (no more than 2 mmHg/sec), noting when the metallic tapping sound becomes muffled (Phase IV diastolic pressure) and when the sound disappears (Phase V diastolic pressure). Typically, the Phase V value is used as the index of diastolic pressure. However, both Phase IV and V diastolic pressures should be noted. During rhythmic exercise, the Phase V pressure tends to decrease because of reduction in peripheral resistance. In some cases, it may even drop to zero.

11. After noting the Phase V pressure, continue deflating the cuff for at least 10 mmHg, making certain that no additional sounds are heard. Then rapidly and completely deflate the cuff.

12. Record all three BP values (Phase I, IV, and V) to the nearest 2 mmHg. Wait at least 30 sec and repeat the measurement. Use the average of the two measurements for each of the three values.

Sources of Measurement Error

Sources of error in measuring BP are numerous (Reeves 1995). You need to be aware of the following sources of error and do as much as possible to control them:

- Inaccurate sphygmomanometer
- Improper cuff width or length
- Cuff not centered, too loose, or over clothing
- Arm unsupported or elbow lower than heart level
- Poor auditory acuity of technician
- Improper rate of inflation or deflation of the cuff pressure
- Improper stethoscope placement or pressure
- Expectation bias and inexperience of the technician
- Slow reaction time of the technician
- Parallax error in reading the manometer
- Background noise
- Client holding treadmill handrails or cycle ergometer handlebars

The following section addresses questions about measuring blood pressure and provides tips for taking more accurate blood pressure measurements during rest or exercise.

■ *Which type of sphygmomanometer—mercury column or aneroid—provides more valid and reliable measures of resting blood pressure?*

For over a century, the mercury column manometer has been considered the gold standard for indirect measurement of blood pressure. Although calibrated, aneroid manometers may yield values similar to those of mercury column manometers, the latter are preferred for a number of reasons. Mercury column manometers are based on gravity, leaving little room for mechanical errors. In contrast, the aneroid manometer is a spring-based device that can fatigue with use and thereby lose its calibration more easily. It can become inaccurate without the technician's awareness. Therefore, aneroid manometers must be calibrated frequently (at least every 6 mo). Often when the aneroid manometer fails the calibration test, it must be returned to the manufacturer for repair.

■ *How can I check the accuracy of an aneroid manometer?*

To check the accuracy of an aneroid manometer against a mercury unit, follow the procedure suggested by Reeves (1995):

- Disconnect the bulbs of both cuffs and reconnect the bulb and dial of the aneroid unit to the cuff of the mercury unit.
- Loosely roll up the cuff, secure the Velcro strips, and hold the cuff steady while gradually inflating it.
- Hold the dial of the aneroid manometer close to the mercury column and compare the two readings at several pressures throughout the measurement scale (e.g., throughout 40-220 mmHg). If the aneroid and mercury manometer pressures differ by more than 2 to 3 mmHg, send the aneroid manometer to the manufacturer for adjustment.

■ *What criteria are used to judge the accuracy of devices that measure blood pressure?*

The Association for the Advancement of Medical Instrumentation (AAMI) and the British Hypertension Society (BHS) have established separate criteria for judging the accuracy of blood pressure devices. Most validation studies use one or both of these sets of criteria. For either set, measured values from the device are compared to those obtained from a mercury sphygmomanometer. To meet AAMI criteria, the measured average blood pressure (systolic and diastolic) should not differ from the mercury standard by more than 5 mmHg and the standard deviation should not exceed 8 mmHg. For the BHS criteria (O'Brien, Waeber, Parati, Staessen, and Myers 2001), differences in both systolic and diastolic blood pressures are graded as A, B, C, or D depending on the cumulative percentage of absolute individual difference scores falling within three categories: 5, 10, and 15 mmHg (see table 2.8). To be recommended, a device must achieve at least a

TABLE 2.8   BHS Validation Criteria for Blood Pressure Measuring Devices[a]

Grade[b]	CATEGORY		
	≤ 5 mmHg	≤ 10 mmHg	≤ 15 mmHg
A	60%	85%	95%
B	50%	75%	90%
C	40%	65%	85%
D	Worse than C		

[a]Values are the cumulative percentage of absolute difference scores between the mercury standard and the test device.

[b]All 3 percentages must be greater than or equal to the values shown for a specific grade to be awarded.

B; A and D denote the greatest and least degree of agreement with the mercury standard.

The European Society of Hypertension (ESH) updated the BHS validation criteria (O'Brien et al. 2002). The ESH protocol, also known as the International Protocol, is more complex. Basically, it categorizes mean differences in blood pressure as follows: 0 to 5 mmHg = very accurate, 6 to 10 mmHg = slightly inaccurate, 11 to 15 mmHg = moderately inaccurate, and >15 mmHg = very inaccurate. The number of comparisons *cumulatively* falling within 5, 10, and 15 mmHg is counted (i.e., the 5 mmHg zone represents all values falling within 0-5 mmHg, the 10 mmHg zone represents all values falling within 0-5 mmHg and 6-10 mmHg, the 15 mmHg zone represents all values falling within 0-5 mmHg, 6-10 mmHg, and 10-15 mmHg). These values are then compared to standards set for each of two phases of the validation process. Devices recommended for clinical use must pass both phases of the validation process. For a detailed description of the International Protocol, see O'Brien and colleagues (2002).

■ *In the future, will the mercury column manometer be banned?*

Because of the toxic effects of mercury on the environment, future use of mercury manometers and thermometers in the United States and European countries may be restricted or even banned. Many hospitals and health care facilities in Europe are voluntarily removing mercury manometers and replacing them with aneroid or automated measuring devices. In Sweden and the Netherlands, the use of mercury in hospital settings is already banned (Beevers, Lip, and O'Brien 2001b). Although no health care agencies in the United States presently forbid mercury manometers, some experts predict that the manometers are destined for the museum shelves (Markandu, Whitcher, Arnold, and Carney 2000; O'Brien 2003). The American Heart Association (AHA) encourages the continued use of mercury manometers until other devices are better validated (Jones, Frohlich, Grim, Grim, and Taubert 2001). The AHA also made the following recommendations for health care and fitness settings that exclusively use aneroid or automated devices:

- Select only devices that satisfy the validation criteria of the AAMI or similar organizations.
- Schedule regular maintenance and calibration.
- Insist on the use of mercury manometers for calibration.

- Ensure regular training of personnel who measure blood pressure.

■ *How accurate are automated blood pressure devices?*

There are many automated devices available for clinical and home use. These automated devices inflate and deflate a cuff that is placed over the brachial artery (upper-arm device), radial artery (wrist device), or digital artery (finger device). The automated electronic manometer assesses oscillations in pressure while the cuff is gradually deflated. The maximum oscillation corresponds to mean arterial pressure, and algorithms, which vary among manufacturers, are used to calculate systolic and diastolic pressures. Unfortunately, most of these devices have not been independently evaluated for accuracy.

In a review of various types of blood pressure devices, only 5 of 23 upper-arm models of automated devices for self-measurement of blood pressure passed both the AAMI and BHS validation criteria and received the recommendation of the ESH (O'Brien et al. 2001). The recommended models, all manufactured by Omron Healthcare, Inc., include the HEM-705CP, HEM-713C, HEM-722C, HEM-735C, and HEM-737 Intellisense. None of the four automated wrist models passed the validation criteria. Although finger devices were not included in this review, Schutte and colleagues (2004) recently reported that the Finometer satisfied the criteria of the AAMI and BHS for measuring the resting blood pressure of Black women. For regular updates on the latest research and recommendations on automated devices, visit www.esh.org.

■ *Can automated devices be used to measure blood pressure during exercise?*

The validity and accuracy of automated devices for measuring exercise blood pressure have not yet been firmly established (Griffin, Roberts, and Heyward 1997). To date, no criteria have been established to evaluate the accuracy of devices for measuring blood pressure under stress (e.g., exercise). The accuracy of some finger devices (i.e., Finapres and Portapres Model 2) designed for continuous, noninvasive, ambulatory blood pressure monitoring has been assessed during incremental cycle ergometer exercise (Blum, Carriere, Kolsters, Mosterd, Schiereck, and Wesseling 1997; Eckert and Horstkotte 2002; Idema, van den Meiracker, and Imholz 1989). In these studies, the mean differences between the automated (Finapres and Portapres Model 2) and the intra-arterial measures of blood pressure during low-intensity (~100 W) exercise ranged from 12 to 22 mmHg for systolic pressure and from –5 to –9.8 mmHg for diastolic pressure. During exercise, these automated finger devices systematically underestimated and overestimated systolic and diastolic blood pressures, respectively, and average differences increased as exercise intensity increased. Therefore, these devices should not be used to measure blood pressure during exercise.

■ How do body position and arm position affect blood pressure measurements?

Posture affects blood pressure; generally, blood pressure increases from lying (supine) to sitting to standing. Usually, resting blood pressure is measured in the sitting position. Regardless of body position, the upper arm must be held or supported horizontally at the level of the heart (right atrium); the midsternal level most closely approximates the level of the right atrium. Raising the arm above heart level underestimates blood pressure, and positioning the arm below heart level tends to overestimate blood pressure. Also, the accuracy of automated wrist devices is greatly affected if the wrist is not held at heart level (Beevers, Lip, and O'Brien 2001a). Generally, the arm should be supported at heart level during the measurement of sitting and standing blood pressure; diastolic blood pressure may increase as much as 10% when the arm is extended and unsupported (Beevers et al. 2001a). Typically, the arm is supported by resting it on a table or by having the technician hold it at the elbow. Even when supine blood pressure is measured, a pillow should be placed under the upper arm to support it at heart level.

■ What is white coat hypertension?

White coat hypertension is a condition describing individuals who have normal blood pressure outside of the clinical environment but who become hypertensive when their blood pressure is measured by a health professional. White coat hypertension appears to be more common in women and in the elderly (Chung and Lip 2003). To confirm this condition, blood pressure should be measured outside of the clinical environment by self-measurement at home or by 24 hr ambulatory blood pressure monitoring. Recent studies suggest that white coat hypertension is not benign (Chung and Lip 2003; Gustavsen, Hoegholm, Bang, and Kristensen 2003). A 10 yr follow-up study of 420 patients with stage 1 or 2 hypertension (of which 18% had white coat hypertension) reported that individuals with white coat hypertension have an increased risk of CVD compared to normotensive individuals (Gustavsen et al. 2003). This finding suggests that white coat

hypertension should be considered when evaluating cardiovascular risk factors.

■ What are miscuffing and cuff hypertension?

Miscuffing (i.e., undercuffing or overcuffing) is a serious source of measurement error caused by using a blood pressure cuff with a bladder that is not appropriately scaled for the client's arm circumference. Experts recommend using a cuff with a bladder width that is 40% of the measured upper-arm circumference and a length that encircles at least 80% of the arm circumference. Undercuffing occurs when the bladder is too small for the arm circumference, leading to the overestimation of blood pressure known as cuff hypertension. Conversely, overcuffing underestimates blood pressure because the bladder is too large for the arm circumference (Beevers et al. 2001a). To avoid these problems, the correct cuff and bladder size must be selected for each client.

■ How can I determine the appropriate cuff size for my client?

To ensure accurate blood pressure readings, you need to select a cuff size appropriate for your client's arm circumference. Generally, four cuff sizes are commercially available: children, standard adult, large adult, and obese (i.e., thigh). To select the proper cuff size, measure your client's arm circumference (see appendix D.4, "Standardized Sites for Circumference Measurements," p. 337, for a description of measuring arm circumference). If arm circumference cannot be measured directly, you can estimate it using gender-specific prediction equations (see Ostchega, Prineas, Dillon, McDowell, and Carroll 2004). Table 2.9 presents recommended cuff and bladder sizes for measured or estimated arm circumferences.

TABLE 2.9 Recommended Cuff and Bladder Sizes for Arm Circumferences

Cuff type	Arm circumference (cm)	Bladder width × length (cm)
Smaller child	≤17	4 × 13
Larger child	18-25	10 × 18
Standard adult	26-33	12 × 26
Larger adult	34-42	16 × 33
Obese adult (thigh cuff)	43-50	20 × 42

Data compiled from Beevers et al. 2001a and Ostchega et al. 2004.

■ *How can I measure exercise blood pressure more accurately?*

Measuring BP during exercise is much more difficult than doing so during rest. You should not attempt to measure exercise BP until you have demonstrated competency and have confidence in your ability to measure resting BP. It is particularly difficult to accurately measure BP when the client is running on the treadmill because of extraneous noise and arm movement during running. Sometimes you will not be able to determine diastolic BP during exercise because of the noise and vibration. Novice technicians should first practice taking BPs during cycle ergometer exercise and then try measuring BP during treadmill exercise. See "Tips for Measuring Exercise Blood Pressure" for pointers on improving your BP measurements during exercise.

Measuring Heart Rate

The average resting heart rate for adults is 60 to 80 beats per minute (bpm), with the average resting heart rate of women typically 7 to 10 bpm higher than that of men. Heart rates as low as 28 to 40 bpm have been reported for highly conditioned endurance athletes, whereas poorly trained, sedentary individuals may have heart rates that exceed 100 bpm.

Do not use resting heart rate as a measure of cardiorespiratory fitness. There is wide variability in resting heart rate within the population, and a low resting heart rate is not always indicative of cardiorespiratory fitness level. In some cases, a low resting heart rate indicates a diseased heart

(McArdle, Katch, and Katch 1996). The following general guidelines may be used to classify resting heart rate:

1. < 60 bpm = **bradycardia** (slow rate)
2. 60 to 100 bpm = **normal rate**
3. > 100 bpm = **tachycardia** (fast rate)

Before you measure resting heart rate, your client should rest for 5 to 10 min in either a supine or a seated position. It is important that you measure resting heart rate carefully because this value is sometimes used in the calculation of target exercise heart rates for submaximal exercise tests, as well as for exercise prescriptions. You can measure heart rate using auscultation, palpation, heart rate monitors, or ECG recordings.

Auscultation

When measuring resting heart rate by auscultation, place the bell of the stethoscope over the third intercostal space to the left of the sternum. The sounds arising from the heart are counted for 30 or 60 sec. The 30-sec count is multiplied by 2 to convert it to beats per minute.

Palpation

With use of the **palpation** technique for determining heart rate, the pulse is palpated at one of the following sites:

■ Brachial artery—on the anteromedial aspect of the arm below the belly of the biceps brachii, approximately 2 to 3 cm (1 in.) above the antecubital fossa

---

Tips for Measuring Exercise Blood Pressure

When measuring exercise BP, take extra precautions to ensure accurate readings:

■ Instruct the client to refrain from grasping the handlebars or handrails of the exercise apparatus during the BP measurement.

■ Position the cuff on the arm so that the tubing protruding from its bladder is superior instead of inferior. This position lessens extraneous noise caused by the tubing contacting the stethoscope during exercise.

■ Limit arm movement during the BP measurement; stabilize the client's arm at heart level by placing and holding it firmly between your arm and trunk.

■ Inflate the cuff well above the anticipated value or reading obtained during the previous stage of the graded exercise test, keeping in mind that systolic BP increases with exercise intensity.

■ Position the manometer so that it is no more than 3 ft (92 cm) away and is at eye level so that you can read the scale easily. Errors will occur if you do not keep your eyes close to the level of the meniscus of the mercury column or perpendicular to the aneroid scale. For mercury column sphygmomanometry, use a model that is mounted on a stand with wheels so that the manometer can be properly positioned during incremental stages of the exercise test. Positioning is particularly important when the client is performing graded treadmill tests that progressively increase the incline of the treadmill.

Heart Rate Determination by Palpation

Follow these procedures when determining heart rate by palpation:

- Use the tips of the middle and index fingers. Do not use your thumb; it has a pulse of its own and may produce an inaccurate count.

- When palpating the carotid site, do not apply heavy pressure to the area. Baroreceptors in the carotid arteries detect this pressure and cause a reflex slowing of the heart rate.

- If you start the stopwatch simultaneously with the pulse beat, count the first beat as zero. If the stopwatch is running, count the first beat as 1. Continue counting either for a set period of time (6, 10, 15, 30, or 60 sec) or for a set number of beats. When the heart rate is counted for less than 1 min, use the following multipliers to convert the count to beats per minute: 6-sec count times 10; 10-sec count times 6; 15-sec, 4; 30-sec, 2. Typically, shorter time intervals (i.e., 6- or 10-sec counts) are used to measure exercise and postexercise heart rates during and immediately following exercise. Because there is a rapid and immediate decline in heart rate when a person stops exercising, the 6- or 10-sec count reflects the individual's actual exercise heart rate more accurately than the longer counts do.

- Carotid artery—in the neck just lateral to the larynx
- Radial artery—on the anterolateral aspect of the wrist directly in line with the base of the thumb
- Temporal artery—along the hairline of the head at the temple

For precautions necessary to be sure your measurement is accurate, refer to "Heart Rate Determination by Palpation."

Heart Rate Monitors and Electrocardiogram (ECG) Recordings

Heart rate also can be measured using heart rate monitors or an ECG monitoring system. Generally, heart rate monitors are designed to detect either the pulse or the ECG electrical signal from the heart, and provide a digital display of the heart rate. Pulse monitors use infrared sensors attached to the client's fingertip, earlobe, or wrist (i.e., heart rate watch) to detect pulsations in blood flow during the cardiac cycle. Chest-strap wire and wireless ECG-type monitors tend to be more accurate and reliable than pulse monitors, especially during vigorous exercise. However, the accuracy of wireless chest-strap monitors may be affected by electrical equipment (such as some treadmills, stair climbers, rowing machines, and video screens) generating radio or magnetic interference. Generally, HR monitors provide an accurate measure of ECG HR during rest and exercise (Vehrs, Drummond, Fellingham, and Brigham 2002).

Most ECG monitoring systems provide a continuous digital display of the heart rate. This value is usually recorded at the top of the ECG strip recording. If your equipment does not provide a digital readout, you can use a heart rate ruler that converts the distance of two cardiac cycles to beats per minute. Alternatively, you can count the heart rate by measuring the distance between four consecutive beats (R-R intervals) using a millimeter ruler. Convert the distance to beats per minute based on the paper speed of the recorder (usually 25 $mm \cdot sec^{-1}$). For example, if the distance for four beats is 60 mm and the distance for 1 min is 1500 mm (i.e., 25 mm × 60 sec), the per minute heart rate is determined by setting up the following equation and solving for x:

$$4 \text{ beats}/60 \text{ mm} = x \text{ (bpm)}/1500 \text{ mm}$$

Cross-multiplying, $60x = 6000$; then $x = 100$ bpm. You can use the sample ECG recordings in appendix A.7, "Sample EGC Tracings" (p. 294), to practice measuring heart rates using this method.

No matter which technique is used to measure heart rate, you should be aware that heart rate fluctuates easily due to temperature, anxiety, exercise, stress, eating, smoking, drinking coffee, time of day, and body position. In a supine position, the resting heart rate is lower than in either a sitting or a standing position.

Twelve-Lead Electrocardiogram

The electrocardiogram is a composite record of the electrical events in the heart during the cardiac cycle. As the heart depolarizes and repolarizes during contraction, an electrical impulse spreads to the tissues surrounding the heart. Electrodes placed on opposite sides of the heart transmit the electrical potential to an ECG recorder.

In addition to providing baseline data, the resting ECG is used to detect such contraindications to exercise testing as evidence of previous myocardial infarction, ischemic ST-segment changes, conduction defects, and left ventricular hypertrophy. The reading and interpretation of ECGs require a high degree of skill and practice. As an exercise technician you can administer the resting 12-lead ECG, but a qualified physician should interpret the results. This chapter includes only basic information about administering an ECG. You should consult other references for more detailed information concerning the reading and interpretation of ECG abnormalities (Adamovich 1984; Conover 1992; Dubin 1980; Goldberger and Goldberger 1981; Goldman 1982).

Electrocardiogram Basics

A typical normal ECG (figure 2.1) is composed of a **P wave** that represents depolarization of the atria. The **PR interval** indicates the delay in the impulse at the atrioventricular node. Electrical currents generated during ventricular depolarization and contraction produce the **QRS complex**. The **T wave** and **ST segment** correspond to ventricular repolarization.

A lead is a pair of electrodes placed on the body and connected to an ECG recorder. An axis is an imaginary line connecting the two electrodes. A standard 12-lead ECG consists of three limb leads, three augmented unipolar leads, and six chest leads. Each of the 12 ECG leads records a different view of the heart's electrical activity. Thus, the tracings from the various leads differ from one another.

Resting 12-Lead Electrocardiogram Procedures

To measure the 12 leads, 10 electrodes are used. The electrodes for the three **limb leads** (I, II, and III) are placed on the right arm, left arm, and left leg. A ground electrode is placed on the right leg. This is electronically equivalent to placing the electrodes at the shoulders and the symphysis pubis. Limb lead I measures the voltage differential between the left and right arm electrodes. Limb leads II and III measure the voltage between the

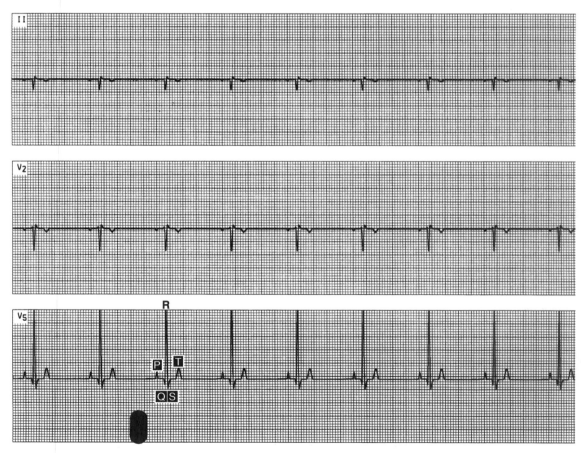

Figure 2.1   Typical normal electrocardiogram.

left leg and right (lead II) and left (lead II) arms. Figure 2.2 shows the three limb leads and three augmented unipolar leads.

The three **augmented unipolar leads** are aVF (feet), aVL (left), and aVR (right). The augmented unipolar lead compares the voltage across one of the limb electrodes with the average voltage across the two opposite electrodes. Lead aVL, for example,

records the voltage across an electrode placed on the left arm and the average voltage across the other two limb electrodes (see figure 2.2).

The six **chest leads** (V_1 to V_6) measure the voltage across a specific area of the chest, with the average voltage across the other three limb leads. Figure 2.3 illustrates electrode placement for the chest leads, V_1 through V_6.

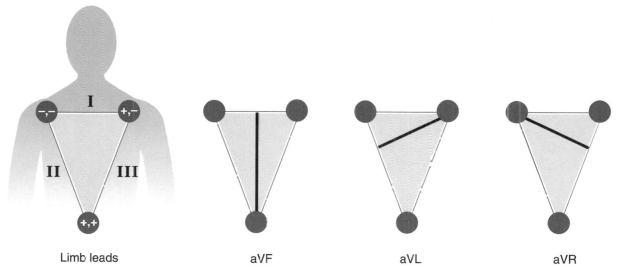

Limb leads   aVF   aVL   aVR

Figure 2.2 Three limb leads and three augmented unipolar leads.

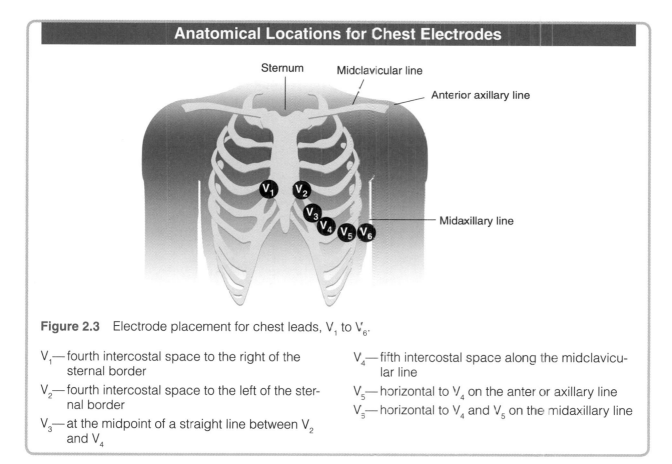

Anatomical Locations for Chest Electrodes

Figure 2.3 Electrode placement for chest leads, V_1 to V_6.

V_1—fourth intercostal space to the right of the sternal border

V_2—fourth intercostal space to the left of the sternal border

V_3—at the midpoint of a straight line between V_2 and V_4

V_4—fifth intercostal space along the midclavicular line

V_5—horizontal to V_4 on the anterior axillary line

V_6—horizontal to V_4 and V_5 on the midaxillary line

During the resting ECG, the client should lie quietly in a supine position on a table. The electrode sites should be shaved if hair is present and should be cleaned with alcohol. Remove the superficial layer of skin at each site by rubbing it with fine-grain emery paper or a gauze pad. Disposable electrodes contain electrode gel and adhesive disks. After applying the electrode, tap it firmly to test for noisy leads. You should always calibrate the ECG recorder prior to use by recording the standard 1-mV deflection per centimeter. Also, to standardize the time base for the ECG, set the paper speed to 25 mm/sec.

The Twelve-Lead Exercise ECG

To avoid poor ECG tracings caused by moving limbs during exercise, the electrode configuration is modified slightly for an exercise 12-lead ECG. The right and left arm electrodes are placed below the right and left clavicles, respectively. The right and left leg electrodes are attached to the right and left sides of the trunk, below the rib cage on the anterior axillary line. The six chest electrodes are positioned as previously described (see figure 2.4).

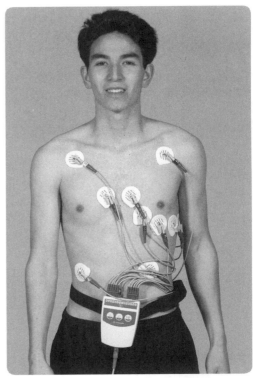

Figure 2.4   Electrode placement for 12-lead exercise electrocardiogram.

Sources for Equipment

Product	Supplier's address
Anaeroid or mercury sphygmomanometer and blood pressure cuffs	W.A. Baum Co. 620 Oak St. Copiague, NY 11726 (888) 281-6061 www.wabaum.com
Automated electronic blood pressure devices	Omron Healthcare, Inc. 300 Lakeview Pkwy. Vernon Hills, IL 60061 (847) 680-6200 www.omronhealthcare.com
Electrocardiograph	GE Marquette Medical Systems P.O. Box 414 Milwaukee, WI 53201 www.gemedicalsystems.com
Heart rate monitors	Creative Health Products 7621 East Joy Rd. Ann Arbor, MI 48105 www.chponline.com

KEY POINTS

- The purpose of the health evaluation is to detect disease and to assess disease risk.
- Important components of the health evaluation are a medical history, CHD risk factor analysis, physical examination, clinical tests, and medical clearance.
- The lifestyle evaluation includes information about the diet, tobacco and alcohol use, physical activity, and psychological stress levels of the individual.
- All clients are required to sign an informed consent prior to taking any physical fitness tests or participating in an exercise program.
- The resting evaluation of cardiorespiratory function includes heart rate, BP, and a 12-lead ECG that is interpreted by a qualified physician.

- Resting BP can be assessed using auscultation or automated BP devices.
- Heart rate may be taken using auscultation, palpation, heart rate monitors, or ECG recordings.
- The 12-lead ECG includes three limb leads (I, II, III), three augmented unipolar leads (aVF, aVR, aVL), and six chest leads (V_1 through V_6).
- A graded maximal exercise test is the best way to assess functional aerobic capacity.
- Unless contraindications to exercise are observed, a maximal exercise test is recommended for men 45 years or older and women 55 years or older before they begin a vigorous exercise program.

KEY TERMS

Learn the definition for each of the following key terms. Definitions of key terms can be found in the glossary on page 379.

augmented unipolar leads	low CHD risk	P wave
auscultation	miscuffing	QRS complex
bradycardia	moderate CHD risk	sphygmomanometer
chest leads	normotensive	ST segment
cuff hypertension	oscillometry	systolic blood pressure
diastolic blood pressure	overcuffing	tachycardia
electrocardiogram	palpation	T wave
high CHD risk	prehypertension	undercuffing
hypertension	PR interval	white coat hypertension
limb leads	pulse pressure	

REVIEW QUESTIONS

In addition to being able to define each of the key terms, test your knowledge and understanding of the material by answering the following review questions.

1. Identify the purpose of each component of the comprehensive health evaluation.
2. At minimum, a pretest health screening should include four items. Name these.
3. Identify cardiovascular, pulmonary, metabolic, and musculoskeletal diseases and/or disorders that warrant referral to a physician for medical clearance (name three signs or symptoms for each category).

(continued)

(continued)

4. Identify the positive and negative risk factors for CHD. Specify the criteria for each of these risk factors.

5. Identify the cutoff values for classifying resting BPs.

6. Identify the cutoff values for classifying TC, LDL-C, HDL-C, and triglycerides.

7. List the three ACSM risk stratification categories and the criterion for each category.

8. Describe the criteria used to determine whether or not an individual needs a physical examination and medical clearance prior to exercise testing or exercise participation.

9. Name three methods for measuring BP. Which one is considered to be the "gold standard" method?

10. Name three sources of error in measurement of BP.

11. Describe three things you should do to ensure accurate BP readings during exercise.

12. Describe the effects of miscuffing on blood pressure readings.

13. What affect does arm position and body posture have on blood pressure readings?

14. Name three methods for measuring heart rate.

15. Identify the component parts of a typical normal ECG tracing. What does each component represent relative to the cardiac cycle?

16. Describe the anatomical locations for placement of the 10 electrodes used to obtain a 12-lead ECG recording.

17. Identify ACSM's guidelines for medical examinations and exercise testing for low-, moderate-, and high-risk individuals.

18. Name three absolute and three relative contraindications to exercise testing.

chapter 3

Principles of Assessment, Prescription, and Exercise Program Adherence

Key Questions

- What are the essential components of a physical fitness profile?

- What are the purposes of physical fitness tests and how can I use the results?

- Several physical fitness tests are available; how do I select the best test for my client?

- Are field tests as good as laboratory tests for measuring physical fitness?

- What is the best way to interpret test results for my client?

- What are the essential elements of an exercise prescription?

- Is one type of exercise better than others for improving each component of physical fitness?

- Does high-intensity exercise improve physical fitness faster than low-intensity exercise?

- Is it safe to exercise every day?

- When should I increase the frequency, intensity, and duration in an exercise prescription? Can these elements be increased simultaneously?

- Do older people benefit as much from exercise as younger people?

- How can I get my clients to stick with their exercise programs?

- Do I need to be professionally certified or licensed in order to work in this field?

Health/fitness professionals need to master the basic principles of physical fitness assessment and exercise prescription. You must know how to use the results of physical fitness tests to plan scientifically sound exercise programs that are individualized to meet your client's needs, interests, and abilities. With your knowledge, leadership, and guidance, your clients can reduce their risk of disease and improve their health and physical fitness levels safely and effectively.

As an exercise specialist, you will have diverse responsibilities, such as

- educating clients about the positive benefits of regular physical activity;

- conducting pretest health evaluations to screen clients for exercise participation (see chapter 2);

- selecting, administering, and interpreting tests designed to assess each component of physical fitness;

- designing individualized exercise programs;

- leading exercise classes;

- analyzing your clients' exercise performance and correcting performance errors;

- educating your clients about the "do's and don'ts" of exercise; and

- motivating your clients to improve their adherence to exercise.

Exercise specialists play many roles: educator, leader, technician, and artist. To be effective in these roles, you must integrate knowledge from many disciplines such as anatomy, physiology, chemistry, nutrition, education, and psychology, as well as refine your exercise testing, prescription, and leadership skills.

This chapter presents principles of exercise testing and prescription, along with information about exercise program adherence and the importance of professional certification for individuals in the field of exercise science.

PHYSICAL FITNESS TESTING

There are several areas that you must understand in order to plan and administer physical fitness tests. These comprise

- the components of physical fitness to be tested;
- purposes of physical fitness testing;
- testing order and the testing environment;
- test validity, reliability, and objectivity;
- prediction equation evaluation; and
- test administration and interpretation.

Components of Physical Fitness

Physical fitness is the ability to perform occupational, recreational, and daily activities without becoming unduly fatigued. As an exercise specialist, one of your primary responsibilities is to assess each of the following physical fitness components:

1. **Cardiorespiratory endurance. Cardiorespiratory endurance** is the ability of the heart, lungs, and circulatory system to supply oxygen and nutrients efficiently to working muscles. Exercise physiologists measure the **maximum oxygen consumption** ($\dot{V}O_2max$), or the rate of oxygen utilization of the muscles during aerobic exercise, in order to assess cardiorespiratory endurance and functional aerobic capacity. Physical fitness evaluations should include a test of cardiorespiratory function during rest and exercise. Graded exercise tests (GXTs) are used for this purpose. Improved cardiorespiratory endurance is one of the most important benefits of aerobic exercise training programs. Chapters 4 and 5 present detailed information about graded exercise testing and aerobic exercise programs.

2. **Musculoskeletal fitness. Musculoskeletal fitness** refers to the ability of the skeletal and muscular systems to perform work. This requires muscular strength, muscular endurance, and bone strength. **Muscular strength** is the maximal force or tension level that can be produced by a muscle group; **muscular endurance** is the ability of a muscle to maintain submaximal force levels for extended periods; **bone strength** is directly related to the risk of bone fracture and is a function of the mineral content and density of the bone tissue. Resistance training is one of the most effective ways to improve the strength of muscles and bones and to develop muscular endurance. Chapters 6 and 7 provide detailed information about assessing musculoskeletal fitness and designing resistance training programs.

3. **Body weight and body composition. Body weight** refers to the size or mass of the individual. **Body composition** refers to body weight in terms of the absolute and relative amounts of muscle, bone, and fat tissues. Aerobic exercise and resistance training are effective in altering body weight and composition. Chapters 8 and 9 discuss body composition assessment techniques and exercise programs for weight management.

4. **Flexibility. Flexibility** is the ability to move a joint or series of joints fluidly through the complete range of motion. Flexibility is limited by factors such as bony structure of the joint and the size and strength of muscles, ligaments, and other connective tissues. Daily stretching can greatly improve flexibility. Chapters 10 and 11 give more information about assessing flexibility and designing stretching programs.

Purposes of Physical Fitness Testing

As mentioned in chapter 2, it is imperative that you carefully screen your clients for exercise testing, classify their disease risk, identify any contraindications to exercise testing, and obtain their informed consent before conducting any physical fitness tests. You can use laboratory and field tests to assess each component of physical fitness and to develop physical fitness profiles for your clients. Results from these tests enable you to identify strengths and weaknesses and to set realistic and attainable goals for your clients. Data from specific tests (e.g., heart rates from a GXT) will help you make accurate and precise exercise prescriptions for each client. Also, you can use baseline and follow-up data to evaluate the progress of exercise program participants.

Testing Order and the Testing Environment

When you administer a complete battery of physical fitness tests in a single session, ACSM (2006) recommends using the following test sequence to minimize the effects of previous tests on subsequent test performance:

- Resting blood pressure and heart rate
- Body composition
- Cardiorespiratory endurance
- Muscular fitness
- Flexibility

Often clients are apprehensive about taking physical fitness tests. Test anxiety may affect the validity and reliability of test results. Therefore, you should put your client at ease by establishing good rapport; projecting a sense of relaxed confidence; and creating a testing environment that is friendly, quiet, private, safe, and comfortable. Room temperature should be maintained at 70 to 74 °F (21 to 23 °C), and the relative humidity should be controlled whenever possible. For pretest health screening and interpretation of the client's test results, the room should have comfortable chairs and a table for completing questionnaires and paperwork, as well as an examination table or bed for the resting evaluation of heart rate, blood pressure, and the 12-lead electrocardiogram. All equipment used for physical testing should be carefully calibrated and prepared before your client arrives for testing. This will ensure valid test data and efficient use of time.

Test Validity, Reliability, and Objectivity

To accurately assess your client's physical fitness status, you must select tests that are valid, reliable, and objective. It is necessary to understand these basic concepts fully in order to evaluate the relative worth of specific physical fitness tests and prediction equations.

Test Validity

With regard to physical fitness testing, test **validity** is the ability of a test to *measure accurately*, with minimal error, a specific physical fitness component. **Reference** or **criterion methods** are used to obtain *direct* measures of physical fitness compo-

nents. However, some physical fitness components cannot always be measured directly, requiring the use of *indirect* measures for estimation of the value of the reference measure. For example, exercise physiologists consider the direct measurement of $\dot{V}O_2$max (i.e., collection and analysis of expired gas samples) during maximal exercise to be the criterion measure of cardiorespiratory fitness. Direct measurement of $\dot{V}O_2$max, however, requires expensive equipment and considerable technical expertise. Therefore in the laboratory setting, $\dot{V}O_2$max is usually estimated using formulas to convert the amount of work output during a GXT to oxygen consumption (see chapter 4). In field settings, prediction equations are used to estimate $\dot{V}O_2$max from a combination of physiological, demographic, and performance predictor variables.

One way in which researchers quantify the validity of physical fitness tests is by calculating the relationship between predicted scores (y') and the criterion scores (y) using correlation coefficients ($r_{y,y'}$). This value, $r_{y,y'}$, is known as the **validity coefficient**. The magnitude of the validity coefficient cannot exceed 1.0. The closer the value is to 1.0, the stronger the validity of the test. Valid physical fitness field tests and prediction equations typically have validity coefficients in excess of $r_{y,y'} = 0.80$.

Because field tests *indirectly* estimate a physical fitness component, there will be a difference between the measured (reference) and predicted values for that component. This difference $(y - y')$ is called the **residual score**. The **standard error of estimate** *(SEE)* is a measure of prediction error and is used to quantify the accuracy of the prediction equation and the validity of the field test. The magnitude of the *SEE* depends on the size of the residual scores and reflects the average degree of deviation of individual data points around the **line of best fit** or **regression line** depicting the linear relationship between the measured and the predicted scores. When individual data points fall close to the regression line, the *SEE* is small (see figure 3.1). A valid field test has a high validity coefficient and a small prediction error.

In addition to test validity, test sensitivity and specificity are often reported. **Sensitivity** refers to the probability of correctly identifying individuals who have risk factors for a specific disease or syndrome (e.g., the probability of correctly diagnosing individuals with CVD risk factors using BMI and waist circumference cutoff values). **Specificity**

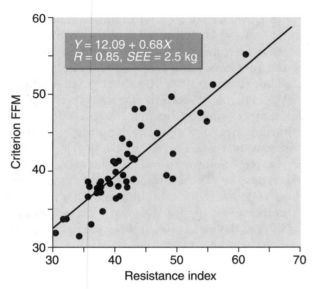

$$Y = 12.09 + 0.68X$$
$$R = 0.85, SEE = 2.5 \text{ kg}$$

Figure 3.1 Line of best fit and *SEE* (prediction error).

is a measure of the ability to correctly identify individuals with *no* risk factors. Given that the sensitivity and specificity of tests are typically less than 1.00 (i.e., < 100% correct), some individuals will be identified as having risk factors even though they have none (**false positive**), and some will be identified as having no risk factors when they do have some (**false negative**).

Test Reliability

Reliability is the ability of a test to yield *consistent* and *stable* scores across trials and over time. For example, the skinfold test is considered to be reliable because a trained skinfold technician obtains similar skinfold values when taking duplicate measurements on the same person. Researchers quantify reliability by calculating the relationship between trial 1 and trial 2 test scores or day 1 and day 2 test scores. This value, $r_{x1,x2}$, is known as the **reliability coefficient**. The magnitude of the reliability coefficient cannot exceed 1.0. In general, physical fitness tests have high reliability coefficients, typically exceeding $r_{x1,x2} = 0.90$.

It is important to know that test reliability affects test validity. Tests with poor reliability also have poor validity because unreliable tests fail to produce consistent test scores. It is possible, however, for a test to have excellent reliability ($r_{x1,x2}$ > 0.90) but poor validity. Even when a test yields stable and precise values across trials or between days, it may not validly measure a specific physical fitness component. For example, researchers reported high test-retest reliability ($r_{x1,x2} = 0.99$)

for the sit-and-reach test, but also noted that this test has poor validity ($r_{y,y'} = 0.12$) as a measure of low back flexibility in women (Jackson and Langford 1989).

Test Objectivity

Objectivity is also known as intertester reliability. Objective tests yield similar test scores for a given individual when the same test is administered by different technicians. Objectivity is quantified by calculating the correlation between pairs of test scores measured on the same individuals by two different technicians. This value, $r_{1,2}$, is known as the **objectivity coefficient**. As with validity and reliability coefficients, the magnitude of the objectivity coefficient cannot exceed 1.0. Most physical fitness tests have high objectivity coefficients ($r_{1,2}$ > 0.90), especially when technicians are highly trained, practice together, and carefully follow standardized testing procedures.

Prediction Equation Evaluation

Although reference measures obtained in the laboratory setting provide the most valid assessment of each physical fitness component, these tests are expensive and time consuming and require considerable technical expertise. In field and clinical settings, you can obtain estimates of these reference measures by selecting valid field tests and prediction equations that have good predictive accuracy. Table 3.1 provides an overview of the types of tests used in laboratory and field settings to assess each physical fitness component.

To select the most appropriate tests for measuring your client's physical fitness, it is important to be able to evaluate the relative worth of the fitness tests and their prediction equations. To do this, you should ask the following questions:

■ *What reference measure was used to develop the prediction equation?*

As mentioned earlier, the reference or criterion measure of a specific physical fitness component is obtained by directly measuring the component. Reference measures are used as the "gold standard" to validate field tests and to develop prediction equations that accurately estimate the reference measure. For example, skinfold prediction equations are developed and cross-validated through comparison of the estimated body density, calculated from the skinfold equation, to the reference measure of body density typically obtained from hydrodensitometry (underwater weighing).

TABLE 3.1 Direct (Reference) and Indirect (Field) Measures of Physical Fitness Components

Physical fitness component	Reference measure	Laboratory or reference method	Indirect measures or field tests	Group prediction error (*SEE* and *TE*)	Individual prediction error*	Chapter
Cardiorespiratory endurance	Direct measurement of $\dot{V}O_2$max (ml $\cdot$ kg^{-1} $\cdot$ min^{-1})	Maximal GXT	Submaximal GXT, distance run/walk tests, step tests	<5.0 ml $\cdot$ kg^{-1} $\cdot$ min^{-1}	±10 ml $\cdot$ kg^{-1} $\cdot$ min^{-1}	4
Body composition	Db (g $\cdot$ cc^{-1}), FFM (kg), or %BF	Hydrodensitometry or dual-energy X-ray absorptiometry	Bioimpedance, skinfold, anthropometry	<0.0080 g $\cdot$ cc^{-1} <3.5 kg FFM (men) <2.8 kg FFM (women) <3.5 %BF	±6.0 kg ±5.0 kg ±7.0%	8
Muscular strength	Maximal force (kg) or torque (Nm)	Isokinetic or 1-RM tests	Submaximal tests (2- to 10-RM value)	<2.0 kg	±4 kg	6
Bone strength	Bone mineral content and bone density	Dual-energy X-ray absorptiometry	Anthropometric measures of bony width	NR	NR	8
Flexibility	ROM at joint (degrees)	X-ray or goniometry	Linear measures of ROM	<6°	±12°	10

Db = total body density; FFM = fat-free mass; %BF = relative body fat; *SEE* = standard error of estimate; *TE* = total error; GXT = graded exercise test; ROM = range of motion; RM = repetition maximum; NR = not reported; Nm = newton -meter.

*95% limits of agreement

Similarly, the validity of the sit-and-reach test for measuring low back flexibility was tested by comparing sit-and-reach scores to range-of-motion values (reference measure) directly measured by X-ray or goniometric methods. Table 3.1 describes reference measures that experts commonly use to assess each physical fitness component. Field tests and prediction equations developed using indirect methods instead of reference methods as a criterion have questionable validity.

■ *How large was the sample used to develop the prediction equation?*

Large randomly selected samples (N = 100 to 400 subjects) generally are needed to ensure that the data are representative of the population for whom the prediction equation was developed. Also, equations based on large samples tend to have more stable regression weights for each predictor variable in the equation.

■ *What is the ratio of sample size to the number of predictor variables in the equation?*

In multiple regression, the correlation between the reference measure of the physical fitness component and the predictors in the equation is represented by the **multiple correlation coefficient (R_{mc})**. The larger the R_{mc} (up to maximum value of 1.00), the stronger the relationship. The size of R_{mc} will be artificially inflated if there are too many predictors in the equation compared to the total number of subjects. Statisticians recommend that there should be a minimum of 20 to 40 subjects per predictor variable. For example, if a skinfold (SKF) prediction equation has three predictors (e.g., triceps SKF, calf SKF, and age), then the minimum sample size needs to be 60 to 120 subjects. Prediction equations that are based on small samples or that have a poor subject-to-predictor ratio are suspect and should not be used.

■ *What were the sizes of the R_{mc} and the standard error of estimate for the prediction equation?*

In general, the R_{mc} for equations predicting physical fitness components exceeds 0.80. This means that at least 64% [$R^2 = 0.80^2 \times 100$] of variance in the reference measure can be accounted for by the predictors in the equation. As you can easily see, the larger the R_{mc}, the greater the amount of shared variance between the reference measure and predictor variables. When you evaluate the relative worth of a prediction equation, it is more important to focus on the size of the

prediction error (*SEE*) than on the R_{mc} because the magnitude of R_{mc} is greatly affected by sample size and variability of the data. Keep in mind that *SEE* reflects the degree of deviation of individual data points (participants' scores) around the line of best fit through the entire sample's data points. In multiple regression, the **line of best fit** is the **regression line** that depicts the linear relationship between the reference measure and all of the predictor variables in the equation. Table 3.1 presents standard values for evaluating prediction errors of physical fitness prediction equations.

■ *To whom is the prediction equation applicable?*

To answer this question, you need to pay close attention to the physical characteristics of the sample used to derive the equation. Factors such as age, gender, race, fitness level, and body fatness need to be examined carefully. Prediction equations are either **population specific** or **generalized**. Population-specific equations are intended only for individuals from a specific homogeneous group. For example, separate skinfold equations have been developed for prepubescent boys and girls (see table 8.3, p. 186). Population-specific equations are likely to systematically over- or underestimate the physical fitness component if they are applied to individuals who do not belong to that population subgroup. On the other hand, there are generalized prediction equations that can be applied to individuals who differ greatly in physical characteristics. Generalized equations are developed using diverse, heterogeneous samples and account for differences in physical characteristics by including these variables as predictors in the equation. For example, the prediction equation for the Rockport walking test (see chapter 4) is a generalized equation because gender and age are predictors in this equation.

■ *How were the variables measured by the researchers who developed the prediction equation?*

It is important to know not only which variables are included in a prediction equation, but also how each one of these predictors was measured by the researchers developing the equation. Although it is highly recommended that standardized procedures be used for all physical fitness testing, this is not always done. For example, the suprailiac skinfold used in the skinfold equations developed by Jackson, Pollock, and Ward (1980) is measured above the iliac crest at the anterior axillary line.

In contrast, the *Anthropometric Standardization Reference Manual* (Lohman, Roche, and Martorell 1988) recommends that the suprailiac skinfold be measured above the iliac crest at the midaxillary line. For most individuals, there will be a difference between skinfold thicknesses measured at these two sites. Thus, larger-than-expected prediction errors may result if physical fitness variables are not measured according to the descriptions provided by the researchers who developed the equation.

■ *Was the prediction equation cross-validated on another sample from the population?*

An equation must be tested on other samples from the population before its validity or predictive accuracy can be determined. For example, the Rockport 1.0-mile walking test was originally developed to assess the cardiorespiratory fitness of women and men ages 20 to 69 years (Kline et al. 1987). Other researchers cross-validated this equation to establish its predictive accuracy for women 65 years of age or older (Fenstermaker, Plowman, and Looney 1992). In general, prediction equations that have not been cross-validated on the original study sample or on additional samples in other studies should not be used.

■ *What were the sizes of the validity coefficient ($r_{y,y'}$) and the prediction errors when this equation was applied to the cross-validation sample (i.e., what is the group predictive accuracy of the equation)?*

An equation with good predictive accuracy has a moderately high validity coefficient ($r_{y,y'}$ > 0.80) and an acceptable prediction error (see table 3.1, Group prediction error). In cross-validation studies, the accuracy of an equation for estimating the reference values of a group is assessed by analyzing two types of prediction error: the *SEE* and the total error *(TE)*. As mentioned, the *SEE* reflects the average deviation of individual data points from the regression line or line of best fit (see figure 3.1). The **total error *(TE)*** is the average degree of deviation of individual data points from the line of identity (see figure 3.2). The **line of identity** has a slope of 1.0 and a y-intercept equal to 0. When an equation closely predicts the actual or measured scores of the cross-validation sample, individual data points fall close to the line of identity (i.e., *TE* is small). Acceptable values for evaluating group prediction errors *(SEE* and *TE)* are presented in table 3.1.

■ *Was the average predicted score similar to the average reference score for the cross-validation sample?*

The prediction equation should yield similar mean values for the actual (measured or reference) and predicted scores of the cross-validation sample. The **constant error (CE)** is the difference between the actual and predicted means. The means are compared using a paired *t*-test and should not differ significantly from each other. A large significant difference indicates a **bias** or systematic difference

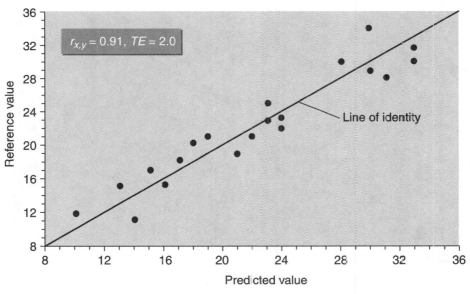

Figure 3.2 Line of identity and total error (prediction error).

(i.e., over- or underestimation) between the original validation sample and the cross-validation sample. This difference is caused by technical error or biological variability between the samples.

■ *How good is the prediction equation for estimating reference values of individual clients (i.e., what is the individual predictive accuracy of the equation)?*

Although a prediction equation may accurately estimate the average reference score for a specific group, it may not necessarily give accurate estimates for all individuals comprising that group. To evaluate how well a prediction equation works for individuals, researchers use the **Bland and Altman method** (1986), which sets **limits of agreement** around the average difference $(\bar{d})$ between the actual and predicted scores for the sample. With this method, difference scores (actual – predicted values) and average scores [(actual + predicted values) / 2] are calculated for each individual in the sample and are plotted on a graph (see figure 3.3). When the difference scores are normally distributed, 95% lie within ± 2 standard deviations from the overall mean difference $(\bar{d})$ for the group. In this case, the standard deviation of the difference scores (S_d) is used to set the upper $(+2S_d)$ and lower $(-2S_d)$ limits of agreement. Smaller 95% limits of agreement indicate that the equation has a better individual predictive accuracy. The limits of agreement estimate how well you will be able to predict your client's actual value when using the equation. In the example in figure

3.3, the predictive accuracy of the equation for estimating the actual %BF of individual clients is approximately $\pm 6\%$ BF (note the upper and lower limits of agreement on the y-axis of the graph).

In summary, you should apply all of the following evaluation criteria when selecting field tests and prediction equations that indirectly assess the physical fitness of your clients:

■ An acceptable method is used to derive reference measures of the physical fitness component.

■ A large sample (N = 100-400) and 20 to 40 subjects per predictor variable are used to develop the equation.

■ The sizes of the multiple correlation and validity coefficients exceed 0.80.

■ The group prediction errors *(SEE* and *TE)* are acceptable (see table 3.1).

■ Demographic characteristics (e.g., age, gender, race, fitness status) of the validation and cross-validation samples are described.

■ The prediction equation is cross-validated in the original study or on independent samples from other studies.

■ The constant error (bias), or difference between the measured and predicted means for the cross-validation sample, is not statistically significant.

■ The 95% limits of agreement are acceptable (see table 3.1).

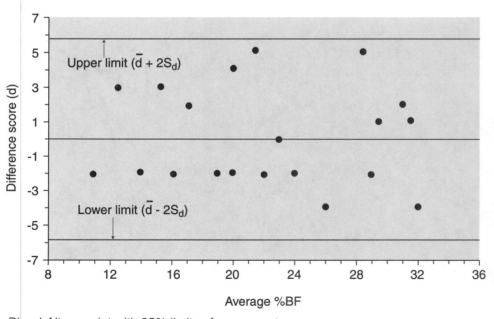

Figure 3.3 Bland-Altman plot with 95% limits of agreement.

Physical Fitness Tests: Administration and Interpretation

To obtain good test results, it is important to prepare your clients for physical fitness testing by giving them appropriate instructions at least one day before the scheduled exercise tests.

Pretest Instructions

Give the client directions to the testing facility and make special arrangements if the facility requires a parking pass. Make sure the client has the following instructions in preparation for the test:

- Wear comfortable clothing, socks, and athletic shoes if available.
- Drink plenty of fluids during the 24-hr period before the test.
- Refrain from eating, smoking, and drinking alcohol or caffeine for 3 hr prior to the test.
- Do not engage in strenuous physical activity the day of the test.
- Get adequate sleep (6 to 8 hr) the night before the test.

Test Administration

Later chapters give detailed procedures for administering laboratory and field tests for each physical fitness component. Your technical skills and expertise in administering these tests are directly related to your mastery of standardized testing procedures and the amount of time you spend practicing testing techniques. For example, to become a proficient skinfold technician, you probably should practice on at least 50 to 100 people (Jackson and Pollock 1985). You also need a great deal of practice in order to measure exercise blood pressures and heart rates accurately and to coordinate the timing of these measurements during a GXT on the treadmill or cycle ergometer. Remember that you cannot obtain valid test scores if you do not follow the standardized testing procedures.

Test Interpretation

After collecting the test data, you must analyze and interpret the results for your client. Computer software programs are available that display and compare the client's test results to normative data. Some graphs display the individual's physical fitness profile so that you and your client can easily pinpoint strengths, as well as physical fitness components in need of improvement.

To classify your client's physical fitness status, you should compare test scores to established norms. For this purpose, age-gender norms are provided for many of the cardiorespiratory fitness, muscular fitness, body composition, and flexibility tests included in this book. For some tests, percentile rankings are used to classify a client's performance. To illustrate the interpretation of a percentile ranking, let's use the example of a 35-year-old male client whose sit-and-reach score ranks in the 60th percentile. This ranking means that his score is better than 60% of the scores of all males the same age taking this test.

When interpreting results for clients, use lay language, rather than highly technical terms and jargon, to explain their test scores. Whenever possible, try to phrase poor results in positive terms. For example, if a female client's body fat level is classified as obese, do not embarrass and alarm her by saying: "Your underwater weighing test indicates that you are obese and need to lose at least 20 pounds to achieve a healthy body fat level in order to reduce your risk of diseases linked to obesity. You need to decrease your caloric intake and increase your caloric expenditure by dieting and exercising. The sooner you start a weight management program, the better."

Instead, you should use a more positive and less intimidating approach when interpreting this result. The following approach is more appropriate, especially for clients with low self-efficacy or motivation to initiate and adhere to an exercise program: "People with more than 32% body fat are at risk for disease. If you wish, I will evaluate your daily calorie intake and suggest healthy foods you like to eat that are low in fat. Also, we can discuss ways to increase your physical activity level. I think we can find some activities that you will enjoy and have time for, so that you'll burn more calories each day. With these changes, you should be able to lower your body fat to a healthy level in a reasonable amount of time."

BASIC PRINCIPLES FOR EXERCISE PROGRAM DESIGN

A number of basic training principles apply to all types of exercise programs, whether they are designed to improve cardiorespiratory fitness, musculoskeletal fitness, body composition, or flexibility.

■ **Specificity-of-Training Principle.** The **specificity principle** states that the body's physiological and metabolic responses and adaptations to exercise training are specific to the type of exercise and the muscle groups involved. For example, physical activities requiring continuous, dynamic, and rhythmical contractions of large muscle groups are best suited for stimulating improvements in cardiorespiratory endurance; stretching exercises develop range of joint motion and flexibility; and resistance exercises are effective for improving muscular strength and muscular endurance. Furthermore, the gains in muscular fitness are specific to the exercised muscle groups, type and speed of contraction, and training intensity.

■ **Overload Training Principle.** To promote improvements in physical fitness components, the physiological systems of the body must be taxed using loads that are greater (**overload principle**) than those to which the individual is accustomed. Overload can be achieved through increases in the frequency, intensity, and duration of aerobic exercise. Muscle groups can be effectively overloaded through increases in the number of repetitions, sets, or exercises in programs designed to improve muscular fitness and flexibility.

■ **Principle of Progression.** Throughout the training program, you must progressively increase the training volume, or overload, to stimulate further improvements (i.e., **progression principle**). The progression needs to be gradual because "doing too much, too soon" may cause musculoskeletal injuries and is a major reason why some individuals drop out of exercise programs.

■ **Principle of Initial Values.** Individuals with low initial physical fitness levels will show greater relative (%) gains and a faster rate of improvement in response to exercise training than individuals with average or high fitness levels (**initial values principle**). For example, during the first month of an aerobic exercise program, the $\dot{V}O_2$max of a client with poor cardiorespiratory endurance capacity may improve 12% or more, whereas a highly trained endurance athlete may improve only 1% or less.

■ **Principle of Interindividual Variability.** Individual responses to a training stimulus are quite variable and depend on a number of factors such as age, initial fitness level, and health status (i.e., **interindividual variability principle**). You therefore must design exercise programs with the specific needs, interests, and abilities of each client in mind and develop personalized exercise

prescriptions that take into account individual differences and preferences.

■ **Principle of Diminishing Returns.** Each person has a genetic ceiling that limits the extent of improvement that is possible due to exercise training. As individuals approach their genetic ceiling, the rate of improvement in physical fitness slows and eventually levels off (i.e., **diminishing return principle**).

■ **Principle of Reversibility.** The positive physiological effects and health benefits of regular physical activity and exercise are reversible. When individuals discontinue their exercise programs (detraining), exercise capacity diminishes quickly, and within a few months most of the training improvements are lost (i.e., **reversibility principle**).

The Art and Science of Exercise Prescription

Traditionally, some exercise specialists have focused on rigidly applying scientific principles of exercise prescription and devoted little or no attention to the *art* of exercise prescription. As an exercise programming artist, you need to be creative, flexible, and able to modify the exercise prescription based on your client's goals, behaviors, and responses to the exercise. Using both a scientific and an artistic approach will enable you to personalize the exercise prescription, increasing the probability of your clients' making long-term commitments to including physical activity and exercise as an indispensable part of their lifestyles.

Basic Elements of the Exercise Prescription

Although prescriptions are individualized for each client, there are basic elements common to all exercise prescriptions. These basic elements include mode, intensity, duration, frequency, and progression.

Mode

As mentioned earlier, the specificity-of-training principle implies that certain types of exercise training are better suited than others to developing specific components of physical fitness. Table 3.2 presents types of training and examples of exercise modes that optimize improvements for each physical fitness component.

TABLE 3.2 Types of Training and Exercise Modes for Improving Physical Fitness Components

Physical fitness component	Type of training	Exercise modes
Cardiorespiratory endurance	Aerobic exercise	Walking, jogging, cycling, rowing, stair-climbing, simulated cross-country skiing, aerobic dance, step aerobics, and elliptical activity
Muscular strength and muscular endurance	Resistance exercise	Free weights, exercise machines, and exercise bands
Bone strength	Weight-bearing aerobic exercise and resistance exercise	Walking, jogging, aerobic dance, step aerobics, stair-climbing, simulated cross-country skiing, free weights, and exercise machines
Body composition	Aerobic exercise and resistance exercise	Same modes as listed for cardiorespiratory endurance and muscular strength
Flexibility	Stretching exercise	Static stretches, PNF stretches, yoga, tai chi, and Pilates

PNF = proprioceptive neuromuscular facilitation.

To promote changes in body composition and bone strength, many experts recommend using more than one type of exercise training. For body composition changes, you should prescribe a combination of aerobic exercise to reduce body fat and resistance exercise to build muscle and bone. Similarly, weight-bearing, aerobic activities and resistance training are both effective for building bone mass for improved bone health.

Intensity

Exercise intensity dictates the specific physiological and metabolic changes in the body during exercise training. As mentioned previously, the initial exercise intensity in the exercise prescription depends on the client's program goals, age, capabilities, preferences, and fitness level and should stress, but not overtax, the cardiopulmonary and musculoskeletal systems. Later chapters provide detailed information and guidelines on selecting exercise intensities for the development of each physical fitness component, as well as for the progression of exercise intensity.

Duration

Duration and intensity of exercise are inversely related; the higher the intensity, the shorter the duration of the exercise. Exercise duration depends not only on the intensity of exercise but also on the client's health status, initial fitness level, functional capability, and program goals. For improved health benefits, ACSM and the Centers for Disease Control and Prevention (CDC) recommend that every individual should accumulate 30 min or more of moderate physical activity on most, but preferably all, days of the week (Pate et al. 1995). This amount of physical activity can be achieved in either one continuous bout of exercise or in multiple bouts of shorter duration throughout the day (e.g., 10-min bouts, three times a day), depending on the client's functional capacity and time constraints.

As the client adapts to the exercise training, the duration of exercise may be slowly increased about every two to three weeks. For older and less fit individuals, ACSM (2006) recommends increasing exercise duration, rather than intensity, in the initial stages of the exercise program. For most clients, the duration of aerobic, resistance, and flexibility exercise workouts should not exceed 60 min. This will lessen the chance of overuse injuries and exercise "burnout."

Frequency

Frequency typically refers to the total number of weekly exercise sessions. Research shows that exercising three days a week on alternate days is sufficient to improve various components of physical fitness. However, frequency is related to the duration and intensity of exercise and varies depending on the client's program goals and preferences, time constraints, and functional capacity. Sedentary clients with poor initial fitness levels may exercise more than once a day. When improved health is the primary goal of the exercise program, ACSM and CDC recommend daily physical activity of moderate intensity. Therefore, when you prescribe daily physical activity for an apparently healthy client, it is important to vary the type of exercise (i.e., aerobic, resistance, and flexibility exercises) or exercise mode (e.g., walking, cycling, and weight-lifting) to lessen the risk of overuse injuries to the bones, joints, and muscles.

Progression of Exercise

Throughout the exercise program, physiological and metabolic changes enable the individual to perform more work. For continued improvements, the cardiopulmonary and musculoskeletal systems must be progressively overloaded through periodic increases in the frequency, intensity, and duration of the exercise.

When applying the principle of progression to an exercise prescription, you should increase the frequency, intensity, and duration gradually, and you should do so one element at a time. A simultaneous increase in frequency, intensity, and duration, or in any combination of these elements, may overtax the individual's physiological systems, thereby increasing the risk of exercise-related injuries and exercise burnout. Generally, for older and less fit clients, it is better to increase exercise duration, instead of exercise intensity, especially during the initial stage of their exercise prescriptions.

Stages of Progression in the Exercise Program

Most individualized exercise programs include initial conditioning, improvement, and maintenance stages. The **initial conditioning stage** typically lasts one to six weeks and serves as a primer to familiarize the client with exercise training. During this stage, you should prescribe stretching exercises, light calisthenics, and low-intensity aerobic or resistance exercises. Have your clients progress slowly by increasing exercise duration first, followed by small increases in exercise intensity. The initial stage of the exercise program may be skipped for some physically active individuals provided that their initial fitness level is good to excellent and that they are accustomed to the exercise modes prescribed for their programs.

The **improvement stage** of the exercise program typically lasts four to eight months, and the rate of progression is more rapid than in the initial conditioning stage. During this stage, the frequency, intensity, and duration are systematically and slowly advanced, one element at a time, until the client's fitness goal is reached.

The **maintenance stage** of the exercise program is designed to maintain the level of fitness achieved by the client at the end of the improvement stage. This stage should continue on a regular, long-term basis. The amount of exercise required to maintain the client's physical fitness level is less than that needed to improve specific fitness components. Thus, the frequency of a specific mode of exercise used to develop any given fitness component can be decreased and that mode replaced with other types of physical activities. By the end of the improvement stage, for example, a client may be jogging five days a week. For maintenance, jogging may be reduced to two or three days a week, and different aerobic activities (e.g., rollerblading and stair-climbing) or other types of exercise and sport activities (e.g., weightlifting or tennis) may be substituted the other three days. Including a variety of enjoyable physical activities during this stage helps to counteract boredom and to maintain the client's interest level.

EXERCISE PROGRAM ADHERENCE

Exercise professionals face the challenge of convincing individuals to start exercising and getting them to make a lifelong commitment to a physically active lifestyle. More than one of every two adults (55%) in the United States do not get the recommended amount of physical activity, and 26% of the adult population report no physical activity at all (Centers for Disease Control 2003b). Exercise specialists play an important role in educating the public about why regular physical activity is absolutely essential for good health and how to exercise safely and effectively.

Of those individuals starting an exercise program, almost 50% will drop out within one year (ACSM 2006). As an exercise specialist, you must help the client to develop a positive attitude toward physical activity and to make a firm commitment to the exercise program. To increase adherence, you need to be aware of factors related to exercise attrition.

Many factors influence regular participation in physical activity and adherence to an exercise program (see table 3.3). Knowing the factors associated with continued participation in physical

TABLE 3.3   Factors Related to Physical Activity Participation and Exercise Program Adherence

Category	Positive factors	Negative factors
Demographic/biological	Education	Age
	Gender[a]	Race[b]
	Socioeconomic status	Overweight/obesity
Psychological/cognitive/emotional	Enjoyment of exercise	Barriers to exercise
	Expected benefits of exercise	Mood disturbance
	Perceived health and fitness	
	Self-efficacy	
	Self-motivation	
Behavioral	Activity history during adulthood	Smoking
	Healthy dietary habits	
Social/cultural	Physician influence	Social isolation
	Support from spouse, family, friends, or peers	
Environmental	Access to exercise facilities	Climate/season
	Satisfaction with exercise facility	Urban location
	Exercise equipment at home	
	Enjoyable scenery	
	Observing others exercising	
	Neighborhood safety	
Program	Exercise leadership/supervision	Initial exercise intensity
	Variety of exercise modes/activities	Perceived effort

[a]Males are more likely to be physically active than females.
[b]Whites are more physically active than non-Whites.
Data compiled from comprehensive reviews of research studies dealing with this topic (Sallis and Owen 1999; Trost et al. 2002).

activity will direct your approach and the steps you take in order to facilitate your clients' adherence to their exercise programs. You should focus on factors that are potentially modifiable such as exercise facilities, program variables (e.g., exercise intensity and perceived exertion), enjoyable scenery while exercising, and support from spouse, family, friends, and peers.

As an exercise specialist, you also need to understand and implement psychological models related to successful behavior change. These models are as follows:

- Behavior modification
- Social cognitive theory
- Stages of motivational readiness for change

With use of the **behavior modification model**, clients become actively involved in the change process by setting realistic short- and long-term goals, developing a plan to achieve these goals, and signing a contract that describes each goal and how it may be achieved. Throughout the exercise program, you should provide your client with feedback and revise the plan as needed. You can help your clients adopt physical activity into their lifestyle by implementing behavior counseling strategies such as having clients keep a diary of their physical activity and developing a social support system for a client. Sometimes it can be effective to give rewards such as T-shirts, certificates, emblems, and pins to recognize the attainment of specific goals, such as walking a total of 50 miles (80.5 km) in one month. Help your client set both short-term and long-term goals that are attainable. For this purpose, you can periodically reevaluate your client's fitness levels to assess improvement. You can state goals in performance or physiological terms. An example of a short-term performance goal is to complete a 3 mile (4.8 km) fun run in less than 33 min. A long-term physiological goal might be to increase maximum oxygen uptake ($\dot{V}O_2$max) by 15% in four months. As the exercise specialist, you must help each individual set realistic goals.

The **social cognitive model**, developed by Bandura (1982), is based on the concepts of self-efficacy and outcome expectation. The likelihood that people will engage in a specific behavior, like exercising regularly, depends on their **self-efficacy** or perception of their ability to perform the task, as well as their confidence in making the behavioral change (Grembowski et al. 1993). To assess self-efficacy, have your clients rate, on a scale of 0% to 100%, their confidence in making the specific behavior change. Individuals with high self-efficacy ratings (≥70%) believe they have the knowledge and skill to exercise successfully. As a result, they are more likely to succeed in making a long-term behavior change. To increase self-efficacy, you should educate your clients so that they fully understand their beliefs and should help them identify specific barriers to engaging in physical activity (Stuhr 1998). Techniques to improve your client's exercise self-efficacy include performance mastery (e.g., teach your clients scientifically sound and safe exercise principles and techniques and allow them to practice these techniques); modeling (e.g., give clients an opportunity to observe role models who are performing the exercise successfully); positive reinforcement (e.g., compliment clients when they perform activities correctly or improve a specific physical fitness component); and emotional arousal (e.g., educate clients about the health benefits of physical activity and exercise). Schlicht, Godin, and Camaione (1999) provide more detailed descriptions of how you can incorporate these techniques into your clients' exercise programs.

The **stages of motivational readiness for change model** is based on the premise that individuals move through a series of stages as they adopt and maintain a new habit (Prochaska and DiClemente 1982). This model has been used to facilitate long-term changes in health behaviors such as smoking, weight management, dietary modification, and stress management (Riebe and Niggs 1998) as well as in physical activity behaviors (Dunn, Marcus, Kampert, Garcia, Kohl, and Blair. 1999; Marcus, Bock, Pinto, Forsyth, Roberts, and Traficante 1998). Your clients' abilities to make a long-term commitment to an exercise program or to daily physical activity are based on their motivational readiness for change. The following example illustrates the five stages of motivational readiness in terms of changing exercise behavior:

1. **Precontemplation:** Client does not exercise and does not intend to start exercising.
2. **Contemplation:** Client is not exercising but intends to start.
3. **Preparation:** Client is exercising but is not meeting the recommended amount of physical activity.
4. **Action:** Client has been performing the recommended amount of exercise regularly for less than six months.
5. **Maintenance:** Client has been exercising regularly at the recommended amount for six months or longer.

Individuals are at different stages of readiness for change; therefore, you need to match intervention strategies to the client's stage and tailor your approach to meet the individual's needs, interests, and concerns. Detailed descriptions of how to plan and deliver physical activity intervention strategies specific to the stages of change are available (see Marcus and Forsyth 2003; Marcus and Lewis 2003).

As an exercise specialist, you need to integrate principles from each of these models and implement strategies to improve your clients' exercise program adherence. The ACSM (2006) recommends program modifications and motivational strategies to increase long-term adherence to an exercise program (see "Strategies to Increase Exercise Program Adherence", p. 49). The key to increasing exercise program adherence lies in the leadership, education, and motivation that you provide. First, you must be a positive role model. You also must be knowledgeable, able to educate clients about exercise and fitness, and able to provide motivation and encourage social support.

CERTIFICATION AND LICENSURE

Exercise professionals need to have extensive knowledge and technical skills in order to be effective. Historically, individuals working in exercise settings, such as health or fitness clubs, were not necessarily required to have specialized education and training in exercise science. Often, the only prerequisites for employment as a health/fitness instructor or exercise trainer were personal experience with exercise and a lean or muscular body. However, survey research indicates that a bachelor's degree in exercise

---

Strategies to Increase Exercise Program Adherence

- Recruiting physician support of the exercise program
- Prescribing moderate-intensity exercise to minimize injury and complications
- Advocating exercising with others
- Offering a variety of exercise and fitness activities that are enjoyable
- Providing positive reinforcement through periodic testing
- Recruiting support of the program from clients' families and friends
- Adding optional recreational games to the conditioning program
- Using progress charts to record exercise achievements
- Establishing a reward system to recognize participant accomplishments
- Providing qualified, exercise professionals who are well trained, innovative, and enthusiastic

---

science and an American College of Sports Medicine (ACSM) or a National Strength and Conditioning Association (NSCA) certification are strong predictors of a personal trainer's knowledge. Contrary to popular belief, experience was *not* related to knowledge (Malek, Nalbone, Berger, and Coburn 2002). These findings suggest that formal education and certification by professional organizations should be required for personal fitness trainers and exercise science professionals.

Professional certification and licensure are two ways to ensure the competency of professionals working in the exercise science field. Although many professional organizations offer certification programs for exercise professionals, Louisiana was the first state in the United States to pass a law requiring licensure of all clinical exercise physiologists (Herbert 1995). This requirement places clinical exercise physiologists on a par with other allied health professionals (e.g., nurses, nutritionists, physical therapists, and occupational therapists) who in many states are required to have licenses to practice. Also, a new law to develop a task force to study the issue of licensure for professional personal trainers has been proposed in Oregon (Herbert 2004). To promote exercise science and physiology as a profession, the American Society of Exercise Physiologists (ASEP) is working with exercise professionals throughout the United States to develop state licensure requirements for exercise physiologists. Also, ASEP has developed

standards of practice for exercise physiologists (American Society of Exercise Physiologists 2004) as well as accreditation standards for universities and colleges offering academic degrees in exercise science (Wattles 2002).

Numerous organizations offer various types and levels (e.g., group exercise leader, personal trainer, health and fitness instructor, exercise physiologist) of certification for exercise science and fitness professionals. This confuses the public in terms of knowing who are and who are not highly trained and qualified as exercise professionals. It also complicates selecting the most appropriate certification for yourself. Some agencies sponsor certification programs primarily for financial gain while others certify professionals in order to promote exercise science as a profession. One way to determine where a specific certification is located on the certification continuum is to check the eligibility requirements for its examinations. Some certification programs are more demanding than others. For example, to be eligible to take the written and practical examinations to become ASEP certified, you must meet all of the following criteria:

- Minimum of a 4 yr academic degree with a major or concentration in exercise physiology or exercise science
- Grades of C or better in 5 of 9 academic courses (exercise physiology, fitness assessment and prescription, exercise metabolism, kinesiology, biomechanics, research design, environmental physiology, nutrition, and exercise for special populations)
- Documentation of a minimum of 400 hr of hands-on experience in exercise physiology (or related) laboratories
- Current membership in ASEP

In contrast, some agencies (e.g., International Sports Science Association and International Fitness Professionals Association, personal fitness trainer certification) do not require formal, academic training; they only require that you attend a 1 or 2 day workshop or seminar before taking the certification exams. To obtain an American Council on Exercise (ACE) certification as a personal trainer, group fitness instructor, lifestyle and weight management consultant, or clinical exercise specialist, ACE recommends self-study for only 3 to 6 mo to prepare for the written portion of the exam. For individuals needing to sharpen their technical skills, ACE suggests attending its 15 hr course before taking the practical portion of the exam. The bottom line is that *all exercise science and fitness certifications are not equal.*

To address the inequality among certification programs, a third-party accrediting agency (i.e., National Commission for Certifying Agencies) is now formally reviewing applications for the accreditation of certification programs. Recently, the ACSM submitted accreditation applications for its Health and Fitness Instructor and Exercise Specialist certifications (American College of Sports Medicine 2004). Likewise, the board of directors of the International Health, Racquet, and Sportsclub Association (IHRSA) recommended that by December 2004 all health clubs belonging to their organization hire only personal fitness trainers certified by a third-party accredited organization or agency (International Dance and Exercise Association 2004). However, not all of the organizations belonging to IHRSA approved this recommendation (Herbert 2004).

In 2003, the National Board of Fitness Examiners (NBFE) was founded as a nonprofit organization with the twin purposes of defining scopes of practice for all fitness professionals and determining standards of practice for various fitness professionals including floor instructors, group exercise instructors, personal fitness trainers, specialists in youth and senior fitness, and medical exercise specialists. The NBFE has established national standards of excellence that every certifying organization and college or university is free to adopt. Potentially, the NBFE standards provide a way to standardize all certifying organizations. Recently, the NBFE developed national board examinations (written and practical) for personal trainers (for additional information, visit www. NBFE.org). To be eligible to sit for the national boards, personal fitness trainers must successfully complete a personal training certification program from an approved NBFE affiliate. Affiliate status is available to qualified groups from the areas of medicine, certification organizations, fitness professionals, health clubs, and higher education. In the future, the national board examinations may be used by certifying organizations, colleges and universities, and state licensing programs to test the knowledge, skill, and competence of fitness professionals (American Fitness Professionals and Associates 2004).

In another effort to provide personal trainers with "a greater degree of public trust and confidence," the Ethics and Safety Compliance Standards (ESCS) has created a seal of approval for personal trainers. To display this seal, trainers are required to follow strict and enforceable protocols concerning safety in preexercise screenings and to conform to a uniform code of conduct established by the ESCS (FMpulse 2004). The ESCS is working through a newly established trade association for certifying agencies (i.e., International Association of Fitness Certifying Agencies, or IAFCA) to obtain industry-wide recognition of its seal.

All of these efforts demonstrate that there is an urgent need to get a handle on certifications for exercise professionals so that we gain control of who is practicing in our field. This will assure the safety of exercise program participants and enable individuals working in the exercise science field to be recognized as "true exercise professionals." Until these issues are resolved and a list of accredited certification agencies and organizations is finalized, you should select a professional certification that matches your level of education and career goals. Table 3.4 compares certifications offered by selected professional organizations. For more information about certification programs, visit the Web sites of professional organizations (addresses are listed in appendix A.9, p. 306).

Many advantages are associated with obtaining either state licensure or certification by professional organizations. You will have a better chance of finding a job in the health/fitness field because many employers are now hiring only professionally certified health/fitness instructors. Certification by reputable, professional organizations upgrades the quality of the typical person working in the field and assures employers and their clientele that employees have mastered the knowledge and skills needed to be competent exercise science professionals. Hence, the likelihood of lawsuits resulting from negligence or incompetence may be lessened. Also, certification and licensure help to validate exercise specialists as health professionals who are equally deserving of the respect afforded to professionals in other allied health professions.

TABLE 3.4 Comparison of Professional Certifications

ELIGIBILITY REQUIREMENTS

Professional organization	Certification	Education	Field	Experience	Scope of practice
American College of Sports Medicine (www.acsm.org)	Health/Fitness Instructor (HFI)	2 or 4 yr degree	Health related		Conduct fitness assessments and prescribe exercise programs for apparently healthy clients
	Health/Fitness Director (HFD)	2 or 4 yr degree	Health related	4000 hr as fitness manager or director	Manage or direct a fitness center or exercise program for apparently healthy clients
	Exercise Specialist (ES)	2 yr degree	Allied health	4000 hr in cardiac rehab or clinical exercise testing	Conduct exercise testing and prescribe exercise programs for clients at increased risk due to cardiopulmonary, metabolic, or musculoskeletal problems
		4 yr degree	Allied health	600 hr in clinical exercise program or clinical exercise testing	Same as above
	Program Director (PD)	Graduate degree	Exercise science, medicine, or allied health	2 yr in managing clinical exercise program	Manage or direct a clinical exercise center or rehabilitation program (e.g., cardiopulmonary rehabilitation)
	Registered Clinical Exercise Physiologist (RCEP)	Graduate degree	Exercise science, exercise physiology, or physiology	1200 hr of clinical experience	Work in the application of physical activity and exercise for clients with clinical and pathological conditions
American Society of Exercise Physiologists (www.asep.org)	Exercise Physiologist Certified (EPC)	4 yr degree	Exercise physiology or exercise science	400 hr in exercise physiology or related laboratories	Measure, examine, analyze, and instruct to evaluate and improve physical fitness components of both apparently healthy and at-risk individuals as well as persons with known disease
Canadian Society for Exercise Physiology (www.csep.ca)	Certified Fitness Consultant (CFC)	College diploma or minimum of 2 yr university training	Exercise science		Conduct a specific fitness assessment* and use results to counsel clients
	Personal Fitness Trainer (PFT)	College diploma or minimum of 2 yr university training	Exercise science		Prescribe exercise programs based on a specific fitness assessment*
	Professional Fitness and Lifestyle Consultant (PFLC)	University undergraduate degree	Exercise science, health, or fitness	Extensive practical experience in fitness assessment, exercise prescription, or fitness counseling	Conduct a variety of fitness assessments, counsel clients, and prescribe exercise programs
	Exercise Therapist (ET)	University undergraduate degree	Exercise science, kinesiology, or related field	750 hr experience in primary (musculoskeletal, cardiorespiratory, or metabolic) and secondary (neuromuscular, aging, psychological, or psychiatric) focus areas	Evaluate and treat asymptomatic and symptomatic populations; prescribe conditioning exercises
National Strength and Conditioning Association (www.nsca-cc.org)	Certified Strength and Conditioning Specialist (CSCS)	4 yr degree	BA or BS in any field		Design and implement safe and effective strength and conditioning programs for athletes

*Certified to conduct only the Canadian Physical Activity and Fitness Lifestyle Assessment (CPAFLA).

KEY POINTS

- The essential components of physical fitness are cardiorespiratory endurance, musculoskeletal fitness, body composition, and flexibility.

- Valid, reliable, and objective laboratory and field tests have been developed to assess each fitness component.

- Test validity refers to the ability of a physical fitness test to accurately measure a specific fitness component.

- Test reliability is the ability of a test to yield consistent and stable scores across trials and over time.

- Objective tests give similar test scores when different technicians administer the test to the same client.

- All physical fitness prediction equations need to be validated and cross-validated to determine their applicability and suitability for use in the field.

- The line of best fit is a regression line depicting a linear relationship between a reference measure and all of the predictor variables in the regression equation.

- The *SEE* is a type of prediction error that reflects the degree of deviation of individual data points around the line of best fit or regression line.

- The *TE* is a type of prediction error that reflects the degree of deviation of individual data points around the line of identity.

- Sensitivity and specificity are measures of the ability of a test to correctly identify individuals with and without risk factors for diseases.

- Use standard evaluation criteria to judge the relative worth of newly developed physical fitness tests and prediction equations.

- The Bland and Altman method evaluates how well a prediction equation works for estimating a physical fitness component of an individual within a group.

- To obtain valid and reliable test results, one must follow standardized testing procedures and have technical skills.

- Established norms for most tests are available and are used to classify physical fitness status based on the client's test scores.

- When interpreting test results to clients, one needs to be positive and to use simple, nontechnical terms.

- To design an effective exercise program, it is necessary to understand and apply training principles. These principles include specificity, overload, progression, initial values, interindividual variability, diminishing returns, and reversibility.

- The basic elements of an exercise prescription are mode, intensity, duration, and frequency.

- The exercise prescription should be individualized to meet the needs, interests, and abilities of the client.

- The three stages of an exercise program are initial conditioning, improvement, and maintenance.

- Throughout the improvement stage of an exercise program, the frequency, intensity, and duration of exercise are increased, one at a time.

- Physical activity participation and exercise adherence are related to demographic, biological, psychological, cognitive, emotional, behavioral, social, cultural, and environmental factors.

- When developing strategies for increasing exercise program adherence, it is important to integrate principles and concepts from the behavior modification, social cognitive, and stages of motivational readiness for change models.

- Professional certification and licensure are two ways to ensure competency of professionals working in the exercise science field.

KEY TERMS

Learn the definition of each of the following key terms. Definitions of terms can be found in the glossary on page 379.

behavior modification model	muscular strength
bias	musculoskeletal fitness
Bland and Altman method	objectivity
body composition	objectivity coefficient
body weight	overload principle
bone strength	physical fitness
cardiorespiratory endurance	population-specific equations
constant error (*CE*)	progression principle
criterion method	reference method
diminishing return principle	regression line
false negative	reliability
false positive	reliability coefficient
flexibility	residual score
generalized prediction equations	reversibility principle
improvement stage	self-efficacy
initial conditioning stage	sensitivity
initial values principle	social cognitive model
interindividual variability principle	specificity
limits of agreement	specificity principle
line of best fit	stages of motivational readiness for change model
line of identity	standard error of estimate
maintenance stage	total error
maximum oxygen consumption	validity
multiple correlation coefficient	validity coefficient
muscular endurance	

REVIEW QUESTIONS

In addition to being able to define each of the key terms, test your knowledge and understanding of the material by answering the following review questions.

1. Define physical fitness. Name and define the four components of physical fitness.

2. What is the recommended sequence of testing for administering a complete physical fitness test battery?

3. Identify the reference or criterion method for each of the four components of physical fitness.

4. Which is more important: test validity or test reliability? Explain your choice.

5. Select one physical fitness component and explain how you can determine the relative worth or predictive accuracy of a field test developed to assess this component.

6. Select one physical fitness component and give an example of how each of the seven training principles can be applied to this component.

7. Identify exercise modes suitable to develop each of the four components of fitness.

8. Identify the three elements of an exercise prescription. For older or less fit clients, which of the elements should be increased first during the initial stage of their exercise programs?

9. Name the three stages of an exercise program. On average, how long should each stage last?

10. Identify three positively related and three negatively related factors associated with physical activity participation.

11. Choose one of the psychological models related to successful behavior change and give specific examples of how this model could be applied to a client undertaking a resistance training program to develop muscular fitness.

12. What are the advantages of becoming a professionally certified exercise scientist?

chapter 4

Assessing Cardiorespiratory Fitness

Key Questions

- How is cardiorespiratory fitness ($\dot{V}O_2$max) assessed?
- What is a graded exercise test?
- How is $\dot{V}O_2$max estimated from graded exercise test and field test data?
- Should all clients be given a maximal graded exercise test? What factors should I consider in determining whether to give my client a maximal or submaximal exercise test?
- How accurate are submaximal exercise tests and field tests in assessing cardiorespiratory fitness?
- What exercise modes are suitable for graded exercise testing?
- What are the standardized testing procedures for graded exercise testing?
- What are the criteria for terminating a graded exercise test?
- Is it safe to give children and older adults a graded exercise test?

One of the most important components of physical fitness is cardiorespiratory endurance. **Cardiorespiratory endurance** is the ability to perform dynamic exercise involving large muscle groups at moderate-to-high intensity for prolonged periods (ACSM 2006). Every physical fitness evaluation should include an assessment of cardiorespiratory function during both rest and exercise.

This chapter presents guidelines for graded exercise testing, as well as maximal and submaximal exercise test protocols and procedures. Although many of the graded exercise test protocols presented in this chapter were developed years ago, these classic protocols are still widely used in research and clinical settings. In addition, each of these protocols meets the current ACSM (2006) guidelines for graded exercise tests. The chapter also addresses graded exercise testing for children and older adults and includes a discussion of cardiorespiratory field tests. All of the test protocols included in this chapter are summarized in appendix B.1, "Summary of Graded Exercise Test and Cardiorespiratory Field Test Protocols," on page 308.

DEFINITION OF TERMS

Exercise physiologists consider directly measured **maximum oxygen uptake** ($\dot{V}O_2$max) the most valid measure of functional capacity of the cardiorespiratory system. The $\dot{V}O_2$max, or rate of oxygen uptake during maximal aerobic exercise, reflects

1. the capacity of the heart, lungs, and blood to transport oxygen to the working muscles; and
2. the utilization of oxygen by the muscles during exercise.

Traditionally, a plateau in oxygen consumption despite increased workload is the criterion used to determine the attainment of $\dot{V}O_2$max during a maximum exercise tolerance test. However, some maximum exercise tolerance tests (see ramp-type protocols, p. 68) elicit a peak rather than a maximum rate of oxygen consumption. $\dot{V}O_2$peak is the highest rate of oxygen consumption measured during the exercise test, regardless of whether or not a $\dot{V}O_2$ plateau was reached. $\dot{V}O_2$peak may be higher, lower, or equal to $\dot{V}O_2$max. For many individuals who do not reach an actual $\dot{V}O_2$ plateau, the $\dot{V}O_2$peak attained during a maximum-effort, incremental test to the limit of tolerance is a valid index of $\dot{V}O_2$max (Day, Rossiter, Coats, Skasick, and Whipp 2003).

Maximal and submaximal $\dot{V}O_2$ is expressed in absolute or relative terms. **Absolute $\dot{V}O_2$** is measured in liters per minute ($L \cdot min^{-1}$) or milliliters per minute ($ml \cdot min^{-1}$) and provides a measure of energy cost for non-weight-bearing activities such as leg or arm cycle ergometry. Absolute $\dot{V}O_2$ is directly related to body size; thus men typically have a larger absolute $\dot{V}O_2$max than women.

Because absolute $\dot{V}O_2$ depends on body size, $\dot{V}O_2$ is typically expressed relative to body weight, that is, in $ml \cdot kg^{-1} \cdot min^{-1}$. **Relative $\dot{V}O_2$max** is used to classify an individual's cardiorespiratory (CR) fitness level or to compare fitness levels of individuals differing in body size. Relative $\dot{V}O_2$ can also be used to estimate the energy cost of weight-bearing activities such as walking, running, and stair-climbing. However, although the relationship between absolute $\dot{V}O_2$max and body mass is strong ($r = 0.86$), it is not perfect ($r = 1.00$). Therefore, when $\dot{V}O_2$max is expressed simply as a linear function of body mass, CR fitness levels of heavier (>75.4 kg) and lighter (<67.7 kg) individuals may be under- or overclassified, respectively (Heil 1997). Some experts propose scaling $\dot{V}O_2$ to an exponential function of body mass (Buresh and Berg 2002; Heil 1997). Heil (1997) suggested using a body mass exponent of 0.67 to compare individuals of similar height, age, and training status and an exponent of 0.75 to compare heterogeneous groups (e.g., older vs. younger or trained vs. sedentary individuals). A current limitation of this exponential approach is that the norms used to classify CR fitness levels were established for relative $\dot{V}O_2$max values expressed as $ml \cdot min^{-1} \cdot kg^{-1}$ and not as $ml \cdot min^{-1} \cdot kg^{0.67 \text{ or } 0.75}$.

Sometimes $\dot{V}O_2$ is expressed relative to the individual's fat-free mass (see chapter 8), that is, as $ml \cdot kgFFM^{-1} \cdot min^{-1}$. For example, your client's improvement in relative $\dot{V}O_2$max following a 16 wk aerobic exercise program may reflect both improved capacity of the cardiorespiratory system (increase in absolute $\dot{V}O_2$max) and weight loss (increase in relative $\dot{V}O_2$ expressed as $ml \cdot kg^{-1} \cdot min^{-1}$ due to a decrease in body weight). Thus, expressing $\dot{V}O_2$max relative to fat-free mass, instead of body weight,

provides you with an estimate of cardiorespiratory endurance that is independent of changes in body weight.

The rate of oxygen consumption can also be expressed as a **gross $\dot{V}O_2$** or **net $\dot{V}O_2$**. Gross $\dot{V}O_2$ is the total rate of oxygen consumption and reflects the caloric costs of both rest and exercise (gross $\dot{V}O_2$ = resting $\dot{V}O_2$ + exercise $\dot{V}O_2$). On the other hand, net $\dot{V}O_2$ represents the rate of oxygen consumption in excess of the resting $\dot{V}O_2$ and is used to describe the caloric cost of the exercise. Both gross and net $\dot{V}O_2$ can be expressed in either absolute (e.g., $L \cdot min^{-1}$) or relative ($ml \cdot kg^{-1} \cdot min^{-1}$) terms. Unless specified as a net $\dot{V}O_2$, the $\dot{V}O_2$ values reported throughout this book refer to gross $\dot{V}O_2$.

GRADED EXERCISE TESTING: GUIDELINES AND PROCEDURES

Exercise scientists and physicians use exercise tests to evaluate functional aerobic capacity ($\dot{V}O_2$max) objectively. The $\dot{V}O_2$max, determined from graded maximal or submaximal exercise tests, is used to classify the cardiorespiratory fitness level of your client (see table 4.1). You can use baseline and follow-up data to evaluate the progress of exercise program participants and to set realistic goals for your clients. You can use the heart rate (HR) and oxygen uptake data obtained during the graded exercise test to make accurate, precise exercise prescriptions.

As discussed in chapter 2, before the start of a vigorous ($>60\%$ $\dot{V}O_2$max) exercise program, ACSM (2006) recommends a graded **maximal exercise test** for

- older men (≥ 45 years) and women (≥ 55 years),
- individuals of any age with moderate risk (two or more coronary heart disease risk factors),
- high-risk individuals with one or more signs/symptoms of cardiovascular and pulmonary disease, and
- high-risk individuals with known cardiovascular, pulmonary, or metabolic disease.

However, you may use **submaximal exercise tests** for low-risk individuals, as well as clients with moderate risk, if they are starting a moderate (40% to 60% $\dot{V}O_2$max) exercise program (ACSM 2006). For medical conditions that are absolute

TABLE 4.1 Cardiorespiratory Fitness Classification: $\dot{V}O_2$max (ml · kg^{-1} · min^{-1})

Age (yr)	Poor	Fair	Good	Excellent	Superior
WOMEN					
20-29	≤35	36-39	40-43	44-49	50+
30-39	≤33	34-36	37-40	41-45	46+
40-49	≤31	32-34	35-38	39-44	45+
50-59	≤24	25-28	29-30	31-34	35+
60-69	≤25	26-28	29-31	32-35	36+
70-79	≤23	24-26	27-29	30-35	36+
MEN					
20-29	≤41	42-45	46-50	51-55	56+
30-39	≤40	41-43	44-47	48-53	54+
40-49	≤37	38-41	42-45	46-52	53+
50-59	≤34	35-37	38-42	43-49	50+
60-69	≤30	31-34	35-38	39-45	46+
70-79	≤27	28-30	31-35	36-41	42+

The Physical Fitness Specialist Manual (2005), The Cooper Institute for Aerobics Research, Dallas, TX. Used with permission.

and relative contraindications to exercise testing, see chapter 2, page 18.

General Guidelines for Exercise Testing

You may use a maximal or submaximal **graded exercise test (GXT)** to assess the cardiorespiratory fitness of the individual. The selection of a maximal or submaximal GXT depends on

- your client's age and risk stratification (low risk, moderate risk, or high risk),
- your reasons for administering the test (physical fitness testing or clinical testing), and
- the availability of appropriate equipment and qualified personnel.

In clinical and research settings, $\dot{V}O_2$max is typically measured directly and requires expensive equipment and experienced personnel. Although $\dot{V}O_2$max can be predicted from maximal exercise intensity with a fair degree of accuracy, submaximal tests also provide a reasonable estimate of your client's cardiorespiratory fitness level and are less costly, time consuming, and risky. Submaximal exercise testing, however, is considered less

sensitive as a diagnostic tool for coronary heart disease (CHD).

In either case, the exercise test should be a multistage, graded test. This means that the individual exercises at gradually increasing submaximal workloads. Many commonly used exercise test protocols require that each workload be performed for 3 min. The GXT measures maximum aerobic capacity ($\dot{V}O_2$max) when the oxygen uptake plateaus and does not increase by more than 150 ml · min^{-1} with a further increase in workload. Other criteria (ACSM 2006) used to indicate the attainment of $\dot{V}O_2$max are the following:

- Failure of the HR to increase with increases in exercise intensity
- Venous lactate concentration exceeding 8 mmol/L
- **Respiratory exchange ratio (RER)** greater than 1.15
- Rating of perceived exertion greater than 17 using the original Borg scale (6-20)

During GXTs, many individuals are unable to attain a true plateau in $\dot{V}O_2$. If the test is terminated before the person reaches a plateau in $\dot{V}O_2$

and an RER greater than 1.15, the GXT is a measure of $\dot{V}O_2$peak rather than $\dot{V}O_2$max. Children, older adults, sedentary individuals, and clients with known disease are more likely than other groups to attain a $\dot{V}O_2$peak rather than a $\dot{V}O_2$max. For CHD screening and classification purposes, bringing a person to at least 85% of the age-predicted maximal HR is desirable, because some electrocardiogram (ECG) abnormalities do not appear until the HR reaches this level of intensity (Pollock, Wilmore, and Fox 1978).

Evidence suggests that maximal exercise tests are no more dangerous than submaximal tests (Rochmis and Blackburn 1971; Shephard 1977), provided you carefully follow guidelines for exercise tolerance testing and monitor the physiological responses of the exercise participant continuously. Shephard (1977) predicted one fatality in every 10 to 20 years for a population of 5 million middle-aged Canadians who undergo maximal exercise testing. For high-risk patients, he estimated 1 fibrillation per 5000 submaximal exercise tests and 1 fibrillation per 3000 maximal exercise tests. For clinical testing, the risk of an exercise test being fatal is approximately 0.4 to 0.5 per 10,000 tests (Atterhog, Jonsson, and Samuelsson 1979; Rochmis and Blackburn 1971), and the risk of myocardial infarction is estimated to be 4 per 10,000 tests (Thompson 1993). The overall risk of exercise testing in a mixed population is 6 cardiac events (e.g., myocardial infarction, death, and dysrhythmias) per 10,000 tests (ACSM 2006).The risk for apparently healthy individuals (without known disease) is very low, with no complications occurring in 380,000 exercise tests done on young individuals (Levine, Zuckerman, and Cole 1998).

General Procedures for Cardiorespiratory Fitness Testing

At least one day before the exercise test, you should give your client pretest instructions (see chapter 3, p. 43). Prior to graded exercise testing, the client should read and sign the informed consent and complete the PAR-Q; see appendix A.1, "Physical Activity Readiness Questionnaire (Par-Q)," p. 278).

Step-by-step procedures, as recommended by ACSM (2006), for administering a GXT are listed below.

Pretest, exercise, and recovery HRs can be measured using the palpation or auscultation techniques (see chapter 2) if a heart rate monitor or ECG recorder is unavailable. Because of extraneous noise and vibration during exercise, it may

---

PROCEDURES FOR ADMINISTERING A GRADED EXERCISE TEST

- Measure the client's resting HR and blood pressure (BP) in the exercise posture (see chapter 2 for these procedures).

- Begin the GXT with a 2- to 3-min warm-up to familiarize clients with the exercise equipment and prepare them for the first stage of the exercise test.

- During the test, monitor HR, BP, and ratings of perceived exertion (RPEs) at regular intervals. Measure exercise HR at least two times during each stage of the test, near the end of the minute. Assess exercise BP and RPE near the end of each exercise stage. Throughout the exercise test, continuously monitor the client's physical appearance and symptoms.

- Discontinue the GXT when the test termination criteria are reached, if the client requests stopping the test, or if any of the indications for stopping an exercise test are apparent (see p. 60).

- Have the client cool down by exercising at a low work rate that does not exceed the intensity of the first stage of the exercise test (e.g., walking on the treadmill at 2 mph [53.6 m · min^{-1}] and 0% grade or cycling on the cycle ergometer at 50 to 60 revolutions per minute [rpm] and zero resistance). Active recovery reduces the risk of hypotension from venous pooling in the extremities.

- During recovery, continue measuring postexercise HR, BP, and RPE every 1 to 2 min for at least 5 min, or longer if there are any abnormal responses. The HR and BP during active recovery should be stable but may be higher than preexercise levels. Continue monitoring the client's physical appearance during recovery.

- If your client has signs of discomfort or if an emergency occurs, use a passive cool-down with the client in a sitting or supine position.

be difficult to obtain accurate measurements of BP, especially when your client is running on the treadmill. To become proficient at taking exercise BP, you need to practice as much as possible.

To obtain **ratings of perceived exertion (RPE)** during exercise testing, you can use either the original (6 to 20) or revised (0 to 10) RPE scale (see table 4.2). These scales allow clients to rate their degree of exertion subjectively during exercise and are highly related to exercise HRs and $\dot{V}O_2$. Both RPE scales take into account the linear rise in HR and $\dot{V}O_2$ during exercise. The revised scale also reflects nonlinear changes in blood lactate and ventilation during exercise. Ratings of 10 on the revised scale and 19 on the original scale usually correspond with the maximal level of exercise. Ratings of perceived exertion are useful in determining the end points of the GXT, particularly for patients

who are taking beta-blockers or other medications that may alter the HR response to exercise. You can teach your clients how to use the RPE scale to monitor relative intensities during aerobic exercise programs.

Test Termination

In a maximal or submaximal GXT, the exercise usually continues until the client voluntarily terminates the test or a predetermined end point is reached. As an exercise technician, however, you must be acutely aware of all indicators for stopping a test. If you notice any of the signs or symptoms listed on page 60, you should stop the exercise test prior to the client's reaching $\dot{V}O_2$max (for a maximal GXT) or the predetermined end point (for a submaximal GXT).

TABLE 4.2   Ratings of Perceived Exertion Scale and Category-Ratio Scale

RPE SCALE		CR10 SCALE	
6 No exertion at all	0 Nothing at all	"No P"
7	0.3	
Extremely light	0.5 Extremely weak	Just noticeable
8	1 Very weak	
9 Very light	1.5	
10	2 Weak	Light
11 Light	2.5 Moderate	
12	3	
13 Somewhat hard	4	
14	5 Strong	Heavy
15 Hard (heavy)	6	
16	7 Very strong	
17 Very hard	8	
18	9	
19 Extremely hard	10 Extremely strong	"Max P"
20 Maximal exertion	11	
	≒	
	● Absolute maximum	Highest possible

Borg RPE scale
© Gunnar Borg, 1970, 1985, 1994, 1998

Borg CR10 scale
© Gunnar Borg, 1981, 1982, 1998

Reprinted, by permission, from G. Borg, 1998, *Borg's Perceived Exertion and Pain Scales* (Champaign, IL: Human Kinetics), 47.

General Procedures for Clinical Exercise Testing

You can use a maximal GXT for diagnostic and functional testing in order to determine safe levels of exercise for clients with or without heart disease. For clinical testing, measure and record the BP, HR, and 12-lead ECG (see chapter 2 for these procedures) in the supine and exercise postures prior to exercise testing. During exercise, continuously monitor the ECG and record the ECG during the last 15 sec of each stage for traditional GXT protocols or during the last 15 sec of each 2 min period for ramp protocols. Monitor the exercise HR continuously and record the HR and RPE during the last 5 sec of each minute. Measure and record the exercise BP during the last 45 sec of each stage for traditional GXT protocols or during the last 45 sec of each 2 min period for ramp protocols (ACSM 2006). In addition, whenever symptoms or ECG changes occur during exercise, record the 12-lead ECG, HR, BP, and RPE. If you notice any of the signs or symptoms listed in "Absolute and Relative Indications for Termination of a Clinical Graded Exercise Test" below, the exercise test should be stopped immediately. ST-segment elevation with a horizontal or downward slope is indicative of severe CHD or coronary spasm. Horizontal or downsloping ST-segment depression ($\geq$1 mm) suggests myocardial ischemia. The onset, duration, and magnitude of the ST-segment depression are related to the severity of the ischemia. Failure of systolic BP to rise, or a significant drop in systolic BP (20 mmHg) during the exercise test, is an indicator of CHD or heart failure (Hanson 1988).

Following the exercise test, monitor the ECG continuously and record the ECG immediately postexercise, then during the last 15 sec of the first min of recovery, and then every 2 min thereafter. During recovery, monitor HR continuously and record it during the last 5 sec of each minute. Measure and record BP immediately postexercise and then every 2 min thereafter. Record the peak exercise RPE immediately after exercise (ACSM 2006).

Absolute and Relative Indications for Termination of a Clinical Graded Exercise Test[a]

Absolute Indications

1. Moderate-to-severe angina
2. Drop in systolic blood pressure of $\geq$10 mmHg from baseline blood pressure despite an increase in workload, when accompanied by other evidence of ischemia
3. Increasing nervous system symptoms (e.g., ataxia, dizziness, or near syncope)
4. Signs of poor perfusion (cyanosis or pallor)
5. Technical difficulties monitoring the electrocardiogram or systolic blood pressure
6. Client's desire to stop
7. Sustained ventricular tachycardia
8. ST elevation ($\geq$1.0 mm) in leads without diagnostic Q waves (other than V_1 or aVR)

Relative Indications

1. Drop in systolic blood pressure of $\geq$10 mmHg from baseline blood pressure despite an increase in workload, in the absence of other evidence of ischemia, or failure of systolic blood pressure to increase with increased workload
2. Increasing chest pain
3. Fatigue, shortness of breath, wheezing, leg cramps, or claudication
4. Hypertensive response (systolic blood pressure >250 mmHg and/or diastolic blood pressure >115 mmHg)
5. Arrhythmias other than sustained ventricular tachycardia, including multifocal preventricular contractions (PVCs), triplets of PVCs, supraventricular tachycardia, heart block, or bradyarrhythmias
6. Development of bundle-branch block or intraventricular conduction delay that cannot be distinguished from ventricular tachycardia
7. ST or QRS changes such as excessive ST-segment depression ($\geq$1 mm horizontal or downsloping ST-segment depression) or marked axis shift

---

[a]For definitions of specific terms, refer to the glossary on page 379.

From Gibbons, R.J. et al. 2002. ACC/AHA 2002 Guideline update for exercise testing. A report of the American College of Cardiology/American Heart Association Task Force on Practice Guidelines (Committee on Exercise Testing). www.acc.org/clinical/guidelines/exercise/dirindex.htm.

If your clients are having difficulty breathing, they should sit down. Even though an active cool-down may decrease hypotension, it is not recommended following a GXT that is given for diagnostic purposes because active cool-down may increase the magnitude of ST-segment depression.

MAXIMAL EXERCISE TEST PROTOCOLS

Many maximal exercise test protocols have been devised to assess aerobic capacity. As the exercise technician, you must be able to select an exercise mode and test protocol that is suitable for your clients given their age, gender, and health and fitness status. Commonly used modes of exercise are treadmill walking or running and stationary cycling. Arm ergometry is useful for persons with paraplegia and clients who have limited use of the lower extremities. Bench stepping is not highly recommended but could be useful in field situations when large groups need to be tested. Whichever mode of exercise you choose, be sure to adhere to "General Principles of Exercise Testing" below.

The exercise test may be continuous or discontinuous. A continuous test is performed with no rest between work increments. Continuous exercise tests can vary in the duration of each

GENERAL PRINCIPLES OF EXERCISE TESTING[a]

1. Typically, you will use either a treadmill or stationary cycle ergometer for graded exercise testing (GXT). All equipment should be calibrated before use.

2. Begin the GXT with a 2- to 3-min warm-up to orient the client to the equipment and prepare the client for the first stage of the GXT.

3. The initial exercise intensity should be considerably lower than the anticipated maximal capacity.

4. Exercise intensity should be increased gradually throughout the stages of the test. Work increments may be 2 METs or greater for apparently healthy individuals and as small as 0.5 MET for patients with disease.

5. Closely observe contraindications for testing and indications for stopping the exercise test. When in any doubt about the safety or benefits of testing, do not perform the test at that time.

6. Monitor the heart rate at least two times, but preferably each minute, during each stage of the GXT. Heart rate measurements should be taken near the end of each minute. If the heart rate does not reach steady state (two heart rates within $\pm$5-6 bpm), extend the work stage an additional minute, or until the heart rate stabilizes.

7. Measure blood pressure and RPE once during each stage of the GXT, in the later portion of the stage.

8. Continually monitor client appearance and symptoms.

9. For submaximal GXTs, terminate the test when the client's heart rate reaches 70% HRR or 85% HRmax, unless the protocol specifies a different termination criterion. Also, stop the test immediately if there is an emergency situation, if the client fails to conform to the exercise protocol, or if the client experiences signs of discomfort.

10. The test should include a cool-down period of at least 5 min, or longer if abnormal heart rate and blood pressure responses are observed. During recovery, heart rate and blood pressure should be monitored each minute. For active recovery, the workload should be no more than that used during the first stage of the GXT. A passive recovery is used in emergency situations and when clients experience signs of discomfort and cannot perform an active cool-down.

11. Exercise tolerance in METs should be estimated for the treadmill or ergometer protocol used, or directly assessed if oxygen uptake is measured during the GXT.

12. The testing area should be quiet and private. The room temperature should be 21 to 23 °C (70 to 72 °F) or less and the humidity 60% or less if possible.

[a]Physician supervision is recommended for maximal exercise tests of moderate or high-risk clients, as well as submaximal exercise tests for high-risk clients.

exercise stage and the magnitude of the increment in exercise intensity between stages. The total test duration should be between 8 and 12 min to increase the probability of the individual's reaching $\dot{V}O_2$max. For most continuous exercise test protocols, the exercise intensity is increased gradually (2 to 3 METs for low-risk individuals) throughout the test, and the duration of each stage is usually 2 to 3 min, allowing most individuals to reach a steady-state $\dot{V}O_2$ during each stage. Across the stages of this type of GXT, the workload may increase linearly or nonlinearly. Each increment in workload is dictated by the specific protocol and does not vary among individuals. Although this type of GXT is widely used in research and clinical settings, it may not be optimal for assessing the aerobic capacity of all individuals, especially those with low exercise tolerance.

Today, continuous ramp-type tests are gaining popularity and are widely used because they can be individualized for the client's estimated exercise tolerance. For example, increments in work rate during a ramp protocol are much higher for endurance-trained athletes than for sedentary individuals (e.g., 30 W/min vs. 10 W/min). Also, each exercise stage for ramp protocols is much shorter (e.g., 20 sec) than that of the traditional continuous GXT protocols (2-3 min). **Ramp protocols** provide continuous and frequent increments in work rate throughout the test so that the $\dot{V}O_2$ increases linearly; they are designed to bring individuals to their limit of exercise tolerance in approximately 10 min. Because of the frequent (e.g., every 10 or 20 sec) increases in work rate, $\dot{V}O_2$ plateaus are rarely observed. However, as previously mentioned, the $\dot{V}O_2$peak from ramp-type protocols appears to be a valid index of $\dot{V}O_2$max even without a plateau in $\dot{V}O_2$ (Day et al. 2003). This ramp approach potentially improves the prediction of $\dot{V}O_2$max given that $\dot{V}O_2$ increases linearly across work rates. Ramp protocols allow some individuals to reach a higher exercise tolerance compared to traditional GXT protocols. However, there are disadvantages. To design an individualized ramp protocol, the maximum work rate for each client must be predetermined or accurately estimated from training records or questionnaires so that you can select a work rate that allows the individual to reach his peak exercise tolerance in approximately 10 min. Also, ramp protocols increase work rate frequently (e.g., 25-30 stages in a 10 min test), requiring more expensive electromagnetically braked cycle ergometers and programmable treadmills that make rapid and smooth transitions between the stages of the

exercise test. Lastly, inexperienced technicians may have difficulty measuring exercise blood pressure during each minute of the ramp protocol.

For **discontinuous tests**, the client rests 5 to 10 min between workloads. The workload is progressively increased until the client reaches maximum exercise tolerance (exhaustion). Typically, each stage of the discontinuous protocol lasts 5 to 6 min, allowing $\dot{V}O_2$ to reach a steady state. On average, discontinuous tests take five times longer to administer than do continuous tests. Similar $\dot{V}O_2$max values are attained using discontinuous and continuous (increasing workload every 2-3 min) protocols (Maksud and Coutts 1971); therefore, continuous tests are preferable in most research and clinical settings.

McArdle, Katch, and Pechar (1973) compared the $\dot{V}O_2$max scores as measured by six commonly used continuous and discontinuous treadmill and cycle ergometer tests. They noted that the $\dot{V}O_2$max scores for the cycle ergometer tests were approximately 6% to 11% lower than for the treadmill tests. Many subjects identified local discomfort and fatigue in the thigh muscles as the major factors limiting further work on both the continuous and discontinuous cycle ergometer tests. For the treadmill tests, subjects indicated windedness and general fatigue as the limiting factors and complained of localized fatigue and discomfort in the calf muscles and lower back.

Treadmill Maximal Exercise Tests

The exercise is performed on a motor-driven treadmill with variable speed and incline (see figure 4.1). Speed varies up to 25 mph, and incline is measured in units of elevation per 100 horizontal units and is expressed as a percentage. The workload on the treadmill is raised through increases in the speed or incline or both. Workload is usually expressed in miles per hour and percent grade.

It is difficult and expensive to measure the oxygen consumption during exercise. Therefore, ACSM (2006) has developed equations (table 4.3) to estimate the metabolic cost of exercise ($\dot{V}O_2$). These equations provide a valid estimate of $\dot{V}O_2$ for steady-state exercise only. When used to estimate the maximum rate of energy expenditure ($\dot{V}O_2$max), the measured $\dot{V}O_2$ will be less than the estimated $\dot{V}O_2$ if steady state is not reached. Also, because maximal exercise involves both aerobic and anaerobic components, the $\dot{V}O_2$max will be overestimated since the contribution of the anaerobic component is not known.

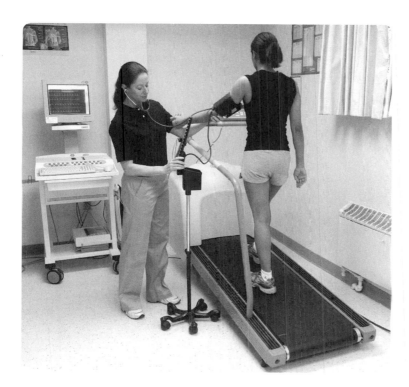

Figure 4.1 Treadmill.

Before using any of the ACSM metabolic equations to estimate $\dot{V}O_2$, make certain that all units of measure match those in the equation (see Converting Units of Measure).

The ACSM metabolic equations in table 4.3 are useful in clinical settings for estimating the total rate of energy expenditure (gross $\dot{V}O_2$) during steady-state treadmill walking or running. The total energy expenditure, in $ml \cdot kg^{-1} \cdot min^{-1}$, is a function of three components: *speed, grade,* and *resting energy expenditures.* For treadmill walking, the oxygen cost of raising one's body mass against gravity (vertical work) is approximately $1.8\ ml \cdot kg^{-1} \cdot m^{-1}$, and $0.1\ ml \cdot kg^{-1} \cdot m^{-1}$ of oxygen is needed to move the body horizontally. For treadmill running, the oxygen cost for vertical work is one-half that for treadmill walking ($0.9\ ml \cdot kg^{-1} \cdot m^{-1}$), whereas the energy expenditure for running on the treadmill ($0.2\ ml \cdot kg^{-1} \cdot m^{-1}$) is twice that for walking. See page 65 for an example of how to take these three factors into account when figuring $\dot{V}O_2$.

The $\dot{V}O_2$ estimated from the ACSM walking equation (see table 4.3) is reasonably accurate for walking speeds between 50 and 100 $m \cdot min^{-1}$ (1.9 to 3.7 mph). However, since the equation is more accurate for walking up a grade than on the level, $\dot{V}O_2$ may be underestimated as much as 15% to 20% during walking on the level (ACSM 2006). For the ACSM running/jogging equations, the $\dot{V}O_2$

CONVERTING UNITS OF MEASURE

- Convert body mass (M) in pounds to kilograms (1 kg = 2.2 lb). For example, 170 lb/2.2 = 77.3 kg.

- Convert treadmill speed (S) in miles per hour to meters per minute (1 mph = 26.8 m/min). For example, 5.0 mph $\times$ 26.8 = 134.0 $m \cdot min^{-1}$.

- Convert treadmill grade (G) from percent to decimal form by dividing by 100. For example, 12%/100 = 0.12.

- Convert METs to $ml \cdot kg^{-1} \cdot min^{-1}$ by multiplying (1 MET = 3.5 $ml \cdot kg^{-1} \cdot min^{-1}$). For example, 6 METs $\times$ 3.5 = 21.0 $ml \cdot kg^{-1} \cdot min^{-1}$.

- Convert $kgm \cdot min^{-1}$ to watts (W) (1 W = 6 $kgm \cdot min^{-1}$) by dividing. For example, 900 $kgm \cdot min^{-1}$/6 = 150 W.

- Convert step height in inches to meters (1 in. = 0.0254 m) by multiplying. For example, 8 in. $\times$ 0.0254 = 0.2032 m.

estimates are relatively accurate for speeds exceeding 134 $m \cdot min^{-1}$ (5 mph) and speeds as low as 80 $m \cdot min^{-1}$ (3 mph) provided that the client is jogging and not walking (ACSM 2006).

Exercise mode gross $\dot{V}O_2$ (ml $\cdot$ kg^{-1} $\cdot$ min^{-1})	Resting $\dot{V}O_2$ (ml $\cdot$ kg^{-1} $\cdot$ min^{-1})	Comments
Walking $\dot{V}O_2 = S^a \times 0.1 + S \times G^b \times 1.8$	+ 3.5	1. For speeds of 50-100 m $\cdot$ min^{-1} (1.9-3.7 mph)
		2. 0.1 ml $\cdot$ kg^{-1} $\cdot$ m^{-1} = O$_2$ cost of walking horizontally
		3. 1.8 ml $\cdot$ kg^{-1} $\cdot$ m^{-1} = O$_2$ cost of walking on incline (% grade of treadmill)
Running $\dot{V}O_2 = S^a \times 0.2 + S \times G^b \times 0.9$	+ 3.5	1. For speeds >134 m $\cdot$ min^{-1} (>5.0 mph)
		2. If truly jogging (not walking), this equation can also be used for speeds of 80-134 m$\cdot$min^{-1} (3-5 mph)
		3. 0.2 ml $\cdot$ kg^{-1} $\cdot$ m^{-1} = O$_2$ cost of running horizontally
		4. 0.9 ml $\cdot$ kg^{-1} $\cdot$ m^{-1} = O$_2$ cost of running on incline (% grade of treadmill)
Leg ergometry $\dot{V}O_2 = W^c/M^d \times 1.8 + 3.5$	+ 3.5	1. For work rates between 50 and 200 watts (300-1200 kgm $\cdot$ min^{-1})
		2. kgm $\cdot$ min^{-1} = kg $\times$ m/rev $\times$ rev/min
		3. Monark and Bodyguard = 6 m/rev; Tunturi = 3 m/rev
		4. 1.8 ml $\cdot$ kg^{-1} $\cdot$ min^{-1} = O$_2$ cost of cycling against external load (resistance)
		5. 3.5 ml $\cdot$ kg^{-1} $\cdot$ min^{-1} = O$_2$ cost of cycling with zero load
Arm ergometry $\dot{V}O_2 = W^c/M^d \times 3.0 + None$	+ 3.5	1. For work rates between 25 and 125 W (150-750 kgm $\cdot$ min^{-1})
		2. kgm $\cdot$ min^{-1} = kg $\times$ m/rev $\times$ rev/min
		3. 3.0 ml $\cdot$ kg^{-1} $\cdot$ min^{-1} = O$_2$ cost of cycling against external load (resistance)
		4. None = due to small mass of arm musculature, no special term for unloaded (zero load) cycling is needed
Stepping $\dot{V}O_2 = F^e \times 0.2 + F \times ht^f \times 1.8 \times 1.33$	+ 3.5	1. Appropriate for stepping rates between 12 and 30 steps/min and step heights between 0.04 m (1.6 in.) and 0.40 m (15.7 in.)
		2. 0.2 ml $\cdot$ kg^{-1} $\cdot$ m^{-1} = O$_2$ cost of moving horizontally
		3. 1.8 ml $\cdot$ kg^{-1} $\cdot$ m^{-1} = O$_2$ cost of stepping up (bench height)
		4. 1.33 includes positive component of stepping up (1.0) + negative component of stepping down (0.33)

[a]S = speed of treadmill in m $\cdot$ min^{-1}; 1 mph = 26.8 m $\cdot$ min^{-1}.
[b]G = grade (% incline) of treadmill in decimal form; e.g., 10% = 0.10.
[c]W = work rate in kgm $\cdot$ min^{-1}; 1 W = 6 kgm $\cdot$ min^{-1}.
[d]M = body mass in kilograms; 1 kg = 2.2 lb.
[e]F = frequency of stepping in steps per minute.
[f]ht = bench height in meters; 1 in. = 0.0254 m.

ACSM WALKING EQUATION

To calculate the gross $\dot{V}O_2$ for a 70-kg subject who is walking on the treadmill at a speed of 3.5 mph and a grade of 10%, follow these steps:

$\dot{V}O_2$ = speed + (grade × speed)
 + resting VO_2 (ml · kg^{-1} · min^{-1})
 = [speed (m · min^{-1}) × 0.1] + [grade (decimal) × speed (m · min^{-1}) × 1.8] + 3.5

1. Convert the speed in mph to m · min^{-1}; 1 mph = 26.8 m · min^{-1}.

   3.5 mph × 26.8 = 93.8 m · min^{-1}

2. Calculate the speed component (S).

   S = speed (m · min^{-1}) × 0.1
    = 93.8 m · min^{-1} × 0.1
    = 9.38 ml · kg^{-1} · min^{-1}

3. Calculate the grade × speed component (G × S). Convert % grade into a decimal by dividing by 100.

   G × S = grade (decimal) × speed × 1.8
    = 0.10 × (93.8 m · min^{-1}) × 1.8
    = 16.88 ml · kg^{-1} · min^{-1}

4. Calculate the total gross $\dot{V}O_2$ in ml · kg^{-1} · min^{-1} by adding the speed, grade × speed, and resting $\dot{V}O_2$ (R).

   $\dot{V}O_2$ = S + (S × G) + R
    = (9.38 + 16.88 + 3.5) ml · kg^{-1} · min^{-1}
    = 29.76 ml · kg^{-1} · min^{-1}

Figure 4.2 illustrates commonly used treadmill exercise test protocols. These protocols conform to the general guidelines for maximal exercise testing. Some of the protocols are designed for a specific population, such as well-conditioned athletes or high-risk cardiac patients. The exercise intensity for each stage of the various treadmill test protocols can be expressed in METs. The MET estimations for each stage of some commonly used treadmill protocols are listed in table 4.4.

Population-specific and generalized equations have been developed to estimate $\dot{V}O_2$max from exercise time for some treadmill protocols (see table 4.5). It is important for exercise technicians to keep in mind that the initial workload in some of the protocols designed for highly trained athletes is too intense (exceeding 2 to 3.5 METs) for the average individual. The Balke and Bruce proto-

cols are well suited for low-risk individuals, and the Bruce protocol is easily adapted for high-risk individuals using an initial workload of 1.7 mph at 0% to 5% grade.

Balke Treadmill Protocol

To administer the Balke and Ware (1959) exercise test protocol (see figure 4.2), set the treadmill speed at 3.4 mph (91.1 m · min^{-1}) and the initial grade of the treadmill at 0% during the first minute of exercise. Maintain a constant speed on the treadmill throughout the entire exercise test. At the start of the second minute of exercise, increase the grade to 2%. Thereafter, at the beginning of every additional minute of exercise, increase the grade by only 1%.

Use the prediction equation for the Balke protocol in table 4.5 to estimate your client's $\dot{V}O_2$max from exercise time. Alternatively, you can use a nomogram (see figure 4.3) developed for the Balke treadmill protocol to calculate the $\dot{V}O_2$max of your client. To use this nomogram, locate the time corresponding to the last complete minute of exercise during the protocol along the vertical axis labeled "Balke time," and draw a horizontal line from the time axis to the oxygen uptake axis. Be certain to plot the exercise time of women and men in the appropriate column when using this nomogram.

Bruce Treadmill Protocol

The Bruce, Kusumi, and Hosmer (1973) exercise test is a multistaged treadmill protocol (see figure 4.2). The workload is increased by changing both the treadmill speed and percent grade. During the first stage (minutes 1 to 3) of the test, the normal individual walks at a 1.7 mph pace at 10% grade. At the start of the second stage (minutes 4 to 6), increase the grade by 2% and the speed to 2.5 mph (67 m · min^{-1}). In each subsequent stage of the test, increase the grade 2% and the speed by either 0.8 or 0.9 mph (21.4 or 24.1 m · min^{-1}) until the client is exhausted. Prediction equations for this protocol have been developed to estimate the $\dot{V}O_2$max of active and sedentary women and men, cardiac patients, and people who are elderly (see table 4.5). As an alternative, you may use the nomogram (see figure 4.4) developed for the Bruce protocol. Plot the client's exercise time for this protocol along the vertical axis labeled "Bruce time," and draw a horizontal line from the time axis to the oxygen uptake. Again, be certain to use the appropriate column for men and women.

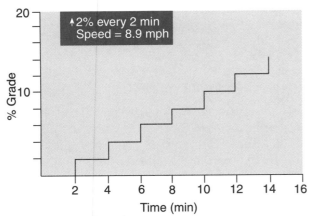

Costill and Fox (1969)
For: highly trained
Warm-up: 10-min walk or run
Initial workload: 8.9 mph, 0%, 2 min

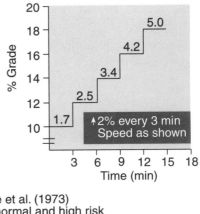

Bruce et al. (1973)
For: normal and high risk
Initial workload: 1.7 mph, 10%, 3 min = normal
1.7 mph, 0-5%, 3 min = high risk

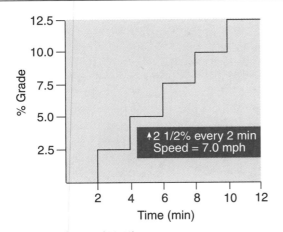

Maksud and Coutts (1971)
For: highly trained
Warm-up: 10-min walking 3.5 mph, 0%
Initial workload: 7 mph, 0%, 2 min

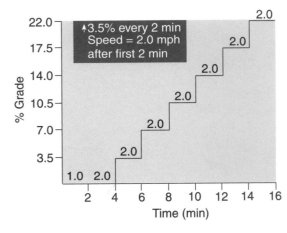

Naughton et al. (1964)
For: cardiac and high risk
Initial workload: 1.0 mph, 0%, 2 min

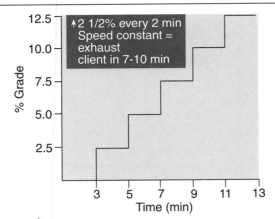

Modified Åstrand (Pollock et al. 1978)
For: highly trained
Warm-up: 5-min walk or jog
Initial workload: 5-8 mph, 0%, 3 min

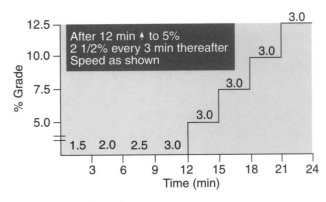

Wilson et al. (1978)
For: cardiac and high risk
Initial workload: 1.5 mph, 0%, 3 min

(continued)

Figure 4.2 Treadmill exercise test protocols.

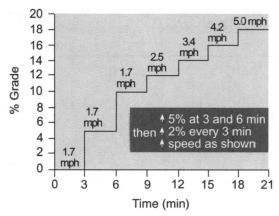

Modified Bruce (Lerman et al. 1976)
For: normal and high risk
Initial workload: 1.7 mph, 0%, 3 min

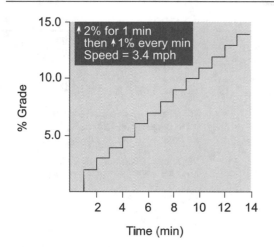

Balke and Ware (1959)
For: normal risk
Initial workload: 3.4 mph, 0%, 1 min

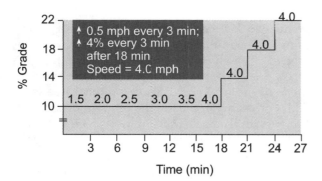

Kattus (1968)
For: cardiac and high risk
Initial workload: 1.5 mph, 10%, 3 min

Figure 4.2 *(continued)*

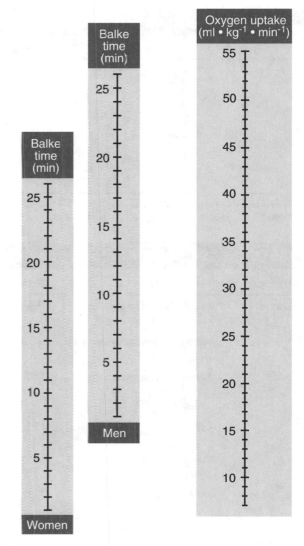

Figure 4.3 Nomogram for Balke graded exercise test.

Reprinted, by permission, from N. Ng, 1995, *Metcalc* (Champaign, IL: Human Kinetics), 30.

Modified Bruce Protocol

The modified Bruce protocol (see figure 4.2) is more suitable than the Bruce protocol for high-risk and elderly individuals. However, with the exception of the first two stages, this protocol is similar to the standard Bruce protocol. Stage 1 starts at 0% grade and a 1.7 mph walking pace. For stage 2, the % grade is increased to 5%. McInnis and Balady (1994) compared physiological responses to the standard and modified Bruce protocols in patients with CHD and reported similar HR and BP responses at matched exercise stages despite the additional 6 min of low-intensity exercise performed using the modified Bruce protocol.

TABLE 4.4 MET Estimations for Each Stage of Commonly Used Treadmill Protocols

Stage[a]	Bruce	Modified Bruce[b]	Balke	Naughton
1	4.6	2.3	3.6	1.8
2	7.0	3.5	4.5	3.5
3	10.2	4.6	5.0	4.5
4	12.1	7.0	5.5	5.4
5	14.9	10.2	5.9	6.4
6	17.0	12.1	6.4	7.4
7	19.3	14.9	6.9	8.3

[a]Percent grade and speed for each stage are illustrated in figure 4.2.
[b]Stage 1 = 0% grade, 1.7 mph; Stage 2 = 5% grade, 1.7 mph.

TABLE 4.5 Population-Specific and Generalized Equations for Treadmill Protocols

Protocol	Population	Reference	Equation
Balke	Active and sedentary men	Pollock et al. 1976	$\dot{V}O_2max = 1.444(time) + 14.99$ $r = 0.92, SEE = 2.50$ ml · kg^{-1} · min^{-1}
	Active and sedentary women[a]	Pollock et al. 1982	$\dot{V}O_2max = 1.38(time) + 5.22$ $r = 0.94, SEE = 2.20$ ml · kg^{-1} · min^{-1}
Bruce[b]	Active and sedentary men	Foster et al. 1984	$\dot{V}O_2max = 14.76 - 1.379(time) +$ $0.451(time^2) - 0.012(time^3)$ $r = 0.98, SEE = 3.35$ ml · kg^{-1} · min^{-1}
	Active and sedentary women	Pollock et al. 1982	$\dot{V}O_2max = 4.38(time) - 3.90$ $r = 0.91, SEE = 2.7$ ml · kg^{-1} · min^{-1}
	Cardiac patients and elderly persons[c]	McConnell and Clark 1987	$\dot{V}O_2max = 2.282(time) + 8.545$ $r = 0.82, SEE = 4.9$ ml · kg^{-1} · min^{-1}
Naughton	Male cardiac patients	Foster et al. 1983	$\dot{V}O_2max = 1.61(time) + 3.60$ $r = 0.97, SEE = 2.60$ ml · kg^{-1} · min^{-1}

[a]For women, the Balke protocol was modified: speed 3.0 mph; initial workload 0% grade for 3 min, increasing 2.5% every 3 min thereafter.
[b]For use with the standard Bruce protocol, not modified Bruce protocol.
[c]This equation is used only for treadmill walking while holding the handrails.
SEE = standard error of estimate.

Note that the prediction equations for the Bruce protocol (see table 4.5) can be used for only the standard, not the modified, Bruce protocol. To estimate $\dot{V}O_2$ for the modified Bruce protocol, use the ACSM metabolic equation for walking (see table 4.3).

Treadmill Ramp Protocols

Kaminsky and Whaley (1998) developed a standardized ramp protocol (i.e., BSU/Bruce ramp protocol) for assessing the functional aerobic capacity of symptomatic, sedentary, and apparently healthy individuals. For this protocol, the treadmill speed increases gradually (in 0.1-0.4 mph, or 2.68-10.72 m · min^{-1}, increments) every minute. The minimum speed is 1.0 mph (26.8 m · min^{-1}); the maximum speed is 5.8 mph (155 m · min^{-1}). The treadmill

grade also increases gradually (by 0%-5%) every minute. The minimum grade is 0%; the maximum grade is 20%. Every 3 min during this ramp protocol, the work rates (i.e., speed and grade) equal those of the traditional Bruce protocol (see table 4.6). For example, during the 6th min of exercise, the treadmill speed (2.5 mph, or 53.6 m · min^{-1}) and grade (12%) are the same for both protocols, allowing comparisons between the two types of protocols. The ramp approach has the advantage of avoiding large, unequal increments in workload. Also, it results in uniform increases in hemodynamic and physiological responses to incremental exercise and more accurately estimates exercise capacity and ventilatory threshold.

Porszasz and colleagues (2003) devised a ramp protocol that increases work rate linearly so that

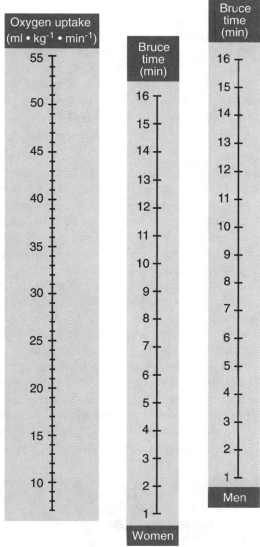

Figure 4.4 Nomogram for standard Bruce graded exercise test.

Reprinted, by permission, from N. Ng, 1995, *Metcalc* (Champaign, IL: Human Kinetics), 32.

TABLE 4.6 Comparison of Work Rates for the Standard Bruce Protocol and the Bruce Ramp Protocol

	SPEED IN MPH[b]		GRADE (%)	
Minute[a]	SB	BR	SB	BR
1	1.7	1.0	10	0
2	1.7	1.3	10	5
3	*1.7*	*1.7*	*10*	*10*
4	2.5	2.1	12	10
5	2.5	2.3	12	11
6	*2.5*	*2.5*	*12*	*12*
7	3.4	2.8	14	12
8	3.4	3.1	14	13
9	*3.4*	*3.4*	*14*	*14*
10	4.2	3.8	16	14
11	4.2	4.1	16	15
12	*4.2*	*4.2*	*16*	*16*
13	5.0	4.5	18	16
14	5.0	4.8	18	17
15	*5.0*	*5.0*	*18*	*18*
16	5.5	5.3	20	18
17	5.5	5.6	20	19
18	5.5	5.8	20	20

SB = standard Bruce protocol; BR = Bruce ramp protocol.
[a]Boldfaced italics identify the times during the two protocols when the work rates are equivalent.
[b]To convert mph to m · min^{-1} multiply by 26.8.

the individual walking on a treadmill reaches exhaustion in approximately 10 min. To linearly increase work rate over time, it is necessary to couple linear increases in walking speed with curvilinear increases in treadmill grade. Because this protocol starts with slow walking (i.e., 0.5-1.0 mph, or 13.4-26.8 m · min^{-1}), it is suitable for individuals with low exercise tolerance as well as for sedentary individuals with a range of exercise tolerances. As with all types of ramp protocols, this protocol is individualized. The peak work rate, a comfortable range of walking speeds, and the increments in treadmill incline or grade are determined for each client.

This protocol compares favorably to cycle ergometer ramp protocols that increment work rate linearly so that maximum exercise tolerance is reached in ~10 min. The slope of the relationship between $\dot{V}O_2$ and work rate, however, is consistently steeper on the treadmill than on the cycle ergometer (Porszasz et al. 2003). This steeper slope reflects additional use of the limbs (i.e., swinging the arms and legs) and frictional force as treadmill speed increases. For each individual, the time course for the grade increments needed to elicit a linear increase in work rate can be calculated with a prediction equation based on the client's body weight, desired initial and final walking speeds, initial grade, and estimated peak work rate (see

Porszasz et al. 2003). These individual variables, along with the prediction equation for increasing grade, can be programmed into the computer of contemporary treadmills. Thus, each individualized ramp protocol is controlled by the computer so that the frequent increases in speed and grade are smooth and rapid.

Cycle Ergometer Maximal Exercise Tests

The cycle ergometer is a widely used instrument for assessing cardiorespiratory fitness. On a friction-type cycle ergometer (see figure 4.5), resistance is applied against the flywheel using a belt and weighted pendulums. The handwheel adjusts the workload by tightening or loosening the brake belt. The workload on the cycle ergometer is raised through increases in the resistance on the flywheel. The power output is usually expressed in kilogram-meters per minute (kgm · min^{-1}) or watts (1 W = 6 kgm · min^{-1}) and is easily measured using the equation:

$$power = force \times distance/time$$

where force equals the resistance or tension setting on the ergometer (kilograms) and distance is the distance traveled by the flywheel rim for each revolution of the pedal times number of revolutions per minute. On the Monark and Bodyguard cycle ergometers, the flywheel travels 6 m per pedal revolution. Therefore, if a resistance of 2 kg is applied and the pedaling rate is 60 rpm, then

$$power = 2 \text{ kg} \times 6 \text{ m} \times 60 \text{ rpm} = 720 \text{ kgm} \cdot \text{min}^{-1},$$
$$\text{or } 120 \text{ W}$$

To calculate the distance traveled by the flywheel of cycle ergometers with varying-sized flywheels, measure the circumference (in meters) of the resistance track on the flywheel and multiply the circumference by the number of flywheel revolutions during one complete revolution (360°) of the pedal (Gledhill and Jamnik 1995).

When you are standardizing the work performed on a friction-type cycle ergometer, the client should maintain a constant pedaling rate. Some cycle ergometers have a speedometer that displays the individual's pedaling rate. Check this dial frequently to make certain that your client is maintaining a constant pedaling frequency throughout the test. If a speedometer is not available, use a metronome to establish your client's pedaling cadence. Controlling the pedaling rate on an electrically braked cycle ergometer (figure 4.6)

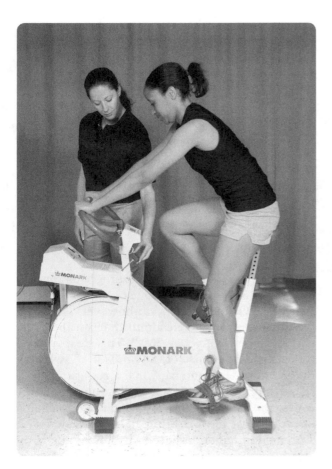

Figure 4.5   Cycle ergometer (mechanically braked).

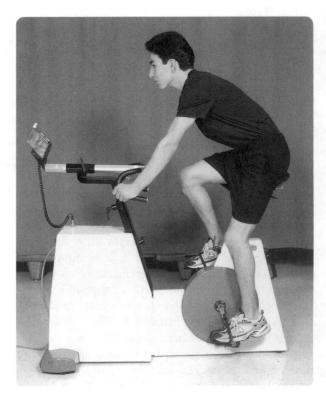

Figure 4.6   Cycle ergometer (electrically braked).

is unnecessary. An electromagnetic braking force adjusts the resistance for slower or faster pedaling rates, thereby keeping the power output constant. This type of cycle ergometer, however, is difficult to calibrate.

Most cycle ergometer test protocols for untrained cyclists use a pedaling rate of 50 or 60 rpm, and power outputs are increased by 150 to 300 $kgm \cdot min^{-1}$ (25 to 50 W) in each stage of the test. However, you can use higher pedaling rates (≥ 80 rpm) for trained cyclists. A pedaling rate of 60 rpm produces the highest $\dot{V}O_2max$ when compared with rates of 50, 70, or 80 rpm (Hermansen and Saltin 1969). Figure 4.7 illustrates some widely used discontinuous and continuous maximal exercise test protocols for the cycle ergometer. Guidelines for use of cycle ergometers are presented below in "Testing with Cycle Ergometers."

To calculate the energy expenditure for cycle ergometer exercise, use the ACSM equations provided in table 4.3. The total energy expenditure or gross $\dot{V}O_2$, in $ml \cdot kg^{-1} \cdot min^{-1}$, is a function of the oxygen cost of pedaling against resistance (power output in watts), the oxygen cost of unloaded cycling (approximately 3.5 $ml \cdot kg^{-1} \cdot min^{-1}$ at 50

TESTING WITH CYCLE ERGOMETERS

The following guidelines are suggested for the use of cycle ergometers (Sinning 1975):

1. Calibrate the cycle ergometer often by hanging known weights from the belt of the flywheel and reading the dial on the handwheel.

2. Always release the tension on the belt between tests.

3. Establish pedaling frequency before setting the workload.

4. Check the load setting frequently during the test because it may change as the belt warms up.

5. Set the metronome so that one revolution is completed for every two beats (e.g., set the metronome at 120 for a test requiring a pedaling frequency of 60 rpm).

6. Adjust the height of the seat so the knee is slightly flexed (about 5°) at maximal leg extension with the ball of the foot on the pedal.

7. Have the client assume an upright, seated posture with hands properly positioned on the handlebars.

to 60 rpm with zero resistance), and the resting oxygen consumption. The cost of cycling against an external load or resistance is approximately 1.8 $ml \cdot kg^{-1} \cdot m^{-1}$. For an example calculation, see "ACSM Leg Ergometry Equation".

Keep in mind that the leg and arm ergometry equations are accurate in estimating $\dot{V}O_2$ only if the client attains a steady state during the maximal GXT. If, for example, the client is able to complete only 1 min of exercise during the last stage of the maximal test protocol, the power output from the previous stage (in which the client reached steady state) should be used to estimate $\dot{V}O_2max$ rather than the power output corresponding to the last stage.

Åstrand Cycle Ergometer Maximal Test Protocol

For the Åstrand (1965) continuous test protocol (see figure 4.7), the initial power output is 300 $kgm \cdot min^{-1}$ (50 W) for women and 600 $kgm \cdot min^{-1}$ (100 W) for men. Because the pedaling rate is 50 rpm, the resistance is 1 kg for women (1 kg × 6 m × 50 rpm = 300 $kgm \cdot min^{-1}$) and 2 kg for men (2 kg × 6 m × 50 rpm = 600 $kgm \cdot min^{-1}$). Have your client exercise at this initial workload for 2 min. Then increase the power output every 2 to 3 min in increments of 150 $kgm \cdot min^{-1}$ (25 W) and 300 $kgm \cdot min^{-1}$ (50 W) for women and men, respectively. Continue the test until the client is

ACSM LEG ERGOMETRY EQUATION

To calculate the energy expenditure of a 62-kg (136 lb) woman cycling at a work rate or power output of 360 $kgm \cdot min^{-1}$, follow these steps:

1. Calculate the energy cost of cycling at the specified power output.

$\dot{V}O_2$ = work rate[a] (W)/body mass (M) × 1.8
= 360 $kgm \cdot min^{-1}$/62 kg × 1.8
= 10.45 $ml \cdot kg^{-1} \cdot min^{-1}$

2. Add the estimated cost of cycling at zero load (i.e., 3.5 $ml \cdot kg^{-1} \cdot min^{-1}$).

$\dot{V}O_2$ = 10.45 $ml \cdot kg^{-1} \cdot min^{-1}$ + 3.5 $ml \cdot kg^{-1} \cdot min^{-1}$
= 13.95 $ml \cdot kg^{-1} \cdot min^{-1}$

3. Add the estimated resting energy expenditure (3.5 $ml \cdot kg^{-1} \cdot min^{-1}$).

$\dot{V}O_2$ = 13.95 $ml \cdot kg^{-1} \cdot min^{-1}$ + 3.5 $ml \cdot kg^{-1} \cdot min^{-1}$
= 17.45 $ml \cdot kg^{-1} \cdot min^{-1}$

[a]work rate is in $kgm \cdot min^{-1}$

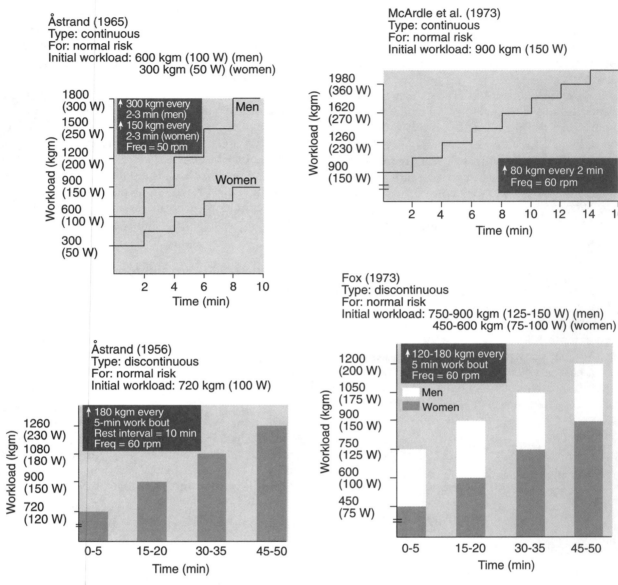

Figure 4.7   Cycle ergometer exercise test protocols.

exhausted or can no longer maintain the pedaling rate of 50 rpm. Use the ACSM metabolic equation for leg ergometry to estimate $\dot{V}O_2$ from your client's power output during the last steady-state stage of the GXT.

Fox Cycle Ergometer Maximal Test Protocol

The Fox (1973) protocol is a discontinuous test consisting of a series of 5-min exercise bouts with 10-min rest intervals. The starting workload is between 750 (125 W) and 900 kgm · min⁻¹ (150 W) for men and 450 (75 W) and 600 kgm · min⁻¹ (100 W) for women. The progressive increments in work depend on the client's HR response and

usually are between 120 and 180 kgm · min⁻¹ (20 and 30 W). The client exercises until exhausted or until no longer able to pedal for at least 3 min at a power output that is 60 to 90 kgm · min⁻¹ (10 to 15 W) higher than the previous workload. You can use the metabolic equations to convert the power output from the last steady-state stage of this protocol to $\dot{V}O_2$max.

Bench Stepping Maximal Exercise Tests

The least desirable mode of exercise for maximum exercise testing is bench stepping. During bench stepping, the individual is performing both positive (up phase) and negative (down phase) work.

Approximately one-quarter to one-third less energy is expended during negative work (Morehouse 1972). This factor, coupled with adjusting the step height and stepping rate for differences in body weight, makes standardization of the work extremely difficult.

General Procedures

Most step test protocols increase the intensity of the work by gradually increasing the height of the bench or stepping rate. The work (W) performed can be calculated using the equation $W = F \times D$, where F is body weight in kilograms and D is bench height times number of steps per minute. For example, a 50-kg woman stepping at a rate of 22 steps/min on a 30-cm (0.30 m) bench is performing $330 \text{ kgm} \cdot \text{min}^{-1}$ of work ($50 \text{ kg} \times 0.30 \text{ m} \times 22 \text{ steps} \cdot \text{min}^{-1}$).

The following equations can be used to adjust the step height and stepping rate for differences in body weight to achieve a given work rate (Morehouse 1972):

step height (cm) = work (kg cm · min⁻¹)/body
weight (kg) × stepping rate

stepping rate = work (kg cm · min⁻¹)
(steps·min⁻¹) ÷ body weight (kg)
              × step height (cm)

For example, if you devise a graded step test protocol that requires a client weighing 60 kg to exercise at a work rate of $300 \text{ kgm} \cdot \text{min}^{-1}$, and the stepping rate is set at 18 steps/min, you need to determine the step height that corresponds to the work rate:

step height = 300 kgm · min⁻¹/60 kg × 18
steps · min⁻¹
= 0.28 m, or 28 cm

Alternatively, you may choose to keep the step height constant and vary the stepping cadence for each stage of the GXT. For example, if the step height is set at 30 cm (0.30 m), and the protocol requires that a client weighing 60 kg exercise at a work rate of $450 \text{ kgm} \cdot \text{min}^{-1}$, you need to calculate the corresponding stepping rate for this client:

stepping rate = 450 kgm · min⁻¹/60 kg × 0.30 m
= 25 steps · min⁻¹

You can calculate the energy expenditure in METs using the ACSM metabolic equation for stepping exercise (see table 4.3). The total gross $\dot{V}O_2$ is a function of step frequency, step height, and the resting energy expenditure. The oxygen cost of the horizontal movement is approximately $0.2 \text{ ml} \cdot \text{kg}^{-1} \cdot \text{m}^1$ for each four-count stepping cycle. The oxygen demand for stepping up is $1.8 \text{ ml} \cdot \text{kg}^{-1} \cdot \text{m}^{-1}$; approximately one-third more must

ACSM STEPPING EQUATION

To calculate the energy expenditure for bench stepping using a 16-in. step height at a cadence of 24 $\text{steps} \cdot \text{min}^{-1}$, use the following procedure:

$\dot{V}O_2$ in ml · kg⁻¹ · min⁻¹ = [frequency (F) in steps · min⁻¹
× 0.2] + (step height in m/step
× F in steps·min⁻¹ × 1.33
× 1.8) + resting VO₂

1. Calculate the $\dot{V}O_2$ for the stepping frequency (F).

   $\dot{V}O_2$ = stepping frequency (F) × 0.20
   = 24 steps · min⁻¹ × 0.20
   = 4.8 ml · kg⁻¹ · min⁻¹

2. Convert the bench height to meters (1 in. = 2.54 cm or 0.0254 m).

   ht = 16 in. × 0.0254 m
   = 0.4064 m

3. Calculate the $\dot{V}O_2$ for the vertical work performed during stepping.

   $\dot{V}O_2$ = bench ht × stepping rate × 1.33 × 1.8
   = 0.4064 m × 24 steps·min⁻¹ × 1.33 × 1.8
   = 23.35 ml · kg⁻¹ · min⁻¹

4. Add resting $\dot{V}O_2$ to the calculated $\dot{V}O_2$ from steps 1 and 3.

   $\dot{V}O_2$ = 4.8 ml · kg⁻¹ · min⁻¹ + 23.35 ml · kg⁻¹ · min⁻¹
   + 3.5 ml · kg⁻¹ · min⁻¹
   = 31.65 ml · kg⁻¹ · min⁻¹

be added (i.e., constant of 1.33 in equation) to account for the oxygen cost of stepping down. For an example of such calculations, see "ACSM Stepping Equation."

Nagle, Balke, and Naughton Maximal Step Test Protocol

Nagle, Balke, and Naughton (1965) devised a graded step test for assessing work capacity. Have your client step at a rate of 30 steps/min on an automatically adjustable bench (2 to 50 cm). Set the initial bench height at 2 cm and increase the height 2 cm every minute of exercise. Use a metronome to establish the stepping cadence (4 beats per stepping cycle). To establish a cadence of 30 steps/min, set the metronome at 120 (30×4). Terminate the test when the subject is fatigued or can no longer maintain the stepping cadence. Use the ACSM metabolic equation for stepping exercise to calculate the energy expenditure ($\dot{V}O_2$max) corresponding to the step height and stepping cadence during the last work stage of this protocol.

SUBMAXIMAL EXERCISE TEST PROTOCOLS

It is desirable to directly determine the functional aerobic capacity of the individual for classifying the cardiorespiratory fitness level and prescribing an aerobic exercise program. However, it is not always practical to do so. The actual measurement of $\dot{V}O_2max$ requires expensive laboratory equipment, a considerable amount of time to administer, and a high level of motivation on the part of the client.

Alternatively, you can use submaximal exercise tests to predict or estimate the $\dot{V}O_2max$ of the individual. Many of these tests are similar to the maximal exercise tests described previously but differ in that they are terminated at some predetermined HR intensity. You will monitor the HR, BP, and RPE during the submaximal exercise test. The treadmill, cycle ergometer, and bench stepping exercises are commonly used for submaximal exercise testing.

Assumptions of Submaximal Exercise Tests

Submaximal exercise tests assume a steady-state HR at each exercise intensity, as well as a linear relationship between HR, oxygen uptake, and work intensity. Although these relationships hold for light-to-moderate workloads, the relationship between oxygen uptake and work becomes curvilinear at heavier workloads.

Another assumption of submaximal testing is that the mechanical efficiency during cycling or treadmill exercise is constant for all individuals. However, a client with poor mechanical efficiency while cycling has a higher submaximal HR at a given workload, and the actual $\dot{V}O_2max$ is underestimated due to this inefficiency (McArdle, Katch, and Katch 1996). As a result, $\dot{V}O_2max$ predicted by submaximal exercise tests tends to be overestimated for highly trained individuals and underestimated for untrained, sedentary individuals.

Submaximal tests also assume that the maximal heart rate (HRmax) for clients of a given age is similar. The HRmax, however, has been shown to vary as much as ± 11 bpm, even after controlling for variability due to age and training status (Londeree and Moeschberger 1984). Also, for submaximal tests, the HRmax is estimated from age. The equation, HRmax = 220 − age, is widely used. The HRmax of approximately 5% to 7% of men and women is more than 15 bpm less than their age-predicted HRmax. On the other hand, 9% to 13% have HRmax values that exceed their age-predicted HRmax by more than 15 bpm (Whaley, Kaminsky, Dwyer, Getchell, and Norton 1992). Because of interindividual variability in HRmax and the potential inaccuracy with use of age-predicted HRmax, there may be considerable error ($\pm 10\%$ to 15%) in estimating your client's $\dot{V}O_2max$, especially when submaximal data are extrapolated to an age-predicted HRmax.

In addition, Tanaka, Monahan, and Seals (2001) noted that the traditional age-predicted HRmax equation (220 − age) overestimates the measured HRmax of younger individuals and increasingly underestimates the actual HRmax of individuals older than 40 yr. Using data from a meta-analysis of 351 studies that included over 18,000 healthy, nonsmoking adults and from a controlled laboratory-based study of 514 healthy adults (18-81 yr), the authors reported that age singly accounts for 80% of the variance in HRmax, independent of gender and physical activity status. They derived the following equation to predict HRmax from age: HRmax = 208 − (0.7 × age). HRmax estimates yielded by this equation differ from those of the traditional equation, particularly in older (>40 yr) adults. For example, the age-predicted HRmax for a 60-year-old client is 166 bpm for the revised equation (208 − 0.7 × 60 = 166 bpm) and 160 bpm for the traditional equation (220 − 60 = 160 bpm).

Because of interindividual variability in HRmax and the potential inaccuracy of age-predicted HRmax equations, the actual HRmax should be measured directly (by ECG or HR monitor) whenever possible. An accurate HRmax is particularly important in situations where

- the exercise test is terminated at a predetermined percentage of either HRmax (% HRmax method) or heart rate reserve [HRR = % (HR_{max} − HR_{rest}) + HR_{rest}],
- your client's $\dot{V}O_2max$ is estimated from submaximal exercise test data that are extrapolated to an age-predicted HRmax, and
- HRmax is used to determine target exercise HRs for aerobic exercise prescriptions (see chapter 5).

Treadmill Submaximal Exercise Tests

Treadmill submaximal tests provide an estimate of functional aerobic capacity ($\dot{V}O_2max$) and assume a linear increase in HR with successive increments in workload. Compared to clients with low cardiorespiratory fitness levels, the well-conditioned individual presumably is able to perform a greater quantity of work at a given submaximal HR.

You can use treadmill maximal test protocols (figure 4.2) to identify the slope of the individual's HR response to exercise. The $\dot{V}O_2$max can be predicted from either one (single-stage model) or two (multistage model) submaximal HRs. Mahar, Jackson, Ross, Pivarnik, and Pollock (1985) reported that the accuracy of the single-stage model is similar to that of the multistage model.

Multistage Model

To estimate $\dot{V}O_2$max with the multistage model, use the HR and workload data from two or more submaximal stages of the treadmill test. Be sure your client reaches steady-state HRs between 115 and 150 bpm (Golding 2000). Determine the slope *(b)* by calculating the ratio of the difference between the two submaximal (SM) workloads (expressed as $\dot{V}O_2$) and the corresponding change in submaximal HRs:

$$b = (SM_2 - SM_1)/(HR_2 - HR_1)$$

Calculate the $\dot{V}O_2$ for each workload using the ACSM metabolic equation (table 4.3), and use the following equation to predict $\dot{V}O_2$max:

$$\dot{V}O_2max = SM_2 + b(HR_{max} - HR_2)$$

If the actual maximal HR is not known, estimate it using the formula 220 – age. See "Protocol: Bruce" for an example that illustrates the use of the multistage model for estimating $\dot{V}O_2$max for a submaximal treadmill test given to a 38-year-old male.

Single-Stage Model

To estimate $\dot{V}O_2$max with the single-stage model, use one submaximal HR and one workload. The steady-state submaximal HR during a single-stage GXT should reach 130 to 150 bpm. "Formulas for Men and Women" have been developed (Shephard 1972).

$SM_{\dot{V}O_2}$ is calculated using the ACSM metabolic equations (see table 4.3). Estimate HR_{max} (if not known) using the formula 220 – age; HR_{SM} is the submaximal HR.

The "Protocol: Balke" example illustrates the use of the single-stage model for estimating $\dot{V}O_2$max for a treadmill submaximal test given to a 45-year-old female.

Protocol: Bruce

Submaximal data:

Stage 2[a]	Stage 1[a]
$\dot{V}O_2$[b] = 24.5 ml · kg^{-1} · min^{-1} (SM$_2$)	16.1 ml · kg^{-1} · min^{-1} (SM$_1$)
HR = 145 bpm (HR$_2$)	130 bpm (HR$_1$)

Maximal HR: 220 – age = 182 bpm

$$\text{Slope } (b) = \frac{(SM_2 - SM_1)}{(HR_2 - HR_1)}$$

$$b = \frac{(24.5 - 16.1)}{(145 - 130)}$$

$$b = \frac{8.4}{15}$$

$$b = 0.56$$

$\dot{V}O_2$**max: SM$_2$ + b(HR$_{max}$ – HR$_2$)**

$$= 24.5 + 0.56(182 - 145)$$
$$= 24.5 + 20.72$$
$$\dot{V}O_2max = 45.22 \text{ ml} \cdot \text{kg}^{-1} \cdot \text{min}^{-1}$$

---

[a]Stages 1 and 2 refer to the last two stages of the GXT completed by the client, and not the first and second stage of the test protocol. For example, if the client completes three stages of the submaximal exercise test protocol, data from stage 2 and stage 3 are used to estimate $\dot{V}O_2$.

[b]$\dot{V}O_2$ is calculated using ACSM metabolic equations (see table 4.3). $\dot{V}O_2$ can be expressed in L · min^{-1}, ml · kg^{-1} · min^{-1}, or METs.

Formulas for Men and Women

Men

$$\dot{V}O_2max = SM_{\dot{V}O_2} \times [(HR_{max} - 61)/(HR_{SM} - 61)]$$

Women

$$\dot{V}O_2max = SM_{\dot{V}O_2} \times [(HR_{max} - 72)/(HR_{SM} - 72)]$$

Protocol: Balke

Submaximal data: Stage 3

$$\dot{V}O_2 = 5.0 \text{ METs } (SM_{\dot{V}O_2})$$
$$HR = 148 \text{ bpm } (HR_{SM})$$

Maximal HR: 220 – age = 175 bpm

$\dot{V}O_2$**max:** $= SM_{\dot{V}O_2} \times [(HR_{max} - 72)/(HR_{SM} - 72)]$
$$= 5 \times [(175 - 72)/(148 - 72)]$$
$$= 5 \times (103/76)$$
$$= 6.8 \text{ METs}$$

Single-Stage Treadmill Walking Test

Ebbeling and colleagues (1991) developed a single-stage treadmill walking test suitable for estimating $\dot{V}O_2$max of low-risk, healthy adults 20 to 59 years of age. For this protocol, walking speed is individualized and ranges from 2.0 to 4.5 mph (53.6 to 120.6 m · min⁻¹) depending on your client's age, gender, and fitness level. Establish a walking pace during a 4-min warm-up at 0% grade. The warm-up work bout should produce a heart rate within 50% to 70% of the individual's age-predicted HRmax. The test consists of brisk walking at the selected pace for an additional 4 min at 5% grade. Record the steady-state HR at this workload, and use it in the following equation to estimate $\dot{V}O_2$max:

$$\dot{V}O_2\text{max} = 15.1 + 21.8(\text{speed in mph})$$
$$(\text{ml} \cdot \text{kg}^{-1} \cdot \text{min}^{-1}) \quad - 0.327(\text{HR in bpm})$$
$$- 0.263(\text{speed} \times \text{age in years})$$
$$+ 0.00504(\text{HR} \times \text{age})$$
$$+ 5.48(\text{gender: female} = 0; \text{male} = 1)$$

Single-Stage Treadmill Walking or Jogging Test

You can also estimate your client's $\dot{V}O_2$max from one 6-min treadmill walk (50% $\dot{V}O_2$max) or run (70% $\dot{V}O_2$max) and steady-state HR from the last 2 min of exercise (Latin and Elias 1993). For the walking protocol, set the treadmill speed at 3.0 mph (80.4 m · min⁻¹) for women and 3.5 mph (93.8 m · min⁻¹) for men, and raise the grade to a level requiring 50% or 60% $\dot{V}O_2$max. For the running protocol, have the client run at a speed requiring about 70% to 80% $\dot{V}O_2$max at 0% grade. Estimate the energy expenditure ($\dot{V}O_2$) of the exercise workload using the ACSM walking or running equation (see table 4.3). Plot the client's energy expenditure in L · min⁻¹ and the steady-state exercise HR in the corresponding columns of the Åstrand-Ryhming nomogram (see figure 4.8). Connect these points with a ruler and read the estimated $\dot{V}O_2$max at the point where the line intersects the $\dot{V}O_2$max column.

Single-Stage Treadmill Jogging Test

You can estimate the $\dot{V}O_2$max of younger adults (18 to 28 years) using a single-stage treadmill jogging test (George, Vehrs, Allsen, Fellingham, and Fisher 1993). For this test, select a comfortable jogging pace ranging from 4.3 to 7.5 mph (115.2 to 201 m · min⁻¹), but not more than 6.5 mph (174.2 m · min⁻¹) for women and 7.5 mph (201 m · min⁻¹) for men. Have the client jog at a constant speed for about 3 min. The steady-state exercise HR should

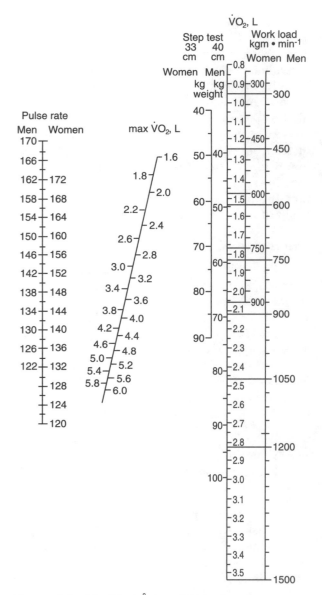

Figure 4.8 Modified Åstrand-Ryhming nomogram.

From "Aerobic Capacity in Men and Women with Special Reference to Age" by I. Åstrand, 1960, *Acta Physiologica Scandinavica* 49 (Suppl. 169), p. 51. Copyright 1960 by *Acta Physiologica Scandinavica*. Reprinted by permission.

not exceed 180 bpm. Estimate $\dot{V}O_2$max using the following equation:

$$\dot{V}O_2\text{max} = 54.07 - 0.1938(\text{BW in kg})$$
$$(\text{ml} \cdot \text{kg}^{-1} \cdot \text{min}^{-1}) \quad + 4.47(\text{speed in mph})$$
$$- 0.1453(\text{HR in bpm})$$
$$+ 7.062(\text{gender: female} = 0; \text{male} = 1)$$

Cycle Ergometer Submaximal Exercise Tests

Cycle ergometer multistage submaximal tests can be used to predict $\dot{V}O_2$max. These tests are either continuous or discontinuous and are based on the assumption that HR and oxygen uptake are linear functions of work rate. The HR response to submaximal workloads is used to predict $\dot{V}O_2$max.

YMCA Cycle Ergometer Submaximal Exercise Test Protocol

The YMCA protocol (Golding 2000) is a cycle ergometer submaximal test for women and men. This protocol uses three or four consecutive 3-min workloads on the cycle ergometer designed to raise the HR to between 110 bpm and 85% of the age-predicted HRmax for at least two consecutive workloads. The pedal rate is 50 rpm, and the initial workload is 150 kgm · min⁻¹ (25 W). Use the HR during the last minute of the initial workload to determine subsequent workloads (see figure 4.9). If the HR is less than 86 bpm, set the second workload at 600 kgm · min⁻¹. If HR is 86 to 100,

the workload is 450 kgm · min⁻¹ for the second stage of the protocol. If the HR at the end of the first workload exceeds 100 bpm, set the second workload at 300 kgm · min⁻¹.

Set the third and fourth workloads accordingly (see figure 4.9). Measure the HR during the last 30 sec of minutes 2 and 3 at each workload. If these HRs differ by more than 5 to 6 bpm, extend the workload an additional minute until the HR stabilizes. If the client's steady-state HR reaches or exceeds 85% of the age-predicted HRmax during the third workload, terminate the test.

Calculate the energy expenditure ($\dot{V}O_2$) for the last two workloads using the ACSM metabolic equations (see table 4.3). To estimate $\dot{V}O_2$max from these data, use the equations for the multistage model to calculate the slope of the line depicting the HR response to the last two workloads. Alternatively, you can graph these data to estimate $\dot{V}O_2$max (see figure 4.10). To do this, plot the $\dot{V}O_2$ for each workload and corresponding HRs. Connect these two data points with a straight edge, extending the line so that it intersects the predicted maximal HR line. To extrapolate $\dot{V}O_2$max, drop a perpendicular line from the point of intersection to the x-axis of the graph. If this is done carefully, the graphing method and multistage method will yield similar estimates of $\dot{V}O_2$max.

Swain Cycle Ergometer Submaximal Exercise Test Protocol

Recently, Swain and colleagues devised a submaximal cycle ergometry protocol for estimating $\dot{V}O_2$ max based on the relationship between heart rate range (HRR) and $\dot{V}O_2$ reserve ($\dot{V}O_2$R) rather than on

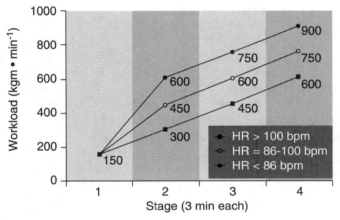

Figure 4.9 YMCA cycle ergometer protocol.

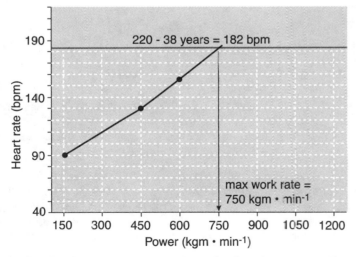

Figure 4.10 Plotting heart rate versus submaximal work rates to estimate maximal work capacity and $\dot{V}O_2$max.

the HR–$\dot{V}O_2$ relationship (Swain, Parrott, Bennett, Branch, and Dowling 2004). This protocol gradually approaches a target HR of 65% to 75% HRR in 1 min stages. This target HR zone is equivalent to 65% to 75% $\dot{V}O_2R$. When the client reaches her target HR, she continues to exercise at that workload for an additional 5 min. The initial work rate and increments in work rate differ depending on the client's body mass and activity level (see figure 4.11). The predictive validity of this test was good $(r = 0.89; SEE = 4.0 \text{ ml} \cdot \text{kg}^{-1} \cdot \text{min}^{-1})$ for estimating the $\dot{V}O_2$max of adults ages 18 to 44. However, more cross-validation studies are needed to determine this test's applicability to older or high-risk clients.

Figure 4.11 illustrates the Swain test protocols for active and inactive clients who weigh < 90 kg or ≥90 kg. To select the appropriate protocol and to calculate your client's estimated $\dot{V}O_2$max, follow the preliminary procedures and general instructions for all clients shown on page 79 (Swain et al. 2004).

Åstrand-Ryhming Cycle Ergometer Submaximal Exercise Test Protocol

The Åstrand-Ryhming protocol (1954) is a single-stage test that uses a nomogram to predict $\dot{V}O_2$max from HR response to one 6-min submaximal workload. A power output is selected that produces a heart rate between 125 and 170 bpm. The initial workload is usually 450 to 600 kgm · min⁻¹ (75 to 100 W) for trained, physically active women and 600 to 900 kgm · min⁻¹ (100 to 150 W) for trained, physically active men. An initial workload of 300 kgm · min⁻¹ (50 W) may be used for unconditioned or older individuals.

During the test, measure the HR every minute and record the average HR during the fifth and sixth minutes. If the difference between these two HRs exceeds 5 to 6 bpm, extend the work bout until a steady-state HR is achieved. If the HR is less than 130 bpm at the end of the exercise bout, increase the workload by 300 kgm · min⁻¹ (50 W) and have the client exercise an additional 6 min.

To estimate $\dot{V}O_2$max for this protocol, use the modified Åstrand-Ryhming nomogram (see figure 4.8). This nomogram estimates $\dot{V}O_2$max (in L · min⁻¹) from submaximal treadmill, cycle

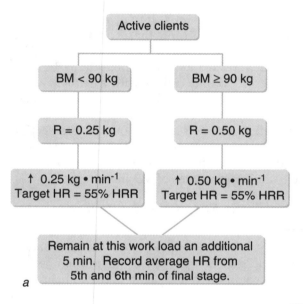

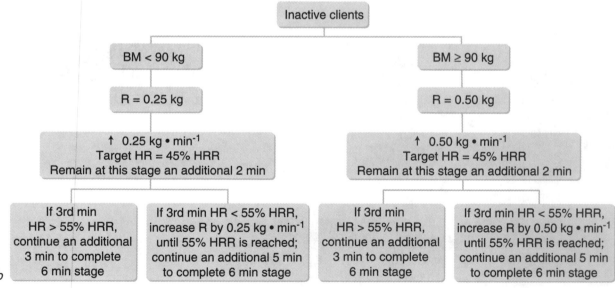

Figure 4.11   Swain cycle ergometer protocol for *(a)* active clients and *(b)* inactive clients.

Preliminary Procedures and General Instructions for Swain Protocol

To select the protocol, follow these steps:

- Measure the body weight and record your client's age.
- Classify your client's activity level as either *active* (>90 min/wk of vigorous activity or >120 min/wk of moderate-intensity exercise) or *inactive* (<90 min/wk of vigorous activity or <120 min/wk of moderate-intensity exercise). Vigorous activities include running, vigorous cycling, or any equivalent; moderate-intensity activities include brisk walking, moderate cycling, or any equivalent.
- Estimate your client's age-predicted HRmax (220 − age). Calculate the target exercise HRs corresponding to 45%, 55%, and 75% HRR (see p. 100 for an example). Target HR = % HRR × (HR_{max} − HR_{rest}) + HR_{rest}.
- Select a protocol based on your client's body weight and activity level. Instruct your client to maintain a 60 rpm pedaling frequency throughout the test.
- Measure exercise HRs during the last 15 sec of each minute of the test. Terminate the test immediately if the target HR corresponding to 75% HRR is exceeded.

To estimate maximum workload and the corresponding $\dot{V}O_2$max from the final 6 min stage of this test use the following steps:

- Calculate the power in watts (W) for the final 6 min workload. $Power_{6-min}$ (W) = resistance (kg) × 60 rpm × 9.81 m/sec².
- Average the 5th and 6th min HRs from the final stage (HR_{6-min}) and calculate the client's age-predicted HRmax using 220 − age.
- Calculate the client's % HRR for the final stage. % HRR = (HR_{6-min} − HR_{rest}) / (HR_{max} − HR_{rest}).
- Estimate the client's maximum workload or power in watts (W) by dividing the power of the final stage, calculated in step 1, by the % HRR calculated in step 3. $Power_{max}$ (W) = $power_{6-min}$ / % HRR.
- Use the ACSM metabolic equation for cycle ergometry to convert maximum power to an estimated $\dot{V}O_2$max. $\dot{V}O_2$max = 7 + [10.8 × $power_{max}$ (W) / body mass in kg].

ergometer, and step test data. For each test mode, the submaximal HR is plotted with either oxygen cost of treadmill exercise ($\dot{V}O_2$ in L·min⁻¹), power output (kgm·min⁻¹) for cycle ergometer exercise, or body weight (kg) for stepping exercise. The correlation between measured $\dot{V}O_2$max and the $\dot{V}O_2$max estimated from this nomogram is r = 0.74. The prediction error is ±10% and ±15%, respectively, for well-trained and untrained individuals (Åstrand and Rodahl 1977). A recent cross-validation study of this protocol and nomogram yielded a validity coefficient of 0.82 and a prediction error of 5.1 ml·kg⁻¹·min⁻¹ for estimating the $\dot{V}O_2$max of adults ages 18 to 44 (Swain et al. 2004).

For clients younger or older than 25 years, you must use the following age-correction factors to adjust the $\dot{V}O_2$max predicted from the nomogram for the effect of age. For example, if the estimated $\dot{V}O_2$max from the nomogram is 3.2 L·min⁻¹ for a 45-year-old client, the adjusted $\dot{V}O_2$max is 2.5 L·min⁻¹ (3.2 × 0.78 = 2.5 L·min⁻¹).

Age-Correction Factors for Åstrand-Ryhming Nomogram

Age	Correction factor
15	1.10
25	1.00
35	0.87
40	0.83
45	0.78
50	0.75
55	0.71
60	0.68
65	0.65

Fox Single-Stage Cycle Ergometer Test Protocol

You can modify the maximal exercise test protocol (see figure 4.7) designed by Fox (1973) to predict $\dot{V}O_2$max ($ml \cdot min^{-1}$). Have your client perform a single workload (i.e., 900 $kgm \cdot min^{-1}$ or 150 W) for 5 min. The standard error of estimate for this test is ± 246 $ml \cdot min^{-1}$, and the standard error of prediction is $\pm 7.8\%$. The correlation between actual and predicted $\dot{V}O_2$max is $r = 0.76$. To estimate $\dot{V}O_2$max, measure the HR at the end of the fifth minute of exercise (HR_5) and use the following equation:

$$\dot{V}O_2\text{max } (ml \cdot min^{-1}) = 6300 - 19.26(HR_5)$$

Bench Stepping Submaximal Exercise Tests

Although there are many step tests available to evaluate cardiorespiratory fitness, few provide equations for predicting $\dot{V}O_2$max. Only step test protocols with prediction equations are included in this section.

Åstrand-Ryhming Step Test Protocol

As mentioned previously, you can use the Åstrand-Ryhming nomogram (see figure 4.8, p. 76) to predict $\dot{V}O_2$max from postexercise HR and body weight during bench stepping. For this protocol, the client steps at a rate of 22.5 steps/min for 5 min. The bench height is 33 cm (13 in.) for women and 40 cm (15.75 in.) for men. Measure the postexercise HR by counting the number of beats between 15 and 30 sec immediately after exercise (convert this 15-sec count to beats per minute by multiplying by 4). Correct the predicted $\dot{V}O_2$max from the nomogram if your client is older or younger than 25 years (using the age-correction factors).

Queens College Step Test Protocol

In a step test to predict $\dot{V}O_2$max devised by McArdle, Katch, Pechar, Jacobson, and Ruck (1972), the client steps at a rate of 22 steps/min (females) or 24 steps/min (males) for 3 min. The bench height is 16.25 in. (41.3 cm). Have your client remain standing after the exercise. Wait 5 sec and then take a 15-sec HR count. Convert the count to beats per minute by multiplying by 4. If you are administering this test simultaneously to more than one client, you should teach your clients how to measure their own pulse rates (see p. 82). To estimate $\dot{V}O_2$max in $ml \cdot kg^{-1} \cdot min^{-1}$, use the equations listed in table 4.7. The standard error of prediction for these equations is $\pm 16\%$.

Additional Modes for Submaximal Exercise Testing

If you are working in the context of a health or fitness club, you may have access to stair climbers and rowing ergometers. You can use some of these exercise machines for submaximal exercise testing of your clients.

Stair-Climbing Submaximal Test Protocols

In light of the popularity of and continued interest in step aerobic training, you may choose to use a simulated stair climbing machine to estimate the aerobic capacity of some clients. The StairMaster 4000 PT and 6000 PT are two step ergometers commonly used in health and fitness settings. The StairMaster 4000 PT has step pedals that go up and down, whereas the 6000 PT model has a revolving staircase. Howley, Colacino, and Swensen (1992) reported that the HR response to increasing submaximal workloads (4.7 and 10 METs) on the StairMaster 4000 PT step ergometer was linear. Also, compared to values with treadmill exercise, the HRs measured during stepping were systematically higher (7 to 11 bpm) at each submaximal intensity. However, the MET values read from the step ergometer were about 20% higher than the measured MET values. To obtain more accurate MET values for each submaximal intensity, use the following equation:

$$\text{actual METs} = 0.556 + 0.745(\text{StairMaster 4000 PT MET value})$$

The StairMaster 4000 PT test protocol, developed by the manufacturer, provides a relatively more accurate estimate of $\dot{V}O_2$max for young women (20-25 yr) who use this device for aerobic training ($r = 0.57$; $SEE = 5.3$ $ml \cdot kg^{-1} \cdot min^{-1}$; $CE = 1.0$ $ml \cdot kg^{-1} \cdot min^{-1}$) as compared to estimates for their untrained counterparts ($r = 0.00$; $SEE = 6.7$ $ml \cdot kg^{-1} \cdot min^{-1}$; $CE = 6.9$ $ml \cdot kg^{-1} \cdot min^{-1}$) (Roy, Smith, Bishop, Hallinan, Wang, and Hunter 2004). This finding illustrates that the exercise testing mode should match the exercise training mode (i.e., application of the specificity principle).

To estimate $\dot{V}O_2$max, measure the steady-state HR and calculate the corrected MET value for each of two submaximal exercise intensities (e.g., 4 and 7 METs). Each stage of the test should last 3 to 6 min in order to produce steady state. Then use either the multistage model formulas (see p. 75) or the graphing method (see figure 4.10) to predict $\dot{V}O_2$max.

TABLE 4.7 Prediction Equations for Cardiorespiratory Field Tests

Field test	Equation[a]	Source
DISTANCE RUN/WALK		
1.0 mile steady-state jog	$\dot{V}O_2max = 100.5 - 0.1636(BW, kg) - 1.438(time, min) - 0.1928(HR, bpm) + 8.344(gender)$[b]	George et al. 1993
1.0 mile run/walk (8-17 years)	$\dot{V}O_2max = 108.94 - 8.41(time, min) + 0.34(time, min)^2 + 0.21(age \times gender)$[b]$ - 0.84(BMI)$[c]	Cureton et al. 1995
1.5 mile run/walk	$\dot{V}O_2max = 88.02 - 0.1656(BW, kg) - 2.76(time, min) + 3.716(gender)$[b]	George et al. 1993
1.5 mile run/walk	$\dot{V}O_2max = 100.16 + 7.30(gender)$[b]$ - 0.164(BW, kg) - 1.273(time, min) - 0.1563(HR, bpm)$	Larsen et al. 2002
12 min run	$\dot{V}O_2max = 0.0268(distance, meters) - 11.3$	Cooper 1968
15 min run	$\dot{V}O_2max = 0.0178(distance, meters) + 9.6$	Balke 1963
1.0 mile walk	$\dot{V}O_2max = 132.853 - 0.0769(BW, lb) - 0.3877(age, years) + 6.315(gender)$[b]$ - 3.2649(time, min) - 0.1565(HR, bpm)$	Kline et al. 1987
STEP TESTS		
Åstrand	Men: $\dot{V}O_2max \ (L \cdot min^{-1}) = 3.744[(BW + 5)/(HR - 62)]$ Women: $\dot{V}O_2max \ (L \cdot min^{-1}) = 3.750[(BW - 3)/(HR - 65)]$	Marley and Linnerud 1976
Queens College	Men: $\dot{V}O_2max = 111.33 - (0.42 \ HR, bpm)$ Women: $\dot{V}O_2max = 65.81 - (0.1847 \ HR, bpm)$	McArdle et al. 1972

[a]All equations estimate $\dot{V}O_2max$ in $ml \cdot kg^{-1} \cdot min^{-1}$ unless otherwise specified.
[b]For gender, substitute 1 for males and 0 for females.
[c]BMI = body mass index or body weight (body weight [BW] in kg)/ht² (in meters).
HR = heart rate.

During the test, clients may hold the handrail lightly for balance but should not support their body weight. If they support their body weight, $\dot{V}O_2max$ will be overestimated (Howley, Colacino, and Swenson 1992). Also, compared to the value with treadmill testing, your client's estimated $\dot{V}O_2max$ may be lower because stair-climbing produces systematically higher HRs at any given submaximal exercise intensity.

Rowing Ergometer Submaximal Test Protocols

Submaximal exercise protocols have been developed for the Concept II rowing ergometer and can be used to estimate your client's $\dot{V}O_2max$. The Hagerman (1993) protocol is designed for noncompetitive or unskilled rowers. Before beginning the test, set the fan blades in the fully closed position and select the small axle sprocket. For this test, select a submaximal exercise intensity (the HR should not exceed 170 bpm) that the client can sustain for 5 to 10 min. Measure the exercise HR at the end of each minute. Continue the rowing exercise until the client achieves a steady-state HR. Use the Hagerman (1993) nomogram (see figure 4.12) to estimate $\dot{V}O_2max$ from the submaximal power output (watts) and the steady-state HR during the last minute of exercise.

FIELD TESTS FOR ASSESSING AEROBIC FITNESS

The maximal and submaximal exercise tests using the treadmill or cycle ergometer are not well suited for measuring the cardiorespiratory fitness of large groups in a field situation. Thus, a number of performance tests such as distance runs have been devised to predict $\dot{V}O_2max$ (see table 4.7). These tests are practical, inexpensive, less time consuming than the treadmill or cycle ergometer tests, easy to administer to large groups, and suitable for personal training settings; they

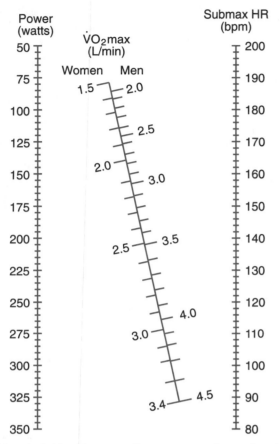

Figure 4.12 Concept II nomogram for estimating $\dot{V}O_2$max in noncompetitive and unskilled male and female rowers.

From "Concept II Rowing Ergometer Nomogram for Prediction of Maximal Oxygen Consumption" by Dr. Fritz Hagerman, Ohio University, Athens, OH. The nomogram is not appropriate for use with non-Concept II ergometers and is designed to be used by noncompetitive or unskilled rowers participating in aerobic conditioning programs. Adapted by permission of CONCEPT II, INC. RR1, Box 1100, Morrisville, VT, (800) 245-5676.

can be used to classify the cardiorespiratory fitness level of healthy men (≤45 years) and women ≤55 years). You cannot use field tests to detect CHD because HR, ECG, and BP are usually not monitored during the performance. Most field tests used to assess cardiorespiratory endurance involve walking, running, swimming, cycling, or bench stepping; they require that clients be able to accurately measure their postexercise HR. Pollock, Broida, and Kendrick (1972) found that with practice, men could learn to measure their own pulse rates accurately. The correlation between manual and electronic measurements of pulse rate ranged between $r = 0.91$ and 0.94. Similar results ($r = 0.95$) were reported for college women for pulse rates measured manually and electronically (Witten 1973). Prior to administering field tests that require the measurement of HR, you should

teach your clients how to measure their pulse rates using the palpation technique described in "How to Measure Your Pulse Rate."

Distance Run Tests

The most commonly used distance runs involve running distances of 1.0 or 1.5 miles (1600 to 2400 m) to evaluate aerobic capacity. Distance run tests are based on the assumption that the more fit individual will be able to run a given distance in less time or to run a greater distance in a given period of time. Using factor analysis, Disch, Frankiewicz, and Jackson (1975) noted that runs greater than 1.0 mile tended to load exclusively on the endurance factor rather than the speed factor.

You should be aware that the relationship between distance runs and $\dot{V}O_2$max has not been firmly established. Although performance on a distance run can be accurately measured, it may not be an accurate index of $\dot{V}O_2$max or a substitute for the direct measurement of $\dot{V}O_2$max. Endurance running performance may be influenced by other factors such as motivation, percent fat (Cureton, Sparling, Evans, Johnson, Kong, and Purvis 1978; Katch, McArdle, Czula, and Pechar 1973), running efficiency (pacing ability), and lactate threshold

---

HOW TO MEASURE YOUR PULSE RATE

1. Use your middle and index fingers to locate the radial pulse on the outside of your wrist just below the base of your thumb. Do not use your thumb to feel the pulse because it has a pulse of its own and may produce an inaccurate count.

2. If you cannot feel the radial pulse, try locating the carotid pulse by placing your fingers lightly on the front of your neck, just to the side of your voice box. Do not apply heavy pressure because this will cause your HR to slow down.

3. Use a stopwatch or the second hand of your wristwatch and count the number of pulse beats for a 6-, 10-, or 15-sec period.

4. Convert the pulse count to beats per minute using the following multipliers: 6-sec count times 10, 10-sec count times 6, and 15-sec count times 4.

5. Remember this value and record it on your scorecard.

(Costill and Fox 1969; Costill, Thomason, and Roberts 1973).

The correlations between distance run tests and $\dot{V}O_2$max tend to vary considerably (r = 0.27 to 0.90) depending on the subjects, sample size, and testing procedures (George et al. 1993; Rikli, Petray, and Baumgartner 1992; Zwiren, Freedson, Ward, Wilke, and Rippe 1991). Generally, the longer the run, the higher the correlation with $\dot{V}O_2$max. On the basis of this observation, it is recommended that you select a test with a distance of at least 1.0 mile (1600 m) or a duration of at least 9 min.

The most widely used distance run tests are the 9 and 12 min runs and the 1.0 and 1.5 mile runs. Some physical fitness test batteries for children and adolescents recommend using either the 9-min or 1.0-mile run tests.

9 or 12 Min Run Tests

To administer the 9 or 12 min run test, use a 400-m track or flat course with measured distances so that the number of laps completed can be easily counted and multiplied by the course distance. Place markers to divide the course into quarters or eighths of a mile so that you can quickly determine the exact distance covered in 9 or 12 min. Instruct your clients to run as far as possible. Walking is allowed, but the objective of these tests is to cover as much distance as possible in either 9 or 12 min. At the end of the test, calculate the total distance covered in meters and use the appropriate equation in table 4.7 to estimate the client's $\dot{V}O_2$max.

1.5 Mile Run/Walk Test

The 1.5 mile run/walk test is conducted on a 400-m track or flat measured area. To measure the course, use an odometer or measuring wheel. For the 1.5 mile run, instruct your clients to cover the specified distance in the fastest possible time. Walking is allowed, but the objective is to cover the distance in the shortest possible time while maintaining a steady exercise pace. Call out the elapsed time (in minutes and seconds) as the client crosses the finish line. You can use a HR monitor to ensure that your client maintains a steady exercise pace during this test. Instruct your clients to keep their target HR between 60% and 90% HRmax. The exercise HR at the end of the test, along with gender, body mass, and elapsed exercise time, can be substituted into the Larsen equation (see table 4.7) to estimate the $\dot{V}O_2$max of young (18-29 yr) adults (Larsen, George, Alexander, Fellingham, Aldana, and Parcell 2002). Cross-validation of this equation yielded a high validity coefficient (r = 0.89) and

small prediction errors (SEE = 2.5 ml·kg⁻¹·min⁻¹; TE = 2.68 ml·kg⁻¹·min⁻¹) for a sample of young military personnel (Taylor, George, Allsen, Vehrs, Hager, and Roberts 2002).

To use the $\dot{V}O_2$max prediction equations for the 1.5 mile run/walk test (see table 4.7), convert the seconds to minutes by dividing the seconds by 60. For example, if a client's time for the test is 12:30, the exercise time is converted to 12.5 min (30/60 sec = 0.5 min).

1.0 Mile Jogging Test

One limitation of distance run tests is that individuals are encouraged to run as fast as possible and give a maximal effort, thereby increasing the risk of cardiovascular and orthopedic injuries. The potential risk is even greater for untrained individuals who do not run or jog regularly and have difficulty selecting a proper jogging pace. To address this problem, George et al. (1993) developed a submaximal 1-mile track jogging test for 18- to 29-year-old women and men that requires only moderate, steady-state exertion.

For this test, instruct your clients to select a comfortable, moderate jogging pace and to measure their postexercise HR immediately following the test. The elapsed time for 1 mile should be at least 8 min for males and 9 min for females, and the postexercise HR (15-sec count × 4) should not exceed 180 bpm. To help establish a suitable pace, precede the timed 1-mile test with a 2- to 3-min warm-up. Use either an indoor or outdoor track for this test. Record the time required to jog 1 mile in minutes, and have your clients measure their postexercise HRs using the palpation technique (radial or carotid sites). Estimate the client's $\dot{V}O_2$max using the prediction equation for the 1.0-mile steady-state jog test (see table 4.7).

Walking Test

The Rockport Walking Institute (1986) has developed a walking test to assess cardiorespiratory fitness for men and women ages 20 to 69 years. Because this test requires only fast walking, it is useful for testing older or sedentary individuals (Fenstermaker, Plowman, and Looney 1992). The test was developed and validated for a large, heterogeneous sample of 86 women and 83 men (Kline et al. 1987). The cross-validation analysis resulted in a high validity coefficient and small standard error of estimate (SEE), indicating that the 1.0-mile walking test yields a valid submaximal assessment of estimated $\dot{V}O_2$max. Other researchers have substantiated the predictive accuracy of this equation for women 65 years of age and older (Fenstermaker et al. 1992).

To administer this test, instruct your clients to walk 1.0 mile as quickly as possible and to take their HR immediately at the end of the test by counting the pulse for 15 sec. It is important that clients know how to take their pulse accurately. The walking course should be a measured mile that is flat and uninterrupted, preferably a 400-m track. Clients should stretch for 5 to 10 min before the test and wear good walking shoes and loose-fitting clothes.

To estimate your client's $\dot{V}O_2max$, use the generalized equation for the 1.0-mile walking test (see table 4.7). Alternatively, you can use the Rockport relative fitness charts (appendix B.2, p. 310) to classify your client's cardiorespiratory fitness level. Locate the walking time and corresponding postexercise HR (bpm) on the appropriate chart for the individual's age and gender. These charts are based on body weights of 125 lb for women and 170 lb for men. If the client weighs substantially more than this, the cardiorespiratory fitness level will be overestimated.

Step Tests

The major advantage of using step tests to assess cardiorespiratory fitness is that they can be administered to large groups in a field situation without requiring expensive equipment or highly trained personnel. Most of these step tests use postexercise and recovery HRs to evaluate aerobic fitness, but they do not provide an estimate of the individual's $\dot{V}O_2max$. Step test protocols and scoring procedures are described in appendix B.3, "Step Test Protocols," page 312.

The validity of step tests is highly dependent on the accurate measurement of pulse rate. Step tests that use recovery HR tend to possess lower validity than those using the time required for the HR to reach a specified level during performance of a standardized workload (Baumgartner and Jackson 1975). The correlation coefficients between step test performance and $\dot{V}O_2max$ range between $r = 0.32$ and 0.77 (Cureton and Sterling 1964; deVries and Klafs 1965; McArdle et al. 1972).

Additional Field Tests

In addition to running, walking, and step tests, cycling and swimming tests have been devised for use in field situations (Cooper 1977). The 12-min cycling test, using a bike with no more than three speeds, is conducted on a hard, flat surface when the wind velocity is less than 10 mph (268 m · min^{-1}). These conditions limit the effect of outside influences on the rider's performance. Five- and ten-speed bikes are not employed unless use of the lower gears can be restricted. Use an odometer to measure the distance traveled in 12 min. In the 12-min swimming test, the client may use any stroke and rest as needed. Norms for the 12-min cycling test and 12-min swimming test are available (Cooper 1977).

Of these two tests, the swimming test is the less preferred because the outcome is highly skill dependent. For example, a skilled swimmer with an average cardiorespiratory fitness level will probably be able to swim farther in 12 min than a poorly skilled swimmer with an above-average cardiorespiratory fitness level. In fact, Conley and colleagues (1991, 1992) reported that the 12-min swim has low validity ($r = 0.34$ to 0.42) as a cardiorespiratory field test for male and female recreational swimmers. Whenever possible, select an alternative field test and avoid using the 12-min swim test.

EXERCISE TESTING FOR CHILDREN AND OLDER ADULTS

You may need to modify the generic guidelines for exercise testing (see "General Principles of Exercise Testing," p. 61) of low-risk adults when you are assessing cardiorespiratory fitness of children and older adults. You must take into account growth, maturation, and aging when selecting exercise testing modes and protocols for these groups.

Assessing Cardiorespiratory Fitness of Children

In the laboratory setting, you can assess the cardiorespiratory fitness of children using either the treadmill or cycle ergometer. Treadmill testing is usually preferable, especially for younger children, because their shortened attention span may not allow them to maintain a constant pedaling rate during a cycle ergometer test. Also, children younger than 8 years or shorter than 50 in. (127 cm) may not be tall enough to use a standard cycle ergometer. To accommodate children, modify the seat height, pedal crank length, and handlebar position.

For treadmill testing, you may choose to use the modified Balke protocol (see table 4.8) because the speed is constant and the intensity is increased by changing the grade. The ACSM (2006) recommends using either the modified Balke protocol or the modified Bruce protocol (i.e., 2 min instead of 3 min stages). Age and gender endurance time norms for children (4-18 yr) for the modified Bruce protocol are available elsewhere (Wessel, Strasburger, and Mitchell 2001). For cycle ergometer testing, you can use the McMaster protocol (see table 4.8). For this protocol, the pedaling frequency is 50 rpm, and increments in work rate are based on the child's height.

Field tests, such as the 1.0-mile (1600 m) run/walk, are widely used to assess the cardiorespiratory fitness of children 5 to 17 years of age. These tests are part of the Physical Best Program (American Alliance for Health, Physical Education, Recreation and Dance 1988), Fitnessgram (Cooper Institute for Aerobics Research 1994), and the President's Challenge Test (President's Council on Physical Fitness and Sports 1997), as well as national physical fitness surveys of children and youth (Ross and Pate 1987). To estimate $\dot{V}O_2$peak of 8- to 17-year-olds for the 1.0-mile run/walk test, you can use a generalized prediction equation (see table 4.7) (Cureton, Sloniger, O'Bannon, Black, and McCormack 1995). For younger children (5 to 7 years of age), the 0.5-mile run/walk test is recommended (Rikli, Petray, and Baumgartner 1992). Criterion-referenced standards for the 1.0-mile test are available elsewhere (American Alliance for Health, Physical Education, Recreation and Dance 1988; Cooper Institute for Aerobics Research 1994).

In Canada and Europe, the multistage 20-meter shuttle run test, developed by Leger and colleagues (1982, 1988), is a popular alternative to distance running/walking field tests to estimate the aerobic fitness of children (8-19 yr) in educational settings. This test has been cross-validated using other samples of European and Canadian children (Anderson 1992; vanMechelen, Holbil, and Kemper 1986).

For this test, children run back and forth continuously on a 20-meter (indoor or outdoor) course. The running speed is set using a sound signal emitted from a prerecorded tape. The starting pace is 8.5 km · hr^{-1} and the speed is increased 0.5 km · hr^{-1} each minute until they can no longer maintain the pace. The maximal aerobic speed at this stage is used, in combination with age, in the following equation to estimate $\dot{V}O_2$max:

TABLE 4.8 Graded Exercise Test Protocols for Children (Skinner 1993)

MODIFIED BALKE TREADMILL PROTOCOL

Activity classification	Speed (mph)	Initial grade (%)	Increment (%)	Duration (min)
Poorly fit	3.0	6	2	2
Sedentary	3.25	6	2	2
Active	5.0	0	2.5	2
Athletes	5.25	0	2.5	2

MCMASTER CYCLE ERGOMETER PROTOCOL

Height (cm)	Initial work rate: kgm · min^{-1} (watts)	Increments: kgm · min^{-1} (watts)	Duration (min)
<120	75 (12.5)	75 (12.5)	2
120-139.9	75 (12.5)	150 (25)	2
140-159.9	150 (25)	150 (25)	2
≥160	150 (25)	300 (50) for boys 150 (25) for girls	2

$$\dot{V}O_2max = 31.025 + 3.238(\text{speed, km} \cdot \text{hr}^{-1})$$
$$(\text{ml} \cdot \text{kg}^{-1} \cdot \text{min}^{-1}) \quad -3.248(\text{age, yr})$$
$$+ 0.1536(\text{age} \times \text{speed})$$

Assessing Cardiorespiratory Fitness of Older Adults

To assess the cardiorespiratory fitness of elderly clients, you can use modified treadmill and cycle ergometer protocols. The following modifications for standard GXT protocols are recommended:

- Extend the warm-up to more than 3 min.
- Set an initial exercise intensity of 2 to 3 METs; work increments should be 0.5 to 1.0 MET (e.g., Naughton treadmill protocol; see table 4.4, p. 68).
- Adjust (reduce) the treadmill speed to the walking ability of your client when needed.
- Extend the duration of each work stage (at least 3 min), allowing enough time for the client to attain steady state.
- Select a protocol likely to produce a total test time of 8 to 12 min.

Select treadmill protocols that increase grade, instead of speed, especially for older clients with poor ambulation. You can modify the standard Balke protocol (see figure 4.2) by having the client walk at 0% grade and 3.0 mph or slower initially and by increasing the duration of each stage to at least 3 min. If elderly clients are more comfortable holding on to the handrails during a treadmill test, you can use the standard Bruce protocol and the McConnell and Clark (1987) prediction equation to estimate their $\dot{V}O_2max$ (see table 4.5). Alternatively, you could use cycle ergometer GXTs for older individuals with poor balance, poor neuromuscular coordination, or impaired vision. You can also use field tests to estimate the cardiorespiratory fitness of your older (60-94 yr) clients. The Senior Fitness Test Battery (Rikli and Jones 2001) includes two measures of aerobic endurance: the 6 min walking test and the 2 min step test.

6 Min Walking Test

Purpose: Assess aerobic endurance.
Application: Measure ability to perform activities of daily living such as walking, stair-climbing, shopping, and sightseeing.
Equipment: You will need a 5 × 20 yd (4.6 × 18.3 m) rectangular walking area, a measuring tape, a stopwatch, four cones, masking tape, index cards, and chairs.
Test Procedures: Use masking tape or chalk to mark 5 yd (4.6 m) lines on a flat, rectangular course. Place cones on the inside corners of the rectangle. Instruct participants to walk (not jog) as fast as possible around the course for 6 min. Partners can keep track of the total number of laps and distance covered by marking the index card each time a lap is completed. Administer one trial; measure total distance to the nearest 5 yd (4.6 m). Test two or more people at a time for motivation.
Scoring: Calculate the total distance covered in 6 min. Each mark on the index card represents 50 yd (45.6 m). Use table 4.9 to determine a client's percentile ranking.
Safety Tips: Place chairs around the outside of the walking course in case a client needs to sit and rest during the test. Select a well-lit, level walking area with a nonslip surface. Discontinue the test if the client shows signs of overexertion. Have the client cool down by stepping in place for 1 min.
Validity and Reliability: The 6 min walking distance was positively related (r = 0.78) to submaximal treadmill walking time (Bruce protocol, time to reach 85% HRmax). This walking test detects the expected performance declines across age groups and discriminates between individuals with high and low physical activity levels and functional ability test scores. The test–retest reliability was r = 0.94.

2 Min Step Test

Purpose: Alternative test of aerobic endurance when time, space, or weather prohibits administering the 6 min walking test.
Application: Measure ability to perform activities of daily living such as walking, stair-climbing, shopping, and sightseeing.
Equipment: You will need a stopwatch, a tape measure, masking tape, and a tally counter to count steps.
Test Procedures: Determine the minimum knee-stepping height of the client by identifying the midpoint between the knee cap (midpatellar level) and iliac crest. Mark this point on the anterior aspect of the client's thigh and on a nearby wall or chair. These marks are used to monitor knee height during the test. Ask the client to step in place for 2 min, lifting the right knee as high as the target level marked on the wall. Use the tally counter to

TABLE 4.9   6 Min Walking Test Norms for Older Adults[a]

Percentile rank	60-64 yr		65-69 yr		70-74 yr		75-79 yr		80-84 yr		85-89 yr		90-94 yr	
	F	M	F	M	F	M	F	M	F	M	F	M	F	M
95	741	825	734	800	709	779	696	762	654	721	638	710	564	646
90	711	792	697	763	673	743	655	716	612	678	591	659	518	592
85	690	770	673	738	650	718	628	686	584	649	560	625	488	557
80	674	751	653	718	630	698	605	661	560	625	534	596	463	527
75	659	736	636	700	614	680	585	639	540	604	512	572	441	502
70	647	722	621	685	599	665	568	621	523	586	493	551	423	480
65	636	710	607	671	586	652	553	604	508	571	476	532	406	461
60	624	697	593	657	572	638	538	586	491	554	458	512	388	440
55	614	686	581	644	561	625	524	571	477	540	443	495	373	422
50	603	674	568	631	548	612	509	555	462	524	426	477	357	403
45	592	662	555	618	535	599	494	539	447	508	409	459	341	384
40	582	651	543	605	524	586	480	524	433	494	394	442	326	366
35	570	638	529	591	510	572	465	506	416	477	376	422	308	345
30	559	626	515	577	497	559	450	489	401	462	359	403	291	326
25	547	612	500	562	482	544	433	471	384	444	340	382	273	304
20	532	597	483	544	466	526	413	449	364	423	318	358	251	279
15	516	578	463	524	446	506	390	424	340	399	292	329	226	249
10	495	556	439	499	423	481	363	394	312	370	261	295	196	214
5	465	523	402	462	387	445	322	348	270	327	214	244	150	160

F = females; M = males.

[a]Values represent distance in yards; to convert yards to meters multiply by 0.91.

Adapted, by permission, from R. Rikli and C. Jones, 2001, *Senior fitness test manual* (Champaign, IL: Human Kinetics).

count the number of times the right knee reaches the target level. If the proper knee height cannot be maintained, ask the client to slow down or stop until he can execute proper form; keep the stopwatch running. Administer one trial.

Scoring: Count the times that the right knee reaches the target level in 2 min. Use table 4.10 to determine your client's percentile ranking.

Safety Tips: Clients with poor balance should stand close to a wall, doorway, or chair for support in case they lose their balance during the test. Spot each client carefully. Have the client cool down after the test by walking slowly for 1 min. Discontinue the test if your client shows signs of overexertion.

Validity and Reliability: The 2 min step test scores were moderately correlated (r = 0.73 - 0.74) with Rockport 1 mi walking scores and treadmill walking (Bruce protocol, time to reach 85% HRmax) in older adults. This step test detected expected performance declines across age groups and discriminated between exercisers and nonexercisers. The test–retest reliability was r = 0.90.

TABLE 4.10   2 Min Step Test Norms for Older Adults[a]

Percentile rank	60-64 yr		65-69 yr		70-74 yr		75-79 yr		80-84 yr		85-89 yr		90-94 yr	
	F	M	F	M	F	M	F	M	F	M	F	M	F	M
95	130	135	133	139	125	133	123	135	113	126	106	114	92	112
90	122	128	123	130	116	124	115	126	104	118	98	106	85	102
85	116	123	117	125	110	119	109	119	99	112	93	100	80	96
80	111	119	112	120	105	114	104	114	94	107	88	95	76	91
75	107	115	107	116	101	110	100	109	90	103	85	91	72	86
70	103	112	104	113	97	107	96	105	87	99	81	87	69	83
65	100	109	100	110	94	104	93	102	84	96	79	84	66	79
60	97	106	96	107	90	101	90	98	81	93	76	81	63	76
55	94	104	93	104	87	98	87	95	78	90	73	78	61	72
50	91	101	90	101	84	95	84	91	75	87	70	75	58	69
45	88	98	87	98	81	92	81	87	72	84	67	72	55	66
40	85	96	84	95	78	89	78	84	69	81	64	69	53	62
35	82	93	80	92	74	86	75	80	66	78	61	66	50	59
30	79	90	76	89	71	83	72	77	63	75	59	63	47	55
25	75	87	73	86	68	80	68	73	60	71	55	59	44	52
20	71	83	68	82	63	76	64	68	56	67	52	55	40	47
15	66	79	63	77	58	71	59	63	51	62	47	50	36	42
10	60	74	57	72	52	66	53	56	46	56	42	44	31	36
5	52	67	47	67	43	67	45	47	37	48	39	36	24	26

F = females; M = males.

[a]Values represent number of times right knee reaches target level.

Adapted, by permission, from R. Rikli and C. Jones, 2001, *Senior fitness test manual* (Champaign, IL: Human Kinetics).

Sources for Equipment

Product	Supplier's address
Cycle ergometer (Lode electronically braked)	Physio-Dyne Instrument Corporation 1095 Broadhollow Rd. Farmingdale, NY 11735 (800) 860-5930 www.physio-dyne.com
Cycle ergometer (Monark)	Monark 948 Greenbay Rd. Winnetka, IL 60093 (800) 359-4609 www.monarkbikes.com

Product	Supplier's address
Cycle ergometer (Bodyguard, Tunturi, Schwinn)	U.S. Fitness Products 3072 Wake Forest Rd. Raleigh, NC 27609 (888) 761-1638 www.usafitness.com
Elliptical trainers	Life Fitness 10601 W. Belmont Ave. Franklin Park, IL 60131 (800) 735-3867 www.lifefitness.com Precor 20031 142nd Ave. NE Woodinville, WA 98072-4002 (800) 786-8404 www.precor.com
Nordic ski machine	Nordic Track 104 Peavey Rd. Chaska, MN 55138 (800) 220-1256 www.nordictrack.com
Rowing ergometer	Concept 2, Inc. 105 Industrial Park Dr. Morrisville, VT 05661 (800) 245-5676 www.concept2.com
Stair climbing machines	StairMaster Sales and Service 1400 NE 136th Ave. Vancouver, WA 98684 (800) 782-4799 www.nautilus.com
Treadmill (Quinton)	Quinton Instrument Co. 3303 Monte Villa Pkwy. Bothell, WA 98021 (800) 426-0337 www.quinton.com

KEY POINTS

- The best way to assess aerobic capacity (cardiorespiratory fitness) is through a GXT in which the functional $\dot{V}O_2max$ is measured.

- Unless contraindications to exercise are observed, you should administer a maximal exercise test to moderate-risk men (≥ 45 years) and women (≥ 55 years) before they begin a vigorous exercise program.

- Before, during, and after a maximal or submaximal exercise test, closely monitor the HR, BP, and RPE.

- Treadmill, cycle ergometer, and bench stepping are the most commonly used modes of exercise for exercise testing.

- The choice of exercise mode and exercise test protocol depends on the age, gender, purpose of the test, and the health and fitness status of the individual.

- Submaximal exercise tests are used to estimate the functional aerobic capacity by predicting the $\dot{V}O_2max$ of the individual. Failure to meet the assumptions underlying submaximal exercise tests produces a $\pm 10\%$ to 20% error in the prediction of $\dot{V}O_2$max from submaximal HR data.

- Field tests are the least desirable way of assessing aerobic capacity and should not be used for diagnostic purposes. However, field tests are useful for assessing the cardiorespiratory fitness of large groups.
- Commonly used field tests include distance runs, walking tests, and step tests.
- Distance runs should last at least 9 min to assess aerobic function. Distance runs usually range between 1 and 2 miles (1600 to 3200 m) or 9 to 12 min.

- The validity of step tests for assessing cardiorespiratory fitness is highly dependent on the accurate measurement of HR and is usually somewhat lower than the validity of distance run tests.
- For children and older adults, select a treadmill protocol that increases grade rather than speed.
- The 6 min walking test or 2 min step test can be used to assess cardiorespiratory fitness of older adults in field settings.

KEY TERMS

Learn the definition for each of the following key terms. Definitions of key terms can be found in the glossary on page 379.

absolute $\dot{V}O_2$
cardiorespiratory endurance
continuous exercise test
discontinuous exercise test
graded exercise test (GXT)
gross $\dot{V}O_2$
maximal exercise test
maximum oxygen uptake ($\dot{V}O_2$max)

net $\dot{V}O_2$
ramp protocols
rating of perceived exertion (RPE)
relative $\dot{V}O_2$max
respiratory exchange ratio (RER)
submaximal exercise test
$\dot{V}O_2$max
$\dot{V}O_2$peak

REVIEW QUESTIONS

In addition to being able to define each of the key terms listed, test your knowledge and understanding of the material by answering the following review questions.

1. What is the most valid and direct measure of functional aerobic capacity?
2. What is the difference between absolute and relative $\dot{V}O_2$?
3. What is the difference between gross and net $\dot{V}O_2$?
4. What is the difference between $\dot{V}O_2$max and $\dot{V}O_2$peak?
5. What factors should you consider when choosing a maximal or submaximal exercise test protocol for your client?

6. Identify the ACSM criteria for attainment of $\dot{V}O_2$max during a GXT.
7. During a GXT, what three variables are monitored at regular intervals?
8. List three reasons for stopping a GXT.
9. What is active recovery, and why is it recommended for graded exercise testing?
10. What is the difference between continuous, discontinuous, and ramp exercise testing protocols?

11. Calculate the gross $\dot{V}O_2$ for a 60-kg woman running on a treadmill at a speed of 6.0 mph and a grade of 10%.

12. Calculate the gross $\dot{V}O_2$ for an 80-kg man cycling on Monark cycle ergometer at a pedaling frequency of 70 rpm and a resistance of 3.5 kg.

13. Calculate the energy expenditure for bench stepping using an 8-in. step and a cadence of 30 steps/min.

14. Name three types of field tests for estimating aerobic capacity.

15. Which type of testing, treadmill or cycle ergometer, should be used for assessing the cardiorespiratory fitness of children?

16. How should standard GXT protocols be modified for testing of older adults?

chapter 5

Designing Cardiorespiratory Exercise Programs

Key Questions

- What are the basic components of an aerobic exercise prescription?
- How is the aerobic exercise prescription individualized to meet each client's goals and interests?
- What methods are used to prescribe and monitor exercise intensity?
- Which exercise modes are best suited for an aerobic exercise prescription?
- How often does a client need to exercise to improve and maintain aerobic fitness?
- How long does a client need to exercise to improve aerobic fitness?
- Is discontinuous aerobic training as effective as continuous training?
- How effective are multimodal, cross-training programs?
- What are the physiological benefits of aerobic exercise training?

Once you have assessed an individual's cardiorespiratory fitness status, you are responsible for planning an aerobic exercise program to develop and maintain the cardiorespiratory endurance of that program participant—a program designed to meet the individual's needs and interests, taking into account age, gender, physical fitness level, and exercise habits. Appendix A.5, "Lifestyle Evaluation," page 288, provides forms that will help you determine your clients' exercise patterns and preferences.

In designing the exercise prescription, keep in mind that some people engage in aerobic exercise to improve their health status or reduce their disease risk, while others are primarily interested in enhancing their physical fitness (VO_2max) levels. Given that the quantity of exercise needed to promote health is less than that needed to develop and maintain higher levels of physical fitness, you must adjust the exercise prescription according to your client's primary goal.

This chapter provides guidelines for writing individualized exercise prescriptions that promote health status as well as develop and maintain cardiorespiratory fitness. The chapter compares various training methods and aerobic exercise modes, and presents examples of individualized exercise programs.

THE EXERCISE PRESCRIPTION

It is important to consider your client's goals and purposes for engaging in an exercise program. The primary goal for exercising may affect the mode, intensity, frequency, duration, and progression of the exercise prescription. For example, the quantity of physical activity needed to achieve health benefits or reduce one's risk of illness and death is less than the amount of activity typically prescribed when the client's goal is to make substantial improvements in cardiorespiratory fitness. When the primary goal for the exercise prescription is improved health, refer to "Guidelines for Exercise Prescription for Improved Health," on page 94.

On the other hand, when the primary goal for the exercise prescription is to improve cardiorespiratory fitness, refer to "ACSM Guidelines for Exercise Prescription for Cardiorespiratory Fitness," below.

Elements of a Cardiorespiratory Exercise Workout

Each exercise workout of the aerobic exercise prescription and program should include the following phases:

- Warm-up
- Endurance conditioning
- Cool-down

The purpose of the warm-up is to increase blood flow to the working cardiac and skeletal muscles, increase body temperature, decrease the chance of muscle and joint injury, and lessen the chance of abnormal cardiac rhythms. During the warm-up, the tempo of the exercise is gradually increased to prepare the body for a higher intensity of exercise performed during the conditioning phase. The warm-up starts with 5 to 10 min of low-intensity (10%-30% $\dot{V}O_2R$) aerobic activity (e.g., brisk walking for clients who jog during their endurance conditioning phase). This is usually followed by 5 to 10 min of static stretching exercises for the legs, lower back, abdomen, hips, groin, and shoulders (for specific exercises, see appendix F.1, "Selected Flexibility Exercises," p. 357).

During the endurance conditioning phase of the workout, the aerobic exercise is performed according to the exercise prescription. This phase usually lasts 20 to 60 min, depending on the exercise intensity, and is followed immediately by the cool-down phase.

GUIDELINES FOR EXERCISE PRESCRIPTION FOR IMPROVED HEALTH

The following guidelines are from the U.S. Department of Health and Human Services (1996).

1. Mode: Select endurance-type physical activities, including formal aerobic exercise training, housework and yard work, and physically active recreational pursuits.

2. Intensity: Prescribe at least moderate-intensity physical activities ($\geq$45% $\dot{V}O_2$max).

3. Frequency: Schedule physical activity for most, preferably all, days of the week.

4. Duration: Accumulate at least 30 min of moderate activity each day. Duration varies according to the type and intensity of activity (see "Examples of Moderate Amounts of Physical Activity," chapter 1, p. 4).

ACSM GUIDELINES FOR EXERCISE PRESCRIPTION FOR CARDIORESPIRATORY FITNESS

These are the ACSM 2006 guidelines:

1. Mode: Select rhythmical aerobic activities that can be maintained continuously and that involve large muscle groups (see "Classification of Aerobic Exercise Modalities," p. 95).

2. Intensity*: Prescribe intensities between 64/70% and 94% of maximal heart rate or between 40/50% and 85% of the oxygen uptake reserve ($\dot{V}O_2R$) or heart rate reserve (HRR). For individuals with very low initial cardiorespiratory fitness, use intensities between 40% and 50% $\dot{V}O_2R$.

3. Frequency: Schedule exercise 3 to 5 days a week.

4. Duration: Schedule 20 to 60 min of continuous or intermittent activity, depending on the exercise intensity.

5. Rate of progression: Adjust the exercise prescription for each client in accordance with the conditioning effect, participant characteristics, new exercise test results, or performance during the exercise sessions. The rate of progression depends on the individual's age, functional capacity, health status, and goals. For apparently healthy adults, the aerobic exercise prescription consists of three stages: initial conditioning, improvement, and maintenance.

*For clients with higher $\dot{V}O_2$max ($>$40 ml $\cdot$ kg^{-1} $\cdot$ min^{-1}), the minimum training intensity should be 45% $\dot{V}O_2R$; for clients with lower $\dot{V}O_2$max ($<$40 ml $\cdot$ kg^{-1} $\cdot$ min^{-1}), training intensities as low as 30% $\dot{V}O_2R$ may be effective (Swain and Franklin 2002).

A cool-down phase immediately after endurance exercise is needed to reduce the risk of cardiovascular complications caused by stopping exercise suddenly. During cool-down, the individual continues exercising (e.g., walking, jogging, or cycling) at a low intensity for about 5 to 10 min. This light activity allows the heart rate (HR) and blood pressure (BP) to return to near baseline levels, prevents the pooling of blood in the extremities, and reduces the possibility of dizziness and fainting. The continued pumping action of the muscles increases the venous return and speeds up the recovery process. Stretching exercises may be repeated during the cool-down phase to reduce the chance of muscle cramps or muscle soreness.

The ACSM (2006) also recommends including recreational activities during or immediately after the endurance conditioning phase. Enjoyable games and sports (e.g., golf and volleyball) may encourage exercise program adherence. Games should be modified to decrease skill requirements, competition, and energy cost.

Modes of Exercise

If the primary goal of the exercise program is to develop and maintain cardiorespiratory fitness, prescribe aerobic activities using large muscle groups in a continuous, rhythmical fashion. In the initial and improvement stages of the exercise program, it is important to closely monitor the exercise intensity. Therefore, you should select modes of exercise that allow the individual to maintain a constant exercise intensity and are not highly dependent on the participant's skill. **Group I activities**, such as walking, cycling, and simulated stair-climbing (see below), are best suited for this purpose.

For **Group II activities** such as aerobic dance, step aerobics, and swimming, the rate of energy expenditure is highly dependent on the participant's skill level. You may prescribe Group II activities in the initial and improvement stages only for skilled individuals who are able to maintain constant exercise intensity while performing the activity. However, you should consider using Group II activities to add variety in the later stages (maintenance stage) of your client's exercise program.

Group III activities such as racquetball, basketball, and volleyball are highly variable in terms of exercise intensity and skill. Incorporate these activities only on a limited basis in the maintenance stage to add variety and fun to the exercise program. It is best that you do not emphasize competitive aspects of these activities, especially for high-risk and symptomatic participants.

In addition to walking, jogging, and cycling, there are other exercise modalities that provide a sufficient cardiorespiratory demand for improving aerobic fitness. Exercise modalities such as bench step aerobics, machine-based stair-climbing, elliptical training, and rowing offer your exercise

---

Classification of Aerobic Exercise Modalities[a]

Group I activities	Group II activities	Group III activities
Cycling (indoors)	Aerobic dancing	Basketball
Jogging	Bench step aerobics	Country and western dancing
Running	Cycling (outdoors)	Handball
Walking	Hiking	Racket sports
Rowing[b]	In-line skating	Volleyball
Stair-climbing[b]	Nordic skiing (outdoors)	Super circuit weight training
Simulated climbing[b]	Rope skipping	
Nordic skiing[b]	Swimming	
Elliptical training[b]	Water aerobics	
Aerobic riding[bc]		

[a]Group I activities provide constant intensity and are not skill dependent; Group II activities may provide constant or variable intensity, depending on skill. Group III activities provide variable intensity and are highly skill dependent.

[b]Machine-based activities.

[c]May not provide adequate training intensity for above-average fitness levels.

program participants a variety of options for their exercise prescription. Many individuals prefer to cross-train to add variety and enjoyment to their aerobic workouts. But are these exercise modes just as effective as traditional Group I activities (walking, jogging, and cycling)? The answer to this question is not simple and depends on the method (% $\dot{V}O_2$max or perceived exertion) used to equate different exercise modalities.

During exercise at a prescribed percentage of $\dot{V}O_2$max, Thomas, Ziogas, Smith, Zhang, and Londeree (1995) noted that six different aerobic exercise modes (treadmill jogging, Nordic skiing, shuffle skiing, stepping, cycling, and rowing) produced relatively similar cardiovascular responses (see figure 5.1), but that cycling resulted in a significantly higher perceived exertion (RPE) compared to the other modes. Likewise, other researchers have reported that compared to the value for treadmill jogging, the relationship between HR and $\dot{V}O_2$ at constant, submaximal intensities was similar for in-line skating (Wallick et al. 1995) and aerobic dancing with arms used extensively above the head or kept below the shoulders (Berry, Cline, Berry, and Davis 1992). In contrast, Parker, Hurley, Hanlon, and Vaccaro (1989) reported that the average steady-state HR during 20 min

of aerobic dancing was significantly higher than that for treadmill jogging when the subjects exercised at the same relative intensity (60% $\dot{V}O_2$max). Likewise, Howley, Colacino, and Swensen (1992) noted that HR response during electronic stepping ergometer exercise was systematically higher than that with treadmill exercise at the same submaximal $\dot{V}O_2$. Also, supporting the body weight during step ergometer exercise significantly reduced the HR and oxygen consumption compared to lightly holding on to the handrails for balance.

When exercise modes are equated using subjective ratings of perceived exertion (RPEs), research suggests that treadmill jogging may be superior to other aerobic exercise modes in terms of total oxygen consumption and rate of energy expenditure (Kravitz, Roberga, and Heyward 1996; Kravitz, Roberga, Heyward, Wagner, and Powers 1997; Zeni, Hoffman, and Clifford 1996). Subjects exercising on seven different modalities at a somewhat hard (RPE = 13 to 14) intensity for 15 to 20 min experienced a greater total oxygen consumption for treadmill jogging compared to stepping, rowing, Nordic skiing, cycling, shuffle skiing, and aerobic riding (Kravtiz, Roberga, et al. 1997; Thomas et al. 1995). Also, the rate of energy expenditure during treadmill exercise was 20% to 40% greater than

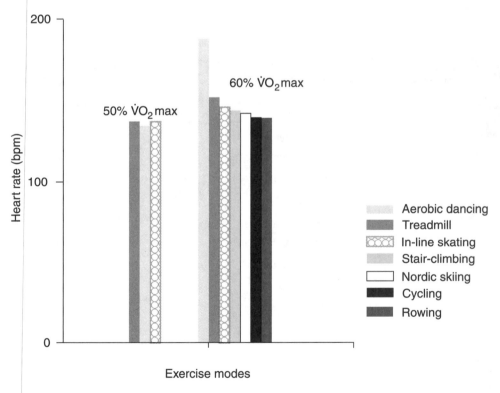

Figure 5.1 Comparison of steady-state heart rate response at submaximal exercise intensities for various aerobic exercise modes.

during stationary cycling (Kravitz, Robergs, et al. 1997; Zeni et al. 1996) and 57% greater than during aerobic riding (Kravitz et al. 1996, Kravitz, Robergs, et al. 1997). In addition, steady-state exercise HRs were higher (see figure 5.2) for treadmill jogging compared to cycling and aerobic riding (Kravitz et al. 1996; Kravitz, Robergs, et al. 1997; Zeni et al. 1996).

When selecting aerobic exercise modes for your client's exercise prescription, you should consider how easily the exercise intensity can be graded and adjusted in order to overload the cardiorespiratory system throughout the improvement stage. For aerobic dance and bench step aerobic exercise, work rates can be progressively increased by means of quicker cadences, different bench heights (Olson, Williford, Blessing, and Greathouse 1991), and upper-body exercise using light (1 to 4 lb) handheld weights (Kravitz, Heyward, Stolarczyk, and Wilmerding 1997). The intensity of in-line skating can be effectively graded by increasing the skating velocity (Wallick et al. 1995). The intensity of rowing, stair-climbing, and simulated whole-body climbing exercise can be incremented progressively using a variety of exercise machines (Brahler and Blank 1995; Howley et al. 1992).

Prescribe rope-skipping activities with caution; the exercise intensity for skipping 60 to 80 skips/min is approximately 9 METs. This value exceeds the maximum MET capacity of most sedentary individuals. Also, the exercise intensity is not easily graded because doubling the rate of skipping increases the energy requirement by only 2 to 3 METs. Town, Sol, and Sinning (1980) reported an average energy expenditure of 11.7 to 12.5 METs for skipping at rates of 125, 135, and 145 skips/min. They concluded that rope skipping is a strenuous exercise that may not be well suited as a form of graded, aerobic exercise.

When selecting exercise modes for your older clients, you need to consider their functional aerobic capacity, musculoskeletal problems, and neuromuscular coordination (impaired vision or balance). Select activities that are enjoyable and convenient. For many older adults, walking is an excellent mode. Stationary cycling and aquatic exercise can be used for individuals with impaired vision or balance. Research suggests that tai chi increases balance, muscular strength, and flexibility, as well as cardiorespiratory fitness ($\dot{V}O_2$peak) of older adults (Chewning, Yu, and Johnson 2000; Lan, Lai, Chen, and Wong 1998).

Intensity of Exercise

Traditionally, exercise intensity has been expressed as a straight percentage of either the individual's maximal aerobic capacity ($\dot{V}O_2$max), peak oxygen

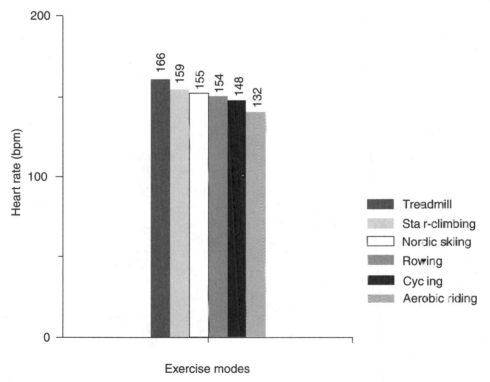

Figure 5.2 Comparison of steady-state heart rate response at somewhat hard intensity (rating of perceived exertion = 13 to 14) for various aerobic exercise modes.

consumption ($\dot{V}O_2$peak), or HRR. However, research has suggested that the %$\dot{V}O_2$max is not equivalent (1:1 ratio) to the %HRR for cycling and treadmill exercise (Swain and Leutholtz 1997; Swain, Leutholtz, King, Haas, and Branch 1998). Therefore, ACSM recently changed its recommendation regarding the method used to calculate exercise intensity for aerobic exercise prescriptions. Instead of expressing relative intensity as a straight percentage of $\dot{V}O_2$max (%$\dot{V}O_2$max), ACSM now recommends using the **percent $\dot{V}O_2$max reserve (% $\dot{V}O_2$R)**. The $\dot{V}O_2$R is the difference between the $\dot{V}O_2$max and resting oxygen consumption ($\dot{V}O_2$rest). With this modification, percent values for the % $\dot{V}O_2$R and %HRR methods for prescribing exercise intensity are approximately equal, thereby improving the accuracy of calculating a target $\dot{V}O_2$, particularly for clients who are engaging in low-intensity aerobic exercise (Swain 1999).

Regardless of the method used, intensity and duration of exercise are indirectly related. In other words, the higher the exercise intensity, the shorter the duration of exercise required and vice versa. Before prescribing the exercise intensity for aerobic exercise, carefully evaluate the individual's initial cardiorespiratory fitness classification, goals for the program, exercise preferences, and injury risks. Your client can improve cardiorespiratory fitness with either lower-intensity, longer-duration exercise or higher-intensity, shorter-duration exercise. For most individuals, low-to-moderate intensities of longer duration are recommended; higher-intensity exercise increases the risk of orthopedic injury and discourages continued participation in the exercise program.

Part of the art of exercise prescription is being able to select an exercise intensity that is adequate to stress the cardiovascular system without overtaxing it. According to ACSM (2006), the initial exercise intensity for apparently healthy adults is 40/50% to 85% $\dot{V}O_2$R. Lower-intensity exercise (30% $\dot{V}O_2$R) may be sufficient to provide important health benefits for sedentary clients and/or older individuals with low initial cardiorespiratory fitness levels. For most individuals, intensities of 60% to 80% $\dot{V}O_2$R are sufficient to improve cardiorespiratory fitness. As a general rule, the more fit the individual, the higher the exercise intensity needs to be to produce further improvement in cardiorespiratory fitness. Exercise intensity can be prescribed using the $\dot{V}O_2$reserve, HR, or RPE method.

$\dot{V}O_2$ Reserve (MET) Method

First, measure the client's functional aerobic capacity ($\dot{V}O_2$max or $\dot{V}O_2$peak) using a graded exercise test (see chapter 4). Express the client's $\dot{V}O_2$max in relative terms, that is, ml·kg^{-1}·min^{-1} or METs (metabolic equivalents). Given that 1 MET approximately equals 3.5 ml·kg^{-1}·min^{-1}, a $\dot{V}O_2$max of 35 ml·kg^{-1}·min^{-1}, for example, would be equivalent to 10 METs (35/3.5 = 10 METs).

Next determine the $\dot{V}O_2$reserve ($\dot{V}O_2$R). As mentioned previously, the $\dot{V}O_2$R is the difference between $\dot{V}O_2$max and $\dot{V}O_2$rest ($\dot{V}O_2$R = $\dot{V}O_2$max – $\dot{V}O_2$rest). The percent of $\dot{V}O_2$R depends on the initial cardiorespiratory fitness level of the client. To calculate the target $\dot{V}O_2$ (in METs) based on the $\dot{V}O_2$R, use the following equation:

$$\text{target } \dot{V}O_2 = [\text{relative exercise intensity (\%)} \times \ VO_2R] + \ VO_2\text{rest}$$

For example, the target $\dot{V}O_2$ corresponding to 50% $\dot{V}O_2$R for a client with a $\dot{V}O_2$max of 10 METs is calculated as follows:

$$
\begin{aligned}
\text{target } \dot{V}O_2 &= [0.50 \times (10 - 1 \text{ MET})] + 1 \text{ MET} \\
&= (0.50 \times 9 \text{ METs}) + 1 \text{ MET} \\
&= 4.5 + 1.0 \text{ METs, or } 5.5 \text{ METs}
\end{aligned}
$$

The exercise intensity (METs) for walking, jogging, running, cycling, and bench stepping activities is directly related to the speed of movement, power output, or mass lifted. Use the ACSM equations (table 4.3, p. 64) to calculate the speed or work rates corresponding to a specific MET intensity for the exercise prescription. For example, to estimate how fast a woman should jog on a level course to be exercising at an intensity of 8 METs, follow these steps:

1. Convert the METs to ml·kg^{-1}·min^{-1}.

$$
\begin{aligned}
\dot{V}O_2 &= 8 \text{ METs} \times 3.5 \text{ ml} \cdot \text{kg}^{-1} \cdot \text{min}^{-1} \\
&= 28 \text{ ml} \cdot \text{kg}^{-1} \cdot \text{min}^{-1}
\end{aligned}
$$

2. Substitute known values into the ACSM running equation and solve for speed.

$$28 \text{ ml} \cdot \text{kg}^{-1} \cdot \text{min}^{-1} = [\text{speed (m} \cdot \text{min}^{-1}) \times 0.2] + 3.5 \text{ ml} \cdot \text{kg}^{-1} \cdot \text{min}^{-1}$$

$$28.0 \text{ ml} \cdot \text{kg}^{-1} \cdot \text{min}^{-1} - 3.5 = \text{speed (m} \cdot \text{min}^{-1}) \times 0.2$$
$$122.5 \text{ m} \cdot \text{min}^{-1} = \text{speed}$$

3. Convert speed to mph.

$$1 \text{ mph} = 26.8 \text{ m} \cdot \text{min}^{-1}$$

$$122.5 \text{ m} \cdot \text{min}^{-1}/26.8 \text{ m} \cdot \text{min}^{-1} = 4.57 \text{ mph}$$

4. Convert mph to minute per mile pace.

$$
\begin{aligned}
\text{pace} &= 60 \text{ min} \cdot \text{hr}^{-1}/\text{mph} \\
&= 60 \text{ min} \cdot \text{hr}^{-1}/4.57 \text{ mph} \\
&= 13.1 \text{ min} \cdot \text{mile}^{-1} \text{ (or } 8.1 \text{ min} \cdot \text{km}^{-1})
\end{aligned}
$$

Average MET values for selected conditioning exercises, sports, and recreational activities are presented in appendix E.4, "Gross Energy Expenditure for Conditioning Exercises, Sports, and Recreational Activities," page 348. Prescribing exercise intensity using only MET values has certain limitations. The caloric costs (i.e., average MET values) of conditioning exercises are only estimates of energy expenditure. The caloric costs of activities, particularly Group II and III activities, vary greatly with the individual's skill level. Although these MET estimates provide a starting point for prescribing exercise intensity, environmental factors such as heat, humidity, altitude, and pollution may alter the HR and RPE responses to exercise. Therefore, you should use the HR or RPE method along with the MET method to ensure that the exercise intensity does not exceed safe limits.

Heart Rate Methods

There are three ways to prescribe exercise intensity for your clients using HR data. Each of these approaches is based on the assumption that HR is a linear function of exercise intensity (i.e., the higher the exercise intensity, the higher the HR).

Heart Rate Versus MET Graphing Method

When a submaximal or maximal graded exercise test (GXT) is administered, the client's steady-state HR response to each stage of the exercise test can be plotted (see figure 5.3). The HRmax is the HR observed at the highest exercise intensity during a maximal GXT. For submaximal GXTs, you can estimate your client's HRmax using 220 − age. From this graph, you can obtain HRs corresponding to given percentages of the estimated functional capacity or $\dot{V}O_2$max. In our example, the functional capacity of the individual is 7.4 METs, and the HRmax is 195 bpm. The HRs corresponding to exercise intensities of 4.8 and 6.4 METs (60% to 85% $\dot{V}O_2$R) are 139 and 175 bpm, respectively. During exercise workouts, the individual should measure the HR using a heart rate monitor or palpation to verify that the appropriate exercise intensity is reached.

It is important to note that the HR response to graded exercise is dependent to some extent on the mode of exercise testing. For example, compared to treadmill testing, exercising on an electronic step ergometer elicits higher HRs, and stationary cycling typically results in somewhat lower HRs

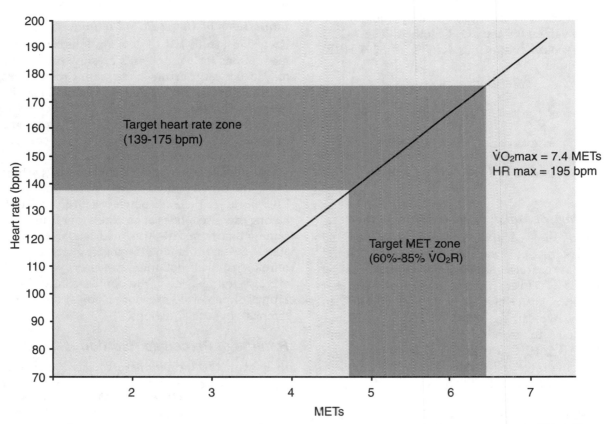

Figure 5.3 Plotting target heart rate zone using graded exercise test data (heart rate vs. METs). HRmax = maximal heart rate; $\dot{V}O_2$R = oxygen reserve.

at the same relative exercise intensities. When using this method to obtain HRs for an exercise prescription, be sure to match the exercise testing and training modes by selecting a testing mode that elicits HR responses that are similar to those obtained for the training mode (see figure 5.1). For example, if your client chooses in-line skating as a training mode, you should administer a treadmill GXT, given that the relationship between HR and $\dot{V}O_2$ at submaximal exercise intensities is similar for these two exercise modes (Berry et al. 1992).

Heart Rate Reserve Method

When HR data from a GXT are not available, you can use the **Karvonen**, or **percent heart rate reserve (%HRR), method** to determine target HRs for your client's exercise prescription. The **heart rate reserve (HRR)** method takes into account the resting heart rate and maximal HR. The HRR is the difference between the maximal HR and resting HR. A percentage of HRR is added to the client's resting HR to determine the target exercise HR:

target HR = [% exercise intensity $\times$ (HR$_{max}$ – HR$_{rest}$)] + HR$_{rest}$

As previously mentioned, the percent values for the HRR method are approximately equal to the percent values for the $\dot{V}O_2R$ method. The ACSM (2006) recommends using 40/50% to 85% HRR. For example, if

maximal HR = 178 bpm,

resting HR = 68 bpm, and

exercise intensity = 60% HRR, then

target exercise HR = 0.60 (178 – 68) + 68
or 134 bpm

Percentage of Maximal Heart Rate Method

You also can use a straight percentage of maximal HR (**percent heart rate maximum; %HRmax**) to estimate exercise intensity and determine target exercise HR. This method is based on the fact that the %HRmax is related to % $\dot{V}O_2R$ and %HRR. In table 5.1, we can see that 55% and 90% HRmax correspond to exercise intensities of 40% and 85% $\dot{V}O_2R$ or HRR. The ACSM (2006) recommends prescribing target HRs between 64/70% and 94% HRmax depending on the fitness level of your client.

With use of this technique, the actual maximal HR must be known or must be predicted either from the HR response to submaximal workloads or

from the formula 220 – age in years. For example, if the age-predicted maximal HR is 180 bpm and the exercise intensity is set at 70% HRmax, the target exercise HR is equal to 126 bpm.

%HR$_{max}$ $\times$ HR$_{max}$ = target HR

0.70 $\times$ 180 bpm = 126 bpm

Compared to the Karvonen (%HRR) method, the %HRmax method tends to give a lower value when the same relative intensity is used. If in our example the client's resting HR is 80 bpm, the target HR using the Karvonen method is 150 bpm [0.70 $\times$ (180 – 80) + 80 bpm] compared to 126 bpm for the %HRmax method.

The ACSM (2006) recommends using the %HRmax method to prescribe exercise intensity for your older clients. The %HRmax provides a more accurate estimate of %$\dot{V}O_2$peak of older adults than the %HRR method; using the %HRR method results in a higher-than-expected percentage of $\dot{V}O_2$max (Kohrt, Spina, Holloszy, and Ehsani 1998). However, you should measure, not predict (220 – age), the client's HRmax, for two reasons. Older individuals (>65 years of age) have large variability in HRmax, and they are more likely to be taking medications that affect peak HR.

Limitations of Heart Rate Methods

Exclusive use of HR to develop intensity recommendations for your client's exercise prescription may lead to large errors in estimating relative exercise intensities (%$\dot{V}O_2R$) for some individuals. This is especially true when HRmax is predicted from age (220 – age) instead of being directly measured. In about 30% of the population, an age-predicted prescription of 60% HRR may be as low as 70% and as high as 80% of the actual HRmax (Dishman 1994). Measured HRmax varies with exercise mode. Therefore, your client's perceived effort may differ among exercise modes even when exercising at the same submaximal HR. Also, medications, emotional states, and environmental factors (e.g., temperature, humidity, and air pollution) can affect your client's exercise training HRs. You should consider using ratings of perceived exertion to adjust the exercise intensity in such situations.

Ratings of Perceived Exertion Method

In light of the limitations associated with using HR for setting exercise intensity, consider using a combination of HR and RPE in developing prescriptions for your clients. You can use RPEs to prescribe and monitor exercise intensity (Birk and Birk 1987). The RPE scales (see table 4.2) are valid

Table 5.1 Comparison of Methods for Prescribing Exercise Intensity for Healthy Adults[a]

	Relative intensity		
Classification	% $\dot{V}O_2R$ or %HRR	%HRmax	RPE (6-20 scale)
Very light	<20	<35	<10
Light	20-39	35-54	10-11
Moderate	40-59	55-69	12-13
Hard	60-84	70-89	14-16
Very hard	≥85	≥90	17-19
Maximal	100	100	20

[a]Based on data from Pollock et al. 1998.

HRR = heart rate reserve; RPE = rating of perceived exertion.

and reliable tools for assessing the level of physical exertion during continuous, aerobic exercise (Birk and Birk 1987; Borg and Linderholm 1967; Dunbar et al. 1992).

During the GXT, the client rates the intensity of each stage of the test using the RPE scale. You can use the intensities (METs) corresponding to ratings of 12 (somewhat hard) and 16 (hard) to set the minimum and maximum training intensities for the exercise prescription. Compared to the %HRR method, RPEs between 12 and 16 closely approximate 40% and 84% HRR, respectively (Pollock et al. 1998). With practice an individual can learn to associate RPE with a specific target exercise HR, especially at higher exercise intensities (Smutok, Skrinar, and Pandolf 1980). Thus, the RPE can be used instead of HR, or in combination with HR, to monitor training intensity and to adjust the exercise prescription for conditioning effects.

One advantage of RPE as a method of monitoring exercise intensity is that your clients do not need to stop exercising in order to check their HRs. For an extensive review of research pertaining to the use of perceived exertion for prescribing exercise intensity, see Dishman 1994.

Monitoring Exercise Intensity

Throughout the aerobic exercise program, carefully monitor exercise intensity in order to ensure your client's safety and to confirm that your client is exercising at or near the prescribed intensity. The HR and RPE methods can be used for this purpose. Teach your clients how to monitor exercise intensity using HR palpation techniques (see chapter 2),

heart rate monitors, and the RPE scale (see table 4.2, page 59).

Some clients may prefer using a talk test to monitor their exertion. The **talk test** is a measure of the client's ability to converse comfortably while exercising and is based on the relationship between exercise intensity and pulmonary ventilation. **Pulmonary ventilation,** or the movement of air into and out of the lungs, increases linearly with exercise intensity ($\dot{V}O_2$) up to a point. At the breaking point, known as the **ventilatory threshold,** pulmonary ventilation increases exponentially relative to the exercise intensity and rate of oxygen consumed. At the ventilatory threshold, the ability to speak during exercise becomes difficult. Studies of college-age students (Persinger, Foster, Gibson, Fater, and Porcari 2004), clinically stable cardiac patients (Voelker, Foster, Skemp-Arlt, Brice, and Backes 2002), and athletes (Recalde et al. 2002) reported that individuals who pass the talk test are exercising at intensities that are within the accepted guidelines for the exercise prescription. Those failing the talk test are exercising at intensities that exceed the prescribed level. The talk test provides a fairly precise and consistent method for monitoring exercise during stationary cycling and treadmill exercise (Persinger et al. 2004).

Frequency of Exercise

The frequency of the exercise sessions depends on your client's caloric goals, health and fitness level, preferences, and time constraints. For health benefits, individuals should exercise at a moderate intensity most, if not all, days of the week.

Individuals with functional capacities >5 METs should exercise at a moderate to vigorous intensity a minimum of three times per week to produce significant changes in cardiorespiratory endurance (ACSM 2006). As the fitness level increases, however, the frequency should be increased to five times per week for continued improvement (Pollock 1973). For individuals with functional capacities <3 METs, multiple daily exercise sessions are advisable.

In terms of improving $\dot{V}O_2$max, the sequence of exercise sessions seems to be less important than the total work performed during the training. Similar improvements were noted for individuals who trained every other day (M-W-F) and three consecutive days (M-T-W) (Moffatt, Stamford, and Neill 1977). The ACSM (2006) recommends exercising on alternate days during the initial stages of training to lessen the chance of bone or joint injury. Also, older adults who can tolerate vigorous exercise should work out at least 2 to 3/wk with a day of rest between each exercise session (ACSM 2006).

Once people reach the desired level of cardiorespiratory fitness, they may maintain it by exercising 2 to 4 days/wk, provided that the intensity and duration of the workouts are similar to those used to achieve the current fitness level (Brynteson and Sinning 1973; Hickson and Rosenkoetter 1981).

Duration of Exercise

As an exercise specialist, you must prescribe an appropriate combination of exercise intensity and duration so that the individual adequately stresses the cardiorespiratory system without overexertion. As mentioned earlier, the intensity and duration of exercise are inversely related (the lower the exercise intensity, the longer the duration of the exercise). The ACSM (2006) recommends 20 to 60 min of continuous or intermittent activity. Apparently healthy individuals usually can sustain exercise intensities of 60% to 85% $\dot{V}O_2$R for 20 to 30 min. To improve aerobic capacity ($\dot{V}O_2$max), exercise of moderate intensity and duration (20-30 min) is recommended for most adults (ACSM 2006). During the improvement stage, duration can be increased every two to three weeks until participants can exercise continuously for 30 min at a moderate to vigorous intensity (ACSM 2006). Poorly conditioned and older individuals may be able to exercise continuously at a low intensity (40% $\dot{V}O_2$R) for only 5 to 10 min. They may need to perform multiple sessions (e.g., four to six 5-min exercise bouts or two to three 10-min exercise bouts) in a given day to accumulate 20 to 30 min of aerobic exercise.

An alternative way of estimating the duration of exercise is to use the caloric cost of the exercise. To achieve health benefits, ACSM (2006) recommends target **caloric thresholds** of 150 to 400 kcal/day, and a minimal weekly caloric threshold of 1000 kcal from physical activity or exercise.

During the initial stage of the exercise program, however, weekly exercise caloric expenditure may be considerably lower (200 to 600 kcal/wk). Throughout the improvement stage, the goal is to increase your client's caloric expenditure from 1000 to 2000 kcal/wk by gradually increasing the frequency, intensity, and duration of the exercise. For example, in order for a 60-kg woman who is exercising at an intensity of 7 METs, five times per week, to reach a weekly net caloric threshold of 1500 kcal/wk, she needs to expend 300 kcal per exercise session (1500 kcal/5 = 300 kcal). You can estimate the net caloric cost of her exercise (kcal · min⁻¹) using the following formula:

$$\text{net cal cost (kcal} \cdot \text{min}^{-1}) = \text{METs} \times 3.5 \times \text{body mass in kg}/200$$

To calculate the net caloric expenditure from her activity, subtract the resting oxygen consumption (1 MET) from the gross $\dot{V}O_2$ ($\dot{V}O_2$ cost of exercise + $\dot{V}O_2$rest) and substitute this value (7 – 1 = 6 METs) into the equation:

$$\text{net cal cost} = 6 \text{ METs} \times 3.5 \times 60 \text{ kg}/200$$
$$= 6.3 \text{ kcal} \cdot \text{min}^{-1}$$

Therefore, she needs to exercise approximately 48 min (300 kcal/6.3 kcal · min⁻¹), five times per week, in order to achieve her weekly caloric expenditure goal of 1500 kcal.

Rate of Progression

Physiological changes associated with aerobic endurance training (see "Physiological Changes Induced by Cardiorespiratory Endurance Training," p. 103) enable the individual to increase the total work performed. The greatest conditioning effects occur during the first six to eight weeks of the exercise program. Aerobic endurance may improve as much as 3% per week during the first month, 2% per week for the second month, and 1% per week or less thereafter (Sharkey 1979). For continued improvements, the cardiorespiratory system must be overloaded through adjustments in the intensity and duration of the exercise to the new level of fitness. The degree and rate of improvement depend on the age, health status, and initial fitness level of the participant. For the average person, aerobic training programs generally produce a 5% to 20% increase in $\dot{V}O_2$max (Pollock 1973). Sedentary, inactive persons may improve as much as 40% in aerobic fitness, while elite athletes may improve only 5% because they begin at a level much closer to their genetic limits. We do not expect older individuals entering the exercise program to improve as quickly as younger individuals even when the initial fitness levels are the same.

Stages of Progression

As discussed in chapter 3, the three stages of progression for cardiorespiratory exercise programs are the **initial conditioning, improvement,** and **maintenance stages** (ACSM 2006).

Initial Conditioning

The initial conditioning stage may last 1 to 6 wk, depending on your client's rate of adaptation to the exercise program. In this stage, each exercise session should include a warm-up, moderate-intensity (40%-60% HRR) aerobic activity, low-intensity muscular fitness exercises, and a cool-down that emphasizes stretching exercises (ACSM 2006). Clients starting a moderate-intensity aerobic conditioning program should exercise a minimum of 3 to 4 days/wk. The duration of the aerobic exercise should be at least 15 to 20 min and progress to 30 min. After clients are able to sustain aerobic activity at 60% HRR for 30 min they may progress to the improvement stage.

Improvement

The improvement stage usually lasts 4 to 8 mo. During this stage, the rate of progression is more rapid. Intensity, duration, and frequency of exercise

---

Physiological Changes Induced by Cardiorespiratory Endurance Training

Increases	Decreases
CARDIORESPIRATORY SYSTEM	
Heart size and volume	Resting heart rate
Blood volume and total hemoglobin	Submaximal exercise heart rate
Stroke volume—rest and exercise	Blood pressure (if high)
Cardiac output—maximum	
$\dot{V}O_2$max	
Oxygen extraction from blood	
Lung volumes	
MUSCULOSKELETAL SYSTEM	
Mitochondria—number and size	
Myoglobin stores	
Triglyceride stores	
Oxidative phosphorylation	
OTHER SYSTEMS	
Strength of connective tissues	Body weight (if overweight)
Heat acclimatization	Body fat
High-density lipoprotein cholesterol	Total cholesterol
	Low-density lipoprotein cholesterol

should always be increased independently. Either duration or frequency should be increased before intensity is increased. Increase the duration no more than 20% per week until your clients are able to sustain moderate-to-vigorous exercise for 20 to 30 min. Frequency should progress from 3 or 4 to 5 days/wk. Once the desired duration and frequency are reached, the exercise intensity may be increased by no more than 5% HRR every sixth exercise session (ACSM 2006).

Rate of progression during this stage depends on a number of factors. Cardiac patients, older adults, and less fit individuals may need more time for the body to adapt to a higher conditioning intensity. In such cases, the exercise duration should be at least 20 to 30 min before the exercise intensity increases (ACSM 2006).

Maintenance

After achieving the desired level of cardiorespiratory fitness, an individual enters the maintenance stage of the exercise program. This stage continues on a regular, long-term basis if the individual has made a lifetime commitment to exercise.

The goal of this stage is to maintain the cardiorespiratory fitness level and the weekly exercise caloric expenditure achieved during the improvement stage. Have your client accomplish this goal by engaging in aerobic activities 2 to 3 days/wk at the intensity and duration that were reached at the end of the improvement stage. Reducing the training frequency from 5 to 2 or 3 days/wk does not adversely affect $\dot{V}O_2$max as long as the training intensity remains the same. However, clients should participate in other activities an additional 2 to 3 days/wk. To this end, a variety of enjoyable activities from Groups II and III may be selected to counteract boredom and to maintain the interest level of the participant. For example, an individual who was running 5 days/wk at the end of the improvement stage may choose to run only 3 days/wk and substitute in-line skating and racquetball on the other 2 days.

AEROBIC TRAINING METHODS AND MODES

Either continuous or discontinuous training methods can improve cardiovascular endurance. **Continuous training** involves one continuous, aerobic exercise bout performed at low-to-moderate intensities without rest intervals. **Discontinuous training** consists of several intermittent low- to

high-intensity aerobic exercise bouts interspersed with rest periods. Research indicates that continuous training and discontinuous training are equally effective in improving cardiorespiratory fitness. When the absolute training intensity and total amount of work performed in both the continuous and discontinuous (intermittent) training programs are equal, the magnitude and rate of change in $\dot{V}O_2$peak over 10 wk are similar for both programs (Morris, Gass, Thompson, Bennett, Basic, and Morton 2002). However, Pollock, Gettman, Milesis, Bah, Durstine, and Johnson(1977) reported that the dropout rate of adults in a high-intensity interval (discontinuous) training program was twice that of those in a continuous jogging program.

Continuous Training

All of the exercise modes listed as Group I and II activities (see p. 95) are suitable for continuous training. One advantage of continuous training is that a prescribed exercise intensity (e.g., 75% HRR) is maintained fairly consistently throughout the duration of the steady-paced exercise. Generally, continuous exercise at low-to-moderate intensities is safer, more comfortable, and better suited for individuals initiating an aerobic exercise program.

Walking, Jogging, and Cycling

The most popular modes of continuous training are walking, jogging or running, and cycling. Exercise programs using walking, jogging, and cycling provide similar cardiovascular benefits (Magel, Foglia, McArdle, Gutin, Pechard, and Katch 1974; Pollock, Cureton, and Greninger 1969; Pollock et al. 1971; Pollock, Dimmick, Miller, Kendrick, and Linnerud 1975; Wilmore, Davis, O'Brien, Vodak, Walder, and Amsterdam 1980). Improvements in $\dot{V}O_2$max are comparable for most commonly used exercise modes. Pollock et al. (1975) compared running, walking, and cycling exercise programs of middle-aged men who trained at 85% to 90% HRmax. All three groups showed significant improvements in $\dot{V}O_2$max. These results indicate that improvement in $\dot{V}O_2$max is independent of the mode of training when frequency, intensity, and duration of exercise are held constant and are prescribed in accordance with sound, scientific principles.

Aerobic Dance

Aerobic dance is a popular mode of exercise for improving and maintaining cardiorespiratory fitness. A number of excellent books provide detailed information about aerobic dance methods and techniques (Kuntzelman 1979; Wilmoth 1986). A typical aerobic dance workout consists of 8 to 10 min of stretching, calisthenics, and low-intensity exercise. This is followed by 15 to 45 min of either high- or low-impact aerobic dancing at the target training intensity. Handheld weights (1 to 4 lb) can be used to increase exercise intensity. Heart rates should be monitored at least six times during the exercise to ensure that the HR stays within the target zone (Russell 1983). The 10-min cool-down period usually includes more stretching and calisthenic-type exercises.

Several studies conducted to assess the cardiorespiratory effect of aerobic dance training have documented average increases in $\dot{V}O_2$max of 10% or greater (Blessing, Wilson, Puckett, and Ford 1987; Milburn and Butts 1983; Parker et al. 1989; Williford, Blessing, Barksdale, and Smith 1988). Milburn and Butts (1983) reported that aerobic dance was as effective as jogging for improving cardiorespiratory endurance when performed at similar intensity, frequency, and duration. The subjects trained 30 min, 4 days/wk for 7 wk, at 83% to 84% HRmax.

Bench Step Aerobics

Health and fitness clubs throughout the United States are promoting bench step training as an effective high-intensity, low-impact aerobic exercise mode. Step training uses whole-body movements on steps or benches, ranging in height from 4 to 12 in. (10.2 to 30.5 cm). Choreographed movement routines are performed to music. A typical bench step aerobic workout consists of 5 to 10 min of warm-up and 20 to 30 min of step training. This is followed by a short (3 to 5 min) cool-down.

Exercise training intensity can be graded through use of variations in stepping cadence or bench height. To reduce the risk of injury while stepping on and off the bench, bench heights of 6 to 8 in. (15.2-20.3 cm) and stepping cadences ranging from 118 to 128 steps/min are recommended. In terms of energy expenditure, increasing bench height is more effective than increasing cadence. In a study comparing the energy expenditure of bench stepping at two different cadences (125 vs. 130 steps/min) and bench heights (6 vs. 8 in., or 15.2 vs. 20.3 cm), there was no significant difference in energy expenditure (kcal/min) for the two different cadences. Increasing bench height from 6 to 8 in. (15.2 to 20.3 cm), however, increased energy expenditure by 1.04 kcal/min (Grier, Lloyd, Walker, and Murray 2002). Thus, the intensity of a typical aerobic stepping routine is more effectively

altered by increasing the step height and not by increasing the stepping cadence.

Studies confirm that continuous step training at bench heights ranging from 6 to 12 in. (15.2 to 30.5 cm) provides an adequate training stimulus that meets ACSM (2006) guidelines for intensity and duration (Olson et al. 1991; Petersen, Verstraete, Schultz, and Stray-Gundersen 1993; Woodby-Brown, Berg, and Latin 1993). Following 8 to 12 wk of step aerobic training, $\dot{V}O_2$max improves as much as 8% to 16% (Kravitz, Cizar, Christensen, and Setterlund 1993 Kravitz, Heyward, et al. 1997; Velasquez and Wilmore 1992). In a study comparing bench step exercise with and without hand weights, use of 2- to 4-lb hand weights did not result in a greater improvement in $\dot{V}O_2$max than step training without hand weights (Kravitz, Heyward, et al. 1997).

Step Ergometry and Stair-Climbing

Step ergometry (machine-based stair-climbing) is a popular exercise mode in health and fitness clubs. Research shows a linear HR response to graded submaximal exercise performed on stair-climbing ergometers. However, the MET levels displayed on the StairMaster 4000 PT overestimate the actual MET intensity of the exercise (Howley, Colacino, and Swensen 1992). When prescribing exercise intensity using this type of stair-climber, be certain to adjust the machine's estimates for each MET level using the following equation:

$$\text{actual METs} = 0.556 + 0.745 \text{(StairMaster MET setting)}$$

Although machine-based stair-climbing provides a training stimulus that meets guidelines for exercise intensity, presently there is no research comparing the effectiveness of stair-climbing training to other aerobic training modes.

Elliptical Training

Elliptical training machines have become popular in the fitness industry. Elliptical trainers are designed for either upper-body or combined upper- and lower-body exercise. The lower-body motion during exercise on an elliptical trainer is a cross between the actions performed with machine-based stair-climbing and upright stationary cycling. With elliptical trainers, the feet move in an egg-shaped or elliptical pattern, and the feet stay in contact with the footpads of the device throughout the exercise. Unlike running or jogging, this form of exercise may provide a high-intensity workout with low-impact forces comparable to walking

(Porcari, Foster, and Schneider 2000). Although there is no research documenting the long-term effects of this type of training on cardiovascular fitness, preliminary data suggest that this exercise modality meets ACSM (2006) guidelines for developing and maintaining cardiorespiratory fitness (Kravitz, Wax, Mayo, Daniels, and Charette 1998; Porcari et al. 2000). Kravitz et al. (1998) reported that the average energy expenditure during forward/backward exercise with no resistance and against resistance for 5 min (125 strides/min) was, respectively, 8.1 and 10.7 kcal · min⁻¹. Exercise intensities ranged between 72.5% and 83.5% HRmax (age-predicted). Compared to treadmill exercise, upper-body elliptical training at self-selected intensities produced similar $\dot{V}O_2$, HR, and RPE responses (Crommett, Kravitz, Wongsathikun, and Kemerly 1999; Porcari et al. 2000). Although there was no difference in $\dot{V}O_2$ between combined upper-/lower-body elliptical training and treadmill exercise, upper-/lower-body elliptical training produced a significantly higher HR and RPE (Crommett et al. 1999).

Aerobic Riding

Aerobic riding involves both upper- and lower-body muscle groups. For this reason, some manufacturers claim that this mode of exercise will automatically burn more calories than lower-body-only exercise modes such as jogging, cycling, and stair-climbing. One study, however, noted that the energy expenditure during 10 min of steady-state exercise at a somewhat hard intensity (RPE = 13) on an aerobic rider was significantly lower than the caloric expenditure for treadmill jogging, stationary cycling, and Nordic skiing (Kravitz, Robergs, et al. 1997). Subjects reported that they felt a similar workout intensity, in terms of RPE, during aerobic riding. Aerobic riding appears to challenge the muscular system (subjects complained of muscular discomfort) more than the cardiovascular system. In fact, the relative submaximal $\dot{V}O_2$ (47% $\dot{V}O_2$max) for aerobic riding was significantly less than that for treadmill jogging (74% $\dot{V}O_2$max), Nordic skiing (68% $\dot{V}O_2$max), and stationary cycling (64% $\dot{V}O_2$max). Thus, aerobic riding may not be suitable for aerobic exercise prescriptions, particularly for individuals with above-average cardiorespiratory fitness.

Water-Based Exercise

Water-based exercise, such as water aerobics or walking in waist-deep water, has been promoted as an effective way to increase the cardiorespi-ratory fitness of young, middle-aged, and older adults. This exercise is especially popular among individuals who are older, overweight, or afflicted with orthopedic disabilities. A typical water-based exercise session includes the following phases:

- Warm-up—20 min of stretching before entering the pool, followed by walking slowly in the water
- Endurance phase—30 min of continuous walking and dancing in the water
- Resistance phase—10 min of resistance exercises performed underwater with dumbbells, barbell-like devices, and leg pads
- Cool-down—10 min of relaxation and floor exercises outside of the pool

In older women (60-75 yr) participating in water-based exercise training 3 days/wk for 12 wk, $\dot{V}O_2$peak increased by 12% while total cholesterol and LDL-C decreased by 11% and 17%, respectively. Also, muscle strength and arm and leg power increased significantly in response to exercising the limbs against the resistance of water (Takeshima et al. 2002).

Discontinuous Training

As mentioned previously, discontinuous training involves a series of low- to high-intensity exercise bouts interspersed with rest or relief periods. All of the exercise modes listed as Group I and II activities (see p. 59) are suitable for discontinuous training. Because of the intermittent nature of this form of training, the exercise intensity and total amount of work performed can be greater than with continuous training, making discontinuous training a versatile method that is widely used by athletes, as well as individuals with low cardiorespiratory fitness. In fact, ACSM (2006) recommends the use of discontinuous (intermittent) training for symptomatic individuals who are able to tolerate only low-intensity exercise for short periods of time (3 to 5 min). Interval training, treading, spinning, and circuit resistance training are examples of intermittent or discontinuous training.

Interval Training

Interval training involves a repeated series of exercise work bouts interspersed with rest or relief periods. This method is popular among athletes because it allows the athlete to exercise at higher relative intensities during the work interval than are possible with longer-duration, continuous training. Interval training programs also can be designed to improve speed and anaerobic endurance, as well as aerobic endurance, simply by means of modifications in the exercise intensity and length of the work and relief intervals.

Each work interval consists of running at a pace such that a distance of 1100 yd is covered in 3 to 4 min. The work interval is followed by a rest-relief interval of 1.5 to 2 min. This sequence is repeated three times. During the rest-relief interval, the individual usually walks or jogs while recovering from the work bout. For aerobic interval training, the ratio of work to rest-relief is usually 1:1 or 1:0.5. Each work interval is 3 to 5 min and is repeated three to seven times. The exercise intensity usually ranges between 70% and 85% $\dot{V}O_2$max. Apply the overload principle by increasing the exercise intensity or length of the work interval, decreasing the length of the rest-relief interval, or increasing the number of work intervals per exercise session. For a discussion of interval training and sample programs, including programs for developing speed and anaerobic endurance, refer to Fox and Mathews 1974.

AN INTERVAL TRAINING PRESCRIPTION TO DEVELOP AEROBIC ENDURANCE

Sets: 1

Repetitions: 3

Distance: 1100 yd

Time: 3 to 4 min

Rest-relief interval: 1.5 to 2 min

Treading and Spinning

Treading and spinning are two examples of interval training that have gained popularity in fitness clubs because of the variety and enjoyment they offer. Treading and spinning are group classes that involve walking, jogging, and running at various speeds and grades on a treadmill (treading) or stationary cycling at various cadences and resistances (spinning). A typical treading or spinning workout consists of 1:1 or 1.5:1 work–recovery intervals or stages that are repeated for a specified duration. For example, a 30 min treading class may consist of six stages. Each stage lasts 5 min (i.e., 3-min work interval and 2-min recovery interval). One can advance the intensity of the work interval by increasing the treadmill speed or grade. During the recovery interval, both the speed and grade of the treadmill are decreased (e.g., 2.5 mph and

0% grade). Instructors individualize and adapt the workouts for their clients by adjusting the duration of the work-recovery intervals and varying the speed and grade.

In one study researchers designed 30-min treading workouts for walkers and runners (Nichols, Sherman, and Abbott 2000). They reported that the average intensity of the walking protocol was 40% to 49% $\dot{V}O_2$max for male and female walkers, respectively. For the running protocol, the average intensity of the work intervals was 76% to 80% $\dot{V}O_2$max for male and female runners, respectively. The researchers suggested that these average intensities, as well as the duration of the workout (30 min), are sufficient to meet ACSM standards for an aerobic exercise prescription. More research is needed to determine the long-term training effects of treading and spinning on cardiorespiratory fitness.

Circuit Resistance Training

Use of circuit resistance training for the development of aerobic fitness, as well as muscular strength and tone, has received much attention. An example of a circuit resistance training program is presented in chapter 7, page 148 (see figure 7.1). Circuit resistance training usually consists of several circuits of resistance training with a minimal amount of rest between the exercise stations (15 to 20 sec). Alternatively, instead of rest, you can have your clients perform 1 to 3 min of aerobic exercise between each station. The aerobic stations may include activities such as stationary cycling, jogging in place, rope skipping, stair-climbing, bench stepping, and rowing. This modification of the circuit is known as super circuit resistance training.

Gettman and Pollock (1981) reviewed the research dealing with the physiological benefits of circuit resistance training. Because it produces only a 5% increase in aerobic capacity as compared to a 15% to 25% increase with other forms of aerobic training, the authors concluded that circuit resistance training should not be used to develop aerobic fitness. Rather, it may be used during the maintenance stage of an aerobic exercise program.

PERSONALIZED EXERCISE PROGRAMS

The aerobic exercise prescription should be individualized to meet each client's training goals and interests. To do this, you need to consider your client's age, gender, physical fitness level, and exercise preferences. This section presents a sample case study and examples of individualized exercise prescriptions to illustrate how the exercise prescription may be personalized for each client.

Case Study

Like any preventive or therapeutic intervention, exercise should be prescribed carefully. You must be able to evaluate your client's medical history, medical condition, physical fitness status, lifestyle characteristics, and interests before designing the exercise program. In addition, to test your ability to extract, analyze, and evaluate all pertinent information needed to design a safe exercise program for your client, many professional certification examinations require that you be able to analyze a case study. For these reasons this section includes a sample case study (see p. 111).

A case study is a written narrative that summarizes client information that you will need to develop an accurate and safe individualized exercise prescription (Porter 1988). Important elements to focus on when reading and analyzing a case study are listed in "Essential Elements of a Case Study" (see p. 109). First, identify the client's coronary heart disease (CHD) risk factors by focusing on information provided about family history of CHD, blood lipid profile (total cholesterol, high- and low-density lipoprotein cholesterol [HDL-C and LDL-C]), blood glucose levels, resting BP, physical activity, body fat level, and smoking. Become familiar with ideal or typical values for various blood chemistry tests so that you will be able to recognize normal or abnormal test results. Remember that each of the following factors place individuals at greater risk for CHD:

- Triglycerides $\geq$150 mg $\cdot$ dl^{-1}
- Total cholesterol $\geq$200 mg $\cdot$ dl^{-1}
- LDL-cholesterol $\geq$130 mg $\cdot$ dl^{-1}
- HDL-cholesterol < 40 mg $\cdot$ dl^{-1}
- Total cholesterol/HDL ratio > 5.0
- Blood glucose $\geq$110 mg $\cdot$ dl^{-1}
- Systolic BP $\geq$140 or diastolic BP $\geq$90 mmHg

Use the demographic data (age and gender) and CHD risk factors to determine the client's CHD risk classification (low, moderate, or high risk). The CHD risk classification dictates how closely the client's exercise program needs to be monitored.

Pay close attention to information about the client's *medical history* and *physical examination*

results. These may reveal signs or symptoms of CHD, particularly if shortness of breath, chest pains, or leg cramps are reported or high BP is detected. It is also important to note the types of medication the client is using. Drugs such as digitalis, beta-blockers, diuretics, vasodilators, bronchodilators, and insulin may alter the body's physiological responses during exercise and could affect the HR and BP responses reported for the GXT. Keep in mind that exercise programs need to be modified for individuals with musculoskeletal disorders such as arthritis, low back pain, osteoporosis, and chondromalacia. Next, be certain to key in on information regarding the client's lifestyle. Factors such as smoking, lack of physical activity, or diets high in saturated fats or cholesterol increase the risk of CHD, atherosclerosis, and hypertension. You often can target these factors for modification; they also help you assess the likelihood of the client's adherence to the exercise program. (See table 3.3, p. 47.)

Examine the BP, HR, and RPE data for the *graded exercise test* used to assess the client's functional aerobic capacity and cardiorespiratory fitness level. You need to be acutely aware of the normal and abnormal physiological responses to graded exercise. After assessing the client's CHD risk and cardiorespiratory fitness level, you can design an aerobic exercise program using a personalized exercise prescription of intensity, frequency, duration, mode, and progression. To write the exercise prescription, use the results from the GXT (HR, RPE, functional MET capacity).

The sample case study on page 111 is provided to test your ability to evaluate risk factors and GXT results and to prescribe an accurate and safe aerobic exercise program for this individual. See the results of the analysis in appendix A.8, "Analysis of Sample Case Study," page 303.

Sample Cycling Program

The sample cycling program on page 112 shows a personalized cycling program for a 27-year-old female who was given a maximal GXT on a stationary cycle ergometer. Her measured $\dot{V}O_2$max is 7.4 METs. The exercise intensity is based on a percentage of her $\dot{V}O_2$ reserve (%$\dot{V}O_2$R), and the target exercise HRs corresponding to 60% (4.8 METs) and 80% $\dot{V}O_2$R (6.1 METs) are 139 bpm and 168 bpm, respectively (see figure 5.3). Thus, the training exercise HR should fall within this HR range. During the initial stage of the exercise program, the woman will cycle at a work rate corresponding to 60% $\dot{V}O_2$R (4.8 METs) for 2 weeks.

During weeks 1 and 2, the exercise duration is increased by 5 min/wk (from 40 to 45 min). During the 3rd week, relative exercise intensity rather than duration is increased by 5% (from 60% $\dot{V}O_2R$ to 65% $\dot{V}O_2R$). The work rate corresponding to an exercise intensity is calculated by using the ACSM formulas for leg ergometry (see table 4.3). For example, the work rate corresponding to 60% $\dot{V}O_2R$ (4.8 METs or 16.8 ml·kg^{-1}·min^{-1}) is calculated as follows:

$$\dot{V}O_2 \ (ml \cdot kg^{-1} \cdot min^{-1}) = W \ / \ M \times 1.8 + 3.5 + 3.5,$$

where W = work rate in kgm·min^{-1} and M = body mass in kg.

$$16.8 = W \ / \ 70 \ kg \times 1.8 + 7.0$$

$$16.8 - 7.0 = W \ / \ 70 \ kg \times 1.8$$

$$9.8 \times 70 \ kg \ / \ 1.8 = 381 \ kgm \cdot min^{-1}.$$

To calculate the resistance setting corresponding to 381 kgm·min^{-1} for a cycling cadence of 50 rpm,

---

Essential Elements of a Case Study

Demographic Factors

Age

Gender

Ethnicity

Occupation

Height

Body weight

Family history of coronary heart disease

Medical History

Present symptoms

Dyspnea or shortness of breath

Angina or chest pain

Leg cramps or claudication

Musculoskeletal problems or limitations

Medications

Past history

Diseases

Injuries

Surgeries

Lab tests

Lifestyle Assessment

Alcohol and caffeine intake

Smoking

Nutritional intake/eating patterns

Physical activity patterns and interests

Sleeping habits

Occupational stress level

Mental status/family lifestyle

Physical Examination

Blood pressure

Heart/lung sounds

Orthopedic problems/limitations

Laboratory Tests (Ideal or Typical Values)

Triglycerides (<150 mg · dl^{-1})

Total cholesterol (<200 mg · dl^{-1})

LDL-cholesterol (<100 mg · dl^{-1})

HDL-cholesterol (>40 mg · dl^{-1})

Total cholesterol/HDL-cholesterol (<3.5)

Blood glucose (60-110 mg · dl^{-1})

Hemoglobin: 13.5-17.5 g · dl^{-1} (men)

11.5-15.5 g · dl^{-1} (women)

Hematocrit: 40-52% (men)

36-48% (women)

Potassium (3.5-5.5 meq · dl^{-1})

Blood urea nitrogen (4-24 mg · dl^{-1})

Creatinine (0.3-1.4 mg · dl^{-1})

Iron: 40-190 μg · dl^{-1} (men)

35-180 μg · dl^{-1} (women)

Calcium (8.5-10.5 mg · dl^{-1})

Physical Fitness Evaluation

Cardiorespiratory fitness (HR, BP, $\dot{V}O_2$max)

Body composition (% body fat)

Musculoskeletal fitness (muscle and bone strength)

Flexibility

divide the work rate by the total distance the flywheel travels: 381 / 50 rpm × 6 = 1.27 kg, or 1.3 kg.

To calculate the net energy cost (kcal · min⁻¹) of cycling, subtract the resting $\dot{V}O_2$ (1 MET) from the gross $\dot{V}O_2$ for each intensity. Convert this net MET value to kcal · min⁻¹ using the following formula:

$$\text{kcal} \cdot \text{min}^{-1} = \text{METs} \times 3.5 \times \text{body mass (kg)}/200$$
$$(\text{e.g.}, 4.8 - 1.0 = 3.8 \text{ METs}; 3.8 \times 3.5 \times 70 \text{ kg}/200$$
$$= 4.7 \text{ kcal} \cdot \text{min}^{-1})$$

In the initial stages of the program, the weekly net energy expenditure is between 752 and 1040 kcal. In the improvement stage, the exercise intensity, duration, and frequency are progressively increased, and the weekly net caloric expenditure ranges between 1040 and 1874 kcal. Only one variable—intensity, duration, or frequency—should be increased at a time. The variable that is increased during each stage of the progression for this exercise program is indicated by boldface. During the improvement stage, this client's net caloric expenditure due to exercise meets the caloric threshold (>1000 kcal per week from physical activity) recommended by ACSM (2006). In the maintenance phase, tennis and aerobic dancing are added to give variety and to supplement the cycling program. The ACSM (2006) guidelines were followed to calculate each component of this exercise prescription.

Sample Jogging Program

The sample jogging program on page 113 is designed for a 29-year-old male who has an excellent cardiorespiratory fitness level. Since a GXT could not be administered, the $\dot{V}O_2$max was predicted from performance on the 12-min distance run test. The maximal HR was predicted using the formula 220 – age. Because this client is accustomed to jogging and his cardiorespiratory fitness level is classified as excellent, he is exempted from the initial stage and enters the improvement stage of the program immediately. During this time (20 wk), the exercise intensity is increased from 70% to 85% of the estimated $\dot{V}O_2R$. The speed corresponding to each MET intensity is calculated using the ACSM formulas for running on a level course (see table 4.3). The intensity, duration, and frequency of the exercise sessions provide a weekly *net* caloric expenditure between 1010 and 2170 kcal. During the first 4 wk of the program, this client's *net* rate of energy expenditure due to exercise is 10.2 kcal · min⁻¹ (8.3 METs × 3.5 × 70 kg/200 = 10.2 kcal · min⁻¹); thus, he will expend approximately 1010 kcal, jogging 33 min at an 11:06 min per mile pace three times per week (33 min × 10.2 kcal · min⁻¹ × 3). The distance

covered is figured by dividing the exercise duration by the running pace: 33 min/11.1 min · mile⁻¹ = 3 miles. During the improvement stage, the frequency of exercise sessions gradually progresses from 3 to 5 days/wk. During the maintenance stage, the running is reduced to 3 days/wk, and handball and basketball are added to the aerobic exercise program. The ACSM (2006) guidelines were followed to calculate each component of this exercise prescription.

Sample Multimodal Exercise Program

Some clients may prefer to engage in a variety of exercise modes (**cross training**) to develop their cardiorespiratory fitness (see "Sample Multimodal Exercise Program" on p. 114). For these cases, it is difficult to systematically prescribe increments in exercise intensity using METs or target HRs. Although MET equivalents for various activities are available (see appendix E.4, pp. 348-352), typically a range of values is given, making it difficult for you to accurately prescribe work rates corresponding to specific intensity recommendations in an exercise prescription. Also, the HR response to a given MET level is highly dependent on the exercise mode.

The degree of muscle mass involved in the activity, as well as whether the body weight is supported during exercise, can affect the HR response to a prescribed exercise intensity. For example, whole-body exercise modes, such as Nordic skiing and aerobic dancing, involve both upper- and lower-body musculature. These produce higher submaximal HRs than lower-body exercise modes (e.g., cycling and jogging). Also, at any given exercise intensity, the HR response during weight-bearing exercise, such as jogging, is greater than that for non-weight-bearing exercise (e.g., cycling).

Therefore, you should use RPEs to progressively increase exercise intensity throughout the improvement stage of a multimodal aerobic exercise program (see table 4.2). To use the RPE safely and effectively, you will need to teach your clients to focus on and learn to monitor important exertional cues such as breathing effort (rate and depth of breathing) and muscular sensations (e.g., pain, warmth, and fatigue).

Guidelines for developing multimodal exercise prescriptions are presented on page 115. For **multimodal exercise programs**, you should set exercise frequency and weekly *net* caloric expenditure goals for each client (see "Sample Multimodal Exercise Program"). Provide your

Sample Case Study

A 28-year-old female police officer (5 ft 5 in. or 165.1 cm; 140 lb or 63.6 kg, and 28% body fat) has enrolled in the adult fitness program. Her job demands a fairly high level of physical fitness—a level she was able to achieve six years ago when she passed the physical fitness test battery used by the police department. Before becoming a police officer, she jogged 20 min, usually three times a week. Since starting her job, she has had little or no time for exercise and has gained 15 lb (6.8 kg). She works 8 hr a day, is divorced, and takes care of two children, ages 7 and 9. At least three times a week, she and the children dine out, usually at fast-food restaurants like Burger King and Taco Bell. She reports that her job, along with the sole responsibility for raising her two children, is quite stressful. Occasionally she experiences headaches and a tightness in the back of her neck. Usually in the evening she has one glass of wine to relax.

Her medical history reveals that she smoked one pack of cigarettes a day for four years while she was in college. She quit smoking three years ago. The past two years she has tried some quick weight-loss diets, with little success. She was hospitalized on two occasions to give birth to her children. She reports that her father died of heart disease when he was 52 and that her older brother has high blood pressure. Recently she had her blood chemistry analyzed because she was feeling light-headed and dizzy after eating. In an attempt to lose weight, she eats only one large meal a day, at dinnertime. Results of the blood analysis were total cholesterol = 220 mg · dl^{-1}; triglycerides = 98 mg · dl^{-1}; glucose = 82 mg · dl^{-1}; high-density lipoprotein cholesterol = 37 mg · dl^{-1}; and total cholesterol/high-density lipoprotein cholesterol ratio = 5.9.

The exercise evaluation yielded the following data:

- Mode/protocol: Treadmill/modified Bruce
- Resting data: HR = 75 bpm; BP = 140/82 mmHg
- End point: Stage 4 (2.5 mph, 12% grade). Test terminated because of fatigue.

Stage	METs	Duration (min)	HR (bpm)	BP (mmHg)	RPE
1	2.3	3	126	145/78	8
2	3.5	3	142	160/78	11
3	4.6	3	165	172/80	14
4	7.0	3	190	189/82	18

Analysis

1. Evaluate the client's CHD risk profile. Be certain to address each of the positive and negative risk factors.
2. Describe any special problems or limitations that need to be considered in designing an exercise program for this client.
3. Were the HR, BP, and RPE responses to the graded exercise test normal? Explain.
4. What is the client's functional aerobic capacity in METs? Categorize her cardiorespiratory fitness level (see table 4.1)
5. Plot the HR versus METs on graph paper.
6. From the graph, determine the client's target heart rate zone for the aerobic exercise program. What HRs and RPEs correspond to 60%, 70%, and 75% of the client's $\dot{V}O_2R$?
7. The client expressed an interest in walking outside on a level track to develop aerobic fitness. Calculate her walking speed for each of the following training intensities: 60%, 70%, and 75% $\dot{V}O_2R$. Use the ACSM equations presented in table 4.3.
8. In addition to starting an aerobic exercise program, what suggestions do you have for this client for modifying her lifestyle?

See Appendix A.8, page 303, for answers to these questions.

Sample Cycling Program

Client data

Age	27 yr
Gender	Female
Body weight	70 kg (154 lb)
Resting heart rate	67 bpm
Maximal heart rate	195 bpm (measured)
$\dot{V}O_2max$	26 ml·kg⁻¹·min⁻¹ (measured) 7.4 METs
Graded exercise test	Cycle ergometer
Initial cardiorespiratory fitness level	Poor

Exercise prescription

Mode	Stationary cycling
Intensity	60-80% $\dot{V}O_2R$ 16.8-21.4 ml · kg⁻¹ · min⁻¹ 4.8-6.1 METs
Exercise heart rates (from figure 5.3)	139 bpm minimum 168 bpm maximum
RPE	10-16
Duration	40-60 min
Frequency	4-5 days/wk

Cycling Program[a]

Phase (weeks)	Intensity % $\dot{V}O_2R$	METs	HR (bpm)	RPE	Power output (W)	Resistance (kg)	Pedal rate (rpm)	Net kcal · min⁻¹	Time (min)	Frequency	Weekly net expenditure (kcal)
Initial											
1	60	4.8	139	10	63	1.3	50	4.7	40	4	752
2	60	4.8	139	10	63	1.3	50	4.7	**45**	4	846
3	**65**	5.2	150	11	73	1.5	50	5.2	45	4	936
4	65	5.2	150	11	73	1.5	50	5.2	**50**	4	1040
Improvement											
5-8	65-**70**	5.2-5.5	150-155	11-12	73-80	1.5-1.6	50	5.2-5.5	50	4	1040-1103
9-12	65-70	5.2-5.5	150-155	11-12	73-80	1.5-1.6	50	5.2-5.5	**55**	4	1144-1210
13-16	70-**75**	5.5-5.8	152-162	12-14	80-86	1.6-1.7	50	5.5-5.9	55	4	1210-1298
17-20	75	5.8	162	14	86	1.7	50	5.9	**60**	4	1416
21-24	75	5.8	162	14	86	1.7	50	5.9	60	**5**	1770
25-28	**80**	6.1	168	16	93	1.9	50	6.2	60	5	1874
Maintenance											
24+											
Cycling	80	6.1	168	16	93	1.9	50	6.2	60	3	1116
Low-impact aerobics	65% HRR	5.0	150	13-14				4.9	60	1	294
Tennis		7.0		16-18				7.4	60	1	440

[a]Values in boldface indicate training variables that were increased during each stage of the exercise progression.

Sample Jogging Program

Client data

Age	29 years
Gender	Male
Body weight	70 kg (154 lb)
Resting heart rate	50 bpm
Maximal heart rate	191 bpm (age-predicted)
$\dot{V}O_2max$	45 ml · kg^{-1} · min^{-1} (predicted) 12.9 METs
Graded exercise test	None
Initial cardiorespiratory fitness level	Excellent

Exercise prescription

Mode	Jogging and running
Intensity	70-85% $\dot{V}O_2R$ 32.5-38.8 ml · kg^{-1} · min^{-1} 9.3-11.1 METs
Exercise heart rates	149 bpm minimum (70% HRR) 170 bpm maximum (85% HRR)
RPE	12-16
Duration	33-35 min
Frequency	3-5 times/wk

Jogging Program[a]

Phase (weeks)	Intensity % $\dot{V}O_2R$	METs	HR (bpm)	RPE	Pace: mph (min/mile)	Distance (miles)	Net kcal/min	Time (min)	Frequency	Weekly net expenditure (kcal)
Improvement										
1-4	70	9.3	149	12	5.4 (11:06)	3.0	10.2	33	3	1010
5-8	70-**80**	9.3-10.5	149-163	12-13	5.4-6.2 (9:40)	3.0-3.4	10.2-11.6	33	3	1010-1148
9-12	70-80	9.3-10.5	149-163	12-13	5.4-6.2 (9:40)	3.0-3.4	10.2-11.6	33	4	1347-1531
13-16	80-**85**	10.5-11.1	163-170	14-16	6.2-6.6 (9:05)	3.4-3.6	11.6-12.4	33	4	1531-1637
17-20	80-85	10.5-11.1	163-170	14-16	6.2-6.6 (9:05)	3.4-3.8	11.6-12.4	33-**35**	5	1914-2170
Maintenance										
21+										
Jogging	85	11.2	170	14-16	6.6 (9:05)	3.8	12.4	35	3	1302
Handball	60	8.0		12-13			9.2	60	1	552
Basketball	60	8.0		12-13			9.2	60	1	552

[a]Values in boldface indicate training variables that are increased during each stage of the exercise progression.

clients with estimates of *net* energy expenditure (kcal · min^{-1}) for each of the aerobic activities they select for their exercise prescriptions. The exercise duration to achieve a specified weekly *net* caloric expenditure goal will vary depending on the activity mode chosen for each exercise session. Any combination of Group I and II activities can be used, provided that the client is able to maintain the prescribed RPE intensity for at least 20 min.

Flexibility is the key to successful multimodal exercise prescriptions. Clients should be free not only to select exercise modes of interest but also to decide on various combinations of frequency and duration as long as they meet the caloric thresholds specified in their exercise prescriptions for each week.

Sample Multimodal Exercise Program

Client data

Age	44 years
Sex	Female
Weight	68 kg (150 lb)
Resting heart rate	70 bpm
Maximal heart rate	170 bpm
$\dot{V}O_2max$ (measured)	30 ml · kg^{-1} · min^{-1} 8.6 METs
Graded exercise test	Treadmill maximal GXT (Bruce protocol)
Initial cardio-respiratory fitness level	Fair

Exercise prescription

Modes and estimates of gross caloric expenditure (METs) and net caloric expenditure (kcal · min^{-1})[a]	Stationary cycling (100 W): 5.5 METs; 5.4 kcal · min^{-1} Step aerobics (6-8 in. step): 8.5 METs; 8.9 kcal · min^{-1} Rowing (100 W): 7.0 METs; 7.1 kcal · min^{-1} Swimming (moderate effort): 7.0 METs; 9.5 kcal · min^{-1} Stair-climbing (machine): 9.0 METs; 7.1 kcal · min^{-1} Hiking: 6.0 METs; 5.9 kcal · min^{-1} Resistance training (free weights/machines): 3.0 METs; 2.4 kcal · min^{-1}
Intensity	RPE: 10 to 16
Duration	20 to 60 min
Frequency	3 to 5 days/wk
Weekly caloric expenditure	500 to 1250 kcal/wk

Multimodal Exercise Program

Phase (weeks)	Intensity (RPE)	Minimal duration (min)	Minimal frequency	Average kcal/workout	Weekly caloric goal (kcal)
Initial					
1-2	10	20	3	133	500
3-4	10	25	3	200	600
Improvement					
5-8	12	25	3	200	700
9-12	12	30	3	233	800
13-16	12-13	30	4	225	900
17-20	14-15	30	4	250	1000
21-24	15-16	30	5	250	1250
Maintenance					
24+	15-16	30	5	250	1250

Examples

Week 21	Activity	Net kcal · min^{-1} estimates	Time (min)	Frequency	Kcal/work out (net)	Activity group[b]
Monday	Stationary cycling	5.4	20	1	108	I
Wednesday	Step aerobics	8.9	20	1	178	II
Friday	Stair-climbing	9.5	30	1	285	I
	Totals*		70	3	571	3
	Goals		60	3	500	3

Week 21	Activity	Net kcal · min^{-1} estimates	Time (min)	Frequency	Kcal/work out (net)	Activity group[b]
Monday	Swimming	7.1	35	1	248	II
Tuesday	Rowing	7.1	35	1	248	I
Wednesday	Stair-climbing	9.5	30	1	285	I
Friday	Resistance training	2.4	40	1	96	III
Sunday	Hiking	5.9	60	1	354	II
	Totals*		200	5	1231	4
	Goals		150	5	1250	4

[a]Gross MET levels for activities from Ainsworth et al. (2000); net energy expenditure in kcal · min^{-1} = net MET level × 3.5 × body mass (kg)/200.

[b]Check all Group I and II activities.

*Compare weekly totals to goals.

The primary advantages of multimodal exercise programs over single-mode (e.g., jogging or cycling) programs for many of your clients are

- greater likelihood of engaging in a safe and effective exercise program,
- overall greater enjoyment of physical activity and exercise,
- better understanding of how their bodies respond to exercise,
- more direct involvement and sense of control in developing and monitoring their exercise programs, and
- increased likelihood of incorporating physical activity and exercise into their lifestyles.

GUIDELINES FOR MULTIMODAL EXERCISE PRESCRIPTIONS

- Modes: Select at least three per week from Group I and II activities.
- Frequency: Three to seven sessions a week. Engage in either Group I or II activities at least three times per week.
- Intensity: Rating of perceived exertion between 10 and 16.
- Duration: At least 15 min, preferably 20 to 30 min. Duration depends on energy cost ($kcal \cdot min^{-1}$) of exercise mode.
- Caloric expenditure: 1000 to 2000 kcal/wk. Group III activities can be used to reach weekly caloric expenditure goal but cannot be counted as one of the required aerobic activities.

KEY POINTS

- Always personalize cardiorespiratory exercise programs to meet the needs, interests, and abilities of each participant.
- The exercise prescription includes mode, frequency, intensity, duration, and progression of exercise.
- Aerobic endurance activities involving large muscle groups are well suited for developing cardiorespiratory fitness. Group I activities such as walking, jogging, and cycling allow the individual to maintain steady-state exercise intensities and are not highly dependent on skill.
- Exercise intensity can be prescribed using the HR, $\dot{V}O_2R$, or RPE methods, or a combination of these methods.

- For the average healthy person, the cardiorespiratory exercise program should be at an intensity of 60% to 85% $\dot{V}O_2max$, a duration of 20 to 60 min, and a frequency of 3-5 days/wk.
- The cardiorespiratory exercise program includes three stages of progression: initial conditioning, improvement, and maintenance.
- Each exercise session includes warm-up, aerobic conditioning exercise, and cooldown.
- Continuous and discontinuous training methods are equally effective for improving cardiorespiratory fitness.
- Multimodal exercise prescriptions use a variety of Group I and II aerobic activities to improve cardiorespiratory endurance.

KEY TERMS

Learn the definition for each of the following key terms. Definitions of key terms can be found in the glossary on page 379.

caloric threshold	maintenance stage
continuous training	multimodal exercise program
cross training	percent heart rate maximum (%HRmax)
discontinuous training	percent heart rate reserve (%HRR) method
Group I aerobic activities	percent $\dot{V}O_2$max reserve (%$\dot{V}O_2$R)
Group II aerobic activities	pulmonary ventilation
Group III aerobic activities	spinning
heart rate reserve (HRR)	super circuit resistance training
improvement stage	talk test
initial conditioning stage	treading
interval training	ventilatory threshold
Karvonen method	$\dot{V}O_2$ reserve ($\dot{V}O_2$R)

REVIEW QUESTIONS

In addition to being able to define each of the key terms, test your knowledge and understanding of the material by answering the following review questions.

1. Name the four components of any aerobic exercise prescription.

2. What are the guidelines for an exercise prescription for improved health?

3. What are the guidelines for an exercise prescription for cardiorespiratory fitness?

4. Identify the three parts of an aerobic exercise workout and state the purpose of each part.

5. To classify an aerobic exercise mode as either a Group I, II, or III activity, what criteria are used?

6. Give three examples each for Group I, II, and III aerobic activities.

7. Describe three methods used to prescribe intensity for an aerobic exercise prescription.

8. Using the $\dot{V}O_2$ reserve method, calculate the target $\dot{V}O_2$ for a client whose $\dot{V}O_2$max is 12 METs and relative exercise intensity is 70% $\dot{V}O_2$R.

9. Which method of prescribing intensity (%HRR or %HRmax) corresponds 1:1 with the %$\dot{V}O_2$R method?

10. What are the limitations of using HR methods to monitor intensity of aerobic exercise?

11. Describe how RPEs can be used to prescribe and monitor the intensity of aerobic exercise.

12. Describe how your clients can use the talk test to monitor exercise intensity during their aerobic exercise workouts.

13. What target caloric thresholds are recommended by ACSM for aerobic exercise workouts and weekly caloric expenditure from physical activity and exercise?

14. What is the recommended frequency of activity and exercise for improved health benefits? For improved cardiorespiratory fitness?

15. Name the three stages of a cardiorespiratory exercise program. For the average individual, what is the typical length (in weeks) of each stage?

16. What is the difference between continuous and discontinuous aerobic exercise training? Give examples of continuous and discontinuous training methods.

17. What are the essential elements of a client case study?

chapter 6

Assessing Muscular Fitness

Key Questions

- How are strength and muscular endurance assessed?
- How does the type of muscle contraction (concentric, eccentric, or isokinetic) affect force production?
- What test protocols can be used to assess a client's muscular fitness?
- What are the advantages and limitations of using free weights and exercise machines to assess muscular strength?
- What are sources of measurement error for muscular fitness tests, and how are they controlled?
- What are the recommended procedures for administering 1-RM strength tests?
- Is it safe to give 1-RM strength tests to children and older adults?
- What tests can be used to assess the functional strength of older adults?

Muscular strength and endurance are two important components of muscular fitness. Minimal levels of muscular fitness are needed to perform activities of daily living, to maintain functional independence as one ages, and to partake in active leisure-time pursuits without undue stress or fatigue. Adequate levels of muscular fitness lessen the chance of developing low back problems, osteoporotic fractures, and musculoskeletal injuries.

This chapter describes a variety of laboratory and field tests for assessing all forms of muscular strength and endurance. In addition, this chapter compares types of exercise machines, addresses factors affecting muscular fitness tests, discusses sources of measurement error, and provides guidelines for testing muscular fitness of children and older adults.

DEFINITION OF TERMS

Muscular strength is defined as the ability of a muscle group to develop maximal contractile force against a resistance in a single contraction. The force generated by a muscle or muscle group, however, is highly dependent on the velocity of movement. Maximal force is produced when the limb is not rotating (i.e., zero velocity). As the speed of joint rotation increases, the muscular force decreases. Thus, *strength for dynamic movements* is defined as the maximal force generated in a single contraction at a specified velocity (Knuttgen and Kraemer 1987). **Muscular endurance** is the ability of a muscle group to exert submaximal force for extended periods.

Both strength and muscular endurance can be assessed for static and dynamic muscular contractions. If the resistance is immovable, the muscle contraction is **static** or **isometric** ("iso," same; "metric," length), and there is no visible movement of the joint. **Dynamic contractions**, in which there is visible joint movement, are either concentric, eccentric, or isokinetic (see figure 6.1, *a* and *b*).

If the resistance is less than the force produced by the muscle group, the contraction is **concentric**, allowing the muscle to shorten as it exerts tension to move the bony lever. The muscle is also

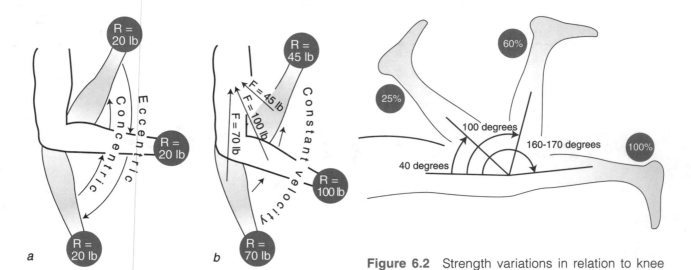

Figure 6.1   Types of muscle contraction.

Figure 6.2   Strength variations in relation to knee joint angle.

capable of exerting tension while lengthening. This is known as **eccentric contraction** and typically occurs when the muscles produce a braking force to decelerate rapidly moving body segments or to resist gravity (e.g., slowly lowering a barbell). Both concentric and eccentric contractions are sometimes called **isotonic** ("iso," same; "tonic," tension). The term "isotonic contraction" is a misnomer because the tension produced by the muscle group fluctuates greatly even though the resistance is constant throughout the range of motion (ROM). This fluctuation in muscular force is due to the change in muscle length and angle of pull as the bony lever is moved, creating a strength curve that is unique for each muscle group (Kreighbaum and Barthels 1981). For example, the strength of the knee flexors is maximal at 160° to 170° (see figure 6.2).

In regular (concentric and eccentric), dynamic exercise, because of the change in mechanical and physiological advantage as the limb is moved, the muscle group is not contracting maximally throughout the ROM. Thus, the greatest resistance that can be used during regular, dynamic exercise is equal to the maximum weight that can be moved at the *weakest* point in the ROM.

Isokinetic contraction (see figure 6.1*b*) is a maximal contraction of a muscle group at a constant velocity throughout the entire range of joint motion ("iso," same; "kinetic," motion). The velocity of contraction is controlled mechanically so that the limb rotates at a set velocity (e.g., $120° \cdot sec^{-1}$). Electromechanical devices vary the resistance to match the muscular force produced at each point in the ROM. Thus, isokinetic exercise machines allow the muscle group to encounter variable but maximal resistances during the movement.

STRENGTH AND MUSCULAR ENDURANCE ASSESSMENT

Measures of static or dynamic strength and endurance are used to establish baseline values before training, monitor progress during training, and assess the overall effectiveness of resistance training and exercise rehabilitation programs. Static strength and muscular endurance are measured using dynamometers, cable tensiometers, and load cells. Free weights (barbells and dumbbells), as well as constant-resistance, variable-resistance, and isokinetic exercise machines, are used to assess dynamic strength and endurance (see table 6.1.). The testing procedures vary depending on the type of test (i.e., strength or endurance) and equipment.

Isometric Muscle Testing Using Dynamometers

You can use isometric dynamometers to measure static strength and endurance of the grip squeezing muscles and leg and back muscles (see figure 6.3). The handgrip dynamometer has an adjustable handle to fit the size of the hand and measures forces between 0 and 100 kilograms (kg), in 1-kg increments. The back and leg dynamometer consists of a scale that measures forces ranging from 0 to 2500 lb in 10-lb increments. Both dynamometers are spring devices. As force is applied to the dynamometer, the spring is compressed and moves the indicator needle a corresponding amount.

TABLE 6.1 Strength Testing Modes

Testing mode	Equipment	Measure*
Static	Isometric dynamometers, cable tensiometers, and load cells	MVC (kg)
Dynamic		
Constant-resistance	Free weights (barbells and dumbbells) and exercise machines	1-RM (lb or kg)
Variable-resistance	Exercise machines	NA
Isokinetic and omnikinetic	Isokinetic and omnikinetic dynamometers	Peak torque (Nm or ft-lb)

*MVC = maximal voluntary contraction; NA = not applicable; Nm = newton-meter; ft-lb = foot-pound.

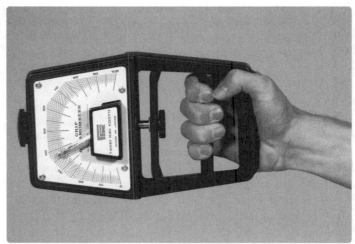

a

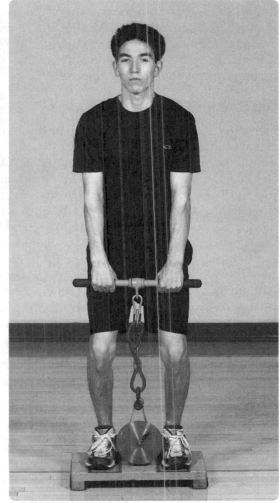

b

Figure 6.3 Dynamometers for measuring static strength and endurance: *(a)* handgrip dynamometer and *(b)* back and leg dynamometer.

Grip Strength Testing Procedures

Before using the handgrip dynamometer, adjust the handgrip size to a position that is comfortable for the individual. Alternatively, you can measure the hand width with a caliper and use this value to set the optimum grip size (Montoye and Faulkner 1964). The individual stands erect, with the arm and forearm positioned as follows (Fess 1992): shoulder adducted and neutrally rotated, elbow flexed at 90°, forearm in the neutral position, and wrist in slight extension (0° to 30°). For some test protocols, however, the client must keep the arm straight and slightly abducted when measuring the grip strength of each hand (Canadian Society for Exercise Physiology 2003). The individual squeezes the dynamometer as hard as possible using one brief maximal contraction and no extraneous body movement. Administer three trials for each hand, allowing a 1-min rest between trials, and use the best score as the client's static strength.

Grip-Endurance Testing Procedures

Once the grip size is adjusted, instruct the client to squeeze the handle as hard as possible and to continue squeezing for 1 min. Record the initial force and the final force exerted at the end of 1 min. The greater the endurance, the less the rate and degree of decline in force. The relative endurance score is the final force divided by the initial force times 100.

Alternatively, you can assess static grip endurance by having your client exert a submaximal force, which is a given percentage of the individual's maximum voluntary contractile (MVC) strength (e.g., 50% MVC). The relative endurance score is the amount of time that this force level is maintained. During the test, the client must watch the dial of the dynamometer and adjust the amount of force exerted as necessary in order to maintain the appropriate submaximal force level.

Leg Strength Testing Procedures

Using the back and leg dynamometer, the individual stands on the platform with trunk erect and the knees flexed to an angle of 130° to 140°. The client holds the hand bar using a pronated grip and positions it across the thighs by adjusting the length of the chain (see figure 6.3*b*). If a belt is available, attach it to each end of the hand bar after positioning the belt around the client's hips. The belt helps to stabilize the bar and to reduce the stress placed on the hands during the leg lift. Without using the back, the client slowly exerts as much force as possible while extending the knees. The maximum indicator needle remains at the peak force achieved. Administer two or three trials with

a 1-min rest interval. Divide the maximum score (in pounds) by 2.2 to convert it to kilograms.

Back Strength Testing Procedures

Using the back and leg dynamometer, the individual stands on the platform with the knees fully extended and the head and trunk erect. The client grasps the hand bar using a pronated grip with the right hand and a supinated grip with the left. Position the hand bar across the client's thighs. Without leaning backward, the client pulls the hand bar straight upward using the back muscles and is instructed to roll the shoulders backward during the pull. Clients should be reminded before lifting to flex the trunk minimally and to keep the head and trunk erect during the test. Administer two trials with a 1-min rest between the trials. Divide the maximum score (in pounds) by 2.2 to convert it to kilograms.

Static Strength Norms

Table 6.2 provides age-gender norms for evaluating the static grip strength of the right and left hands combined. Grip strength norms for each hand are presented in table 6.3. You can also use norms developed for men and women to assess your client's static strength for each dynamometric test item (see table 6.3). Calculate your client's total strength score by adding the right grip, left grip, leg strength, and back strength scores. Before doing this, convert the leg and back strength scores (measured in pounds) to kilograms. To calculate the relative strength score, divide the total strength score by body mass (expressed in kilograms).

TABLE 6.2   Age–Gender Norms for Combined Isometric Grip Strength

| | GRIP STRENGTH (KG)* | | | | | | | | | | | |
| | 15-19 YR | | 20-29 YR | | 30-39 YR | | 40-49 YR | | 50-59 YR | | 60-69 YR | |
Rating	M	F	M	F	M	F	M	F	M	F	M	F
Excellent	≥108	≥68	≥115	≥70	≥115	≥71	≥108	≥69	≥101	≥61	≥100	≥54
Very good	98-107	60-67	104-114	63-69	104-114	63-70	97-107	61-68	92-100	54-60	91-99	48-53
Good	90-97	53-59	95-103	58-62	95-103	58-62	88-96	54-60	84-91	49-53	84-90	45-47
Fair	79-89	48-52	84-94	52-59	84-94	51-57	80-87	49-53	76-83	45-48	73-83	41-44
Needs improvement	≤78	≤47	≤83	≤51	≤83	≤50	≤79	≤48	≤75	≤44	≤72	≤40

*Combined right- and left-hand grip strength scores.
M = males; F = females.

Source: The Canadian Physical Activity, Fitness and Lifestyle Approach: CSEP-Health & Fitness Program's Health-Related Appraisal and Counselling Strategy, 3rd Edition © 2003. Adapted with permission of the Canadian Society for Exercise Physiology.

TABLE 6.3	Static Strength Norms					
Classification	Left grip (kg)	Right grip (kg)	Back strength (kg)	Leg strength (kg)	Total strength (kg)	Relative strength*
MEN						
Excellent	>68	>70	>209	>241	>587	>7.50
Good	56-67	62-69	177-208	214-240	508-586	7.10-7.49
Average	43-55	48-61	126-176	160-213	375-507	5.21-7.09
Below average	39-42	41-47	91-125	137-159	307-374	4.81-5.20
Poor	<39	<41	<91	<137	<307	<4.81
WOMEN						
Excellent	>37	>41	>111	>136	>324	>5.50
Good	34-36	38-40	98-110	114-135	282-323	4.80-5.49
Average	22-33	25-37	52-97	66-113	164-281	2.90-4.79
Below average	18-21	22-24	39-51	49-65	117-163	2.10-2.89
Poor	<18	<22	<39	<49	<117	<2.10

*Relative strength is determined by dividing total strength by body mass (kg).

For persons over age 50, reduce scores by 10% to adjust for muscle tissue loss due to aging. Data from Corbin et al. (1978).

Isometric Muscle Testing Using Cable Tensiometers

You can use cable tensiometry to assess the static strength of 38 different muscle groups throughout the body. Standardized testing procedures have been described elsewhere in detail and should be followed closely to ensure the validity and reliability of the test results (Clarke 1966). The instrumentation includes a tensiometer, steel cables, testing table, wall hooks, straps, and goniometer. Attach one end of the cable to the wall or table hooks and, using a strap, attach the other end to the body part to be tested. Always position the cable at a right angle to the pulling bony lever. Use a goniometer to measure the appropriate joint angle. Place the tensiometer on a taut cable. As the individual exerts force on the cable, the riser of the tensiometer is depressed and a maximum indicator needle registers the static strength score. Tensiometers measure forces ranging between 0 and 400 lb (0 to 181.8 kg). However, the larger tensiometers are less accurate in the lower range; therefore, you should use a small tensiometer, which measures forces between 0 and 100 lb (0 to 45.4 kg), to obtain greater accuracy in the lower range.

Cable tensiometry tests can be used to assess strength impairment at specific joint angles and to monitor progress during rehabilitation. As with all forms of static strength testing, you should be aware that strength is specific to the joint angle and muscle group being tested. Therefore, test at least three to four muscle groups to provide an adequate estimation of static strength.

Test batteries and norms have been developed for males and females 9 years old through college age (Clarke 1975; Clarke and Monroe 1970). The test battery for males of all ages includes the same three strength tests: shoulder extension, knee extension, and ankle plantar flexion. For elementary and junior high school girls, the test battery includes shoulder extension, hip extension, and trunk flexion. The three test items in the battery developed for senior high school and college women are shoulder flexion, hip flexion, and ankle plantar flexion.

Dynamic Muscle Testing Using Constant-Resistance and Variable-Resistance Modes

Although either a constant-resistance or a variable-resistance exercise mode can be used to assess dynamic (concentric and eccentric) muscle strength and endurance, you will be better served if you use either free weights or constant-resistance exercise machines.

A major disadvantage of free weights, dumbbells, and constant-resistance exercise machines, however, is that they measure dynamic strength only at the weakest point in the ROM. The reason is that the resistance cannot be varied to account for fluctuations in muscular force caused by the changing mechanical (angle of pull of muscle) and physiological (length of muscle) advantage of the musculoskeletal system during the movement.

In an attempt to overcome this deficiency, equipment manufacturers have designed variable-resistance machines that vary the resistance during the ROM. Variable-resistance machines have a moving connection (i.e., lever, cam, or pulley) between the resistance and the point of force application. As the weight is lifted, the mechanical advantage of the machine decreases. Therefore, more force must be applied to continue moving the resistance. The variable-resistance mode of exercise attempts to match the force capability of the musculoskeletal system throughout the ROM. However, many variable-resistance exercise machines fail to match the strength curves of different muscle groups. Also, with variable-resistance machines, it is difficult to assess the client's maximal force or strength because the resistance is modified by the levers, pulleys, and cams, causing the movement velocity to vary. Variable-resistance exercise machines, therefore, have limited usefulness for maximal testing. Still, these types of machines are well suited for resistance training.

Although free weights and constant-resistance exercise machines are generally recommended for muscular fitness testing, there are advantages and limitations to each of these modalities. Compared to exercise machines, free weights require more neuromuscular coordination in order to stabilize body parts and maintain balance during lifting of the barbell or dumbbell. While exercise machines may reduce the need for spotting during the test, these machines limit the individual's range of joint motion and plane of movement. Also, some exercise machines have relatively large weight plate increments so that you must attach smaller weights to the weight stack in order to measure your client's strength accurately.

Lastly, some machines cannot accommodate individuals with short limbs; you may need to use child-sized machines to standardize their starting positions for testing. Clients with long limbs or large body and limb circumferences (e.g., some bodybuilders or obese clients) also may have difficulty using standard exercise machines. Body size and weight increments are less of a problem with free weights.

Recently, new constant- and variable-resistance exercise machines have been developed. These **free-motion machines** have adjustable seats, lever arms, and cable pulleys that can be set to exercise muscle groups in multiple planes. Also, these machines can accommodate smaller or larger individuals, are easy to get in and out of, and have smaller weight increments (5 lb or 2.3 kg) than do older standard machines (typically 10 lb or 4.5 kg). When using free-motion exercise machines for muscular fitness testing, take care to adjust the plane of movement and the seat so that you simulate the starting and ending body positions that were used to develop test norms for older constant-resistance machines. If you use free-motion machines to monitor the progress of your clients, make certain that you use the same settings (i.e., seat and plane-of-movement adjustments) for each test session.

Dynamic Strength Tests

Dynamic strength is usually measured as the one-repetition maximum (1-RM), which is the maximum weight that can be lifted for one complete repetition of the movement. The 1-RM strength value is obtained through trial and error.

Although 1-RM strength tests can be safely administered to individuals of all ages, you should take precautions to decrease the risk of injury when clients attempt to lift maximal loads. Be cer-

STEPS FOR 1-RM MAXIMUM TESTING

The following basic steps are recommended for 1-RM testing.

1. Have your client warm up by completing 5 to 10 repetitions of the exercise at 40% to 60% of the estimated 1-RM.

2. During a 1-min rest, have the client stretch the muscle group. This is followed by three to five repetitions of the exercise at 60% to 80% of the estimated 1-RM.

3. Increase the weight conservatively, and have the client attempt the 1-RM lift. If the lift is successful, the client should rest 3 to 5 min before attempting the next weight increment. Follow this procedure until the client fails to complete the lift. The 1-RM typically is achieved within three to five trials.

4. Record the 1-RM value as the maximum weight lifted for the last successful trial.

tain that your client warms up before attempting the lift and starts with a weight that is below the individual's expected 1-RM. When you administer these tests, you should spot your clients and closely monitor their lifting technique and breathing.

The ACSM (2006) recommends the bench press and leg press (upper plate of constant-resistance exercise machine) for assessing strength of the upper and lower body, respectively. To determine **relative strength**, divide the 1-RM values by the client's body mass. Norms for men and women are provided in tables 6.4 and 6.5.

Another test of dynamic strength includes six test items: bench press, arm curl, latissimus pull, leg press, leg extension, and leg curl. For

each exercise, express and evaluate the 1-RM as a percentage of body mass. For example, if a 120-lb (54.5 kg) woman bench presses 60 lb (27.2 kg), her strength-to-body mass ratio is 0.50 (60 divided by 120), and she scores 3 points for that exercise. Follow this procedure for each exercise; then add the total points to determine the overall strength and fitness category of the individual. Strength-to-body mass ratios with corresponding point values for college-age men and women are presented in table 6.6.

Dynamic Muscle Endurance Tests
You can assess your client's dynamic muscle endurance by having the individual perform as

TABLE 6.4 Age-Gender Norms for 1-RM Bench Press (1-RM/BM)

Percentile rankings* for men	AGE				
	20-29	30-39	40-49	50-59	60+
90	1.48	1.24	1.10	0.97	0.89
80	1.32	1.12	1.00	0.90	0.82
70	1.22	1.04	0.93	0.84	0.77
60	1.14	0.98	0.88	0.79	0.72
50	1.06	0.93	0.84	0.75	0.68
40	0.99	0.88	0.80	0.71	0.66
30	0.93	0.83	0.76	0.68	0.63
20	0.88	0.78	0.72	0.63	0.57
10	0.80	0.71	0.65	0.57	0.53

Percentile rankings* for women	AGE					
	20-29	30-39	40-49	50-59	60-69	70+
90	0.54	0.49	0.46	0.40	0.41	0.44
80	0.49	0.45	0.40	0.37	0.38	0.39
70	0.42	0.42	0.38	0.35	0.36	0.33
60	0.41	0.41	0.37	0.33	0.32	0.31
50	0.40	0.38	0.34	0.31	0.30	0.27
40	0.37	0.37	0.32	0.28	0.29	0.25
30	0.35	0.34	0.30	0.26	0.28	0.24
20	0.33	0.32	0.27	0.23	0.26	0.21
10	0.30	0.27	0.23	0.19	0.25	0.20

*Descriptors for percentile rankings: 90 = well above average; 70 = above average; 50 = average; 30 = below average; 10 = well below average.

Data for women provided by the Women's Exercise Research Center, The George Washington University Medical Center, Washington, D.C., 1998.
Data for men provided by The Cooper Institute for Aerobics Research, *The Physical Fitness Specialist Manual.* Author: Dallas, TX. 2005.

TABLE 6.5	Age–Gender Norms for 1-RM Leg Press (1-RM/BM)				
Percentile rankings* for men	**AGE**				
	20-29	**30-39**	**40-49**	**50-59**	**60+**
90	2.27	2.07	1.92	1.80	1.73
80	2.13	1.93	1.82	1.71	1.62
70	2.05	1.85	1.74	1.64	1.56
60	1.97	1.77	1.68	1.58	1.49
50	1.91	1.71	1.62	1.52	1.43
40	1.83	1.65	1.57	1.46	1.38
30	1.74	1.59	1.51	1.39	1.30
20	1.63	1.52	1.44	1.32	1.25
10	1.51	1.43	1.35	1.22	1.16

Percentile rankings* for women	**AGE**					
	20-29	**30-39**	**40-49**	**50-59**	**60-69**	**70+**
90	2.05	1.73	1.63	1.51	1.40	1.27
80	1.66	1.50	1.46	1.30	1.25	1.12
70	1.42	1.47	1.35	1.24	1.18	1.10
60	1.36	1.32	1.26	1.18	1.15	0.95
50	1.32	1.26	1.19	1.09	1.08	0.89
40	1.25	1.21	1.12	1.03	1.04	0.83
30	1.23	1.16	1.03	0.95	0.98	0.82
20	1.13	1.09	0.94	0.86	0.94	0.79
10	1.02	0.94	0.76	0.75	0.84	0.75

*Descriptors for percentile rankings: 90 = well above average; 70 = above average; 50 = average; 30 = below average; 10 = well below average.

Data for women provided by the Women's Exercise Research Center, The George Washington University Medical Center, Washington, D.C., 1998.
Data for men provided by The Cooper Institute for Aerobics Research, *The Physical Fitness Specialist Manual.* Author: Dallas, TX. 2005.

many repetitions as possible using a weight that is a set percentage of the body weight or maximum strength (1-RM). Pollock, Wilmore, and Fox (1978) recommend using a weight that is 70% of the 1-RM value for each exercise. Although norms for this test have not been established, these authors suggest, on the basis of their testing and research findings, that the average individual should be able to complete 12 to 15 repetitions.

The YMCA (Golding 2000) recommends using a bench press test to assess dynamic muscular endurance of the upper body. For this absolute endurance test, use a flat bench and barbell. The client performs as many repetitions as possible at a set cadence of 30 repetitions per minute. Use a metronome to establish the exercise cadence. Male clients lift an 80-lb (36.4 kg) barbell, whereas female clients use a 35-lb (15.9 kg) barbell. Terminate the test when the client is unable to maintain the exercise cadence. Table 6.7 presents norms for this test.

Alternatively, you can use a test battery consisting of seven items to assess dynamic muscular endurance. Select the weight to be lifted using a set percentage of the individual's body mass. The client lifts this weight up to a maximum of 15 repetitions. Table 6.8 provides percentages for each test item, as well as the scoring system and norms for college-age men and women.

TABLE 6.6 Strength-to-Body Mass Ratios for Selected 1-RM Tests						
Bench press	Arm curl	Lat pull-down	Leg press	Leg extension	Leg curl	Points
MEN						
1.50	0.70	1.20	3.00	0.80	0.70	10
1.40	0.65	1.15	2.80	0.75	0.65	9
1.30	0.60	1.10	2.60	0.70	0.60	8
1.20	0.55	1.05	2.40	0.65	0.55	7
1.10	0.50	1.00	2.20	0.60	0.50	6
1.00	0.45	0.95	2.00	0.55	0.45	5
0.90	0.40	0.90	1.80	0.50	0.40	4
0.80	0.35	0.85	1.60	0.45	0.35	3
0.70	0.30	0.80	1.40	0.40	0.30	2
0.60	0.25	0.75	1.20	0.35	0.25	1
WOMEN						
0.90	0.50	0.85	2.70	0.70	0.60	10
0.85	0.45	0.80	2.50	0.65	0.55	9
0.80	0.42	0.75	2.30	0.60	0.52	8
0.70	0.38	0.73	2.10	0.55	0.50	7
0.65	0.35	0.70	2.00	0.52	0.45	6
0.60	0.32	0.65	1.80	0.50	0.40	5
0.55	0.28	0.63	1.60	0.45	0.35	4
0.50	0.25	0.60	1.40	0.40	0.30	3
0.45	0.21	0.55	1.20	0.35	0.25	2
0.35	0.18	0.50	1.00	0.30	0.20	1

Total points	Strength fitness category[a]
48-60	Excellent
37-47	Good
25-36	Average
13-24	Fair
0-12	Poor

[a]Based on data compiled by author for 250 college-age men and women.

Dynamic Muscle Testing Using Isokinetic and Omnikinetic Exercise Modes

Isokinetic dynamometers provide an accurate and reliable assessment of strength, endurance, and power of muscle groups (see figure 6.4). The speed of limb movement is kept at a constant preselected velocity. Any increase in muscular force produces an increased resistance rather than increased acceleration of the limb. Thus, fluctuations in muscular force throughout the ROM are matched by an equal counterforce or accommodating resistance.

Isokinetic dynamometers measure muscular torque production at speeds of 0° to 300° · sec^{-1}. From the recorded output, you can evaluate peak

TABLE 6.7   Muscular Endurance Norms for Bench Press[a]

Percentile	18-25	26-35	36-45	46-55	56-65	>65
	AGE GROUP (yr)					
Men						
95	49	48	41	33	28	22
75	34	30	26	21	17	12
50	26	22	20	13	10	8
25	17	16	12	8	4	3
5	5	4	2	1	0	0
Women						
95	49	46	41	33	29	22
75	30	29	26	20	17	12
50	21	21	17	12	9	6
25	13	13	10	6	4	2
5	2	2	1	0	0	0

[a]Score is number of repetitions completed in 1 min using 80-lb barbell for men and 35-lb barbell for women.

Data from YMCA of the USA, 2002, *YMCA Fitness Testing and Assessment Manual* 4th ed. (Champaign, IL: Human Kinetics).

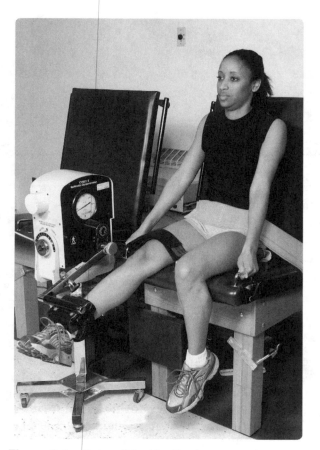

Figure 6.4   Cybex II isokinetic dynamometer.

torque, total work, and power. Some less expensive isokinetic dynamometers lack this recording capability but are suitable for training and rehabilitation exercise.

Omnikinetic exercise dynamometers provide maximum overload at every joint angle throughout the ROM at whatever speed the individual is capable of generating. This testing system provides an accommodating resistance that adjusts to both the force and velocity output of the individual and is not limited to a preset velocity of limb movement. Thus, at any one setting, the individual maximally overloads both the force and velocity production capabilities of the contractile elements. The stronger the individual, the faster the speed of limb movement at any given setting. Also, increasing limb velocity results in increased resistance. Even as the muscle fatigues, the individual receives optimal overload with each repetition because the limb speed and resistance decrease. Theoretically, movement at slower speeds will allow recruitment of motor units that were not contributing to the total force production in earlier repetitions performed at faster speeds. Thus, self-accommodating, variable-resistance–variable-velocity exercise devices assess the isokinetic strength and endurance of both fast-twitch and slow-twitch motor units in the muscle group.

TABLE 6.8	Dynamic Muscular Endurance Test Battery		

	% BODY MASS TO BE LIFTED		
Exercise	**Men**	**Women**	**Repetitions (max = 15)**
Arm curl	0.33	0.25	_____
Bench press	0.66	0.50	_____
Lat pull-down	0.66	0.50	_____
Triceps extension	0.33	0.33	_____
Leg extension	0.50	0.50	_____
Leg curl	0.33	0.33	_____
Bent-knee sit-up			_____
		Total repetitions (max = 105) =	_____

Total repetitions	**Fitness category[a]**
91-105	Excellent
77-90	Very good
63-76	Good
49-62	Fair
35-48	Poor
<35	Very poor

[a]Based on data compiled by author for 250 college-age men and women.

Table 6.9 summarizes isokinetic and omnikinetic test protocols for assessing strength, endurance, and power. For detailed descriptions of isokinetic test protocols and test norms, see Perrin 1993. Appendix C.1, "Average Strength, Endurance, and Power Values for Isokinetic (Omni-Tron) Tests" (p. 316), provides omnikinetic performance norms for young and middle-aged men and women, as well as male and female weight trainers.

Calisthenic-Type Strength and Muscular Endurance Tests

In certain field situations, you may not have access to dynamometers, free weights, or exercise machines to assess muscular fitness. As an alternative, you may use calisthenic-type strength and endurance tests to assess your client's strength and muscular endurance.

Dynamic Strength Tests

You can measure dynamic strength using calisthenic-type exercises by determining the maximum weight, in excess of body mass, that an individual can lift for one repetition of the movement. Because strength is related to the size and body mass of the individual, Johnson and Nelson (1986) recommend using relative strength scores. For each test, attach weight plates (2 1/2, 5, 10, and 25 lb or 1, 2.3, 4.5, and 11.4 kg) to the individual. The relative strength score is the amount of additional weight divided by the body mass. For example, if a 150-lb (68.2 kg) man successfully performs one pull-up with a 30-lb (13.6 kg) weight attached to the waist belt, his relative strength score is 0.20 (30 lb/150 lb). Test protocols and performance norms for the pull-up, dip strength, sit-up, and bench squat are described elsewhere (Johnson and Nelson 1986).

Dynamic Endurance Tests

You can assess dynamic muscular endurance by measuring the maximum number of repetitions of various calisthenic exercises. Pull-up, push-up, and trunk-curl (partial curl-up) tests are widely used for this purpose.

Pull-Up Tests

Pull-up tests may be used to measure the dynamic endurance of the arm and shoulder girdle muscles for individuals who are able to lift their body

TABLE 6.9   Isokinetic and Omnikinetic Test Protocols

Isokinetic tests	Speed setting	Protocol	Measure*
Strength	$30°$ or $60° \cdot sec^{-1}$	2 submax practice trials, followed by 3 maximal trials	Peak torque (ft-lb or Nm)
Endurance	$120°$ to $180° \cdot sec^{-1}$	1 maximal trial	Number of repetitions until torque reaches 50% of initial torque value
Power	$120°$ to $300° \cdot sec^{-1}$	2 submax practice trials, followed by 3 maximal trials	Peak torque (ft-lb or Nm)

Omnikinetic tests	Resistance setting	Protocol	Measure*
Strength	10	3 submax trials at resistance setting 2, followed by 5 maximal trials	Peak torque (ft-lb)
Endurance	3	3 practice trials at resistance setting 2, followed by 20 maximal repetitions	Total work output (ft-lb)
Power	6	3 submax trials, followed by 1 maximal trial	Peak torque or total work (ft-lb)

*ft-lb = foot-pound; Nm = Newton-meter; 1 ft-lb = 0.138 Nm.

weight. For clients who are unable to perform even one pull-up, you can use modified pull-up and flexed-arm hang tests. Baumgartner (1978) developed a modified pull-up that uses an incline board (at a $30°$ angle to the floor) with a pull-up bar at the top. A modified scooter board slides along garage-door tracks attached to the incline board (Baumgartner, East, Frye, Hensley, Knox, and Norton 1984). While lying prone on the scooter board, the client pulls up until his chin is over the pull-up bar. Detailed testing procedures, equipment designs, and performance norms for children, adolescents, and college-age women and men are available (see Baumgartner 1978; Baumgartner et al. 1984).

The flexed-arm hang test is scored as the amount of time that the client maintains the flexed-arm hanging position (i.e., supporting the body weight with the chin over the pull-up bar). Traditionally, a pronated grip on the pull-up bar is used (i.e., overgrip); however, variations of the flexed-arm hang test include using a supinated grip (i.e., undergrip). Although the flexed-arm hang tests isometric endurance of the arm and shoulder girdle musculature, it has been used for more than three decades as a measure of upper-body strength. A recent study of college women showed that flexed-arm hang time relates more to relative strength (1-RM/body mass) than to absolute strength (1-RM) or to dynamic muscle endurance (measured as repetitions to failure at 70% 1-RM)

(Clemons, Duncan, Blanchard, Gatch, Hollander, and Doucer 2004).

Push-Up Tests

The ACSM (2006) and CSEP (2003) recommend using a push-up test to assess endurance of the upper-body musculature. To start, clients lie prone on the mat with their legs together and hands pointing forward under the shoulders. Clients push up from the mat by fully extending the elbows and by using either the toes (for males) or the knees (for females) as the pivot point. The upper body should be kept in a straight line and the head should be kept up. The client returns to the down position, touching the chin to the mat. The stomach and thighs should not touch the mat. Clients perform as many consecutive repetitions (no rest between repetitions) as possible; there is no time limit. Repetitions not meeting the stated criteria should not be counted. Terminate the test when the client strains forcibly or is unable to maintain proper push-up technique over two consecutive repetitions and record the total number of correctly executed repetitions. Table 6.10 provides age-gender norms for the push-up test.

Trunk-Curl Tests

Abdominal muscle endurance tests (e.g., trunk curls, partial curl-ups, and sit-ups) are commonly included in health-related fitness test batteries to identify clients at risk for low back pain or injury due

TABLE 6.10   Age–Gender Norms for Push-Up Test

	AGE (YR)					
	15-19	**20-29**	**30-39**	**40-49**	**50-59**	**60-69**
Men						
Excellent	≥39	≥36	≥30	≥25	≥21	≥18
Very good	29-38	29-35	22-29	17-24	13-20	11-17
Good	23-28	22-28	17-21	13-16	10-12	8-10
Fair	18-22	17-21	12-16	10-12	7-9	5-7
Needs improvement	≤17	≤16	≤11	≤9	≤6	≤4
Women						
Excellent	≥33	≥30	≥27	≥24	≥21	≥17
Very good	25-32	21-29	20-26	15-23	11-20	12-16
Good	18-24	15-20	13-19	11-14	7-10	5-11
Fair	12-17	10-14	8-12	5-10	2-6	2-4
Needs improvement	≤11	≤9	≤7	≤4	≤1	≤1

Source: The Canadian Physical Activity, Fitness & Lifestyle Approach: CSEP-Health & Fitness Program's Health-Related Appraisal and Counselling Strategy, 3rd edition. © 2003. Reprinted with permission of the Canadian Society for Exercise Physiology.

to weak abdominals. However, the validity of these tests as measures of abdominal strength or endurance and as predictors of low back pain is questionable. Most trunk-curl tests are poorly related to abdominal strength ($r_{x,y}$ = –0.21 to 0.36) and only moderately related to abdominal endurance ($r_{x,y}$ = 0.46 to 0.50) (Knudson 2001; Knudson and Johnston 1995). Also, Jackson and colleagues (1998) found no relationship between sit-up test scores and incidence of low back pain. Keep these findings in mind when interpreting the results of these tests.

Trunk-curl tests differ in duration (60-120 sec), cadence (20-25 rep/min), and difficulty. The ACSM (2006) and CSEP (2003) recommend using a timed (1 min) curl-up test with a cadence of 25 rep/min to assess the endurance of the abdominal muscles. For this test, the client lies supine on a mat with the knees flexed to 90°, the legs hip-width apart, and the arms fully extended at the sides with the middle finger of both hands touching a piece of masking tape (the zero mark). Place a second piece of masking tape 10 cm beyond the zero mark and set the metronome to 50 bpm (25 curl-ups per min). Shoes should be worn for this test. Instruct clients to slowly lift their shoulder blades off the mat in time with the metronome. Clients should flex their trunks (curl up) until their fingertips touch the 10 cm mark or their trunk makes a 30° angle with the mat. During the curl-up, the palms of the hands and the heels of the feet must

remain in contact with the mat. On the return, the shoulder blades and head must contact the mat and the fingertips of both hands must touch the zero mark. Score the curl-up test as the total number of consecutive repetitions up to a maximum of 25 in 1 min. Table 6.11 provides age-gender norms for the partial curl-up test.

Other trunk-curl tests use a bench (0.46 m or 18 in. high) to protect the lower back by isolating the abdominal muscles. For these tests, the lower legs rest on the top of the bench and the back of the thighs contacts the bench. Instruct your clients to cross their arms so that each hand holds the opposite elbow. During each curl, their forearms must touch the thighs (concentric phase) and their shoulder blades must touch the floor (eccentric phase). The score is the number of correct repetitions completed in 60, 90, or 120 sec. Use a longer duration (90 or 120 sec) for very fit clients and athletes; use 60 sec for individuals of low or average fitness (Knudson and Johnston 1998).

SOURCES OF MEASUREMENT ERROR IN MUSCULAR FITNESS TESTING

The validity and reliability of strength and muscular endurance measures are affected by client

TABLE 6.11   Age–Gender Norms for Partial Curl-Up Test

	AGE (YR)					
	15-19	20-29	30-39	40-49	50-59	60-69
Men						
Excellent	25	25	25	25	25	25
Very good	23-24	21-24	18-24	18-24	17-24	16-24
Good	21-22	16-20	15-17	13-17	11-16	11-15
Fair	16-20	11-15	11-14	6-12	8-10	6-10
Needs improvement	≤15	≤10	≤10	≤5	≤7	≤5
Women						
Excellent	25	25	25	25	25	25
Very good	22-24	18-24	19-24	19-24	19-24	17-24
Good	17-21	14-17	10-18	11-18	10-18	8-16
Fair	12-16	5-13	6-9	4-10	6-9	3-7
Needs improvement	≤11	≤4	≤5	≤3	≤5	≤2

Source: The Canadian Physical Activity, Fitness & Lifestyle Approach: CSEP-Health & Fitness Program's Health-Related Appraisal and Counselling Strategy, 3rd edition. © 2003. Reprinted with permission of the Canadian Society for Exercise Physiology.

factors, equipment, technician skill, and environmental factors. You must control each of these factors to ensure the accuracy and precision of muscular fitness scores.

Client Factors

Before measuring your client's strength or muscular endurance, familiarize the individual with the equipment and testing procedures. Clients with limited or no prior weightlifting experience need time to practice each lift to control for the effects of learning on performance. You should give even experienced weightlifters time to practice so that you can correct any improper lifting techniques prior to testing.

Muscular fitness tests require clients to give a maximal effort. Therefore, clients should get adequate sleep before performing these tests, and you should restrict the use of drugs and medications that may adversely affect their performance. It is also important that you motivate your clients during testing by encouraging them to do their best and giving them positive feedback after each trial. Adequate rest between trials is necessary in order for clients to obtain scores that truly represent their maximal effort.

Equipment

The design of testing equipment may also affect your client's test scores. Most of the dynamic

strength and muscular endurance protocols and norms presented in this chapter were developed using constant-resistance exercise machines. Therefore you should not use free weights and variable-resistance machines when administering these tests. It is also important to calibrate the equipment and make sure that it is in proper working condition prior to testing. Inspection and maintenance of equipment will increase accuracy and decrease risk of accidents. When selecting exercise machines, make sure that the equipment can be properly adjusted to accommodate varying limb lengths and body sizes. Use equipment specifically designed for smaller individuals when testing children and smaller adults.

Technician Skill

All strength testing should be done by qualified, trained technicians who are knowledgeable about proper lifting and spotting techniques and familiar with standardized testing procedures. Explain and demonstrate the proper lifting technique and then correct any performance errors you see as the client practices. During the test, clients may inadvertently "cheat" by moving extraneous body parts to help lift the weight. Carefully observe the client during the test, focusing on the grip used and the starting position. The type of grip (pronated vs. supinated) has a substantial effect on performance. For example, using a narrow grip instead of a wide grip during a lat pull-down exercise increases the amount of weight that can be lifted. Likewise, the client will be able to produce more force during an arm curl using a supinated grip compared to a pronated grip. The client's starting position may also affect strength scores. During the bench press, for example, eccentric movement (i.e., lowering the weight) prior to the concentric phase of the lift will increase maximal muscular force due to the stretch reflex and the tendency for the client to "bounce" the weight off the chest. To obtain accurate assessments of your client's strength, it is important to standardize starting positions and to follow all testing procedures carefully.

Environmental Factors

Factors such as room temperature and humidity may affect test scores. The room temperature should be 70° to 74° F (21° to 23° C) to maximize subject comfort during testing. Ideally, you want a quiet, clean environment with limited distractions (not an overcrowded weight room, for example). When assessing improvements due to training, remember to pretest and posttest your client at the same time of day to control for diurnal variations in strength.

ADDITIONAL CONSIDERATIONS FOR MUSCULAR FITNESS TESTING

This section addresses a number of additional factors and questions regarding the testing and evaluation of your client's muscular fitness.

■ *How can I estimate my client's 1-RM?*

Although 1-RM tests can be safely administered to clients of all ages, sometimes it is preferable to estimate the 1-RM. 1-RM testing can be time consuming, especially for a large group of clients. Some clients may take 15 min to complete a 1-RM test (multiple attempts and rests). Also, the 1-RM may be underestimated for clients with little or no exercise experience because they are unaccustomed to or may be apprehensive about lifting heavy loads. In these cases, it may be more suitable and practical to estimate 1-RM.

You can estimate the 1-RM of your clients from submaximal muscle endurance tests. Research demonstrates a strong relationship between muscle endurance (measured as the number of repetitions to fatigue) and the percentage of 1-RM lifted (Brzycki 1993). Muscular strength (1-RM) therefore can be predicted from muscular endurance tests

with a fair degree of accuracy (Ball and Rose 1991; Braith, Graves, Leggett, and Pollock 1993; Invergo, Ball, and Looney 1991; Kuramoto and Payne 1995; Mayhew, Ball, Arnold, and Bowen 1992). The most frequently used prediction equations are based on the number of repetitions to fatigue in one set. For example, the Brzycki (1993) equation can be used to estimate 1-RM of men. This equation can be used for any combination of submaximal weights and repetitions to fatigue providing that the repetitions to fatigue do not exceed 10.

$$1\text{-RM} = \text{weight lifted (lb)}/[1.0278 - (\text{reps to fatigue} \times 0.0278)]$$

For example, if your client completes seven repetitions to fatigue during a bench press exercise using a 100-lb barbell, the estimated 1-RM is calculated as follows:

$$1\text{-RM} = 100 \text{ lb}/[1.0278 - (7 \text{ reps} \times 0.0278)]$$

$$= 120 \text{ lb } (54.5 \text{ kg})$$

Brzycki (2000) also suggested using a prediction equation based on the number of repetitions to fatigue obtained in *two* submaximal sets to estimate 1-RM. Any two submaximal sets can be used as long as the number of reps to fatigue does not exceed 10. For example, you can determine your client's 5-RM value, or, the maximum weight that can be lifted for five reps (e.g., 120 lb for five reps) and the 10-RM value (e.g., 80 lb for 10 reps) and use them in the following equation:

$$\text{Predicted 1-RM} = [(SM_1 - SM_2)/(REP_2 - REP_1)] \times (REP_1 - 1) + SM_1$$

$$= [(120 - 80)/(10 - 5)] \times (5 - 1) + 120$$

$$= 152 \text{ lb}$$

In this equation, SM_1 and REP_1 represent the heavier submaximal weight (120 lb) and the respective number of repetitions (5 reps) completed, and SM_2 and REP_2 correspond to the lighter submaximal weight (80 lb) and the respective number of repetitions (10 reps) performed.

Alternatively, you can use the average number of repetitions corresponding to various percentages of 1-RM (see table 6.12). This technique and the Brzycki (1993) equation yield similar 1-RM estimates for lifts between 2-RM and 10-RM. To estimate the 1-RM from 2-RM to 10-RM values, divide the weight lifted by the respective %1-RM, expressed as a decimal (%1-RM/100). For example, a client lifting 100 lb (45.4 kg) for 8 repetitions would have an estimated 1-RM of 125 lb (56.7 kg):

$$1\text{-RM} = 100 \text{ lb}/0.80 \text{ or } 125 \text{ lb } (56.7 \text{ kg})$$

Also, gender-specific prediction equations can be used to estimate upper-body strength (i.e., the 1-RM bench press) from the YMCA bench press test (see p. 126) in younger clients (22-36 yr) (Kim, Mayhew, and Peterson 2002):

For men

Predicted 1-RM (kg) = (1.55 × YMCA test repetitions) + 37.9, $r = 0.87$ and *SEE* = 8.0 kg.

For women

Predicted 1-RM (kg) = (0.31 × YMCA test repetitions) + 19.2, $r = 0.87$ and *SEE* = 3.2 kg.

For example, if a 25-year-old female's YMCA bench press test score is 30 reps, her estimated 1-RM bench press strength is calculated as follows:

Predicted 1-RM (kg) = (0.31 × 30 reps) + 19.2 = 28.5 kg (62.8 lb).

■ *How is muscle balance assessed?*

Muscle strength is important for joint stability; however, a strength imbalance between opposing muscle groups (e.g., quadriceps femoris and hamstrings) may compromise joint stability and increase the risk of musculoskeletal injury. For this reason, experts recommend maintaining a balance in strength between agonist and antagonistic muscle groups.

Muscle balance ratios differ among muscle groups and are affected by the force-velocity of muscle groups at specific joints. To control limb velocity during muscle balance testing, you will do best to use isokinetic dynamometers. In field settings, however, you may obtain a crude index of muscle balance by comparing 1-RM values of muscle groups. Based on isokinetic tests of peak torque production at slow speeds (30° to 60° · sec^{-1}), the following muscle balance ratios are recommended for agonist and antagonistic muscle groups:

Muscle groups	Muscle balance ratio
Hip extensors and flexors	1:1
Elbow extensors and flexors	1:1
Trunk extensors and flexors	1:1
Ankle inverters and everters	1:1
Shoulder flexors and extensors	2:3
Knee extensors and flexors	3:2
Shoulder internal and external rotators	3:2
Ankle plantar flexors and dorsiflexors	3:1

TABLE 6.12 Average Number of Repetitions and %1-RM Values

Repetitions	% 1-RM[a]
1	100
2	95
3	93
4	90
5	87
6	85
7	83
8	80
9	77
10	75

[a]These values may vary slightly for different muscle groups and ages.

Data from Baechle, Earle, and Wathen (2000).

Muscle balance between other pairs of muscle groups is also important. The difference in strength between contralateral (right vs. left sides) muscle groups should be no more than 10% to 15%, and the strength-to-body mass (BM) ratio of the upper-body (bench press 1-RM/BM) should be at least 40% to 60% of the lower-body relative strength (leg press 1-RM/BM). If you detect imbalances, prescribe additional exercises for the weaker muscle groups.

■ *Can strength or muscular endurance be assessed by a single test?*

Strength and endurance are specific to the muscle group, the type of muscular contraction (static or dynamic), the speed of muscular contraction (slow or fast), and the joint angle being tested (static contraction). There is no single test to evaluate total body muscle strength or endurance. Minimally, the strength test battery should include a measure of abdominal, lower-extremity, and upper-extremity strength. In addition, if the individual trains dynamically, select a dynamic, not static, test to assess strength or endurance levels before and after training.

You should also use caution in selecting test items to measure muscle strength. The maximum number of sit-ups, pull-ups, or push-ups that an individual can perform measures muscular endurance, yet maximum-repetition tests have been included in some strength test batteries. This may lead to misinterpretation of the test results.

■ *Should absolute or relative measures be used to classify a client's muscle strength?*

There is a direct relationship between body size and muscle strength. Generally, larger individuals have more muscle mass, and therefore greater strength compared to smaller individuals with less muscle mass.

Because strength directly relates to the body mass and lean body mass of the individual, you should express the test results in relative terms (e.g., 1-RM/BM). This is especially true in comparing your client's score to group norms and in comparing groups or individuals differing in body size and composition (e.g., men vs. women or older vs. younger adults).

Use relative strength scores for assessing individual improvement from training. As a result of resistance training, some individuals may gain body weight while others may lose weight, especially if they are using resistance training as part of a program for weight gain or loss. If you compare the client's relative strength scores (from pre- and posttest training), you will be able to evaluate the change in strength that is independent of a change in body weight.

■ *How can the influence of strength on muscular endurance be controlled?*

Performance on some endurance tests (e.g., pull-ups and push-ups) is highly dependent on the strength of the individual. It is recommended that you use relative endurance tests that are proportional to the body mass or maximum strength of the individual to assess muscle endurance. You cannot use a pull-up test to assess muscular endurance if the individual is not strong enough to lift the body weight for one repetition of that exercise. Therefore, select a modified or submaximal (percentage of body weight) endurance test.

■ *Are there comprehensive norms that can be used to classify muscular fitness levels of diverse population subgroups?*

Strength norms for women (20 to 82 years) were developed for the bench press (1-RM), leg press (1-RM), static grip strength, and push-up tests (Brown and Miller 1998). These norms are based on data obtained from 304 independent-living women attending wellness classes at a university medical center. However, there is a lack of up-to-date endurance norms for men and strength/endurance norms for older men. New norms need to be established for this population in particular.

MUSCULAR FITNESS TESTING OF OLDER ADULTS

It is important to accurately assess the muscular fitness of older individuals. Adequate strength in the upper and lower body lessens risk of falls and injuries associated with falling, reduces age-related loss of bone mineral, maintains lean body tissue, improves glucose utilization, and prevents obesity. Moderate-to-high levels of muscular strength enable older adults to maintain their functional independence and to perform activities of daily living as well as fitness and recreational activities. The following sections address tests that you can use to assess the muscular strength and physical performance of older clients.

Strength Testing of Older Adults

Experts agree that it is safe to administer 1-RM tests to older adults if proper procedures (see "Steps for 1-RM Maximum Testing," p. 122) are followed (Shaw, McCully and Posner 1995). The risk of injury is low, with only 2.4% of older adults (55-80 yr) experiencing an injury during 1-RM assessment (Salem, Wang, and Sigward 2002; Shaw et al. 1995). Salem and colleagues (2002) suggested that at least one pretesting session (i.e. a practice 1-RM test session) is necessary to establish stable baseline 1-RM values for older adults.

Alternatively, you can estimate the 1-RM of older clients from submaximal muscular endurance tests. Kuramoto and Payne (1995) developed prediction equations to estimate 1-RM from a submaximal endurance test in middle-aged and older women. For this endurance protocol, the client completes as many repetitions as possible using a weight equivalent to 45% of her body mass. To estimate 1-RM, use the following equations:

Middle-aged women (40-50 yr)

1-RM = (1.06 × weight lifted in kg) + (0.58 × reps) − (0.20 × age) − 3.41,

r = 0.94 and *SEE* = 1.85 kg.

Older women (60-70 yr)

1-RM = (0.92 × weight lifted in kg) + (0.79 × reps) − 3.73,

r = 0.90 and *SEE* = 2.04 kg.

Knutzen, Brilla, and Caine (1999) tested the validity of selected 1-RM prediction equations for older women (mean age = 69) and men (mean age = 73). On average, these prediction equations underestimated the actual 1-RM for 11 different constant-resistance machine exercises. For exercises such as the biceps curl, the lateral row, the bench press, and ankle plantar and dorsiflexion, the predicted values were on average 0.5 to 3.0 kg less than the actual 1-RM values. However, larger differences (as much as a 10 kg underestimation) were noted for the triceps press-down, the supine leg press, and the hip flexion, extension, abduction, and adduction exercises. The Brzycki (1993) equation gave a closer estimate of actual 1-RMs for hip exercises (extension, flexion, adduction, and abduction) compared to the other equations evaluated; the Wathen (1994a) equation, 1-RM = 100 × weight lifted / [48.8 + 53.8$^{-0.075 \text{(reps)}}$], most closely estimates 1-RM for all upper-body exercises, the leg press, and dorsiflexion exercises. The authors concluded that the actual and predicted 1-RM are close enough to warrant using these prediction equations to determine resistance training intensities (i.e., % 1-RMs) for older adults. In addition, given that the predicted 1-RM values were consistently less than the actual 1-RM values, the resistance training intensity will not likely exceed the prescribed value.

Functional Fitness Testing of Older Adults

Functional fitness is the ability to perform everyday activities safely and independently without undue fatigue (Rikli and Jones 2001). Functional fitness is multidimensional, requiring aerobic endurance, flexibility, balance, agility, and muscular strength. Older individuals with moderate-to-high functional fitness have the ability to perform normal activities of daily living (ADL) such as getting out of a chair or car, climbing stairs, shopping, dressing, and bathing, and these individuals are able to stay strong, active, and independent as they age.

The Senior Fitness Test (Rikli and Jones 2001) assesses the physical capacity and functional fitness of older adults (60-94 yr). This test battery includes two measures of muscular strength: (a) an arm (biceps) curl for upper-body strength (figure 6.5) and (b) a 30 sec chair stand for lower-body strength (figure 6.6).

Arm-Curl Test

Purpose: Assess upper-body strength.

Application: Measure ability to perform ADLs such as lifting and carrying groceries, grandchildren, and pets.

Equipment: You will need a folding or straight-back chair, a stopwatch, and a 5 lb (2.27 kg) dumbbell for women or an 8 lb (3.63 kg) dumbbell for men.

Test Procedures: The client sits in the chair with his back straight and his feet flat on the floor. He holds the dumbbell in his dominant hand using a neutral (handshake) grip and lets his arm hang down at his side (see figure 6.5). For each repetition, the client curls the weight by fully flexing the elbow while supinating the forearm and returns the weight to the starting position by fully extending the elbow and pronating the forearm. Instruct your client to keep his upper arm in contact with his trunk during the test. Have your client perform as many repetitions as possible in 30 sec. Administer 1 trial.

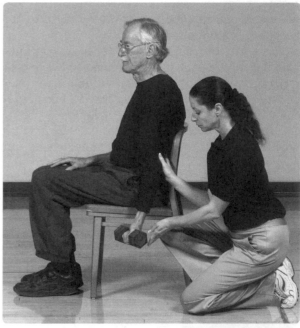

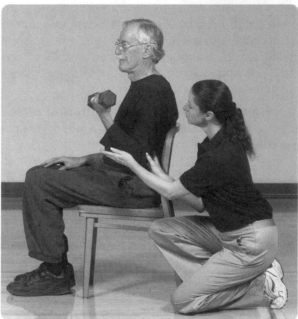

Figure 6.5 Arm-curl test for older adults.

TABLE 6.13 Arm-Curl Test Norms for Older Adults*

Percentile rank	60-64 YR F	60-64 YR M	65-69 YR F	65-69 YR M	70-74 YR F	70-74 YR M	75-79 YR F	75-79 YR M	80-84 YR F	80-84 YR M	85-89 YR F	85-89 YR M	90-94 YR F	90-94 YR M
95	24	27	22	27	22	26	21	24	20	23	18	21	17	18
90	22	25	21	25	20	24	20	22	18	22	17	19	16	16
85	21	24	20	24	19	23	19	21	17	20	16	18	15	16
80	20	23	19	23	18	22	18	20	16	20	15	17	14	15
75	19	22	18	21	17	21	17	19	16	19	15	17	13	14
70	18	21	17	21	17	20	16	19	15	18	14	16	13	14
65	18	21	17	20	16	19	16	18	15	18	14	15	12	13
60	17	20	16	20	16	19	15	17	14	17	13	15	12	13
55	17	20	16	19	15	18	15	17	14	17	13	14	11	12
50	16	19	15	18	14	17	14	16	13	16	12	14	11	12
45	16	18	15	18	14	17	13	16	12	15	12	13	10	12
40	15	18	14	17	13	16	13	15	12	15	11	13	10	11
35	14	17	14	16	13	15	12	14	11	14	11	12	9	11
30	14	17	13	16	12	15	12	14	11	14	10	11	9	10
25	13	16	12	15	12	14	11	13	10	13	10	11	8	10
20	12	15	12	14	11	13	10	12	10	12	9	10	8	9
15	11	14	11	13	10	12	9	11	9	12	8	9	7	8
10	10	13	10	12	9	11	8	10	8	10	7	8	6	8
5	9	11	8	10	8	9	7	9	6	9	6	7	5	6

F = females; M = males.

* Values represent number of repetitions in 30 sec.

Adapted, by permission, from R. Rikli and C. Jones, 2001, *Senior fitness test manual* (Champaign, IL: Human Kinetics).

Scoring: Count the number of repetitions executed in 30 sec. If the forearm is more than halfway up when the time expires, count the move as a complete repetition. Use table 6.13 to determine your client's percentile ranking.

Safety Tips: Before testing, demonstrate the exercise for your client. Have your client perform 1 or 2 repetitions of the exercise without a dumbbell to check body position and lifting technique. Stop the test if the client complains of pain.

Validity and Reliability: Arm-curl test scores were moderately related ($r_{x,y}$ = 0.84 for men and 0.79 for women) to combined 1-RM values for the chest, upper back, and biceps (criterion-related validity). Average arm-curl test scores of physically active older adults were significantly greater than those of sedentary older adults (construct validity). Test–retest reliability was r = 0.81.

30 Sec Chair Stand Test

Purpose: Assess lower-body strength.
Application: Measure ability to perform ADLs such as climbing stairs; getting out of a chair, bathtub, or car; and walking.

Equipment: You will need a folding or straight-back chair (seat height = 17 in. or 43.2 cm) and a stopwatch.

Test Procedures: Place the chair against a wall to prevent slipping. Instruct your client to sit erect in the chair with his feet flat on the floor and his arms crossed at the wrists and held against his chest (see figure 6.6). For each repetition, the client rises to a full stand and then returns to the fully seated starting position. Have your client perform as many repetitions as possible in 30 sec. Administer 1 trial.

Scoring: Count the number of repetitions executed in 30 sec. If the client is more than halfway up when the time expires, count the move as a full stand. Use table 6.14 to determine your client's percentile ranking.

Safety Tips: Brace the chair against a wall, watch for balance problems, and stop the test if the client complains of pain. Before testing, demonstrate the movement slowly to show proper form. Have your client perform 1 or 2 repetitions to check body position (fully standing and fully seated) for the test.

TABLE 6.14   30 Sec Chair Stand Test Norms for Older Adults*

Percentile rank	60-64 YR F	60-64 YR M	65-69 YR F	65-69 YR M	70-74 YR F	70-74 YR M	75-79 YR F	75-79 YR M	80-84 YR F	80-84 YR M	85-89 YR F	85-89 YR M	90-94 YR F	90-94 YR M
95	21	23	19	23	19	21	19	21	18	19	17	19	16	16
90	20	22	18	21	18	20	17	20	17	17	15	17	15	15
85	19	21	17	20	17	19	16	18	16	16	14	16	13	14
80	18	20	16	19	16	18	16	18	15	16	14	15	12	13
75	17	19	16	18	15	17	15	17	14	15	13	14	11	12
70	17	19	15	18	15	17	14	16	13	14	12	13	11	12
65	16	18	15	17	14	16	14	16	13	14	12	13	10	11
60	16	17	14	16	14	16	13	15	12	13	11	12	9	11
55	15	17	14	16	13	15	13	15	12	13	11	12	9	10
50	15	16	14	15	13	14	12	14	11	12	10	11	8	10
45	14	16	13	15	12	14	12	13	11	12	10	11	7	9
40	14	15	13	14	12	13	12	13	10	11	9	10	7	9
35	13	15	12	13	11	13	11	12	10	11	9	9	6	8
30	12	14	12	13	11	12	11	12	9	10	8	9	5	8
25	12	14	11	12	10	11	10	11	9	10	8	8	4	7
20	11	13	11	11	10	11	9	10	8	9	7	7	4	7
15	10	12	10	11	9	10	9	10	7	8	6	6	3	6
10	9	11	9	9	8	9	8	8	6	7	5	5	1	5
5	8	9	8	8	7	8	6	7	4	6	4	4	0	3

F = females; M = males.

*Values represent number of repetitions.

Adapted, by permission, from R. Rikli and C. Jones, 2001, *Senior fitness test manual* (Champaign, IL: Human Kinetics).

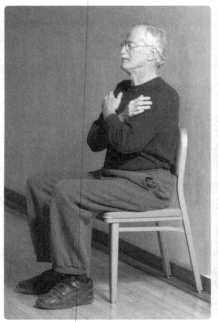 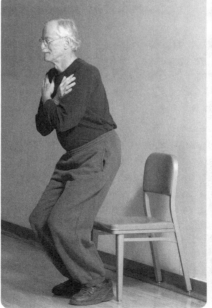 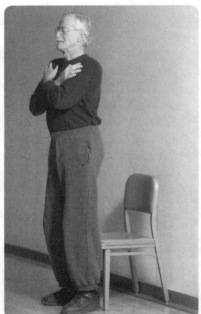

Figure 6.6   30 sec chair stand test for older adults.

Validity and Reliability: Scores for the chair stand test were moderately related to the 1-RM leg press (criterion-related validity) in older men ($r_{x,y} = 0.78$) and women ($r_{x,y} = 0.71$). Average scores were lower for older adults (80+ yr) than for relatively younger adults (60-69 yr) and higher for physically active older adults compared to sedentary older adults (construct validity). Test–retest reliability was $r = 0.86$ and $r = 0.92$ for older men and women, respectively.

MUSCULAR FITNESS TESTING OF CHILDREN

In the past, experts questioned whether or not it was safe to use 1-RM tests to evaluate children. A major concern was the risk of growth plate fractures when the children attempted to lift heavy weights. Experts now agree that it is safe to administer 1-RM tests to children (6-12 yr) if appropriate procedures are followed (Faigenbaum, Milliken, and Westcott 2003).

Results from 1-RM tests may be used to establish baselines for evaluating the progress of children in resistance training programs. You can also use these values to plan a personalized resistance training program for each child, to identify muscle imbalances, and to provide motivation. One shortcoming of 1-RM testing is that it must be closely supervised (one on one) to ensure safety, which limits its usefulness in physical education classes and youth sport programs. Also, child-sized exercise machines must be used; the safety of 1-RM testing using other modes (e.g., dumbbells or barbells) has not been adequately established.

1-RM Testing Guidelines for Children

The following steps are recommended for 1-RM testing of children (Faigenbaum, Milliken, and Westcott 2003):

1. Have a certified, experienced exercise professional administer and closely supervise (one on one) all tests.

2. Before testing, familiarize the children with proper lifting techniques (i.e., proper breathing and controlled movements), allow them to practice these techniques, and answer any questions they may have.

3. Have the child warm up by performing 10 min of low-to-moderate intensity aerobic exercise and stretching.

4. Use dynamic, constant-resistance exercise machines designed specifically for children or individuals with small body frames.

5. Before the 1-RM lift instruct the child to perform 6 repetitions with a relatively light load followed by 3 repetitions with a heavier load. Then gradually increase the weight and have the child attempt the 1-RM lift. Allow at least 2 min of rest between the series of single repetitions with increasing loads. Follow this procedure until the child fails to complete the full range of motion of the exercise for at least two attempts. The 1-RM is typically achieved within 7 to 11 trials.

6. Record the 1-RM as the maximum weight lifted for the last successful trial.

7. After testing, have the child stretch the exercised muscle groups for 5 min.

Sources for Equipment

Product	Supplier's address
Aquatic exercise equipment	Hydro-Fit, Inc. 160 Madison St. Eugene, OR 97402 (800) 346-7295 www.hydrofit.com
Body Masters (constant and variable resistance)	Body Masters Sports Industries, Inc. 700 E. Texas Ave. Rayne, LA 70578 (800) 325-8964 www.body-masters.com

(continued)

Sources for Equipment *(continued)*

Product	Supplier's address
Cable tensiometer (static)	Pacific Scientific Co., Inc. 110 Fordham Rd. Wilmington, MA 01887 (888) 772-6284 www.pacsci.com
CAM II (variable resistance)	Keiser Corp. 2470 S. Cherry Ave. Fresno, CA 93706 (800) 888-7009 www.keiser.com
Cybex II, Orthotron (isokinetic)	Cybex International 10 Trotter Dr. Medway, MA 02053 (508) 533-4300 www.ecybex.com
Exercise/stability balls	FitBALL USA 14215 Mead St. Longmont, CO 80504 (800) 752-2255 www.fitball.com
Free-motion machines (constant and variable resistance)	FreeMotion Fitness 1096 Elkton Dr., Ste. 600 Colorado Springs, CO 80907 (877) 363-8449 www.freemotionfitness.com
Free weights (constant resistance)	York Barbell Co. Box 1707 3300 Board Rd. York, PA 17405 (800) 358-9675 www.yorkbarbell.com
Handgrip dynamometer (static)	Creative Health Products 5148 Saddle Ridge Rd. Plymouth, MI 48170 (800) 742-4478 www.chponline.com
Leg/back dynamometer (static)	Best Priced Products P.O. Box 1174 White Plains, NY 10602 (800) 824-2939 www.best-priced-products.com
Nautilus (variable resistance)	Nautilus Health and Fitness Group 1886 Prairie Way Louisville, CO 80027 (800) 864-1270 www.nautilusgroup.com
Resistance bands/tubing	Creative Health Products 5148 Saddle Ridge Rd. Plymouth, MI 48170 (800) 742-4478 www.chponline.com

Total Gym machines (variable resistance)

Total Gym/EFI
7755 Arjons Dr.
San Diego, CA 92126
(800) 541-4900
www.totalgym.com

Universal Gym machines
(constant and variable resistance)

Universal Gym Equipment
4130 Thomas Dr. SW
Cedar Rapids, IA 52404
(800) 843-3906
www.universalgym.com

KEY POINTS

- Strength is the ability of a muscle group to exert maximal contractile force against a resistance in a single contraction.

- Muscular endurance is the ability of a muscle group to exert submaximal force for an extended duration.

- Both strength and muscular endurance are specific to the muscle group and to the type of muscle contraction—static, concentric, eccentric, or isokinetic.

- The greatest resistance that can be used during dynamic, concentric muscular contraction with a constant-resistance exercise mode is equal to the maximum weight that can be moved at the weakest point in the ROM.

- Dynamometers, cable tensiometers, and load cells are used to measure static strength and endurance.

- Constant-resistance modes of exercise (free weights and exercise machines) are used to assess dynamic (i.e., concentric and eccentric) strength and endurance.

- The accommodating-resistance mode of exercise is used to assess isokinetic and omnikinetic strength, endurance, and power.

- Free-motion machines allow muscle groups to be exercised in multiple planes.

- Calisthenic-type exercise tests provide a crude index of strength and endurance but can be used when other equipment is not available.

- Strength should be expressed relative to the body mass or lean body mass of the individual.

- Muscular endurance tests should take into account the body mass or maximal strength of the individual.

- Test batteries should include a minimum of three to four items that measure upper-body, lower-body, and abdominal strength or endurance.

- It is important to follow standardized testing procedures and to control for extraneous variables (e.g., motivation level, time of testing, isolation of body parts, and joint angles) when assessing strength and muscular endurance.

- It is safe to give 1-RM strength tests to children and older adults if appropriate testing procedures are followed.

- Although strength can be predicted from submaximal endurance tests, 1-RM assessments are preferable.

- Use the arm-curl test and the 30 sec chair stand test to assess the functional strength of older clients.

KEY TERMS

Learn the definition of each of the following key terms. Definitions of terms can be found in the glossary on page 379.

accommodating-resistance exercise

activities of daily living (ADL)

concentric contraction

constant-resistance exercise

dynamic contraction

eccentric contraction

free-motion machines

functional fitness

isokinetic contraction

isometric contraction

isotonic contraction

muscular endurance

muscular strength

omnikinetic exercise

one-repetition maximum (1-RM)

relative strength

static contraction

variable-resistance exercise

REVIEW QUESTIONS

In addition to being able to define each of the key terms, test your knowledge and understanding of the material by answering the following review questions.

1. During dynamic movement, why does muscle force production fluctuate throughout the ROM?

2. Name two methods for assessing static strength and muscular endurance.

3. How do constant-resistance, variable-resistance, accommodating-resistance, and free-motion exercise machines differ?

4. Why are strength test scores typically expressed relative to the client's body mass?

5. Describe the recommended procedures for administering 1-RM strength tests.

6. Identify three sources of measurement error for muscular fitness testing. What can you do to control for these potential errors?

7. Is it safe to give 1-RM tests to children and older adults?

8. Describe two tests that can be used to assess the functional strength of older adults.

9. Why is it important to assess muscle balance?

10. In terms of the specificity principle, explain why a single test cannot be used to adequately assess your client's overall strength. Minimally, what muscle groups should be tested to evaluate overall strength?

11. Identify the test items recommended by ACSM for assessing your client's upper- and lower-body strength.

12. For certain clients, you may choose not to administer 1-RM strength tests. Describe how you could obtain an *estimate* of their strength instead.

chapter 7

Designing Resistance Training Programs

Key Questions

- How do training principles specifically apply to the design of resistance training programs?

- How are resistance training programs modified to optimize the development of strength, muscular endurance, muscle tone, or muscle size?

- What factors do I need to consider when designing individualized exercise prescriptions?

- Is resistance training recommended for children, adolescents, and older adults?

- What methods can be used to design advanced resistance training programs?

- What are the outcomes and health benefits derived from resistance training?

- What is the cause of delayed-onset muscle soreness, and can it be prevented?

Muscular strength and endurance are important to the overall health and physical fitness of your clients, enabling them to engage in physically active leisure-time pursuits, to perform activities of daily living more easily, and to maintain functional independence later in life. Resistance training is a systematic program of exercise for development of the muscular system. Although the primary outcome of resistance training is improved strength and muscular endurance, a number of health benefits are also derived from this form of exercise. Resistance exercise builds bone mass, thereby counteracting the loss of bone mineral (osteoporosis) and risk of falls as one ages. This form of training also lowers blood pressure in hypertensive individuals, reduces body fat levels, and may prevent the development of low back syndrome.

While resistance training has long been widely used by bodybuilders, powerlifters, and competitive athletes to develop strength and muscle size, participation in weightlifting by individuals of all ages and levels of athletic interest has increased dramatically over the past 20 years. The popularity and widespread appeal of weightlifting exercise for general muscle conditioning challenge exercise specialists and personal trainers to develop resistance training programs that can meet the diverse needs of their clients.

This chapter shows you how to apply basic training principles (see chapter 3) to the design of resistance training programs for novice, intermediate, and advanced weightlifters. The chapter also presents guidelines for developing general muscle toning and conditioning, strength and muscular endurance, and muscle size. The chapter addresses various models of periodization, functional training exercise progressions, and guidelines for youth resistance training.

TYPES OF RESISTANCE TRAINING

Muscular fitness can be improved using various types of resistance training—static (isometric), dynamic (concentric and eccentric), and isokinetic. Although there are general guidelines for designing static, dynamic, and isokinetic resistance training programs, each exercise prescription should be individualized to meet the specific needs and goals of your client.

Static (Isometric) Training

In 1953, Hettinger and Muller reported that people produce significant gains in static strength (5% per week) by holding one 6-sec contraction at two-thirds of maximum intensity, 5 days/wk. This type of training became popular in the late 1950s and early 1960s because the exercises could be performed anywhere and at any time with little or no equipment. A major disadvantage is that strength gains are specific to the joint angle used during training (Gardner 1963). Thus, to increase strength throughout the range of motion, the exercise needs to be performed at a number of different joint angles (e.g., 30°, 60°, 90°, 120°, and 180° of knee flexion).

Static exercise is widely used in rehabilitation programs to counteract strength loss and muscle atrophy, especially in cases in which the limb is temporarily immobilized. This type of training, however, is contraindicated for coronary-prone and hypertensive individuals because the static contraction may produce large increases in intrathoracic pressure. This reduces the venous return to the heart, increases the work of the heart, and causes a substantial rise in blood pressure.

After further research, Hettinger and Muller modified their original exercise prescription. Table 7.1 presents the general guidelines for designing training programs for static strength and endurance development. For descriptions and illustrations of static exercises for various muscle groups, see appendix C.2, "Isometric Exercises," page 318.

Dynamic Resistance Training

In recent years, the popularity of dynamic resistance training has risen in the United States. This type of training is suitable for developing muscular fitness of men and women of all ages, as well as children. Dynamic resistance training involves concentric and eccentric contractions of the muscle group performed against a constant or variable resistance. For this type of training, people typically use free weights (barbells and dumbbells) and constant- or variable-resistance machines.

Several important concepts used to prescribe dynamic resistance training programs are intensity, repetitions, set, training volume, and order of exercises (Fleck and Kraemer 1997). Intensity is expressed either as a percentage of the individual's one-repetition maximum (%1-RM) or as the **repetition maximum (RM)**, which is the maximum weight that the person can lift for a given number of repetitions of an exercise (e.g., 8-RM equals the maximum weight that the person can lift for eight repetitions). For the number of repetitions (i.e., 1- to 10-RM) corresponding to various percentages of 1-RM (i.e., 75 to 100% 1-RM), see table 6.12, page 132. The %1-RM values and average number of repetitions for intensities less than 75% 1-RM are as follows:

60% 1-RM = 15- to 20-RM

65% 1-RM = 14-RM

70% 1-RM = 12-RM

Intensity is inversely related to repetitions. In other words, individuals are able to perform more **repetitions** using lighter resistance or weights and fewer repetitions using heavier resistance. A **set** consists of a given number of consecutive repetitions of the exercise. **Training volume** is the total amount of weight lifted during the workout and is calculated by summing the products of the weight lifted, repetitions, and sets for each exercise.

The optimal training stimulus for developing muscular strength or endurance is controversial. Some research supports the conventional prescription of **high intensity-low repetition** resistance exercise for strength development and **low intensity-high repetition** exercise for muscular endurance (Kraemer et al. 2002; Kraemer and Ratamess 2004). Contrary to this traditional approach, the ACSM (2006) supports the position that muscular strength and endurance develop *simultaneously* over a wide range of repetitions (3 to 20) provided that

---

TABLE 7.1   Guidelines for Designing Static (Isometric) Training Programs

Type	Intensity	Duration	Repetitions	Frequency (days/week)	Length of program
Static strength	100% MVC*	5 sec/contraction	5-10	5	4 wk or more
Static endurance	60% MVC or less	Until fatigued	1/session	5	4 wk or more

*Maximal voluntary contraction.

the resistance exercise (whether 3-6, 8-12, or 12-15 repetitions) is performed at a high intensity (i.e., to the point of muscular fatigue or failure). To develop the strength and muscular endurance of healthy individuals, the ACSM (2006) recommends 8 to 12 repetitions performed at high intensity. Table 7.2 summarizes the ACSM (2006) guidelines for the resistance training of healthy populations.

Although this training stimulus may be sufficient for beginner and novice lifters, experts recommend that resistance training programs be tailored to the specific goals of intermediate and advanced lifters (Kraemer et al. 2002; Kraemer and Ratamess 2004). You can design programs to optimize the development of muscle strength, size (hypertrophy), endurance, or power by varying the intensity, repetitions, sets, and frequency of training. Tables 7.3 to 7.5 present guidelines for designing programs for novice, intermediate, and advanced weightlifters. For descriptions of dynamic resistance training exercises, see appendix C.3, "Dynamic Resistance Training Exercises," page 322.

Intensity

As previously mentioned, the %1-RM and RM are widely used to estimate intensity for resistance training programs. The ACSM (2006), however, has stated that the %1-RM does not accurately estimate intensity because the number of repetitions performed at a given %1-RM varies among muscle groups and individuals. Still, many experts endorse the %1-RM to prescribe intensity (Kraemer et al. 2002).

The mean optimal intensity for developing strength ranges between 60% and 100% 1-RM. At these intensities, most individuals are able to perform 1 to 12 repetitions (1-RM to 12-RM). The client's experience with resistance training dictates the optimal intensity for developing strength. Generally, you should prescribe intensities of 60% to 70% 1-RM for novice lifters, 70% to 85% 1-RM for intermediate lifters, and 80% to 100% 1-RM for advanced lifters (Kraemer et al. 2002; Kraemer and Ratamess 2004). Recent meta-analyses support these recommendations. Rhea, Alvar, Burkett, and Ball (2003) reported that the optimal intensity for strength gains in untrained (< 1 yr of resistance training) and trained (> 1 yr) lifters differs (60% 1-RM and 80% 1-RM, respectively). For competitive athletes (college and professional), the optimal training intensity is 85% 1-RM (Peterson, Rhea, and Alvar 2004). Keep in mind that these

---

TABLE 7.2   ACSM Guidelines for Resistance Training of Healthy Populations

Goal	Intensity	Repetitions	Sets	Frequency	Number of exercises[c]
Total body strength and muscular endurance	High[a] (RPE = 19-20)	Variable[b] (3-20), typically 8-12	1	2-3 nonconsecutive days	8-10

[a]To point of momentary muscular fatigue or failure.
[b]Any common range of repetitions (3-6, 8-12, 12-15, 15-20) that can be performed at a moderate pace (~3 sec for concentric phase and ~3 sec for eccentric phase) for the exercise set.
[c]Perform a different exercise for a specific muscle group every 2 to 3 sessions.

ACSM 2006

TABLE 7.3   Guidelines for Resistance Training Programs for Novice Lifters

Goal	Intensity	Volume	Velocity	Frequency	Rest interval
Strength	60-70% 1-RM	1-3 sets of 8-12 reps	Slow to moderate	2-3 days/wk	2-3 min MJ; 1-2 min SJ
Hypertrophy	70-85% 1-RM	1-3 sets of 8-12 reps	Slow to moderate	2-3 days/wk	1-2 min
Endurance	50-70% 1-RM	1-3 sets of 10-15 reps	Slow	2-3 days/wk	1-2 min
Power	>80% 1-RM for strength; 30-60% 1-RM for speed	1-3 sets of 3-6 reps	Moderate	2-3 days/wk	2-3 min for core exercises

MJ = multijoint exercise; SJ = single-joint exercise.

Kraemer et al. 2002

TABLE 7.4   Guidelines for Resistance Training Programs for Intermediate Lifters

Goal	Intensity	Volume	Velocity	Frequency	Rest interval
Strength	70-80% 1-RM	1-3 sets of 6-12 reps	Moderate	2-3 days/wk for whole-body workouts; 3-4 days/wk for split workouts	2-3 min MJ; 1-2 min SJ
Hypertrophy	70-85% 1-RM	1-3 sets of 1-12 reps	Slow to moderate	2-4 days/wk	1-2 min
Endurance	50-70% 1-RM	1-3 sets of 10-15 reps	Slow for medium reps; moderate for high reps	2-4 days/wk	<1 min
Power	>80% 1-RM for strength; 30-60% 1-RM for speed	1-3 sets of 3-6 reps	Fast	2-4 days/wk	2-3 min MJ; 1-2 min SJ

MJ = multijoint exercise; SJ = single-joint exercise.

Kraemer et al. 2002

TABLE 7.5   Guidelines for Resistance Training Programs for Advanced Lifters

Goal	Intensity	Volume	Velocity	Frequency	Rest interval
Strength	80-100% 1-RM, periodized	Multiple sets of 1-12 reps, periodized	Slow to fast	4-6 days/wk	2-3 min MJ; 1-2 min SJ
Hypertrophy	70-100% 1-RM	3-6 sets of 1-12 reps,[a] periodized	Slow to moderate	4-6 days/wk	2-3 min MJ; 1-2 min SJ
Endurance	30-80% 1-RM	Multiple sets of 10-25 reps	Slow for 10-15 reps; moderate to fast for 15-25 reps	4-6 days/wk	<1 min for 10-15 reps; 1-2 min for 15-25 reps
Power	85-100% 1-RM for strength; 30-60% 1-RM for speed	3-6 sets of 1-6 reps, periodized	Fast	4-6 days/wk	2-3 min MJ; 1-2 min SJ

MJ = multijoint exercise; SJ = single-joint exercise.
[a]Greater emphasis on 6-RM to 12-RM.
For power, emphasize MJ exercises. For strength, hypertrophy, and endurance, use both MJ and SJ exercises; perform MJ before SJ exercises. Exercise larger muscle groups before smaller muscle groups.

Kraemer et al. 2002

intensities are averages. Throughout the strength training program, intensity needs to be varied for continued improvement.

To develop muscular endurance, prescribe an intensity of <60% 1-RM. Although low-to-moderate intensity best suits muscle endurance and toning, it also brings some strength gains. The degree and rate of strength gain, however, will be less than that experienced with a program designed to optimize strength development (specificity principle).

Sets

The optimal number of sets for improving muscular strength is controversial and depends on your client's goal; 1 to 2 sets for children and older adults and 1 to 3 sets for novice and intermediate lifters are recommended (Kraemer et al. 2002). Some studies suggest that single sets (1 set per exercise) are just as effective as multiple sets (2-3 sets per exercise) for increasing the strength of untrained and recreational lifters during the first 3 to 4 mo of resistance training (Feigenbaum and Pollock 1999; Hass, Garzarella, DeHoyas, and Pollock. 2000). A major advantage of single-set programs is that they require much less time for a training session than do multiple-set programs (20 vs. 50 min), potentially increasing your client's compliance. The ACSM (2006) recommends prescribing one set performed to the point of volitional fatigue for each exercise (see table 7.2)

However, the results of a recent meta-analysis of 140 strength training studies do not support prescribing single-set programs to develop the strength of untrained and trained recreational lifters (Rhea, Alvar, et al. 2003). Traditionally, a *set* refers to the number of consecutive repetitions performed for a specific *exercise;* however, Rhea, Alvar, and colleagues (2003) noted that the total number of sets performed for a specific *muscle group* is a better indicator of training stress than sets per exercise. Using this definition of sets, they reported that an average of 4 sets during each training session optimizes strength development in untrained and trained lifters. For single-set programs, the authors suggest prescribing multiple exercises for a specific muscle group in order to reach the goal of 4 sets.

Multiple sets using periodization are recommended for serious athletes, powerlifters, and bodybuilders engaging in advanced strength training and hypertrophy programs (Kraemer et al. 2002). To optimize the strength gains of collegiate and professional athletes, an average of 8 sets per muscle group is recommended (Peterson et al. 2004).

Frequency

Muscular fitness may improve from exercising just 1 day/wk, especially in clients with below-average muscular fitness. Recent research, however, suggests that the optimal frequency of strength training for untrained individuals is 3 days/wk. For healthy populations, the ACSM (2006) recommends 2 to 3 nonconsecutive days per week. For advanced lifters, 4 to 6 training sessions per week and split routines are recommended (Kraemer et al. 2002). To optimize the strength gains of trained recreational lifters and competitive athletes, each *muscle group* should be exercised twice a week (Rhea, Alvar, et al. 2003; Peterson et al. 2004). Advanced lifters and competitive athletes who train 4 to 6 days/wk can accomplish this goal by using split routines (see p. 146, "Variations in Frequency"). You should prescribe 48 hr of rest between workouts to allow the muscles to recuperate and to prevent injury from overtraining.

Volume

Training volume is the sum of the repetitions performed during each training session multiplied by the resistance used (Kraemer et al. 2002). Throughout the resistance training program, volume and intensity must be systematically increased (progression principle) to avoid plateaus and to ensure continued strength improvements. You can alter training volume by changing the number of exercises performed for each session, the number of repetitions performed for each set, or the number of sets performed for each exercise. Several models of periodized training can be used to systematically vary volume and intensity (see p. 147, "Periodization").

Order of Exercises

A well-rounded resistance training program should include at least one exercise for each of the major muscle groups in the body. In this way, **muscle balance**—that is, the ratio of strength between opposing muscle groups (agonists vs. antagonists), contralateral muscle groups (right vs. left side), and upper- and lower-body muscle groups can be maintained. Order the exercises so that your client first executes multijoint exercises—such as the seated leg press, bench press, and lat pull-down—that involve larger muscles (e.g., gluteus maximus, pectoralis major, and latissimus dorsi) and more muscle groups. Then have your client progress to single-joint exercises for smaller muscle groups (see table 7.6). To avoid muscle fatigue in novice weight lifters, arrange the exercises so that successive exercises do not involve the same muscle group. This allows time for the muscle to recover.

Dynamic Resistance Training Methods

You can use a variety of methods to design dynamic resistance training programs. The majority of these methods are best suited for advanced programs. Each uses a different approach for prescribing sets, order of exercises, or frequency of workouts.

Variations for Sets

You can use either a single set or multiple sets of exercise. For multiple sets, you may choose to have your client consecutively perform a designated number of sets (usually three or more) at a constant intensity (e.g., 10-RM) for each exercise. Alternatively, you may have your client perform one set of three different exercises for the same muscle group. For example, instead of three consecutive

Body segment	Type of exercise*	Joint actions	Exercise
1. Hips and thighs	Multijoint	Hip extension and knee extension	Seated leg press
2. Chest	Multijoint	Shoulder horizontal flexion and elbow extension	Flat bench press
3. Upper and midback	Multijoint	Shoulder extension/adduction and elbow flexion	Lat pull-down
4. Legs	Single joint	Knee extension	Leg extension
5. Shoulders and upper arms	Multijoint	Shoulder abduction and elbow flexion	Upright row
6. Lower back	Multijoint	Trunk extension and hip extension	Back extension
7. Upper arms	Single joint	Elbow extension	Triceps push-down
8. Leg	Single joint	Knee flexion	Leg curl
9. Upper arms	Single joint	Elbow flexion	Arm curl
10. Calves	Single joint	Ankle plantar flexion	Toe raise
11. Forearms	Single joint	Wrist flexion and extension	Wrist curl
12. Abdomen	Single joint	Trunk flexion	Curl-up

TABLE 7.6   Example of Exercise Order for a Basic Resistance Training Program

*Multijoint exercises involving larger muscle groups are followed by single-joint exercises for smaller muscle groups.

sets of barbell curls for the elbow flexors, you may prescribe one set of incline dumbbell curls, one set of hammer curls, and one set of barbell curls. This adds variety to the program and changes the training stimulus because different muscles or parts of a muscle are used to perform each of these exercises.

A client performing multiple sets of a given exercise may choose to lift the same weight for each set or to vary the intensity of each set by lifting progressively heavier (light-to-heavy sets) or lighter (heavy-to-light sets) weights. **Pyramiding** is a light-to-heavy system in which the client performs as many as six sets of each exercise. In the first set, the client lifts a relatively lighter weight for 10 to 12 repetitions (10- to 12-RM). In subsequent sets the individual lifts progressively heavier weights (i.e., 8-RM, 6-RM, and 4-RM). Because this involves such a large volume of work, you should prescribe the pyramid system for experienced weightlifters only. Bodybuilders commonly use this system to develop muscle size.

Variations for Order and Number of Exercises

Exercise scientists generally recommend ordering the exercises so that large muscle groups are exercised at the beginning of the workout with progression to smaller muscle groups later in the workout. To maximize the overload of muscle groups, however, some clients may choose to pre-exhaust muscle groups by reversing this order. To do this, the individual fatigues smaller muscles by using single-joint exercises prior to performing multijoint exercises.

When you prescribe two or more exercises for a specific muscle group, instruct the average individual to alternate muscle groups so that the muscle can rest and recover between exercises. For example, your client should not perform leg press and leg extension exercises consecutively because the quadriceps femoris is used in both of these exercises. Instead, intersperse one or more exercises using different muscle groups between these two exercises.

In contrast, many advanced weightlifters prefer to do **compound sets** or **tri-sets** in order to completely fatigue a targeted muscle group. To use this training system, the client performs two (compound sets) or three (tri-sets) exercises consecutively for the same muscle group, with little or no rest between the exercises. Many bodybuilders also use a training system called **supersetting**. For supersets, the client exercises agonistic and antagonistic muscle groups consecutively without resting. For example, to superset the quadriceps femoris and hamstrings, follow a leg extension set immediately with a leg curl set.

Variations for Frequency

Traditionally for advanced resistance training programs, exercise scientists have recommended resistance training three times per week on alternate days (e.g., M-W-F) to allow the muscles time to recover. For individuals who want to resistance train 4 to 6 days/wk, prescribe a **split routine**. With a split routine, you are targeting different muscle groups on consecutive days, thereby allowing at least one day of recovery for each muscle group. For example, a bodybuilder may exercise the chest and shoulders on Monday and Thursday, the hips and legs on Tuesday and Friday, and the back and arms on Wednesday and Saturday.

Periodization

Periodization systematically varies the intensity and volume of resistance training. The goal of periodization is twofold: (1) to maximize the response of the neuromuscular system (i.e., gains in strength, endurance, power, and hypertrophy) by systematically changing the training or exercise stimulus and (2) to minimize overtraining and injury by planning rest and recovery. The training stimulus may be varied by manipulations in one or more of the following program variables:

- Training volume (number of sets, repetitions, or exercises)
- Training intensity (amount of resistance)
- Type of contraction (concentric, eccentric, or isometric)
- Training frequency

Given the number of program variables, there are numerous possibilities for designing periodized programs. At present, researchers are trying to identify combinations that optimize the training stimulus for developing strength and muscular endurance (Rhea, Ball, Phillips, and Burkett 2002; Rhea, Phillips, et al. 2003).

The recommended amounts of rest between sets and exercises depend on exercise intensity; a lower intensity requires shorter rests and vice versa (see "Exercise Intensity and Recommended Rest Periods," below). In strength or power training, rests should last at least 3 to 5 min to allow resynthesis of adenosine triphosphate (ATP) and creatine phosphate (CP) and to prevent excessive accumulation of muscle and blood lactate (Kraemer 2003).

Three common periodization models are linear periodization (LP), reverse linear periodization (RLP), and undulating periodization (UP). All periodized training programs are divided into periods, or cycles; however, the duration and the training stimulus differ depending on the model used.

Classic Linear Periodization Model

The classic **linear periodization (LP)** model is divided into three types of cycles. The **macrocycle** (usually 9-12 mo) is divided into **mesocycles** that last 3 to 4 mo. Mesocycles are subdivided into **microcycles** lasting 1 to 4 wk. Within and between cycles, training intensity increases as training volume decreases. For example, a 3 mo (12 wk) mesocycle can be divided into three 4 wk microcycles as follows: during wk 1-4, 3 sets are performed at 12-RM or 70% 1-RM; during wk 5-8, 3 sets are performed at 10-RM or 75% 1-RM; and during wk 9-12, 3 sets are performed at 8-RM or 80% 1-RM (see "Sample Linear Periodized (LP) Resistance Training Program for Intermediate Lifter," p. 154). The training intensity increases from 70% 1-RM (12-RM) to 80% 1-RM (8-RM) while the training volume systematically decreases due to the progressive reduction in the number of repetitions (from 12 to 8) performed during each microcycle.

Reverse Linear Periodization Model

The **reverse linear periodization (RLP)** model reverses the progression of the LP training stimulus. Between and within cycles, training intensity decreases as training volume increases. The RLP configuration of the mesocycles and microcycles is as follows: wk 1-4, 3 sets at 80% 1-RM (8-RM); wk 5-8, 3 sets at 75% 1-RM (10-RM); and wk 9-12, 3 sets at 70% 1-RM (12-RM). As you can see, the training intensity decreases from 80% to 70% 1-RM (8-RM to 12-RM) as the training volume increases (from 8 to 12 reps) during the three progressive microcycles.

Undulating Periodization Models

Compared to those in LP and RLP, the microcycles for **undulating periodization (UP)** are considerably shorter (biweekly, weekly, or even daily) so that they frequently change the training stimulus (intensity and volume). Your client may progress from high volume–low intensity to low volume–high intensity in the same week. For example, in a 3 days/wk UP program, the individual may perform 3 sets of 8-RM (high volume–low intensity) on day 1, 3 sets of 6-RM on day 2, and 3 sets of 4-RM on

Exercise Intensity and Recommended Rest Periods (Kraemer 2003)

Intensity	Length of rest
>13-RM ~ <65% 1-RM	<1 min
11-RM to 13-RM ~ 65 to 74% 1-RM	1-2 min
8-RM to 10-RM ~ 75 to 80 % 1-RM	2-3 min
5-RM to 7-RM ~ 76 to 87% 1-RM	3-5 min
<5-RM ~ >87% 1-RM	>5 min

day 3 (low volume–high intensity). In subsequent microcycles (each week) this training stimulus could be repeated or it could be varied to change the order of the training stimulus (e.g., day 1 = 4-RM, day 2 = 6-RM, and day 3 = 8-RM). One advantage of the UP program is that the training volume and intensity change frequently, subjecting the exercising muscles to a different training stimulus on a daily or weekly basis. As such, UP may avoid plateaus in training and maintain the client's interest and motivation for long-term resistance training.

Circuit Resistance Training

Circuit resistance training is a method of dynamic resistance training designed to increase strength, muscular endurance, and cardiorespiratory endurance (Gettman and Pollock 1981). Circuit resistance training compares favorably with the traditional resistance training programs for increasing muscle strength, especially if low-repetition, high-resistance exercises are used (Gettman, Ayres, Pollock, and Jackson 1978; Wilmore et al. 1978).

A circuit resistance training program usually has 10 to 15 stations per circuit (see figure 7.1). The circuit is repeated two to three times so that the total time of continuous exercise is 20 to 30 min. At each exercise station, select a resistance that fatigues the muscle group in approximately 30 sec (as many repetitions as possible at approximately 40% to 55% of 1-RM). Include a 15- to 20-sec rest period between exercise stations. Circuit resistance training is usually performed 3 days/wk for at least 6 wk. This method of training is ideal for clients with a limited amount of time for exercise. As mentioned in chapter 5, you can add aerobic exercise stations to the circuit between each weightlifting station (i.e., super circuit resistance training) to obtain additional cardiorespiratory benefits.

Functional Training

In recent years, functional training has gained popularity and recognition, especially in health and fitness clubs. Its goal is to train and develop muscles so that performing everyday activities is easier, safer, and more efficient (Yoke and Kennedy 2004). **Functional training** is a system of exercise progressions for specific muscle groups that uses a six step approach developed by Yoke and Kennedy (2004). The difficulty (strength) and skill (balance and coordination) levels of specific

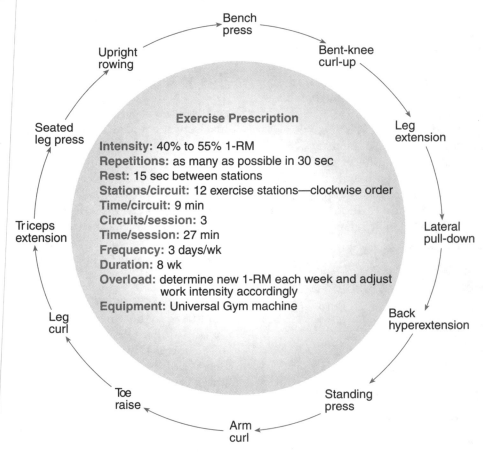

Exercise Prescription

Intensity: 40% to 55% 1-RM
Repetitions: as many as possible in 30 sec
Rest: 15 sec between stations
Stations/circuit: 12 exercise stations—clockwise order
Time/circuit: 9 min
Circuits/session: 3
Time/session: 27 min
Frequency: 3 days/wk
Duration: 8 wk
Overload: determine new 1-RM each week and adjust work intensity accordingly
Equipment: Universal Gym machine

Figure 7.1 Sample circuit resistance training program. 1-RM = one-repetition maximum.

exercises are rated, with 1 representing the least difficult exercises (requiring less strength and skill) and 6 the most difficult exercises (requiring more strength and skill). As the difficulty of the exercises progresses, greater strength, balance, core stability, and coordination are required. The hardest exercises (6 rating) require the most **core stability**, or the ability to maintain the ideal alignment of the neck, spine, scapulae, and pelvis while performing an exercise or a sport skill. To maintain proper postural alignment, the strength of the core muscle groups (erector spinae and abdominal prime movers and stabilizers) needs to be developed (**core strengthening**). Because core stability is dynamic, changing with body position during exercise, isolated core strengthening does not automatically increase core stability unless it is accompanied by motor skill training (Yessis 2003). Functional exercise progressions are designed to develop the strength and function of all muscle groups, not just core muscles. For an outline and example of functional exercise progressions, see "Functional Exercise Progressions: Six-Step Approach and Example," page 150.

It is not necessary for every client to progress to the most difficult levels (5 and 6) on the exercise continuum. Safety is of utmost importance. Be certain that your clients are able to perform exercises with proper form and postural alignment for the duration of the set before progressing to the next level. Your clients' ability to perform each level of exercise depends on their fitness and skill levels. Level 6 exercises are designed to challenge competitive athletes or very fit individuals with excellent balance, strength, motor skill, and core stability. Although functional training potentially adds variety and challenge to workouts, research is needed to compare its effectiveness to that of conventional strength and muscular endurance training. Improvements in strength, endurance, balance, flexibility, and coordination as well as in functional performance of everyday tasks need to be evaluated. For more information, detailed descriptions, and illustrations of functional exercise progressions for all muscle groups, see Yoke and Kennedy (2004).

Isokinetic Training

Isokinetic exercise combines the advantages of dynamic (full range of motion) and static (maximum force exerted) exercise. Since the resistance is accommodating, isokinetic training overcomes the problems associated with using either a constant- or variable-resistance exercise mode. You can use isokinetic training to increase strength, power, and muscular endurance. Isokinetic training involves dynamic, shortening contractions of the muscle group against an accommodating resistance that matches the force produced by the muscle group throughout the entire range of motion. The speed of the movement is controlled mechanically by the isokinetic exercise device. Isokinetic dynamometers are used for isokinetic training. If this equipment is not available, exercises can be done with a partner who offers accommodating resistance to the movement. The speed of the movement, however, is not precisely controlled.

Isokinetic training is done at speeds that vary between 24° and 300° · sec^{-1}, depending on the needs of the individual. The carryover effect appears to be greater when a person trains at faster speeds (180° to 300° · sec^{-1}) as compared to slower speeds (30° to 60° · sec^{-1}). In some studies, strength gains have been limited to velocities at or below the training velocity (Lesmes, Costill, Coyle, and Fink 1978; Moffroid and Whipple 1970). Other researchers have reported significant strength gains at all testing velocities (30° to 300° · sec^{-1}) for high-velocity training groups (240° to 300° · sec^{-1}) (Coyle et al. 1981; Jenkins, Thackaberry, and Killian 1984). Additional research is needed to settle this issue. Table 7.7 presents general guidelines for designing isokinetic training programs for the development of strength and endurance.

A major advantage of isokinetic training over traditional forms of training is that little or no muscle soreness results because the muscles do not contract eccentrically. Isokinetic training is not the best choice, however, when the goal of training is an increase in muscle size. Eccentric contractions are apparently essential for muscle hypertrophy (Cote et al. 1988; Hather, Tesch, Buchanan, and Dudley 1991). Cote et al. (1988) reported no change in muscle fiber cross-sectional area during isokinetic training even though the strength of the quadriceps femoris increased 54%.

DEVELOPING RESISTANCE TRAINING PROGRAMS

Before designing a resistance training program for your client, review training principles and determine how each of these principles can be incorporated into your client's program. The training program needs to be individualized. By varying the combination of intensity, duration, and frequency of exercise, you can develop programs that meet the unique goals and needs of each client. Be sure to follow guidelines and recommendations for resistance training programs (see tables 7.2-7.5, p. 143-144), as well as specific recommendations and precautions, when developing resistance training programs for children and older adults.

Application of Training Principles to Resistance Exercise

To develop effective resistance training programs, you must apply each of the training principles presented in chapter 3 (see p. 43-44). This section

Functional Exercise Progressions: Six-Step Approach and Example

Step	Aim	Body position/resistance	Example for knee extensors
1. Isolate and educate	Teach client to focus on individual muscle action and to selectively contract or isolate the specific muscle group	Lying supine or prone on bench or floor	Lying supine with knees bent, hips flexed to 45°, and arms at sides, client extends the knee one leg at a time.
2. Add resistance	Increase resistance by using exercise machines, longer lever length, or elastic tubing	Sitting on bench or floor	Sitting upright on a bench with elastic tubing attached to the ankle, client extends the knee one leg at a time.
3. Add functional training positions	Decrease supporting base to require greater use of stabilizing muscles	Sitting or standing	Supported at low back level by a stability ball pressed against the wall, with pelvis and spine in neutral position, feet shoulder-width apart and far enough away from wall so that knees flex no more than 90° during exercise, client squats, not allowing hips to drop below the knees.
4. Combine increased function with resistance	Overload core stabilizers in functional positions	Using exercise machines, free weights, or elastic exercise bands to increase resistance	With exercise band attached to ankles, client stands in upright, neutral spine position, balancing on support leg with exercise leg flexed at hip and knee slightly flexed. Client flexes the hip while extending the knee of the exercise leg.
5. Exercise multiple muscle groups with increased resistance and core challenge	Increase demand on strength, balance, coordination, and core stability	Using multijoint exercise machines to increase resistance	Using seated, lying, or standing leg-press machine, client extends hips and knees simultaneously.
6. Add balance, increased function, speed, or rotation	Increase demand on balance, speed, and joint rotation	Using smaller or moving base of support such as stability balls and balance boards or discs; using free weights (barbells or dumbbells) to increase resistance	Standing in upright position with one hand on wall or support bar and holding dumbbell in other hand, client extends hip and places one leg on stability ball. Client rolls the back leg backward on the ball, flexing the knee (no more than 90°) of the opposite leg while keeping the pelvis and spine in a neutral position and the shoulders and hips squared. Client returns to starting position by extending the knee of exercising leg and rolling opposite leg forward on top of the ball.

TABLE 7.7 Guidelines for Designing Isokinetic Training Programs						
Type	Intensity	Repetitions	Sets	Speed	Frequency	Length of program
Isokinetic strength	Maximum contraction	2-15	3	24-180° · sec^{-1}	3-5 days/wk	6 wk or more
Isokinetic endurance	Maximum contraction	Until fatigued	1	≥180° · sec^{-1}	3-5 days/wk	6 wk or more

reviews some of the more pertinent training principles and outlines how these principles are applied to the design of resistance training programs.

Specificity Principle

The development of muscular fitness is specific to the muscle group that is exercised, the type of contraction, and training intensity. To increase the dynamic strength of the elbow flexors, for example, you must select exercises that involve the concentric and eccentric contraction of that particular muscle group. For strength, the person performs exercises at a high intensity with low repetitions; exercising at a low intensity with high repetitions stimulates the development of muscular endurance.

Strength and endurance gains are also specific to the speed and range of motion used during the training. With isometric training, strength gains at angles other than the training angle are typically 50% less than those at the exercised angle (Gardner 1963). Similarly, as previously noted, strength gains in isokinetic training may be limited to velocities at or below the training velocity (Lesmes et al. 1978; Moffroid and Whipple 1970).

Overload Principle

To promote strength and endurance gains, the muscle group must be exercised at workloads that are greater than normal for the client. The exercise intensity should be at least 60% of maximum to stimulate the development of strength (McArdle, Katch, and Katch 1996). More rapid strength gains may be achieved, however, by exercising the muscle at or near maximum (80% to 100%) resistance. To stimulate endurance gains, intensities as low as 30% of maximum may be used; however, at low intensities the muscle group should be exercised to the point of fatigue.

Progression Principle

Generally, throughout the resistance training program, you must periodically increase the training volume, or total amount of work performed, to continue overloading the muscle so that the person can make further improvements in strength

and muscular endurance. The progression needs to be gradual because doing too much too soon may cause musculoskeletal injuries and excessive muscle soreness. Typically you progressively overload muscle groups by increasing the resistance or amount of weight lifted. As clients adapt to the training stimulus, they will be able to perform more repetitions at the prescribed resistance. Thus, the number of repetitions a client is able to perform will indicate when it is necessary to increase the resistance throughout the training program.

Additional Principles

Individuals with lower initial strength will show greater relative gains and a faster rate of improvement in response to resistance training than those starting out with higher strength levels (principles of initial values and interindividual variability). However, the rate of improvement slows, and eventually plateaus, as clients progress through the program and move closer to their genetic ceiling (principle of diminishing returns). Also, when the individual stops resistance training, the physiological adaptations and improvements in muscle structure and function are reversed (principle of reversibility). Using periodization techniques (see "Periodization" on p. 147), you can lessen the effects of detraining on athletes and maintain strength gains during the competitive period by manipulating the intensity and volume of the resistance training exercise (see Wathen 1994b).

General Procedures and Sample Resistance Training Programs

After assessing your client's muscular fitness, you can individualize the resistance training exercise prescription to meet the needs and interests of each client by using the steps outlined on p. 152.

The first example, on page 153, describes a beginning resistance training program developed for an older man (70 yr) with no previous weightlifting experience. The primary goal for this program is to develop adequate muscular fitness so that the client can retain functional independence. This program follows the guidelines suggested by ACSM (2006) for designing resistance training programs for older adults. During the first 4 wk of training, low-intensity (30% to 40% 1-RM), high-repetition (15 to 20 repetitions) exercises familiarize the client with weightlifting exercise and reduce the chance of injury and excessive muscle soreness. The client gradually increases the resistance so that by the end of this phase, the exercise intensity is 50% 1-RM. After 8 wk, the intensity starts at 50% 1-RM and gradually increases to 75% 1-RM. The client does 1 to 2 sets of 10 to 15 repetitions for each exercise. To overload the muscles during this phase, he increases the resistance gradually, but only after he is able to complete 15 or more repetitions at the prescribed relative intensity. This program includes multijoint exercises using exercise machines only (no free weights). The client exercises two times a week, allowing at least two days of rest between each workout.

The second program (see p. 154) is for a 25-year-old woman whose primary goal is to improve muscle strength. This client is an experienced weightlifter. Results from her 1-RM tests indicated that her upper-body strength (particularly the shoulder flexor and forearm flexor muscle groups) is below average. Therefore, two exercises are prescribed for each of the weaker muscle groups. The strength of all other muscle groups is average or above average; therefore, only one exercise is prescribed for each of these muscle groups. Given her initial strength levels and weightlifting experience, the prescription is for three sets of each exercise; and the exercise intensity is set at 70% to 80% 1-RM. To maximize the development of strength. The client completes about eight repetitions at the prescribed intensity for each microcycle. She devotes 50 to 60 min, 3 days/wk, to her workouts.

The third example (see p. 155) illustrates an advanced resistance training program developed for an experienced weightlifter (28-year-old male with superior strength) whose long-term goal is competitive bodybuilding. He engages in a high-volume undulating periodized training program. The intensity (70%-85% 1-RM) and moderate repetitions (6 to 12 reps) vary systematically throughout each macro- and microcycle to maximize the development of muscle size. To achieve a high training volume, he performs three exercises for each muscle group and 3 to 4 sets of each exercise. To effectively overload the muscles, he performs three exercises for each muscle group consecutively (tri-sets) with little or no rest between the sets. He lifts weights 6 days/wk, splitting the routine so that he is not exercising the same muscle groups on consecutive days. With this routine, each muscle group is exercised two times a week.

Several excellent references deal with the design of advanced resistance training programs (Baechle 1994; Bompa, Di Pasquale, and Cornacchia 2003; Fleck and Kraemer 1997; Zatsiorsky 1995).

Designing Resistance Training Programs for Children

Children and adolescents can safely participate in resistance training if special precautions and recommended guidelines are carefully followed (ACSM 2006). Because children are anatomically and physiologically immature, high-resistance

---

STEPS FOR DEVELOPING A RESISTANCE TRAINING PROGRAM

These steps were used to design the sample dynamic resistance training programs on pages 153-155.

1. In consultation with your clients, identify the primary goal of the program (i.e., strength, muscular endurance, muscle size, or muscle toning) and ask clients how much time they are willing to commit to this program.

2. Based on your client's goal, time commitment, and access to equipment, determine the type of resistance training program (i.e., dynamic, static, or isokinetic).

3. Using results from your client's muscular fitness assessment, identify specific muscle groups that need to be targeted in the exercise prescription.

4. In addition to core exercises for the major muscle groups, select exercises for those muscle groups targeted in step 3.

5. For novice weightlifters, order the exercises so the same muscle group is not exercised consecutively.

6. Based on your client's goals, determine appropriate starting loads, repetitions, and sets for each exercise.

7. Set guidelines for progressively overloading each muscle group.

Sample Resistance Training Program for Older Adult

Client data

Age	70 yr	*Intensity*	30-50% 1-RM for first 8 weeks; 50-75% 1-RM thereafter
Gender	Male		
Body weight	160 lb (72.7 kg)	*Frequency*	2 days/wk; at least 48 hr between workouts
Program goal	Muscle fitness and functional independence	*Duration*	16 wk or longer
		Overload	Increase reps first; only increase resistance when able to complete >15 reps
Time commitment	20-30 min/workout		
Equipment	Exercise machines	*Rest*	2-3 min between exercises

Training program

Exercise[a]	1-RM (lb)*	Weeks[b]	Intensity[c] (%1-RM)	Weight* (lb)	Reps	Sets	Muscle groups
Leg press (seated)	180	1-4	30-40	55-70	15-20	1	Hip extensors, knee extensors
		5-8	40-50	72-90	15-20	1	
		9-12	50-60	90-110	10-15	1	
		13-16	60-75	110-135	10-15	1	
Chest flys (seated)	90	1-4	30-40	30-36	15-20	1	Shoulder flexors and adductors
		5-8	40-50	36-45	15-20	1	
		9-12	50-60	45-54	10-15	1	
		13-16	60-75	54-68	10-15	1	
Leg curl (seated)	45	1-4	30-40	13-18	15-20	1	Knee flexors
		5-8	40-50	18-22	15-20	1	
		9-12	50-60	22-27	10-15	1	
		13-16	60-75	27-34	10-15	1	
Lat pull-down	100	1-4	30-40	30-40	15-20	1	Shoulder extensors and adductors, elbow flexors
		5-8	40-50	40-50	15-20	1	
		9-12	50-60	50-60	10-15	1	
		13-16	60-75	60-75	10-15	1	
Shoulder press (seated)	50	1-4	30-40	15-20	15-20	1	Shoulder flexors and abductors, elbow extensors
		5-8	40-50	20-25	15-20	1	
		9-12	50-60	25-30	10-15	1	
		13-16	60-75	30-38	10-15	1	
Heel (calf) raises (seated)	90	1-4	30-40	27-36	15-20	1	Ankle plantar flexors
		5-8	40-50	36-45	15-20	1	
		9-12	50-60	45-54	10-15	1	
		13-16	60-75	54-68	10-15	1	
Abdominal curls	–	1-4	–	Body weight	5-10	1-2	Trunk flexors
		5-8			10-15	1-2	
		9-12			15-20	1-2	
		13-16			20-25	1-2	

[a]Multijoint exercise machines are used for most exercises. Seated and lying (instead of standing) positions are recommended to stabilize the body during lifting. Exercises should be done in the order listed.

[b]During first 2 wk, closely monitor and supervise workouts. Initial training lasts 8 wk.

[c]Intensity is gradually increased every 2 wk, only after client is able to do more than the prescribed number of repetitions at each target intensity.

*1 lb = 0.45 kg.

Client data

Age	25 yr	Cycles	3; each microcycle = 4 wk
Gender	Female	Intensity	70-80% 1-RM
Body weight	155 lb (70.4 kg)	Repetitions	8-12
Program goal	Muscle strength	Sets	3
Time commitment	50-60 min/workout	Rest	1-2 min for 70% 1-RM; 2-3 min for 75-80% 1-RM
Equipment	Variable-resistance machines and free weights	Frequency	3 days/wk, alternate days
		Duration	12 wk or longer

LP training program

Exercise[a]	1-RM (lb)[b]	Cycle 1 wk 1-4			Cycle 2 wk 5-8			Cycle 3 wk 9-12			Sets	Muscle groups
		Int	Wt[b]	Rep	Int	Wt[b]	Rep	Int	Wt[b]	Rep		
Leg press	200	70	140	12	75	150	10	80	160	8	3	Hip extensors, knee extensors
Bench press*	100	70	70	12	75	75	10	80	80	8	3	Shoulder flexors and adductors, elbow extensors
Leg curl (lying)	80	70	55	12	75	60	10	80	65	8	3	Knee flexors
Lat pull-down	140	70	100	12	75	105	10	80	110	8	3	Shoulder extensors and adductors, elbow flexors
Dumbbell fly* (flat bench)	40	70	25	12	75	30	10	80	35	8	3	Shoulder flexors and adductors
Heel (calf) raise (standing)	160	70	110	12	75	120	10	80	130	8	3	Ankle plantar flexors
Abdominal curl	—									25	3	Trunk flexors
Arm curl* (incline bench)	40	70	25	12	75	30	10	80	35	8	3	Elbow flexors
Lateral raise (dumbbell)	25	70	15	12	75	15-20	10	80	20	8	3	Shoulder abductors
Triceps press-down	60	70	40	12	75	45	10	80	50	8	3	Elbow extensors
Hammer curl* (dumbbells)	40	70	25	12	75	30	10	80	35	8	3	Elbow flexors

Int = %1-RM; Wt = weight lifted; Rep = number of repetitions.

[a]Do exercises in order listed, using larger muscle groups first. Perform multijoint exercises before single-joint exercises. Other exercises that work the same muscle groups may be substituted to add variety to the program (see appendix C.3, "Dynamic Resistance Training Exercises," p. 322).

[b]1 lb = 0.45 kg; weight is to nearest 5 lb increment for most exercises.

*Two exercises are prescribed for each of the weaker muscle groups (shoulder flexors and elbow flexors) identified from her strength assessment.

Sample Undulating Periodized (UP) Resistance Training Program for Bodybuilder

Client data

Age	28 yr	*Mesocycles*	4; each mesocycle = 1 mo
Gender	Male	*Microcycles*	4; each microcycle = 1 wk
Body weight	190 lb (86.2 kg)	*Intensity*	70-85% 1-RM
Program goal	Hypertrophy	*Repetitions*	6-12
Time commitment	90 min/workout	*Sets*	3-4
Equipment	Free weights and exercise machines	*Rest*	1 min between tri-sets
		Frequency	6 days/wk, split routine
		Duration	24 wk or longer

UP mesocycles and microcycles

	Intensity	Volume
Month 1		
Week 1	70% 1-RM	3-4 sets; 12 reps
Week 2	75% 1-RM	3-4 sets; 10 reps
Week 3	80% 1-RM	3-4 sets; 8 reps
Week 4	85% 1-RM	3-4 sets; 6 reps
Month 2		
Week 1	75% 1-RM	3-4 sets; 10 reps
Week 2	80% 1-RM	3-4 sets; 8 reps
Week 3	85% 1-RM	3-4 sets; 6 reps
Week 4	70% 1-RM	3-4 sets; 12 reps
Month 3		
Week 1	80% 1-RM	3-4 sets; 8 reps
Week 2	85% 1-RM	3-4 sets; 6 reps
Week 3	70% 1-RM	3-4 sets; 12 reps
Week 4	75% 1-RM	3-4 sets; 10 reps
Month 4		
Week 1	85% 1-RM	3-4 sets; 6 reps
Week 2	80% 1-RM	3-4 sets; 8 reps
Week 3	75% 1-RM	3-4 sets; 10 reps
Week 4	70% 1-RM	3-4 sets; 12 reps

(continued)

Split routine using tri-sets

Exercises	1RM (lb)[c]	Muscles
Monday & Thursday[a]		
Chest[b]		
Flat bench press (barbell)	250	Pectoralis major (midsternal portion); triceps brachii
Incline dumbbell fly	80	Pectoralis major (clavicular portion); anterior deltoid
Decline bench press (barbell)	180	Pectoralis major (lower sternal portion)
Shoulders[b]		
Upright row (barbell)	140	Middle deltoid
Front dumbbell raises	80	Anterior deltoid
Posterior cable pull (horizontal plane)	100	Posterior deltoid
Tuesday & Friday[a]		
Hips and thighs[a]		
First tri-set		
Squats (Smith machine)	300	Gluteus maximus; quadriceps femoris; upper hamstrings
Leg extension (machine)	150	Quadriceps femoris
Leg curl (standing, unilateral, machine)	90	Hamstrings (mid-to-lower portions)
Second tri-set		
Leg press (seated)	400	Gluteus maximus; quadriceps femoris; upper hamstrings
Leg curl (lying)	130	Hamstrings (mid-to-lower portions)
Glut-ham raise	—	Gluteus maximus; hamstrings
Leg and calves[b]		
Standing calf (heel) raise	250	Gastrocnemius; soleus
Ankle flexion exercise (seated)	90	Tibialis anterior
Seated calf raise	180	Soleus; gastrocnemius
Wednesday & Saturday[a]		
Back[b]		
Lat pull-down (wide grip)	225	Latissimus dorsi (lateral portions); biceps brachii; brachialis
Seated row (narrow grip)	240	Latissimus dorsi (midportion); biceps brachii; brachialis
Dumbbell row	90	Latissimus dorsi (midportion); biceps brachii; brachialis
Elbow flexors[b]		
Standing barbell curl	130	Biceps brachii; brachialis; brachioradialis
Preacher curl (dumbbells)	100	Biceps brachii (mid portion); brachialis
Hammer curl (dumbbells)	80	Brachioradialis; brachialis
Elbow extensors[b]		
Lying triceps extension (barbell)	120	Triceps brachii (long head)
Triceps push-down (cables)	150	Triceps brachii (short and lateral heads)
Triceps pull-down with lateral flair (cables)	130	Triceps brachii (lateral head)

[a]Other exercises that work same muscles may be substituted on the second day to add variety to the program (see appendix C.3, "Dynamic Resistance Training Exercises," p. 322).

[b]For tri-sets, the 3 exercises listed are performed consecutively without rest, and then the tri-set is repeated for the prescribed number of sets for that muscle group (1 min rest between sets).

[c]1 lb = 0.45 kg.

training programs are not typically recommended for them. Most experts agree that to lessen the risk of injury (e.g., epiphyseal growth plate fractures) to developing bones and joints, exercise intensity should not exceed 80% 1-RM, which equates to 8 to 15 repetitions per set. Faigenbaum, Westcott, Loud, and Long (1999) reported that high repetition–moderate intensity training (1 set, 13-RM to 15-RM) was more effective than low repetition–high intensity training (1 set, 6-RM to 8-RM) for improving the strength and muscle endurance of children (5-12 yr) during the initial training phase (8 wk). Strength gains in resistance-trained children result from neural adaptations (e.g., increased activation of motor units and coordination) rather than from hypertrophy (Guy and Micheli 2001). In addition, resistance training positively affects the bone mineral density of the femoral neck in adolescent girls ages 14 to 17 yr (Nichols, Sanborn, and Love 2001). There is no evidence that children lose flexibility when they resistance train (Guy and Micheli

2001). Resistance training is safe and beneficial for youth, especially when the established training guidelines are followed (see "Youth Resistance Training Guidelines," below).

Designing Resistance Training Programs for Older Adults

Resistance training provides many health benefits, especially for older adults. The primary goal of the resistance training program is to develop sufficient muscular fitness so that older adults may carry out activities of daily living without undue stress or fatigue and may retain their functional independence.

In addition to increasing strength and muscular endurance, resistance training may improve the performance of functional tasks such as lifting and reaching, rising from the floor or a chair to a standing position, stair-climbing, and walking (Henwood and Taaffe 2003; Messier, Royer, Craven, O'Toole,

Youth Resistance Training Guidelines

- Provide qualified instruction and supervision.
- Provide an exercise environment that is safe and free of hazards.
- Teach clients about the benefits and risks of strength training.
- Design a comprehensive program that focuses on developing muscular fitness and motor skills.
- Begin each workout with a 5 to 10 min warm-up.
- Select 8 to 10 multijoint exercises for major muscle groups; include exercises for the abdominals and lower back.
- Use equipment that is appropriate for the size, strength, and maturity of the child.
- Start with 1 light set of 10 to 15 repetitions for each exercise.
- Slowly progress to 2 or 3 sets at 60% to 80% 1-RM, or 8-RM to 15-RM, depending on the child's needs and goals; as strength improves, increase the number of repetitions before increasing resistance.
- Increase resistance gradually and only when the child can perform the specified number of repetitions with good form.
- Reduce the resistance for prepubescent children who cannot perform a minimum of 8 repetitions with good form.
- Prescribe low-repetition (<8 reps) exercises for mature adolescents only.
- Focus on correct exercise technique (slow and smooth movements and breathing) instead of amount of weight lifted.
- Train 2 to 3 times per week on nonconsecutive days.
- Closely supervise the child in the event of a failed repetition.
- Monitor progress (e.g., use workout logs), listen to the child's concerns, and answer questions.
- Systematically vary the training program to keep it fresh and challenging by adding new exercises, changing the number of sets and repetitions, and incorporating calisthenics as well as exercises using elastic tubing and fitness balls.
- Focus on participation and provide positive reinforcement.

Adapted from ACSM (2006) and Faigenbaum (2003)

Burns, and Ettinger 2000; Schot, Knutzen, Poole, and Mrotek 2003; Vincent et al. 2002). Also, the postural sway and balance of older, osteoarthritic adults were improved by participation in either long-term resistance training or aerobic walking (Messier et al. 2000). Improved strength and balance may help prevent falls and injuries in older adults.

The ACSM (2006) recommends moderate-intensity (RPE = 12-13) exercise to improve the muscular fitness of older adults; prescribe 1 set of 10 to 15 repetitions for 8 to 10 different exercises. Vincent and colleagues (2002) noted long-term (6 mo) improvements in the strength and muscular endurance of older adults (60-83 yr) who participated in either a low-intensity (1 set at 50% 1-RM) or a high-intensity (1 set at 80% 1-RM) resistance training program 3 days/wk. Likewise, Hunter and colleagues (2001) reported that isometric and dynamic muscle strength gains are similar for older adults (>60 yr) engaging in either a nonperiodized, high-intensity program (2 sets at 80% 1-RM, 3 days/wk) or an undulating periodized (UP) program varying training volume each day (2 sets at 50%, 65%, or 80% 1-RM, 3 days/wk). Some evidence suggests that training 1, 2, or 3 days a week at 80% 1-RM produces similar strength gains in older (65-79 yr) men and women (Taaffe, Duret, Wheeler, and Marcus 1999).

In addition to the general guidelines for designing resistance training programs for healthy adults (see table 7.2), ACSM (2006) recommends these guidelines and precautions:

- During the first 8 wk of training, use minimal resistance for all exercises.
- Instruct older adults about proper weightlifting and breathing techniques.
- Trained exercise leaders who have experience working with older adults should closely supervise and monitor the client's weightlifting techniques and resistance training program during the first few exercise sessions.
- Prescribe multijoint, rather than single-joint, exercises.
- Use exercise machines to stabilize body position and control the range of joint motion. Avoid using free weights with older adults.
- Each exercise session should be approximately 20 to 30 min and should never exceed 60 min.
- Older adults should rate their perceived exertion during exercise. Ratings of perceived exertion (RPEs) should be between 12 and

13 (somewhat hard).

- Prescribe 1 set of 10 to 15 repetitions for 8 to 10 different exercises for the major muscle groups.
- Allow at least 48 hr of rest between the exercise workouts.
- Discourage clients with arthritis from lifting weights when they are actively experiencing joint pain or inflammation.
- When clients are returning to resistance training following a layoff of more than 3 wk, they should start with a low resistance that is less than 50% of the weight they were lifting prior to the layoff.

COMMON QUESTIONS ABOUT RESISTANCE TRAINING

Because of the popularity of resistance training, there is an overwhelming amount of information about the subject in professional journals as well as in popular magazines and newspapers. This section presents common questions exercise professionals may have about designing resistance training programs and addresses questions and concerns that your clients may pose.

Program Design

- *Which resistance training method, nonperiodized or periodized, is better?*

The answer depends on your client's initial training status and goals. During the first stage (4 wk) of resistance training, both nonperiodized and periodized multiple-set programs increase the muscular fitness of untrained and novice lifters (Baker, Wilson, and Carlyon 1994); however, a varied training stimulus is needed for continued improvements in muscle strength and endurance during long-term (>4 wk) training (Fleck 1999; Marx et al. 2001). Periodized training is highly recommended for intermediate and advanced lifters; nonperiodized training may be more appropriate for clients just starting a weightlifting program or primarily interested in maintaining strength and muscle tone. Varying workouts daily (undulating periodized training) helps prevent boredom and maintain exercise compliance.

■ *Which periodization model is best?*

The answer depends on your client's training goal. One research team conducted two studies to assess the effectiveness of different types of periodized programs (LP, RLP, and daily UP) for increasing the strength and local muscular endurance of young, resistance-trained women and men (Rhea et al. 2002; Rhea, Phillips, et al. 2003). The researchers reported that daily UP was superior to LP for developing the strength of young men who trained 3 days/wk for 12 wk. For endurance gains, there were no statistically significant differences in LP, RLP, and daily UP training. Analysis of effect sizes, however, indicated that RLP was more effective than either LP or daily UP for increasing the muscular endurance of women and men who trained 2 days/wk for 15 wk.

■ *Is single-set training as effective as multiple-set training?*

Some research suggests that single-set training is as effective as multiple-set training for increasing the strength of untrained individuals during the initial stage of resistance training. For long-term training, however, multiple sets elicit greater strength gains for trained men and women (Marx et al. 2001; Wolfe, LeMura, and Cole 2004). For a comprehensive quantitative meta-analysis of studies comparing single- and multiple-set programs, see Wolfe and colleagues (2004). Paulsen, Myklested, and Reestad (2003) noted that the best method depends on the muscle groups exercised. They reported that multiple sets were superior to single sets for increasing leg strength, whereas both were equally effective for increasing the upper-body strength of untrained men during the initial phase (6 wk) of training.

■ *Is vibration training an effective way to increase the muscular strength of my clients?*

Vibration loading has been used to prevent bone mineral loss in astronauts and to enhance the rehabilitation of injuries such as sprains and tendinitis. Recently, the potential of using whole-body mechanical vibration as a method (vibration training) for increasing strength, balance, and bone integrity has been investigated (Roelants, Delecluse, Goris, and Verschueren 2004; Torvinen et al. 2002). Research has demonstrated that whole-body vibration improves the explosive power of physically active individuals (Bosco et al. 1999), the balance of older adults (Runge, Rehfeld, and Resnicek 2000), and the bone formation of postmenopausal women (Rubin, Recker, Cullen, Ryaby, and McLeod 1998). A power-plate vibration machine applies a low-amplitude, high-frequency (25-40 Hz) current to a platform on which the client stands (erect, relaxed, on heels, shifting weight from one leg to the other) or performs exercises such as push-ups, triceps dips, squats, light jumping, and static stretching.

Vibration loading produces small changes in muscle length that stimulate a **tonic vibration reflex**. This reflex activates muscle spindles and alpha motor neurons, causing the muscles to contract (Torvinen et al. 2002). Torvinen and colleagues examined the long-term (4 mo) effects of vibration training combined with unloaded static and dynamic exercises on strength, power, and balance. They noted that the greatest relative gains in isometric leg-extension strength and in leg power (measured by the vertical jump) occurred after the first 2 mo of training. Gains in strength and power during the last 2 mo of training were minimal. Thus, it appears that vibration training elicits a neural response and adaptation (recruitment of motor units through the activation of muscle spindles) similar to that observed during the early stages of conventional resistance training. When compared to a standard fitness program (combined aerobic and resistance training) and to conventional resistance training (exercise machines) in women, vibration training during unloaded static and dynamic exercises produced similar gains in isometric, isokinetic, and dynamic strength over 3 to 4 mo (Delecluse, Roelants, and Verschueren 2003; Roelants et al. 2004). Vibration training warrants further study, especially to determine its applicability in improving strength, flexibility, and possibly even balance in elderly individuals in order to prevent falls.

■ *Are abdominal training devices more effective than traditional calisthenic exercises for strengthening abdominal muscles?*

Currently, there is little scientific evidence justifying manufacturers' claims that abdominal training devices improve strength more effectively than simply performing calisthenic exercises without these devices (e.g., curl-ups). These devices purportedly overload the abdominals by adding resistance (e.g., abdominal belts) and isolate the abdominal musculature by supporting the head, neck, or back. However, studies using electromyography (EMG) show that exercising with these devices does not increase the muscle activity of the abdominal prime movers (rectus abdominis and external abdominal oblique muscles) more than exercising without the devices (American Council on Exercise 1997; Demont, Lephart, Giraldo, Giannantonio, Yuktanandana, and Fu

1999; Francis, Kolkhorst, Pennuci, Pozos, and Buono 2001). Although research does not support the use of abdominal trainers, they can add variety to conventional abdominal exercises and may even improve some clients' adherence to the abdominal exercise regimen.

To progressively overload (increase the training stimulus of) the abdominal muscles, you can have your client modify body position (e.g., perform abdominal curls on a decline bench rather than on a flat bench), hold a weight across the chest, or change arm positions. Abdominal exercises become more difficult as the arms move from along the sides to behind the head to overhead.

■ *Does performing the curl-up on a labile (moveable) surface increase the challenge for the abdominal muscles?*

Another way to increase the training stimulus for developing abdominal muscular fitness is to perform curl-up exercises on a labile surface. Vera-Garcia, Grenier, and McGill (2000) studied the EMG activity of the abdominal muscles (upper and lower rectus abdominis and internal and external abdominal oblique muscles) during four types of curl-ups: curl-ups on a stable bench, curl-ups on a gym ball with feet flat on the floor, curl-ups on a gym ball with feet on a bench, and curl-ups on a wobble board. Curl-ups performed on labile surfaces (gym ball and wobble board) doubled the EMG activity of the rectus abdominis and quadrupled the activity of the external oblique muscles. In terms of maintaining whole-body stability, the curl-up on the gym ball with the feet flat on the floor was the most demanding, as evidenced by increased EMG activity in all the abdominal muscles. Curl-ups with the upper body supported on the wobble board produced the most EMG activity in the upper rectus abdominis. Although exercising on a labile surface increases abdominal muscle activity and coactivation, it also increases loads on the spine. In rehabilitation programs, curl-ups on moveable surfaces should only be used with clients who can tolerate higher spinal loads (Vera-Garcia et al. 2000).

Client Concerns

■ *Is it OK to lift weights every day?*

During weightlifting, you are exercising your muscles at greater-than-normal workloads, producing microscopic tears in the muscle cells and connective tissues. Your body responds by producing new muscle proteins, which causes muscle growth and increased strength. For these changes to occur, you need to rest the exercised muscles between workouts. Most people show substantial improvements in strength when they lift weights every other day, just 2 to 3 times a week. If you lift weights every day, you run the risk of overtraining your muscles. Overtraining may cause muscle strains, tendinitis, bursitis, and other muscle and joint injuries. Experienced weightlifters who work out every day split their exercise routine so that they do not exercise the same muscle groups on consecutive days. A split routine reduces the risk of excessive muscle soreness and overuse injuries if you lift weights every day.

■ *Can I use calisthenic exercises like push-ups and pull-ups to improve my strength?*

You can use calisthenic exercises to increase your strength. Exercise professionals often prescribe push-ups and pull-ups in addition to free-weight and machine exercises to strengthen the chest, arm, and back muscles. When you do calisthenics, your body weight provides the resistance. If you are unable to lift your body weight, you will need to modify the calisthenic exercise. For example, doing push-ups with your body weight supported by your knees and hands is easier than doing standard push-ups with your body fully extended and your weight supported by your hands and feet. As your strength improves, you may increase the difficulty of the push-up by placing your hands wider than shoulder-width apart.

If you are unable to lift your body weight, you can modify pull-ups by using a spotter. As you pull up, assist your movement by extending your knees as the spotter supports your lower legs or ankles. To increase the difficulty of a pull-up, place your hands wider than shoulder-width apart and use an overhand (pronated) grip instead of an underhand (supinated) grip.

■ *I have followed my exercise prescription closely, but over the last several weeks I haven't seen any change in my strength. What should I do?*

At the beginning of your program, your strength gains were dramatic and rapid because your initial strength level was less than it is now. As your muscles adapt to the training stimulus, you may reach a plateau, or a point where you can't seem to improve further. It may be helpful if you periodically alter the training stimulus more frequently (weekly or even daily) by changing your combination of intensity, repetitions, and sets (ask your personal trainer about a periodized program). For example, if you are presently doing high intensity–low repetition exercises during each workout, you may want to decrease your intensity (from 80% to 70% 1-RM) and increase your repetitions (from 6-8 to 10-12) for several days. Selecting different exercises for the muscle groups may also help.

■ *Will I become muscle bound and lose flexibility if I lift weights?*

It is a common misconception that resistance training decreases joint flexibility. Studies of elite bodybuilders and powerlifters indicate that these athletes have excellent flexibility. Also, one study showed that resistance training actually increased the flexibility of elderly women. The key to remaining flexible during resistance training is to perform each exercise throughout the entire range of motion. Also, statically stretching the muscle groups before and after each workout may help you maintain flexibility.

■ *Will resistance training help me lose weight and fat?*

Resistance training positively alters your body composition and preserves your lean body tissues. Although your body weight may not change, your lean body mass (muscle and bone) increases and your body fat decreases. Given that muscle tissue is more metabolically active (burns more calories) than fat tissue, the increase in muscle size and lean body mass helps maintain your resting metabolic rate when you are on a weight-loss diet. Exercise science and nutrition professionals recommend using resistance training combined with aerobic exercise to maximize the loss of body fat and to maintain lean body tissues.

■ *Will my strength improve if I train aerobically at the same time that I am resistance training?*

If you concurrently participate in aerobic and resistance training, your muscle growth and strength improvement may be lessened because of the increased energy demands and protein requirements of endurance training. Although this possibility is an important consideration for competitive bodybuilders and power athletes, your decision to participate in both forms of training depends on your overall exercise program goal. If your goal is improved health or weight loss, experts recommend including both aerobic and resistance training in your program.

■ *Are protein and amino acid supplements necessary to maximize muscle growth and strength during resistance training?*

Provided that your diet is well balanced and nutritionally sound, you do not need protein or amino acid supplements. Although the protein needs of resistance-trained individuals (1.6-1.8 g/kg each day) are higher than the recommended dietary allowance for inactive individuals (0.8 g/kg each day), in most cases a well-balanced diet containing 12% to 25% protein will meet increased protein needs during weightlifting.

However, amino acid supplementation is especially popular among strength-trained athletes. Studies show that ingesting amino acids or a protein–carbohydrate supplement (e.g., 6 g of essential amino acids and 35 g sucrose) immediately before and after exercise stimulates protein synthesis and maximizes the anabolic (protein-building) response of skeletal muscle tissue to resistance training (Rasmess et al. 2003). Tipton and colleagues (2001) noted that ingesting an amino acid–carbohydrate supplement immediately before resistance exercise is more effective than ingesting the supplement immediately after exercise in terms of increasing the net protein balance in skeletal muscle. In a study of elderly men who resistance trained over 12 wk, Esmarck, Andersen, Olsen, Richter, Mizuno, and Kjaer (2001) noted that those who took a protein–carbohydrate supplement immediately after exercise (within 5 min) had greater gains in muscle hypertrophy, lean body mass, and muscular strength than those who ingested the supplement 2 hr after the training session. These studies show that the timing of amino acid supplementation is critical in optimizing muscle growth in response to resistance training.

■ *Will creatine supplements enhance strength and muscle size during resistance training?*

Over 300 studies have tested the effects of creatine supplementation on performance. Overall, the data suggest that creatine supplementation can improve the performance of high-intensity exercise lasting less than 30 sec (Branch 2003; Rawson and Clarkson 2003). Studies demonstrate that creatine supplementation combined with resistance training increases muscular strength, body mass, fat-free mass, muscle fiber size, and training volume in healthy young adults as well as in older women and men (Brose, Parise, and Tarnopolsky 2003; Nissen and Sharp 2003). Creatine supplements increase muscle creatine; however, there is much interindividual variability in the response (Rawson and Clarkson 2003). Theoretically, an increase in muscle creatine enhances training volume and decreases the amount of recovery time needed between sets and exercises The increased training stimulus improves the physiological adaptation to resistance training for some individuals (i.e., they experience a greater gain in muscle mass and strength).

■ *Is it safe to take creatine supplements?*

Although there are anecdotal reports associating creatine supplementation with muscle cramping, gastrointestinal distress, and soft-tissue injuries (Poortmans and Francaux 2000), short-term and long-term creatine supplementation does not appear to adversely affect kidney, liver, or cardiovascular function (Volek 1999) or markers of health status such as muscle and liver enzymes, lipid profiles, and electrolytes (Kreider et al. 2003).

One reported side effect of creatine supplementation is increased stiffness in the musculotendinous unit, which theoretically predisposes individuals to muscle strains and tears. To address this concern, Watsford and colleagues (2003) studied changes in stiffness following 28 days of creatine supplementation and reported that creatine ingestion does not increase the stiffness of the series elastic components in the musculotendinous unit of the triceps surae (the gastrocnemius and soleus). These findings suggest that the muscle strains and tears reportedly associated with creatine supplementation are not caused by a change in the elasticity (stiffness) of the musculotendinous system. Also, when compared to a placebo group, subjects taking creatine supplements showed no differences in markers of exercise-induced muscle damage following eccentric exercise (Rawson, Gunn, and Clarkson 2001).

■ *Do β-hydroxy-β-methylbutyrate (HMB) supplements increase lean body mass and muscle strength?*

In a meta-analysis of dietary supplements, Nissen and Sharp (2003) reported that HMB is one of only two supplements (the other being creatine) that significantly increase the lean body mass and muscular strength of individuals engaging in resistance training. Analysis of nine studies that used control groups to assess HMB supplementation (3 g/day) indicated that, on average, lean body mass and muscular strength increased 0.28% and 1.40% per week, respectively, for the treatment groups. The effect sizes for net gains in lean body mass (*ES* = 0.15) and strength (*ES* = 0.19) were significant. HMB supplementation during 3 to 8 wk of resistance training did not adversely affect hematology or liver and kidney function but positively affected cardiovascular risk factors (decreased total cholesterol, LDL-cholesterol, and systolic blood pressure) (Nissen and Sharp 2003).

EFFECTS OF RESISTANCE TRAINING PROGRAMS

Resistance training improves muscular fitness by increasing both strength and muscular endurance. This section addresses the morphological, neurological, and biochemical effects of resistance training.

Morphological Effects of Resistance Training on the Musculoskeletal System

Resistance training leads to morphological adaptations in skeletal muscles and bone. Structural changes in muscle fibers account for a large portion of the strength gains resulting from resistance training. Increases in bone mineral content and bone density improve bone health. The following questions deal with these adaptations.

■ *What is exercise-induced muscle hypertrophy?*

One effect of strength training is an increase in the size of the muscle tissue. This adaptation, known as **exercise-induced hypertrophy**, results from an increase in the total amount of contractile protein, the number and size of myofibrils per fiber, and the amount of connective tissue surrounding the muscle fibers (Goldberg, Etlinger, Goldspink, and Jablecki 1975).

■ *Is it possible to increase the number of muscle fibers by resistance training?*

Heavy resistance training has been reported to produce an increase in the number of muscle fibers (i.e., hyperplasia) in animals due to longitudinal splitting and satellite cell proliferation (Antonio and Gonyea 1993; Edgerton 1970; Gonyea, Ericson, and Bonde-Petersen 1977). Such processes, however, have not been clearly demonstrated in human skeletal muscle tissue (Taylor and Wilkinson 1986; Tesch 1988). Although some data suggest that human skeletal muscle has the potential to increase muscle fiber number (Alway, Grumbt, Gonyea, and Stray-Gundersen 1989; Sjostrom, Lexell, Eriksson, and Taylor 1992), hyperplasia probably contributes less than 5% to overall muscle growth in response to heavy resistance training (Kraemer,

Summary of Effects of Resistance Training

Morphological Factors

- Muscle hypertrophy due to increase in contractile proteins, number and size of myofibrils, connective tissues, and size of type II muscle fibers
- No change in relative amounts of type I and II muscle fibers
- Little or no change in the number of muscle fibers (<5%)
- Increase in size and strength of ligaments and tendons
- Increase in bone density and bone strength
- Increase in muscle capillary density

Neural Factors

- Increase in motor unit activation and recruitment
- Increase in discharge frequency of motor neurons
- Decrease in neural inhibition

Biochemical Factors

- Minor increase in ATP and CP stores
- Minor increase in CPK, myosin ATPase, and myokinase activity
- Decrease in mitochondrial volume density
- Increase in testosterone, growth hormone, IGF-I, and catecholamines during resistance training exercises

Additional Factors

- Little or no change in body mass
- Increase in fat-free mass
- Decrease in fat mass and relative body fat
- Improved bone health increases with exercise intensity.

Fleck, and Evans 1996). The major factor contributing to exercise-induced hypertrophy for humans apparently is an increase in the size of existing muscle fibers.

▪ *Does resistance training alter muscle fiber type from slow-twitch to fast-twitch?*

Although strength training produces greater hypertrophy in fast-twitch (type II) muscle fibers than in slow-twitch (type I) fibers (Tesch 1988; Thorstensson, Hulten, vonDobeln, and Karlsson 1976), there is no evidence to support the conversion of slow-twitch to fast-twitch fibers (Costill, Coyle, Fink, Lesmes, and Witzmann 1979; Dons, Bollerup, Bonde-Petersen, and Hancke 1979; Mikesky, Giddings, Matthews, and Gonyea 1991). Resistance training does not alter the percentage of type I and II muscle fibers. However, heavy resistance training affects the proportion of fibers comprising subgroups of type II muscle fibers, increasing the percentage of type IIB (fast-twitch—glycolytic) muscle fibers while decreasing the percentage of type IIA (fast-twitch—oxidative) fibers in both men and women (Deschenes and Kraemer 2002; Kraemer et al. 1995; Staron et al. 1994).

▪ *Is the relationship between muscle size and strength the same for men and women?*

Muscle strength is directly related to the cross-sectional area of the muscle tissue. Ikai and

Fukunaga (1968) noted that the static strength per unit of cross-sectional area of the elbow flexors was similar for young men and women. These values ranged between 4.5 and 8.9 kg/cm^2; average values were 6.2 and 6.7 kg/cm^2 for women and men, respectively. Cureton, Collins, Hill, and McElhannon (1988) also reported that the dynamic strength per unit of cross-sectional area (CSA) was similar for men and women. Posttraining ratios of elbow flexor/extensor strength to upper arm CSA were 1.65 kg/cm^2 and 1.85 kg/cm^2, respectively, for men and women. Likewise, the posttraining ratios for leg strength to thigh CSA were 1.10 kg/cm^2 for men and 0.90 kg/cm^2 for women.

▪ *How much do women's muscles hypertrophy in response to resistance training?*

In the past, it was believed that resistance training produced less muscle hypertrophy in women than in men even though their relative strength gains were similar, but muscle hypertrophy was assessed indirectly using anthropometric and body composition measures. Cureton et al. (1988), however, using computerized tomography to directly assess muscle hypertrophy in a heavy resistance training program (70% to 90% 1-RM, 3 days/wk for 16 wk), found significant increases in CSA of the upper arms of women (5 cm^2 or 23%) as well as men (7 cm^2 or 15%). Although the absolute change was slightly larger in men, the relative degree of hypertrophy was similar for men and women.

Today experts agree that the relative increases in fiber size are similar for women and men when the training stimulus is the same (Deschenes and Kraemer 2002). In addition, periodized resistance training is particularly effective for increasing muscle size in women. Kraemer and colleagues (2004) recently compared the effects of total- and upper-body periodized training programs on muscle hypertrophy in young women. Over 6 mo of training, the total-body periodized program produced greater and more consistent gains in overall (upper- and lower-body) muscle size compared to upper-body periodized training. An intensity range of 3-RM to 8-RM produced greater muscle hypertrophy than did a range of 8-RM to 12-RM.

■ Is it possible for older adults to increase the size of their muscles by resistance training?

Electromyographic evidence led Moritani and deVries (1979) to conclude that increased strength in older men who engaged in resistance training was highly dependent on neural changes, such as increased frequency of motor neuron discharge and recruitment of motor units. Because of studies such as this, it was long believed that strength gains from resistance training in older individuals were due primarily to neural adaptation rather than muscle hypertrophy.

However, Frontera, Meredith, O'Reilly, Knuttgen, and Evans (1988) reported that resistance training produces muscle hypertrophy in men ages 60 to 72 yr. The men trained in a high-intensity program for the knee extensors and flexors (3 sets at 80% 1-RM) for 12 wk. Computerized tomography revealed significant increases in total thigh area (4.8%), total muscle area (11.4%), and quadriceps area (9.3%). The relative increase in total muscle area was similar to values reported for young men (Luthi et al. 1986). Research also shows significant increases in muscle size in older women, as well as in very old (87 to 96 yr) men and women, due to high-intensity (80% 1-RM) resistance training (Charette et al. 1991; Fiatarone, Marks, Ryan, Meredith, Lipstiz, and Evans 1991).

Exercise-induced hypertrophy appears to be an important mechanism underlying strength gains in older women and men. This implies that older adults can effectively counter age-related loss in muscle mass by participating in a vigorous resistance training program.

■ Does resistance training improve bone health and joint integrity?

Resistance training has beneficial effects on bone health that may decrease the risk of osteoporosis and bone fractures, particularly in women. This form of training may help to achieve the highest possible peak bone mass in premenopausal women and may aid in maintaining and increasing bone in postmenopausal women and older adults (Layne and Nelson 1999). Bone mineral density of the lumbar spine and femur in premenopausal women significantly increased after 12 to 18 mo of strength training (Lohman et al. 1995). Also, lumbar bone mineral density of early-postmenopausal women was improved following 9 mo of strength training (Pruitt, Jackson, Bartels, and Lehnhard 1992). However, in a study of older women (65 to 79 yr), 12 mo of high-intensity (80% 1-RM) and low-intensity (40% 1-RM) resistance training did not significantly improve the bone mineral density of the lumbar spine and hip (Pruitt, Taaffe, and Marcus 1995). Still, evidence suggests that resistance training and higher-intensity weight-bearing activities (not walking) may slow the decline in bone loss even if there is no significant increase in bone mineral density. Improvements in bone mineral density appear to be site specific; the greater changes occur in bones to which the exercising muscles attach. Experts agree that resistance training has a more potent effect on bone health than do weight-bearing aerobic exercises such as walking and jogging (Layne and Nelson 1999).

Resistance training also improves the size and strength of ligaments and tendons (Edgerton 1973; Fleck and Falkel 1986; Tipton, Matthes, Maynard, and Carey 1975). These changes may increase joint stability, thereby reducing the risk of sprains and dislocations.

Biochemical Effects of Resistance Training

The morphological changes in skeletal muscles due to resistance training are caused by hormones. This section addresses questions regarding hormonal responses to resistance exercise, as well as changes in the metabolic profile of skeletal muscles.

■ What causes the increase in muscle size with resistance training?

Exercise-induced hypertrophy occurs through hormonal mechanisms. Anabolic (protein-building) hormones such as testosterone, growth hormone, and insulin-like growth hormone increase in response to heavy resistance exercise and interact to promote protein synthesis. The magnitude of testosterone and growth hormone release, however, appears to be related to the size of the muscle groups used, the exercise intensity (%1-RM), and the length of rest between sets, with larger increases observed for high-intensity (5- to 10-RM) exercise and short (1 min) rest periods involving large muscle groups (Kraemer et al. 1991). In men, high-intensity resistance training produces significant increases in testosterone and growth hormone, but testosterone appears to be the principal muscle-building hormone (Deschenes and Kraemer 2002). Levels of catecholamines (norepinephrine, epinephrine, and dopamine), which augment the release of testosterone and insulin-like growth factor, also increase in men in response to heavy resistance exercise (Kraemer, Noble, Clark, and Culver 1987). In women, growth hormone is likely the most potent muscle-building hormone (Deschenes and Kraemer 2002).

■ *Does resistance training alter the metabolic profile of skeletal muscles?*

Although high-intensity resistance training results in substantial increases in muscle proteins, it appears to have little or no effect on muscle substrate stores and enzymes involved with the generation of adenosine triphosphate (ATP). Although stores of ATP and creatine phosphate (CP) may increase significantly in response to strength training (MacDougall, Sale, Moroz, Elder, Sutton, and Howalk 1979), the changes are not large enough to have practical significance. Strength training produces only minor alterations in myosin adenosinetriphosphatase (ATPase) activity (Tesch 1992) and other ATP turnover enzymes, such as creatine phosphokinase (CPK), in response to strength training (Costill et al. 1979; Komi, Viitasalo, Rauramaa, and Vihko 1978; Thorstensson et al. 1976). Strength training using heavy resistance and explosive exercises results in decreased activities for hexokinase, myofibrillar ATPase, and citrate synthase (Tesch 1988).

■ *Does resistance training decrease aerobic capacity and endurance performance?*

The mitochondrial volume density following heavy resistance training has been reported to decrease as a consequence of a disproportionate increase of contractile protein in comparison with mitochondria. In theory, this could be detrimental to aerobic capacity and endurance performance. A review of studies of this phenomenon, however, concluded that participation in heavy resistance training does not negatively affect aerobic power (Dudley and Fleck 1987; Sale, MacDougall, Jacobs, and Garner 1987). Also, capillary density has been shown to increase, which in turn enhances the potential to remove lactate produced by the muscles during moderate-intensity, high-volume resistance exercise (Kraemer et al. 1996).

Neurological Effects of Resistance Training

In addition to muscle hypertrophy, neural adaptations significantly contribute to strength gains, especially during the initial stages of resistance training. This section addresses questions regarding neural adaptations to short- and long-term resistance training.

■ *What changes in neural function occur in response to resistance training?*

The nervous system responds to resistance training by increasing the activation and recruitment of motor units (the alpha motor neuron and all of the muscle fibers it innervates) and by decreasing the cocontraction of antagonistic muscle groups (Sale 1988). Recruiting additional motor units as well as increasing the frequency of firing results in greater muscular force production. Some evidence suggests that the central drive from higher neural centers (e.g., motor cortex of brain) changes and that the amounts of neurotransmitters and postsynaptic receptors at the neuromuscular junction increase (Deschenes and Kraemer 2002). These changes facilitate the activation and recruitment of additional motor units, thereby increasing force production.

■ *At what stage during resistance training does neural adaptation occur?*

In the past, it was believed that neural adaptations are primarily responsible for strength gains *only* during the initial stage (first 2-8 wk) of resistance training. At about 8 to 10 wk of resistance training, muscle hypertrophy contributes more than neural adaptation to strength gains, but hypertrophy eventually levels off (Sale 1988). Evidence suggests that muscle hypertrophy is finite and may be limited to no more than 12 mo (Deschenes and Kraemer 2002). Given that long-term resistance training (>6 mo) continues to increase strength without hypertrophy, experts now believe that a secondary phase of neural adaptation is most likely responsible for strength gains occurring between 6 and 12 mo of training (Deschenes and Kraemer 2002).

MUSCULAR SORENESS

Muscular soreness may develop as a result of resistance training because isolated muscle groups are being overloaded beyond normal use. **Acute-onset muscle soreness** occurs during or immediately following the exercise and is usually caused by ischemia and the accumulation of metabolic waste products in the muscle tissue. The pain and discomfort may persist up to 1 hr after the cessation of the exercise.

In **delayed-onset muscle soreness (DOMS)**, the pain occurs 24 to 48 hr after exercise. Although the causes of DOMS are not known (Armstrong 1984; Smith 1991), it appears to be related to the type of muscle contraction. Eccentric exercise produces a greater degree of delayed muscular soreness than either concentric or isometric exercise (Byrnes, Clarkson, and Katch 1985; Schwane, Johnson, Vandenakker, and Armstrong 1983; Talag 1973). Little or no muscular soreness occurs with isokinetic exercise (Byrnes, Clarkson, and Katch 1985). This most likely relates to the fact that isokinetic exercise devices offer no resistance to the recovery phase of the movement and therefore the muscle does not contract eccentrically.

Theories of Delayed-Onset Muscle Soreness

Although the precise causes of DOMS remain unclear, several theories have been proposed. The more widely recognized theories suggest that exercise, particularly eccentric exercise, causes damage to skeletal muscle cells and connective tissues, producing an acute inflammation.

Connective Tissue Damage

Abraham (1977) extensively studied the factors related to DOMS produced by resistance training. He suggested that DOMS most likely results from disruption in the connective tissue of the muscle and its tendinous attachments. Abraham noted that urinary excretion of hydroxyproline, a specific by-product of connective tissue breakdown, was higher in subjects who experienced muscular soreness than in those who did not. Because a significant rise in urinary hydroxyproline levels indicates an increase in both collagen degradation and synthesis, he concluded that more strenuous exercise damages the connective tissue, which increases the degradation of collagen and creates an imbalance in collagen metabolism. To com-pensate for this imbalance, the rate of collagen synthesis increases.

Skeletal Muscle Damage

Researchers have assessed skeletal muscle damage induced through exercise; much of this research has focused on the effects of eccentric exercise on muscle damage and soreness. Eccentric exercise injures both the contractile and cytoskeletal components of myofibrils as well as the excitation coupling system. Friden, Sjostrom, and Ekblom (1983) observed structural damage to myofibrillar Z bands resulting from eccentric exercise. Proske and Morgan (2001) pointed out that disruption of the sarcomere organization within the skeletal muscle is most likely the cause of the decreased active tension and force production that follows a series of intense, eccentric contractions. More research is needed to assess the effects of high- and low-impact eccentric exercise (e.g., downhill running and eccentric cycle exercise) on muscle injury (Friden 2002).

Researchers also have examined markers of muscle damage such as serum CPK, lactate dehydrogenase, and myoglobin. Schwane et al. (1983) noted a significant increase in plasma CPK levels produced by downhill running. They suggested that the mechanical stress from eccentric exercise causes cellular damage that results in an enzyme efflux. Clarkson, Byrnes, McCormick, Turcotte, and White (1986) reported similar increases in serum CPK levels following concentric (37.6%), eccentric (35.8%), and isometric (34%) arm curl exercises. They concluded that muscle damage occurred with all three types of contraction; however, the subjects perceived greater muscle soreness with eccentric and isometric exercises. Likewise, Byrnes et al. (1985) observed that both concentric and eccentric resistance training elevated serum CPK levels but that individuals who trained concentrically did not develop DOMS.

Armstrong's Model of Delayed-Onset Muscle Soreness

On the basis of an extensive literature review, Armstrong (1984) proposed the following model of the development of DOMS:

1. The structural proteins in muscle cells and connective tissue are disrupted by high mechanical forces produced during exercise, especially eccentric exercise.

2. Structural damage to the sarcolemma alters the permeability of the cell membrane, allowing a net influx of calcium from the interstitial space. Abnormally high levels of calcium inhibit cellular respiration, thereby lessening the cell's ability to produce ATP for active removal of calcium from the cell.

3. High calcium levels within the cell activate a calcium-dependent proteolytic enzyme that degrades Z discs, troponin, and tropomyosin.

4. This progressive destruction of the sarcolemma (postexercise) allows intracellular components to diffuse into the interstitial space and plasma. These substances attract monocytes and activate mast cells and histocytes in the injured area.

5. Histamine, kinins, and potassium accumulate in the interstitial space because of the active phagocytosis and cellular necrosis. These substances, as well as increased tissue edema and temperature, may stimulate pain receptors resulting in the sensation of DOMS.

Acute Inflammation Theory

Smith (1991) suggested that acute inflammation, in response to muscle cell and connective damage caused by eccentric exercise, is the primary mechanism underlying DOMS. Many of the signs and symptoms of acute inflammation, such as pain, swelling, and loss of function, are also present with DOMS. Based on research about acute inflammation and DOMS, Smith proposed the following sequence of events:

1. Connective tissue and muscle tissue disruption occurs during eccentric exercise, especially when the individual is not accustomed to eccentric exercise.

2. Within a few hours, neutrophils in the blood are elevated and migrate to the site of injury for several hours postinjury.

3. Monocytes also migrate to the injured tissues at 6 to 12 hr postinjury.

4. Macrophages synthesize prostaglandins (series E).

5. The prostaglandins sensitize type III and IV pain afferents, resulting in the sensation of pain in response to intramuscular pressure caused by movement or palpation.

6. The combination of increased pressure and hypersensitization produces the sensation of DOMS.

Prevention of Muscular Soreness

To prevent muscular soreness due to resistance training, you should prescribe warm-up and cool-down exercises for your clients. For many years, slow static stretching exercises were recommended to warm up major muscle groups at the start of the resistance training workout. It was believed that this form of stretching prevented muscle injury and soreness (deVries 1961). However, evidence suggests that stretching prior to physical activity does not prevent injury (Pope, Herbert, Kirwan, and Graham 2000). Instead of performing static stretching, your client should warm up by completing 5 to 10 repetitions of the exercise at a low intensity (e.g., 40% 1-RM). Have clients use slow static stretching as part of the cool-down segment of the resistance training workout.

Using a gradual progression of exercise intensity at the beginning of a resistance training program also may help to prevent muscular soreness. McArdle et al. (1996) suggest using 12- to 15-RM during the beginning phases of strength training. Make sure that your clients gradually increase exercise intensity throughout the resistance training program. Avoiding eccentric contractions during dynamic resistance training also may lessen the chance of muscular soreness. An assistant or exercise partner should return the weight to the starting position.

KEY POINTS

- The specificity principle states that muscular fitness development is specific to the muscle group, type of contraction, training intensity, speed, and range of movement.

- The overload principle states that the muscle group must be exercised at greater-than-normal workloads to promote muscular strength and endurance development.

- For non-periodized resistance training programs, the training volume must be progressively increased to overload the muscle groups for continued gains in strength and muscular endurance.

- In most programs, resistance training exercises should be ordered so that successive exercises do not involve the same muscle group. For advanced programs, however, exercises for the same muscle group should be done consecutively.

- Dynamic resistance training can be used to develop muscular strength, power, size, or endurance by modifying the intensity, repetitions, sets, and frequency of the exercise.

- Periodization programs can result in greater changes in strength than non-periodized resistance training programs.

- Strength and endurance gains resulting from resistance training are due to morphological, neurological, and biochemical changes in the muscle tissue.

- Eccentric exercise produces a greater degree of DOMS than either concentric, isometric, or isokinetic exercise.

- Little or no muscular soreness is produced by isokinetic training.

- The precise cause of DOMS is unknown; however, connective tissue and muscle damage, as well as acute inflammation, has been proposed as a possible cause.

KEY TERMS

Learn the definition of each of the following key terms. Definitions of terms can be found in the glossary on page 379.

acute-onset muscle soreness
β-hydroxy-β-methylbutyrate (HMB)
compound sets
core stability
core strengthening
delayed-onset muscle soreness (DOMS)
exercise-induced hypertrophy
functional training
high intensity–low repetitions
linear periodization (LP)
low intensity–high repetitions
macrocycle
mesocycle
microcycle

muscle balance
periodization
pyramiding
repetition maximum (RM)
repetitions
reverse linear periodization (RLP)
set
split routine
supersetting
tonic vibration reflex
training volume
tri-sets
undulating periodization (UP)
vibration training

REVIEW QUESTIONS

In addition to being able to define each of the key terms, test your knowledge and understanding of the material by answering the following review questions.

1. What are the health benefits of resistance training?

2. Name three general types of resistance training. Which one is best suited for physical therapy rehabilitation programs?

3. What is the major advantage of isokinetic training compared to traditional forms of resistance training?

4. Describe the ACSM guidelines for designing resistance training programs for healthy adults. What modifications are necessary when you are planning resistance training programs for children and older adults?

5. Describe how the basic exercise prescriptions for strength training and muscular endurance training programs differ.

6. Describe how you can increase training volume for advanced strength training and hypertrophy programs.

7. Describe two methods of varying sets for advanced strength training programs.

8. Explain two methods that an advanced weightlifter can use to completely fatigue a targeted muscle group.

9. Describe three periodization models. How do they differ?

10. Explain how the specificity, overload, and progression principles are applied in designing resistance training programs.

11. Explain what causes the exercise-induced hypertrophy resulting from resistance training. In the time course of a resistance training program, when is this morphological adaptation most likely to occur?

12. What neural adaptations account for initial strength gains during resistance training? When are these changes most likely to be observed during the time course of resistance training?

13. Describe the potential effects of resistance training on bone health.

14. Describe one theory of DOMS. What can you instruct your clients to do to help prevent and relieve muscle soreness caused by resistance training?

15. What will you tell your clients if they ask about supplementing their resistance training with creatine?

chapter 8

Assessing Body Composition

Key Questions

- Why is it important to measure body composition, and how are body composition measures used by health and fitness professionals?

- What are the standards for classifying body fat levels?

- What is the difference between two-component and multicomponent body composition models?

- What are the guidelines and limitations of the hydrostatic weighing method?

- Is air displacement plethysmography as accurate as hydrostatic weighing?

- Is dual-energy X-ray absorptiometry considered to be a "gold standard" method for measuring body composition?

- What are the guidelines, limitations, and sources of measurement error for the skinfold method?

- What is bioelectrical impedance analysis? What factors affect the accuracy of this method?

- Can circumferences and skeletal diameters be used to accurately assess body composition?

- What anthropometric indices can be used to identify at-risk individuals?

- Is near-infrared interactance a viable alternative to skinfolds and bioimpedance analysis for measuring body composition in field settings?

Body composition is a key component of an individual's health and physical fitness profile. Obesity is a serious health problem that reduces life expectancy by increasing one's risk of developing coronary artery disease, hypertension, type 2 diabetes, obstructive pulmonary disease, osteoarthritis, and certain types of cancer. Too little body fat also poses a health risk because the body needs a certain amount of fat for normal physiological functions. Essential lipids, such as phospholipids, are needed for cell membrane formation; nonessential lipids, like triglycerides found in adipose tissue, provide thermal insulation and store metabolic fuel (free fatty acids). In addition, lipids are involved in the transport and storage of fat-soluble vitamins (A, D, E, and K) and in the functioning of the nervous system, the menstrual cycle, and the reproductive system, as well as in growth and maturation during pubescence. Thus, too little body fatness, as found in individuals with eating disorders (anorexia nervosa), exercise addiction, and certain diseases such as cystic fibrosis, can lead to serious physiological dysfunction.

This chapter describes standardized testing procedures for reference (hydrostatic weighing, air displacement plethysmography, and dual X-ray absorptiometry) and field (skinfold, bioimpedance, and anthropometry) methods for assessing body composition. For each method, you will learn to identify potential sources of measurement error, as well as ways to minimize these errors.

CLASSIFICATION AND USES OF BODY COMPOSITION MEASURES

To classify level of body fatness, the relative body fat (%BF) is used. Table 8.1 presents recommended

TABLE 8.1   Percent Body Fat Standards for Adults, Children, and Physically Active Adults

RECOMMENDED %BF LEVELS FOR ADULTS AND CHILDREN

	NR*	Low	Mid	Upper	Obesity
Males					
18-34 years	<8	8	13	22	>22
35-55 years	<10	10	18	25	>25
55+ years	<10	10	16	23	>23
6-17 years	<5	5-10	11-25	26-31	>31
Females					
18-34 years	<20	20	28	35	>35
35-55 years	<25	25	32	38	>38
55+ years	<25	25	30	35	>35
6-17 years	<12	12-15	16-30	31-36	>36

RECOMMENDED %BF LEVELS FOR PHYSICALLY ACTIVE ADULTS

	Low	Mid	Upper
Males			
18-34 years	5	10	15
35-55 years	7	11	18
55+ years	9	12	18
Females			
18-34 years	16	23	28
35-55 years	20	27	33
55+ years	20	27	33

*NR = not recommended; %BF = percent body fat.
Data from Lohman, Houtkooper, and Going (1997).

%BF standards for men, women, and children, as well as physically active adults. The minimal, average, and obesity fat values vary with age, gender, and activity status. For example, the average or median %BF values for adult men and women (18 to 34 yr) are 13% for men and 28% for women; the minimal fat values are 8% and 20%, respectively; and the standard for obesity is >22% BF for men and >35% BF for women.

In addition to classifying your client's %BF and disease risk, body composition measures are useful for

- estimating a healthy body weight and formulating nutritional recommendations and exercise prescriptions (see chapter 9);
- estimating competitive body weight for athletes participating in sports that use body weight classifications for competition (e.g., wrestling and bodybuilding);

- monitoring the growth of children and adolescents and identifying those at risk because of under- or overfatness; and
- assessing changes in body composition associated with aging, malnutrition, and certain diseases, and assessing the effectiveness of nutrition and exercise interventions in counteracting these changes.

BODY COMPOSITION MODELS

In order to make the most valid assessment of body composition for your client, it is necessary to understand the underlying theoretical models. You may recall that the body is composed of water, protein, minerals, and fat. The two-component model of body composition (Brozek, Grande, Anderson, and Keys 1963; Siri 1961) divides the body into a fat component and a **fat-free body (FFB)** component. The FFB consists of all residual chemicals and tissues including water, muscle (protein), and bone (mineral). The **two-component model** of body composition makes the following five assumptions:

1. The density of fat is 0.901 g·cc⁻¹.
2. The density of the FFB is 1.100 g·cc⁻¹.
3. The densities of fat and the FFB components (water, protein, mineral) are the same for all individuals.
4. The densities of the various tissues composing the FFB are constant within an individual, and their proportional contribution to the lean component remains constant.
5. The individual being measured differs from the reference body only in the amount of fat; the FFB of the reference body is assumed to be 73.8% water, 19.4% protein, and 6.8% mineral.

This two-component model has served as the foundation for the **hydrodensitometry** (underwater weighing) method. With use of the assumed proportions of water, mineral, and protein and their respective densities, equations were derived to convert the individual's total body density (Db) from hydrostatic weighing into relative body fat proportions (%BF). Two commonly used equations are the Siri (1961) equation, %BF = (4.95/Db − 4.50) × 100, and the Brozek, Grande, Anderson, and Keys (1963) equation, %BF = (4.57/Db − 4.142) × 100. These two equations yield similar %BF estimates for body densities ranging from 1.0300 to 1.0900 g/cc. For example, if a client's measured Db is 1.0500 g·cc⁻¹, the %BF estimates, obtained by plugging this value into the Siri and Brozek equations, are 21.4% and 21.0%, respectively.

Generally, two-component model equations provide accurate estimates of %BF as long as the basic assumptions of the model are met. However, there is no guarantee that the FFB composition of an individual within a certain population subgroup will exactly match the values assumed for the reference body. Researchers have reported that FFB density varies with age, gender, ethnicity, level of body fatness, and physical activity level, depending mainly on the relative proportion of water and mineral composing the FFB (Baumgartner, Heymsfield, Lichtman, Wang, and Pierson 1991; Williams, Going, Massett, Lohman, Bare, and Hewitt 1993). For example, the average FFB density of Black women and Black men (~1.106 g·cc⁻¹) is greater

than 1.10 g·cc⁻¹ because of their higher mineral content (~7.3% FFB) and/or relative body protein (Cote and Adams 1993; Ortiz et al. 1992; Wagner and Heyward 2001). Because of this difference in FFB density, the body fat of Blacks will be systematically underestimated when two-component model equations are used to estimate %BF. In fact, negative %BF values were reported for professional football players whose measured Db exceeded 1.10 g·cc⁻¹ (Adams, Mottola, Bagnall, and McFadden 1982). Likewise, the FFB density of White children is estimated to be only 1.086 g·cc⁻¹ because of their relative lower mineral (5.2% FFB) and higher body water values (76.6% FFB) compared to the reference body (Lohman, Boileau, and Slaughter 1984). Also, the average density of the FFB of elderly White men and women is 1.098 g·cc⁻¹ because of the relatively low body mineral value (6.2% FFB) in this population (Heymsfield et al. 1989). Thus, the relative body fat of children and persons who are elderly will be systematically overestimated using two-component model equations.

For certain population subgroups, therefore, scientists have applied **multicomponent models** of body composition based on measured total body water and bone mineral values. With the multicomponent approach, you can avoid systematic errors in estimating body fat by replacing the reference man with population-specific reference bodies that take into account the age (e.g., for children, for persons who are elderly), gender, and ethnicity of the individual. Table 8.2 provides population-specific formulas for converting Db to %BF. You will note that population-specific conversion formulas do not yet exist for all age groups within each ethnic group. You may have to use the age-specific conversion formula developed for White males and females in these cases. Also, you can use the population-specific conversion formulas for anorexic and obese females only when it is obvious that your client is either anorexic or obese.

REFERENCE METHODS FOR ASSESSING BODY COMPOSITION

In many laboratory and clinical settings, **densitometry** and dual-energy X-ray absorptiometry are used to obtain reference measures of body composition. For densitometric methods, total **body density (Db)** is estimated from the ratio of body mass to body volume (Db = BM/BV). Body volume can be measured using either hydrostatic weighing or air displacement plethysmography.

TABLE 8.2 Population-Specific Two-Component Model Formulas for Converting Body Density to Percent Body Fat

Population	Age	Gender	%BF[a]	FFB$_d$ (g · cc^{-1})*
Ethnicity				
African American	9-17	Female	(5.24 / Db) − 4.82	1.088
	19-45	Male	(4.86 / Db) − 4.39	1.106
	24-79	Female	(4.85 / Db) − 4.39	1.106
American Indian	18-62	Male	(4.97 / Db) − 4.52	1.099
	18-60	Female	(4.81 / Db) − 4.34	1.108
Asian				
Japanese Native	18-48	Male	(4.97 / Db) − 4.52	1.099
		Female	(4.76 / Db) − 4.28	1.111
	61-78	Male	(4.87 / Db) − 4.41	1.105
		Female	(4.95 / Db) − 4.50	1.100
Singaporean (Chinese, Indian, Malay)		Male	(4.94 / Db) − 4.48	1.102
		Female	(4.84 / Db) − 4.37	1.107
White	8-12	Male	(5.27 / Db) − 4.85	1.086
		Female	(5.27 / Db) − 4.85	1.086
	13-17	Male	(5.12 / Db) − 4.69	1.092
		Female	(5.19 / Db) − 4.76	1.090
	18-59	Male	(4.95 / Db) − 4.50	1.100
		Female	(4.96 / Db) − 4.51	1.101
	60-90	Male	(4.97 / Db) − 4.52	1.099
		Female	(5.02 / Db) − 4.57	1.098
Hispanic		Male	NA	NA
	20-40	Female	(4.87 / Db) − 4.41	1.105
Athletes				
Resistance trained	24 ± 4	Male	(5.21 / Db) − 4.78	1.089
	35 ± 6	Female	(4.97 / Db) − 4.52	1.099
Endurance trained	21 ± 2	Male	(5.03 / Db) − 4.59	1.097
	21 ± 4	Female	(4.95 / Db) − 4.50	1.100
All sports	18-22	Male	5.12 / Db) − 4.68	1.093
	18-22	Female	4.97 / Db) − 4.52	1.099
Clinical populations				
Anorexia nervosa	15-44	Female	(4.96 / Db) − 4.51	1.101
Obesity	17-62	Female	(4.95 / Db) − 4.50	1.100
Spinal cord injury (paraplegic/quadriplegic)	18-73	Male	(4.67 / Db) − 4.18	1.116
		Female	(4.70 / Db) − 4.22	1.114

FFB$_d$ = fat-free body density; Db = body density; %BF = percent body fat; NA = no data available for this population subgroup.
[a]Multiply value by 100 to calculate %BF.
*FFB$_d$ based on average values reported in selected research articles.
Reprinted, by permission, from V. Heyward and D. Wagner, 2004, *Applied body composition assessment,* 2nd ed. (Champaign, IL: Human Kinetics), 9.

Hydrostatic Weighing

Hydrostatic weighing (HW) is a valid, reliable, and widely used laboratory method for assessing total Db. Hydrostatic weighing provides an estimate of total **body volume (BV)** from the water displaced by the body's volume. According to **Archimedes' principle**, weight loss under water is directly proportional to the volume of water displaced by the body volume. For calculating Db, body mass is divided by body volume. The total Db is a function of the amounts of muscle, bone, water, and fat in the body.

Using Hydrostatic Weighing

Determine BV by totally submerging the body in an underwater weighing tank or pool and measuring the **underwater weight (UWW)** of the body. To measure UWW, you can use either a chair attached to an HW scale (see figure 8.1) or a platform attached to load cells (see figure 8.2). Given that the weight loss under water is directly proportional to the volume of water displaced by the body's volume, the BV is equal to the body mass (BM) minus the UWW (see figure 8.3). The net UWW is the difference between the UWW and the weight of the chair or platform and its supporting equipment (i.e., **tare weight**). The BV must be corrected for the volume of air remaining in the lungs after a maximal expiration (i.e., **residual volume or RV**), as well as the volume of air in the gastrointestinal tract (GV). The GV is assumed to be 100 ml.

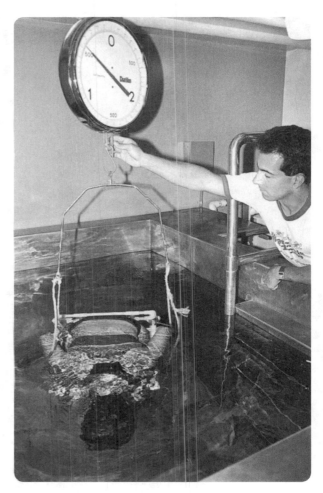

Figure 8.1 Hydrostatic weighing using scale and chair.

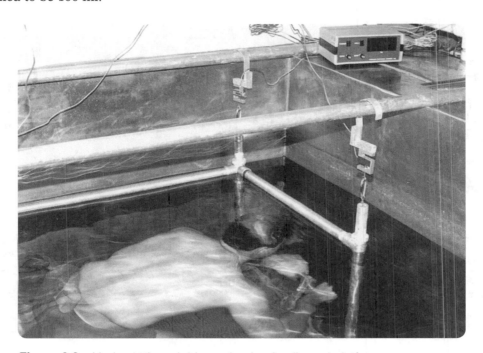

Figure 8.2 Hydrostatic weighing using load cells and platform.

Hydrostatic Weighing Data

Name _____   Date _____

Gender _____

Ethnicity _____

Body mass (BM) _____ lb _____ kg   Age _____

I. Measured RV: Estimated RV (select one equation from Appendix D.1, p. 330):
     (average 2 trials within 100 ml)

     Trial 1 _____ Trial 2 _____ Trial 3 _____

     Average measured RV = _____ L   Estimated RV = _____ L

II. Water temperature _____ °C

     Water density _____ g · cc⁻¹

Temperature (°C)	Density ($g \cdot cc^{-1}$)
33	0.9947
34	0.9944
35	0.9941
36	0.9937
37	0.9934

III. Gross underwater weight (in kg)

     Trial 1 _____   Trial 6 _____

     Trial 2 _____   Trial 7 _____

     Trial 3 _____   Trial 8 _____

     Trial 4 _____   Trial 9 _____

     Trial 5 _____   Trial 10 _____

     Average (3 trials within 0.1 kg)   _____ kg

IV. Tare weight (chair, platform, and supporting
     equipment)   _____ kg

V. Net underwater weight
    gross UWW _____ – tare weight _____ =   _____ kg

VI. Body volume (BV)
     [(BM in kg – net UWW in kg) / water density] – (RV + GV)
     Note. GV assumed value = 100 ml or 0.1 L   BV = _____ L

VII. Body density = BM (kg) / BV (L)
     (carry out to 5 or 6 decimal places)   Db = _____ g · cc⁻¹

VIII. % body fat (select conversion formula from table 8.2)   BF = _____ %

IX. Fat weight = BM × % BF (decimal)
     _____ × _____   FW = _____ kg

X. Fat-free mass = BM – FW
     _____ – _____   FFM = _____ kg

Comments and observations:

Figure 8.3 Hydrostatic weighing data collection form.

From Vivian H. Heyward, 2006, *Advanced Fitness Assessment and Exercise Prescription*, 5th ed. (Champaign, IL: Human Kinetics).

The RV is commonly measured using helium dilution, nitrogen washout, or oxygen dilution techniques. The RV is measured in liters and must be converted to kilograms (kg) in order to correct UWW. This is easy to do because 1 L of water weighs approximately 1 kg; therefore, the water weight per liter of RV is 1 kg. The BV is corrected by subtracting the equivalent weight of the RV and the GV (100 ml or 0.1 kg). Since water density varies with water temperature, the BV is corrected for water density (see figure 8.3). Under normal circumstances, the water temperature of the underwater weighing tank or swimming pool will be between 34 and 36 °C. The resulting equation for BV is

$$BV = [(BM - net\ UWW)/density\ of\ water] - (RV + GV)$$

Calculate body density (Db in $g \cdot cc^{-1}$) by dividing BM by BV: Db = BM/BV. After you calculate Db, you can convert it into **percent body fat (%BF)** by using the appropriate population-specific conversion formula (see table 8.2).

You should adhere to the following guidelines when using the HW technique:

Guidelines for Hydrostatic Weighing

Pretest Client Guidelines

- Do not eat or engage in strenuous exercise for at least 4 hr before your scheduled appointment.
- Avoid ingesting any gas-producing foods or beverages (e.g., baked beans or diet soda) for at least 12 hr before your test.
- Bring a towel and a tight-fitting, lightweight swimsuit.

Testing Procedure Guidelines

- Carefully calibrate the body weight scale and underwater weighing scale. To determine the accuracy of the autopsy scale, hang calibrated weights from the scale and check the corresponding scale values. To calibrate a load cell system, place weights on the platform and check the recorded values.
- Measure the underwater weight of the chair or platform and of the supporting equipment and weight belt; the total is the **tare weight.**
- Measure your client's dry weight (weight in air) to the nearest 50 g.
- Check and record the water temperature of the tank just before the test; it should range between 34 and 36 °C. Use the constant values in figure 8.3 (see p. 176) to determine the density of the water at that temperature.
- Instruct your client to enter the tank slowly, so that the water stays calm. Have the client gently submerge without touching the chair or weighing platform and rub his hands over his body to eliminate air bubbles from his swimsuit, skin, and hair.

- Have the client kneel on the underwater weighing platform or sit in the chair. Your client may need to wear a scuba diving weight belt to facilitate the kneeling or sitting position. If RV is being measured simultaneously, insert the mouthpiece at this time. If RV is measured outside of the tank, administer the RV test *before* the client changes clothes and showers.
- Have the client take a few normal breaths and then exhale maximally while slowly bending forward to submerge the head. Check to make certain that the client's head and back are completely underwater and that the arms and feet are not touching the sides or bottom of the tank. Instruct the client to continue exhaling until RV is reached. The client needs to remain as still as possible during this procedure. A relaxed and motionless state underwater will aid an accurate reading of UWW.
- Record the highest stable weight with the client fully submerged at RV; then signal to the client that the trial is completed.
- Administer as many trials as needed to obtain 3 readings within ±100 g. Most clients achieve a consistent and maximal UWW in 4 or 5 trials (Bonge and Donnelly 1989). Average the 3 highest trials and record this value as the gross UWW (Bonge and Donnelly 1989).
- Determine the net UWW by subtracting the tare weight from the gross UWW. The net UWW is used to calculate body volume (see figure 8.3, p. 176).

In addition to the HW testing guidelines, following the suggestions made in "Tips for Minimizing Error in Hydrostatic Weighing" below may improve the accuracy of your underwater weighing measurements.

Special Considerations

Some clients may have difficulty performing the HW test using these standardized procedures. Accurate test results are highly dependent on the client's skill, cooperation, and motivation. The following section addresses the use of modified HW procedures, as well as other questions and concerns about the use of this method.

■ *What should I do when my client is unable to blow out all of the air from the lungs or remain still while under water?*

You will likely come across clients who are uncomfortable expelling all of the air from their lungs during HW. In such cases, you can weigh these individuals at functional residual capacity (FRC) or total lung capacity (TLC) instead of RV. Thomas and Etheridge (1980) underwater-weighed 43 males, comparing the body densities measured at FRC (taken at the end of normal expiration while the person was submerged) and at RV (at the end of maximal expiration). The two methods yielded similar results. Similarly, Timson and Coffman (1984) reported that Db measured by HW at TLC (vital capacity + RV) was similar (less than 0.3% BF difference) to that measured at RV if TLC was measured in the water. However, when the TLC was measured out of the water, the method significantly overestimated Db. When using these modifications of the HW method, you must still measure RV in order to calculate the FRC or TLC of your client. Also, be certain to substitute the appropriate lung volume (FRC or TLC) for RV in the calculation of BV.

Because of their lower Db, clients with greater amounts of body fat are more buoyant than leaner individuals; therefore, they have more difficulty remaining motionless while under the water. To correct this problem, place a weighted scuba belt around the client's waist. Be certain to include the weight of the scuba belt when measuring and subtracting the tare weight of the HW system.

■ *What should I do when my clients are afraid to put their face in the water or are not flexible enough to get their backs and heads completely submerged?*

Occasionally, you will encounter clients who are extremely fearful of being submerged, who dislike facial contact with water, or who are unable to bend forward to assume the proper body position for HW. In such cases, a satisfactory alternative would be to weigh your clients at TLC while their heads remain above water level. Donnelly et al. (1988) compared this measure (i.e., TLCNS or total lung capacity with head not submerged) to the criterion Db obtained from HW at RV for 75 men and 67 women. Vital capacity was measured with the subject submerged in the water to shoulder level. Regression analysis yielded the following equations for predicting Db at RV, using the Db determined at TLCNS as the predictor:

Males

Db at RV = 0.5829(Db at TLCNS) + 0.4059

r = 0.88, *SEE* = 0.0067 g · cc^{-1}

Tips for Minimizing Error in Hydrostatic Weighing

- Make sure that your clients adhere to all pretesting guidelines.
- Before each test session, check the calibration of the BW and UWW scales or load cells and carefully calibrate the gas analyzers used to measure RV.
- Precisely measure BW to ±50 g, UWW to ±100 g, and RV to ±100 ml.
- Coach the client to maximally exhale and remain motionless under the water.
- Steady the underwater weighing apparatus as the client submerges, but remove your hand from the scale before actually reading the UWW.
- If possible, use a load cell system and measure RV and UWW simultaneously.
- Carry the calculated Db value out to 5 decimal places. Rounding off a Db of 1.07499 g · cc^{-1} to 1.07 g · cc^{-1} corresponds to a difference of 2.2% BF when converted with the Siri (1961) two-component model formula.
- If you are estimating %BF from Db with a two-component model, use the appropriate population-specific conversion formula (see table 8.2).

Females

$$Db \text{ at } RV = 0.4745(Db \text{ at } TLCNS) + 0.5173$$

$$r = 0.85, \ SEE = 0.0061 \text{ g} \cdot \text{cc}^{-1}$$

The correlations (r) between the actual Db at RV and the predicted Db at RV were high, and the standard errors of estimate (*SEE*) were within acceptable limits. These equations were cross-validated for an independent sample of 20 men and 20 women. The differences between the Db from HW at RV and the predicted Db from weighing at TLCNS were quite small (less than 0.0014 g · cc^{-1} or 0.7% BF). This method may be especially useful for HW of older adults, obese individuals with limited flexibility, and people with physical disabilities.

■ *Will the accuracy of the HW test be affected if I estimate RV instead of measuring it?*

Several prediction equations have been developed to estimate RV based on the individual's age, height, gender, and smoking status (see appendix D.1, "Prediction Equations for Residual Volume" p. 330). However, these RV prediction equations have large prediction errors (*SEE* = 400 to 500 ml). When RV is measured, the precision of the HW method is excellent (≤1% BF). However, this precision error increases substantially (±2.8% to 3.7% BF) when RV is estimated (Morrow, Jackson, Bradley, and Hartung 1986). Therefore, always measure RV when you are using the HW method.

■ *When is the best time during the menstrual cycle to hydrostatically weigh my female clients?*

Some women, particularly those whose body weight fluctuates widely during their menstrual cycles, may have significantly different estimates of Db and %BF when weighed hydrostatically at different times in their cycles. Bunt, Lohman, and Boileau (1989) reported that changes in total body water values due to water retention during the menstrual cycle partly explain the differences in body weight and Db during a menstrual cycle. On the average, the relative body fat of the women was 24.8% BF at their lowest body weights, compared to an average of 27.6% BF at their peak body weights during their menstrual cycles. Because their low and peak body weights occurred at different times during the menstrual cycle (varied from 0 to 14 days prior to the onset of the next menses), the effect of total body water fluctuations cannot be routinely controlled by using the same day of the menstrual cycle for all women. However, when you are monitoring changes in body composition over time or establishing healthy body weight for a female client, it is recommended that you hydrostatically weigh her at the same time within her menstrual cycle and outside of the period of her perceived peak body weight.

Air Displacement Plethysmography

Air displacement plethysmography (ADP) is a method used to measure body volume and density that uses air displacement instead of water displacement to estimate volume. Because ADP is quick (usually 5-10 min) and requires minimal client compliance and minimal technician skill, it may prove to be an alternative to hydrostatic weighing. The ADP method requires a whole-body plethysmograph such as the Bod Pod. The Bod Pod is a large, egg-shaped fiberglass chamber that uses air displacement and pressure–volume relationships to measure body volume (see figure 8.4).

The Bod Pod system consists of two chambers: a front chamber in which the client sits during the measurement and a rear reference chamber. A molded fiberglass seat forms the wall between the two chambers, and a moving diaphragm mounted in this wall oscillates during testing (figure 8.5). The oscillating diaphragm creates small volume changes between the two chambers. These changes

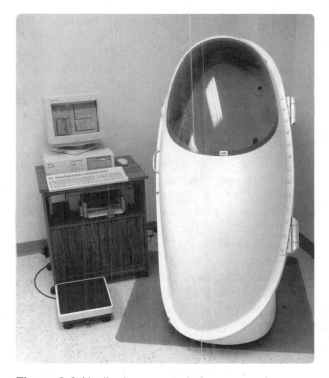

Figure 8.4 Air displacement plethysmograph.

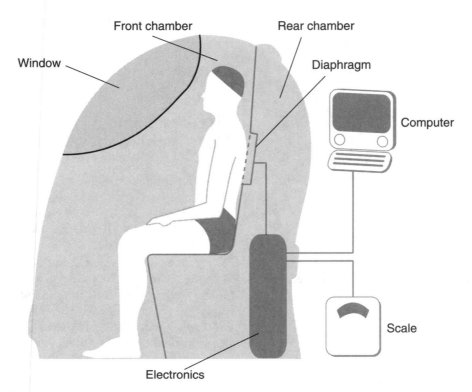

Figure 8.5 Two-chamber Bod Pod system.

are equal in magnitude but opposite in sign, and they produce small pressure fluctuations. The pressure-volume relationship is used to calculate the volume of the front chamber when it is empty and when the client is sitting in it. Body volume is calculated as the difference in the volume of the chamber with and without the client inside.

The principle underlying ADP centers on the relationship between pressure and volume. At a constant temperature (isothermal condition), volume (V) and pressure (P) are inversely related. According to **Boyle's law,**

$$P_1 / P_2 = V_2 / V_1,$$

where P_1 and V_1 represent one paired condition of pressure and volume and P_2 and V_2 represent another paired condition. P_1 and V_1 correspond to the pressure and volume of the Bod Pod when it is empty; P_2 and V_2 represent the pressure and volume of the Bod Pod when the client is in the chamber.

One assumption of the ADP method is that the Bod Pod controls the isothermal effects of clothing, hair, thoracic gas volume, and body surface area in the enclosed chamber. Bod Pod clients are tested while wearing minimal clothing (a swimsuit) and a swim cap to compress the hair. An estimate of the **body surface area**, calculated from the height and weight of the client, is used to correct for the

isothermal effects at the body's surface. **Thoracic gas volume (TGV)**, or the volume of air in the lungs and thorax, is either directly measured or estimated by the Bod Pod to account for the isothermal conditions in the lungs.

Numerous studies have assessed the accuracy of the Bod Pod for measuring Db. Several researchers reported only small differences in average Db (≤ 0.002 g · cc^{-1}) measured by the Bod Pod and HW (Fields et al. 2001; Vescovi et al. 2001; Yee et al. 2001). Others have reported slightly higher and statistically significant differences (0.003-0.007 g · cc^{-1}) in adults (Collins et al. 1999; Demerath et al. 2002; Dewit, Fuller, Fewtrell, Elia, and Wells 2000; Millard-Stafford et al. 2001; Wagner, Heyward, and Gibson 2000). Also, several studies reported "good" group prediction errors (*SEE* ≤ 0.008 g · cc^{-1}) in adults (Fields, Hunter, and Goran 2000; Nunez et al. 1999; Wagner et al. 2000). Compared to multicomponent body composition models, the Bod Pod and HW methods have similar predictive accuracy (Fields, Wilson, Gladden, Hunter, Pascoe, and Goran 2001). Because the Bod Pod is more accommodating than HW, there is much interest in establishing the validity of the ADP method for estimating %BF in clinical populations and special populations such as children and older adults (Heyward and Wagner 2004).

Using the ADP Method

The Bod Pod is user friendly, providing computer prompts for each step of the procedure. ADP is faster and easier than HW; researchers reported better compliance with ADP and a preference for ADP over HW among participants, including among children (Demerath et al. 2002; Dewit et al. 2000; Lockner, Heyward, Baumgartner, and Jenkins 2000). Before the scheduled appointment, give your client pretesting instructions. These instructions are the same as those for HW (see p. 177), except for the addition of bringing a swim cap. For step-by-step instructions for Bod Pod testing, see "Testing Procedures for the Bod Pod" below.

Testing Procedures for the Bod Pod

- Instruct the client to change into a swimsuit and to completely void the bladder and bowels.
- Measure the client's height to the nearest centimeter and body weight to the nearest 5 g using the Bod Pod scale. These measures are used to calculate body surface area.
- Perform the two-point calibration: (a) base-line calibration with the chamber empty and (b) phantom calibration with a 50 L calibration cylinder. Be careful when handling the calibration cylinder; a dent in the cylinder alters its volume.
- Instruct your client to sit in the chamber and close the door tightly. During this 20 sec test, ask your client to breathe normally.
- Open the door and then close it tightly; repeat the 20 sec test. If the two tests disagree by more than 150 ml, perform additional tests until two results agree within 150 ml; average these and use them to calculate raw BV.
- Open the door and connect the client to the system's breathing circuit to begin the TGV measurement.
- Close the door. After a few tidal volume (normal) breathing cycles, the airway is occluded by the Bod Pod. Instruct your client to perform the puffing maneuver. If the computer-calculated figure of merit (indicating similar pressure signals in the airway and chamber) is not met, repeat this step.

Special Considerations for ADP Method

Accurate test results from the Bod Pod depend on a number of factors. The following questions address these factors.

■ *How are the test results affected if my client has excess body hair?*

As mentioned earlier, isothermal air trapped in body hair may affect test results. For clients with beards, %BF may be underestimated by 1%; when scalp hair is exposed (no swim cap), relative body fat is underestimated by about 2.3% BF (Higgins, Fields, Hunter, and Gower 2001). Wearing a tight-fitting swim cap and shaving excess facial and body hair ensure the most accurate estimate of body volume and Db.

■ *Can I use the Bod Pod to measure the body composition of children?*

During the 20 sec test, the client must remain very still, as the body volume estimate from the ADP method can vary if the client moves during testing. Fields and Goran (2000) commented that it took twice as long to measure children compared to adults, primarily because children move during the test. As a result, the test–retest reliability of the Bod Pod is lower in children ($r = 0.90$) than in adults ($r = 0.96$) (Demerath et al. 2002).

Also, several researchers commented that body size may affect Bod Pod estimates, with the largest effects seen in the smallest clients (Demerath et al. 2002; Lockner et al. 2000; Nunez et al. 1999). The ideal chamber-to-client volume ratio may be exceeded for clients who have a small body, especially children (Fields and Goran 2000). This area requires further investigation.

■ *Is it absolutely necessary that my client wear a swimsuit and swim cap during the Bod Pod test?*

The original investigators of the Bod Pod recognized that the isothermal effect of clothing leads to an underestimation of body volume; they recommended that clients wear only a swimsuit and swim cap during testing to minimize this effect (Dempster and Aitkens 1995; McCrory, Gomez, Bernauer, and Mole 1995). More clothing leads to a larger layer of isothermal air and a greater underestimation of body volume. For example, wearing a hospital gown instead of a swimsuit lowers %BF by about 5% (Fields et al. 2000). Thus, the clothing recommendation needs to be followed.

■ *Do I need to measure my client's TGV or can I use a predicted TGV?*

Although McCrory and colleagues (1998) reported an insignificant difference (54 ml) between measured and predicted TGV, the *SEE* was large (442 ml). Some researchers have reported larger mean differences (344-400 ml) and *SEE*s

(650 ml) (Collins et al. 1999; Lockner et al. 2000). Given that only 40% of the TGV value is used to calculate body volume, using a predicted TGV has a relatively smaller effect on Db and %BF compared to using a predicted RV for the HW method. Nevertheless, a measured TGV maximizes accuracy.

■ *If I use both hydrostatic weighing and the Bod Pod to measure my client's body composition, which test should I give first?*

The Bod Pod manufacturer recommends testing clients under resting conditions and when the body is dry. Although there are no published studies indicating the amount of error that may occur by violating these guidelines, experts suggest adhering to these recommendations (Fields, Goran, and McCrory 2002). Thus, if a test battery includes both HW and ADP, administer the Bod Pod test first. If doing so is not possible, make certain that your client is completely dry and fully recovered from the HW test before you administer the Bod Pod test.

■ *Which model and equation should I use to convert Db to %BF?*

Using a multicomponent model and a population-specific conversion formula increases the group and individual accuracy of %BF estimates. The default equation in the Bod Pod software is the Siri (1961) two-component model formula for non-Black adults. A formula for Blacks is also available. In field settings, these two-component conversion formulas may be appropriate for some clients with certain demographic characteristics. For other clients you may need to select an appropriate population-specific, two-component model formula (see table 8.2, p. 174).

Dual-Energy X-Ray Absorptiometry

Dual-energy X-ray absorptiometry (DXA) is gaining recognition as a reference method for body composition research (see figure 8.6). This method yields estimates of bone mineral, fat, and lean soft-tissue mass. Dual-energy X-ray absorptiometry is an attractive alternative to HW because it is safe and rapid (a total-body scan takes 10-20 min), requires minimal client cooperation, and, most importantly, accounts for individual variability in bone mineral content.

The basic principle underlying DXA technology is that the attenuation of X-rays with high and low photon energies is measurable and dependent on the thickness, density, and chemical composition of the underlying tissue. The

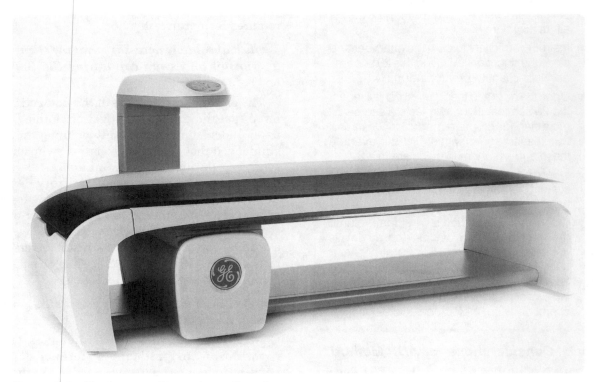

Figure 8.6 Dual-energy X-ray absorptiometer.
© 2006 General Electric Company

attenuation, or weakening, of X-rays through fat, lean tissue, and bone varies due to differences in the densities and chemical compositions of these tissues. The attenuation ratios for the high and low X-ray energies are thought to be constant for all individuals (Pietrobelli, Formica, Wang, and Heymsfield 1996).

It is difficult to assess the validity of the DXA method because each of the three manufacturers of DXA instruments (see "Sources for Equipment," p. 206) has developed its own models and software over the years. As many researchers and some clinicians have discovered, body composition results vary with manufacturer, model, and software version. Thus, some of the variability reported in DXA validation studies may be due to the different DXA scanners and software versions. As such, experts who have reviewed DXA studies have called for more standardization among manufacturers (Genton, Hans, Kyle, and Pichard 2002; Lohman 1996).

Some researchers have reported that the predictive accuracy of DXA is better than that of HW (Fields and Goran 2000; Friedl, DeLuca, Marchitelli, and Vogel 1992; Prior et al. 1997; Wagner and Heyward 2001; Withers et al. 1998). However, the opposite finding (that HW is more accurate than DXA) has also been reported (Bergsma-Kadijk, Baumeister, and Deurenberg 1996; Goran, Toth, and Poehlman 1998; Millard-Stafford et al. 2001). In a review of the DXA studies using recently developed software, Lohman and colleagues concluded that DXA estimates of %BF are within 1% to 3% of multicomponent model estimates (Lohman, Harris, Teixeira, and Weiss 2000). Although some body composition prediction equations have been developed and validated with DXA as the reference method, further research is needed before DXA can be firmly established as the best reference method.

Using the DXA method

The DXA method requires minimal client cooperation and minimal technical skill. However, to use the scanner to get precise and accurate DXA scans, proper training by the manufacturer is essential. Also, many states require that a licensed X-ray technician perform the scan. For general procedures for DXA testing, see "Basic Testing Procedures for DXA".

Basic Testing Procedures for DXA

- Before testing, calibrate the DXA scanner with a calibration marker provided by the manufacturer.
- Measure your client's height and weight with the client wearing minimal clothing and no shoes.
- Carefully place the client in a supine position on the scanner bed for a head-to-toe, anteroposterior scan.
- Use a skeletal anthropometer to accurately determine body thickness (see "Sagittal Abdominal Diameter" on page 202.
- Set the scanner for a whole-body scan at medium speed, which usually takes about 20 min. For clients with sagittal abdominal diameters exceeding 27 cm, use a slow scan, which typically takes 40 min.

Special Considerations

The accuracy of DXA results depends on a number of factors. The following questions address some of these factors.

■ *Will my client's body size and hydration state affect the test results?*

The DXA method should not be used to assess the body composition of clients whose body dimensions exceed the length or width of the scanning bed. Research has reported that normal fluctuations in hydration have little effect on DXA estimates (Lohman et al. 2000).

■ *For client comfort and compliance, is DXA better than other reference methods?*

Compared to other reference methods, DXA requires little client participation. The client does not need to perform the breathing maneuvers that are required for measuring RV for hydrostatic weighing and TGV for air displacement plethysmography.

■ *How do the various DXA machines and software versions affect test results?*

As mentioned previously, variability among DXA technologies is a major source of error. Although all DXA equipment uses the same underlying physical principles, the instruments differ in their generation of the high- and low-energy beams (filter or switching voltage), imaging geometry (pencil beam or fan beam), X-ray detectors, calibration methodology, and algorithms (Genton et al. 2002). Recent software versions have improved the accuracy of

DXA over that of the early 1990s (Kohrt 1998; Lohman et al. 2000; Tothill and Hannan 2000); however, the accuracy of recent DXA devices and software still needs to be determined (Genton et al. 2002). Because of technological differences, you should use the same DXA device and software version for longitudinal assessments or cross-sectional comparisons of body composition.

■ *Is the DXA method safe for my clients, given that it uses X-rays to measure body composition?*

DXA is considered to be safe for estimating body composition. The average skin dose of radiation is low, similar to a typical weekly exposure of environmental background radiation (Lukaski 1993). Still, DXA tests are not recommended for pregnant women.

FIELD METHODS FOR ASSESSING BODY COMPOSITION

In field settings, you can use more practical methods to estimate your client's body composition. Your choices include bioelectrical impedance, skinfold, and other types of anthropometric prediction equations. To use these methods and equations appropriately, you need to understand the basic assumptions and principles, as well as the potential sources of measurement error for each method. You must closely follow standardized testing procedures, and you must practice in order to perfect your measurement techniques for each method. For more detailed information about these field methods and how they are applied to various population subgroups, see Heyward and Wagner (2004).

Skinfold Method

A **skinfold** (SKF) indirectly measures the thickness of subcutaneous adipose tissue. When you use the SKF method to estimate total Db in order to calculate relative body fat (%BF), certain basic relationships are assumed:

■ **The SKF is a good measure of subcutaneous fat.** Research has demonstrated that the subcutaneous fat, assessed by SKF measurements at 12 sites, is similar to the value obtained from magnetic resonance imaging (Hayes, Sowood, Belyavin, Cohen, and Smith 1988).

■ **The distribution of fat subcutaneously and internally is similar for all individuals within each gender.** The validity of this assumption is questionable. There are large interindividual differences in the patterning of subcutaneous adipose tissue within and between genders (Martin, Ross, Drinkwater, and Clarys 1985). Older subjects of the same gender and Db have proportionately less subcutaneous fat than their younger counterparts. Also, lean individuals have a higher proportion of internal fat, and the proportion of fat located internally decreases as overall body fatness increases (Lohman 1981).

■ **Because there is a relationship between subcutaneous fat and total body fat, the sum of several SKFs can be used to estimate total body fat.** Research has established that SKF thicknesses at multiple sites measure a common body fat factor (Jackson and Pollock 1976; Quatrochi et al. 1992). It is assumed that approximately one-third of the total fat is located subcutaneously in men and women (Lohman 1981). However, there is considerable biological variation in subcutaneous, intramuscular, intermuscular, and internal organ fat deposits (Clarys, Martin, Drinkwater, and Marfell-Jones 1987), as well as essential lipids in bone marrow and the central nervous system. Age, gender, and degree of fatness all affect variation in fat distribution (Lohman 1981).

■ **There is a relationship between the sum of SKFs (ΣSKF) and Db.** This relationship is linear for homogeneous samples (population-specific SKF equations) but nonlinear over a wide range of Db (generalized SKF equations) for both men and women. A linear regression line depicting the relationship between the ΣSKF and Db will fit the data well only within a narrow range of body fatness values. Thus, you will get an inaccurate estimate if you use a population-specific equation to estimate the Db of a client who is not representative of the sample used to develop that equation (Jackson 1984).

■ **Age is an independent predictor of Db for both men and women.** Using age and the quadratic expression of the sum of skinfolds (ΣSKF^2) accounts for more variance in Db of a heterogeneous population than using the ΣSKF^2 alone (Jackson 1984).

Using the Skinfold Method

Skinfold prediction equations are developed using either linear (population specific) or quadratic (generalized) regression models. There are well over 100 population-specific equations for predicting Db from various combinations of SKFs, circumferences, and bony diameters (Jackson and Pollock 1985). These equations were developed for relatively homogeneous populations and are assumed to be valid only for individuals having similar characteristics, such as age, gender, ethnicity, or level of physical activity. For example, an equation derived specifically for 18- to 21-year-old sedentary men would not be valid for predicting the Db of 35- to 45-year-old sedentary men. Population-specific equations are based on a linear relationship between SKF fat and Db (linear model); however, research shows that there is a curvilinear relationship (quadratic model) between SKFs and Db across a large range of body fatness (see figure 8.7). Population-specific equations will tend to underestimate %BF in fatter subjects and overestimate it in leaner subjects.

Using the quadratic model, Jackson and colleagues (Jackson and Pollock 1978; Jackson, Pollock, and Ward 1980) developed generalized equations applicable to individuals varying greatly in age (18 to 60 years) and body fatness (up to 45% BF). These equations also take into account the effect of age on the distribution of subcutaneous and internal fat. An advantage of the generalized equations is that you can use one equation, instead of several, to accurately estimate your clients' %BF.

Most equations use two or three SKFs to predict Db. Experts recommend using equations that have SKF measures from a variety of sites, including both upper- and lower-body sites (Martin et al. 1985). The Db is then converted to %BF using the appropriate population-specific conversion formula (see table 8.2). Table 8.3 presents commonly used population-specific and generalized SKF prediction equations. Select the appropriate SKF equation and population-specific conversion formula in table 8.2 to estimate %BF based on physical demographics (e.g., age, gender, ethnicity, and physical activity level) of your client. Using these equations, you can accurately estimate the %BF of your clients within the recommended value, ±3.5% BF (Lohman 1992).

Alternatively, nomograms exist for some SKF prediction equations. The nomogram in figure 8.8 was specifically developed for the Jackson sum of three SKF equations. To use this nomogram, plot the sum of three skinfolds (Σ3SKF) and age in the

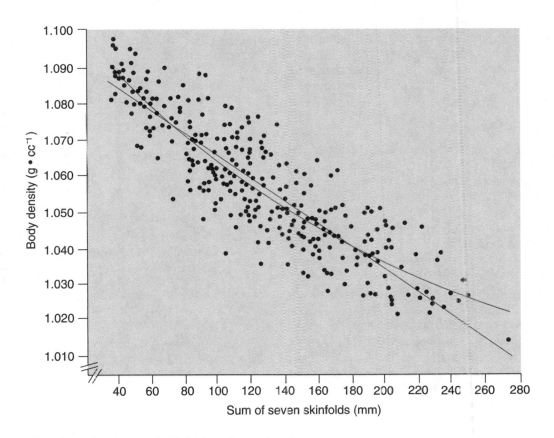

Figure 8.7 Relationship of sum of skinfolds to body density.

Reprinted, by permission, from A.S. Jackson and M.L. Pollock, 1978, "Generalized equations for predicting body density of men," *British Journal of Nutrition* 40: 502.

TABLE 8.3　Skinfold Prediction Equations

SKF sites	Population subgroups	Equation	Reference
Σ7SKF (chest + abdomen + thigh + triceps + subscapular + suprailiac + midaxilla)	Black or Hispanic women, 18-55 years	Db (g · cc^{-1})^a = 1.0970 − 0.00046971(Σ7SKF) + 0.00000056(Σ7SKF)^2 − 0.00012828(age)	Jackson et al. (1980)
	Black men or male athletes, 18-61 years	Db (g · cc^{-1})^a = 1.1120 − 0.00043499(Σ7SKF) + 0.00000055(Σ7SKF)^2 − 0.00028826(age)	Jackson and Pollock (1978)
Σ4SKF (triceps + anterior suprailiac + abdomen + thigh)	Female athletes, 18-29 years	Db (g · cc^{-1})^a = 1.096095 − 0.0006952(Σ4SKF) + 0.0000011(Σ4SKF)^2 − 0.0000714(age)	Jackson et al. (1980)
Σ3SKF (triceps + suprailiac + thigh)	White or anorexic women, 18-55 years	Db (g · cc^{-1})^a = 1.0994921 − 0.0009929(Σ3SKF) + 0.0000023(Σ3SKF)^2 − 0.0001392(age)	Jackson et al. (1980)
(chest + abdomen + thigh)	White men, 18-61 years	Db (g · cc^{-1})^a = 1.109380 − 0.0008267(Σ3SKF) + 0.0000016(Σ3SKF)^2 − 0.0002574(age)	Jackson and Pollock (1978)
Σ2SKF (triceps + calf)	Black or White boys, 6-17 years	%BF = 0.735(Σ2SKF) + 1.0	Slaughter et al. (1988)
	Black or White girls, 6-17 years	%BF = 0.610(Σ2SKF) + 5.1	Slaughter et al. (1988)

ΣSKF = sum of skinfolds (mm).

^{a}Use population-specific conversion formulas to calculate %BF (percent body fat) from Db (body density).

appropriate columns and use a ruler to connect these two points. The corresponding %BF is read at the point where the connecting line intersects the %BF column on the nomogram.

Although nomograms are potential time-savers, you should be aware that this nomogram is based on a two-component body composition model, using the Siri equation to convert Db to %BF. In general, use this nomogram only to calculate %BF of clients with an estimated fat-free body density of 1.100 g · cc^{-1} (see table 8.2).

Skinfold Technique

It takes a great deal of time and practice to develop your skill as a SKF technician. Following standardized procedures (p. 188) will increase the accuracy and reliability of your measurements.

You will also be able to increase your skill as a SKF technician by following the recommendations (p. 188) made by experts in the field (Jackson and Pollock 1985; Lohman, Pollock, Slaughter, Brandon, and Boileau 1984; Pollock and Jackson 1984).

In addition to perfecting your technical skills, you should develop your interpersonal skills when administering SKF and other anthropometric tests. For suggestions about developing interpersonal skills (Habash 2002), see "Tips for Developing Interpersonal Skills".

Tips for Developing Interpersonal Skills

- Before the scheduled test session, instruct your clients to wear loose clothing that allows easy access to the measurement sites, such as shorts and a T-shirt or two-piece exercise gear.

- Often clients are apprehensive about having their SKFs measured, particularly when they are meeting you for the first time. During the testing, put your client at ease by establishing good rapport (e.g., talk about some unrelated topic), projecting a sense of relaxed confidence, and creating a test environment that is friendly, private, safe, and comfortable.

- Perform the test in an uncluttered private room that holds a small table for calipers, pens, and clipboards and a chair for clients who are unstable standing or need to rest during the testing.

- Some clients feel more comfortable having their SKFs measured by a technician of the same gender. If this is not feasible, you could ask your clients if they would like another person of the same gender to observe the test.

- Educate your clients about the SKF test by talking about the purpose and use of the measurements, pointing to the SKF sites on your body, and demonstrating on yourself how the SKF is measured.

- Limit your verbal and facial reactions while collecting SKF data.

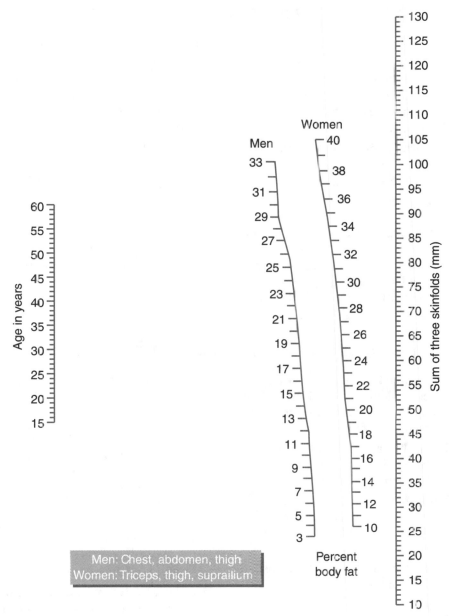

Figure 8.8 Nomogram to estimate percent body fat of college-age men and women using the Jackson sum-of-three skinfold equations.

From "A Nomogram for the Estimate of Percent Body Fat From Generalized Equations" by W.B. Baun and M.R. Baun, 1981. Reprinted with permission from *Research Quarterly for Exercise and Sport*, 52, p. 382. Copyright 1981 by American Alliance for Health, Physical Education, and Dance, 1900 Association Drive, Reston, VA 20191.

Sources of Measurement Error

The accuracy and precision of SKF measurements and the SKF method are affected by the technician's skill, the type of SKF caliper, and client factors. The following questions and responses address these sources of measurement error.

■ *Is there high agreement among SKF values when the measurements are taken by two different technicians?*

A major source of measurement error is differences between SKF technicians. Objectivity, or between-technician reliability, is improved when SKF technicians follow standardized testing procedures, practice taking SKFs together, and mark the SKF site (Pollock and Jackson 1984). A major cause of low intertester reliability is improper location and measurement of the SKF sites (Lohman, Pollock, Slaughter, Brandon, and Boileau 1984).

The amount of between-technician error depends on the SKF site, with larger errors reported for the abdomen (8.8%) and thigh (7.1%) sites than for the triceps (~3.0%), subscapular (~3.0-5.0%), and suprailiac (~4%) sites (Lohman, Pollock et al. 1984).

STANDARDIZED PROCEDURES FOR SKINFOLD MEASUREMENTS

1. Take all SKF measurements on the right side of the body.
2. Carefully identify, measure, and mark the SKF site, especially if you are a novice SKF technician (see appendix D.2, "Standardized Sites for Skinfold Measurements," p. 331).
3. Grasp the SKF firmly between the thumb and index finger of your left hand. Lift the fold 1 cm (0.4 in.) above the site to be measured.
4. Lift the fold by placing the thumb and index finger 8 cm (~3 in.) apart on a line that is perpendicular to the long axis of the SKF. The long axis is parallel to the natural cleavage lines of the skin. For individuals with extremely large SKFs, you will need to separate your thumb and finger more than 8 cm in order to lift the fold.

5. Keep the fold elevated while you take the measurement.
6. Place the jaws of the caliper perpendicular to the fold, approximately 1 cm below the thumb and index finger and halfway between the crest and the base of the fold. Release the jaw pressure slowly.
7. Take the SKF measurement 4 sec after the pressure is released. The ACSM (2006) recommends that you wait only 1 to 2 sec before reading the caliper.
8. Open the jaws of the caliper to remove it from the site. Close the jaws slowly to prevent damage or loss of calibration.

RECOMMENDATIONS FOR SKINFOLD TECHNICIANS

- Be meticulous when locating the anatomical landmarks used to identify the SKF site, when measuring the distance, and when marking the site with a surgical marking pen.
- Read the dial of the caliper to the nearest 0.1 mm (Harpenden or Holtain), 0.5 mm (Lange), or 1 mm (plastic calipers).
- Take a minimum of two measurements at each site. If values vary from each other by more than ±10%, take additional measurements.
- Take SKF measurements in a rotational order (circuits) rather than taking consecutive readings at each site.
- Take the SKF measurements when the client's skin is dry and lotion free.

- Do not measure SKFs immediately after exercise because the shift in body fluid to the skin tends to increase the size of the SKF.
- Practice taking SKFs on 50 to 100 clients.
- Avoid using plastic calipers if you are an inexperienced SKF technician. Instead use metal calipers.
- Train with skilled SKF technicians and compare your results.
- Use a SKF training videotape that demonstrates proper SKF techniques (Lohman 1987; Human Kinetics 1995).
- Seek additional training through workshops held at state, regional, and national conferences or through distance education courses (Human Kinetics 1999).

■ *Are the anatomical descriptions for specific SKF sites the same for all SKF equations?*

In the past, for some SKF sites, the anatomical location and direction of the fold have varied. For example, Behnke and Wilmore (1974) recommend measuring the abdominal SKF using a horizontal fold adjacent to the umbilicus; Jackson and Pollock (1978), however, recommend measuring a vertical fold taken 2 cm (0.8 in.) lateral to the umbilicus. Inconsistencies such as this have led to confusion and lack of agreement among SKF technicians. As a result, groups of experts in the field of anthropometry have developed standard-

ized testing procedures and detailed descriptions for identification and measurement of SKF sites (Harrison et al. 1988; Ross and Marfell-Jones 1991). Appendix D.2, "Standardized Sites for Skinfold Measurements" (p. 331), summarizes some of the most commonly used sites, as described in the *Anthropometric Standardization Reference Manual*.

Although the objective is to have all SKF technicians follow standardized procedures and recommendations for site location and SKF measurements, you may not be able to do so under all circumstances. For example, if you are using the generalized equations of Jackson and Pollock (1978) and Jackson et al. (1980), the chest, midaxillary, subscapular, abdominal, and suprailiac SKFs will be located at sites that differ from those described in the *Anthropometric Standardization Reference Manual*. The descriptions for the sites used in these equations are presented in appendix D.3, "Skinfold Sites for Jackson's Generalized Skinfold Equations," page 336.

■ *How many measurements do I need to take at each SKF site?*

A lack of intratechnician reliability or consistency of measurements by the SKF technician is another source of error for the SKF method. You need to practice your SKF technique on 50 to 100 clients to develop a high degree of skill and proficiency (Jackson and Pollock 1985). Take a minimum of two measurements at each site using a rotational order. If values vary from each other by more than ±10%, take additional measurements and average the two trials that meet this criterion. Use this average value in the SKF prediction equation. The ±10% value for duplicate measurements at each site is recommended as the standardized procedure in the *Anthropometric Standardized Reference Manual*.

However, if you are preparing to take an ACSM certification examination, you will need to modify this standardized procedure slightly by using the ACSM-recommended criterion for duplicate SKF measurements. The ACSM (2006) also suggests taking at least two measurements at each site in rotational order; however, these two measurements at a given site need to be within 1 to 2 mm of each other. If you take more than two measurements to meet this criterion, average the two trials that are within ±1 to 2 mm of each other and use this value in the prediction equation to estimate Db and %BF. On the other hand, some researchers suggest taking three SKF measurements at each site and using the median (middle score) instead of the mean (average) (Ward and Anderson 1998).

■ *What types of SKF calipers are available and how do they differ?*

There is a variety of high-quality metal and plastic calipers for measuring SKF thickness (see figure 8.9). When choosing a caliper, you need to consider factors such as cost, durability, accuracy, and precision as well as consider which type of caliper was used for developing a specific SKF equation. Table 8.4 and figure 8.10 compare some of the basic characteristics of selected SKF calipers.

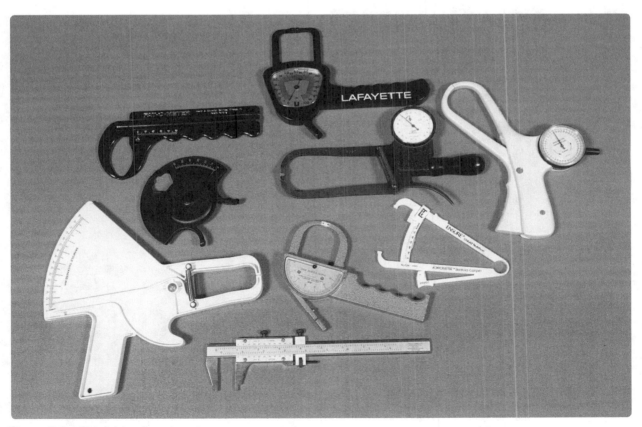

Figure 8.9 Skinfold calipers.

TABLE 8.4 Comparison of High-Quality Metal Calipers and Plastic SKF Calipers

Caliper type	Average pressure (g/mm²)	Range (mm)	Scale precision (mm)	Accuracy	Durability	Cost (approximate)	Unique features	Supplier[c]
METAL								
Harpenden (HA)	8.2	0-55	0.2	HA < LNG[a]	Excellent	$305		Creative Health Products
Lange (LNG)	8.4	0-60	0.5	LNG > HA[a]	Excellent	$180		Creative Health Products
Lafayette (LF)	7.5	0-100	0.5	LF > LNG[a]	Excellent	$440	Measurement range 0-100 mm	Creative Health Products
Skyndex (SKN)	7.3		0.5	SKN < LNG[a]; SKN ≅ HA[a]	Excellent	$450*	Skyndex I: built-in computer, Durnin & Womersley and Jackson & Pollock equations; Syndex II: digital readout but no computer	Creative Health Products
Holtain (HO)			0.2	HO < HA, LNG[b]	Excellent	$300		Pfister Import-Export
PLASTIC								
Accu-Measure (AM)	NR	0-60	1.0	NR	Fair	$20	Can be used for self-assessment of body fat	Accu-Measure
Body Caliper (BC)	NR	0-60	1.0	BC ≅ HA[b]	Good	$59	Measurement scale on both sides of caliper; suitable for right- or left-handed technician	The Caliper Company
Fat-O-Meter (F)	5.6	0-40	2.0	F ≅ LNG[b]	Poor	$15		Creative Health Products
Fat Track (FT)	NR	0-60	0.1	NR	Good	$50	Can be used for self-assessment of body fat; digital readout; Jackson & Pollock equations	Accu-Measure
McGaw (MG)	12.0	0-40	2.0	MG ≅ HA[b], MG < LNG[b]	Fair	$5		None available
Ross Adipometer (RA)	12.0	0-60	2.0	RA ≅ HA[b], RA < LNG[b]	Fair	$7		Ross Products Division
Slim Guide (SG)	7.5	0-80	1.0	SG ≅ HA ≅ SKN[a], SG < LNG[a]	Good	$25		Creative Health Products

[a]Determined by comparing dynamic compression of foam-rubber models of human skinfolds.
[b]Determined by comparing skinfold thicknesses of individuals measured by a technician; thus, any differences include not only instrument error but also error associated with technician skill and client factors.
[c]For supplier's address, see list on page 206.
*This price is for Skyndex I; Skyndex II caliper without the computer is $285.
NR = not reported.

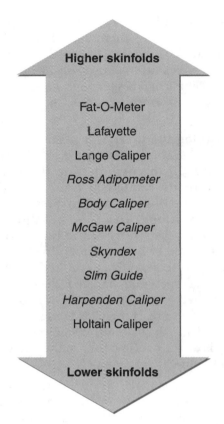

Figure 8.10 Relative ranking of values measured by various types of skinfold calipers. Calipers in italics give similar skinfold readings.

High-quality metal calipers are accurate and precise throughout the range of measurement. The Harpenden, Lange, Holtain, and Lafayette calipers exert constant pressure ($\sim$7-8 g/mm^2) over their range (0-60 mm). Calipers should not have tension that varies by more than 2.0 g/mm^2 throughout the range of measurement or exceeds 15 g/mm^2 (Edwards et al. 1955). Excessive tension and pressure cause client discomfort (pinching sensation) and significantly reduce the SKF measurement (Gruber, Pollock, Graves, Colvin, and Braith 1990). High-quality calipers also have excellent scale precision (e.g., 0.2 and 1.0 mm, respectively, for Harpenden and Lange).

Although the Harpenden and Lange SKF calipers have similar pressure characteristics, a number of researchers reported that SKFs measured with Harpenden calipers are significantly smaller than those measured with Lange calipers (Gruber et al. 1990; Lohman, Pollock et al. 1984; Schmidt and Carter 1990). This difference translates into a systematic underestimation ($\sim$1.5% BF) of average %BF by the Harpenden calipers (Gruber et al. 1990). Even though the pressure is similar for the

Lange (8.37 g/mm^2) and Harpenden (8.25 g/mm^2) calipers (Schmidt and Carter 1990), researchers noted that opening the jaws of the Harpenden caliper requires three times more force. Therefore, it is likely that the Harpenden compresses adipose tissue to a greater extent, resulting in SKF measurements smaller than those the Lange caliper yields.

■ *Are plastic SKF calipers as accurate as high-quality metal calipers?*

Compared to high-quality calipers, some plastic calipers have less scale precision ($\sim$2 mm), do not exert constant tension throughout the range of measurement, and have a smaller range of measurement (0-40 mm). Despite these differences, some plastic calipers compare well (see table 8.4) with more expensive, high-quality metal calipers (Cataldo and Heyward 2000). Given that the type of caliper is a potential source of measurement error, follow these suggestions to minimize error:

■ Use the same caliper when monitoring changes in your client's SKF thicknesses.

■ Use the same type of caliper as was used in the development of the specific SKF prediction equation you have selected. If the same type of caliper is not available, use one that gives similar readings (see figure 8.10).

■ Periodically check the accuracy of your caliper and calibrate if needed.

■ *Will my client's hydration level affect the SKF measurements?*

Skinfold measurements may also be affected by compressibility of the adipose tissue and hydration levels of your clients (Ward, Rempel, and Anderson 1999). Martin, Drinkwater, and Clarys (1992) reported that variation in SKF compressibility may be an important limitation of the SKF method. In addition, an accumulation of extracellular water (edema) in the subcutaneous tissue—caused by factors such as peripheral vasodilation or certain diseases—may increase SKF thicknesses (Keys and Brozek 1953). This suggests that you should not measure SKFs immediately after exercise, especially in hot environments. Also, most of the weight gain experienced by some women during their menstrual cycles is caused by water retention (Burt et al. 1989). This theoretically could increase SKF thicknesses, particularly on the trunk and abdomen; but there are no empirical data to support or refute this hypothesis.

■ *Should SKFs be measured on the right or left side of the body?*

There are only small differences (1 to 2 mm) between SKF thicknesses on the right and left sides of the body for the typical individual. The standard practice in the United States, as well as in European and developing countries, however, is to take SKF measurements on the right side of the body, as recommended in the *Anthropometric Standardization Reference Manual* (Lohman, Roche, and Martorell 1988) and by the International Society for the Advancement of Kinanthropometry (Norton et al. 2000).

■ *Should I use SKFs to measure the body fat of obese clients?*

It is difficult, even for highly skilled SKF technicians, to measure the SKF thickness of extremely obese individuals accurately. Sometimes the client's SKF thickness exceeds the maximum aperture of the caliper, and the jaws of the caliper may slip off the fold during the measurement, resulting in a potentially embarrassing and awkward situation for you and your client. Therefore, avoid using the SKF method to measure body fat of extremely obese clients.

Bioelectrical Impedance Method

Bioelectrical impedance analysis (BIA) is a rapid, noninvasive, and relatively inexpensive method for evaluating body composition in field settings. With this method, a low-level electrical current is passed through the client's body, and the **impedance** (Z), or opposition to the flow of current, is measured with a BIA analyzer. You can estimate the individual's total body water (TBW) from the impedance measurement because the electrolytes in the body's water are excellent conductors of electrical current. When the volume of TBW is large, the current flows more easily through the body with less resistance (R). The resistance to current flow is greater in individuals with large amounts of body fat, since adipose tissue, with its relatively low water content, is a poor conductor of electrical current. Because the water content of the FFB component is relatively large (~73% water), **fat-free mass** (FFM) can be predicted from TBW estimates. Individuals with large FFM and TBW have less resistance to current flowing through their bodies than those with a smaller FFM.

Bioelectrical impedance indirectly estimates FFM and TBW. Therefore, the following assumptions are made about the geometric shape of the body and the relationship of impedance to the length and volume of the conductor.

■ **The human body is shaped like a perfect cylinder with a uniform length and cross-sectional area.** Of course, this assumption is not entirely true. Because the body segments are not uniform in length or cross-sectional area, resistance to the flow of current through these body segments will differ.

■ **Assuming the body is a perfect cylinder, at a fixed signal frequency (e.g., 50 kHz), the impedance (Z) to current flow through the body is directly related to the length (L) of the conductor (height) and inversely related to its cross-sectional area [$Z = \rho(L/A)$, where p is the specific resistivity of the body's tissues and is assumed to be constant].** To express this relationship in terms of Z and the body's volume, instead of its cross-sectional area, the equation is multiplied by L/L: $Z = \rho(L/A)(L/L)$. $A \times L$ is equal to volume (V), so rearranging this equation yields $V = \rho L^2/Z$. Thus, the volume of the FFM or TBW of the body is directly related to L^2, or height squared (ht^2), and indirectly related to Z.

■ **Biological tissues act as conductors or insulators, and the flow of current through the body will follow the path of least resistance.** Because the FFM contains large amounts of water (~73%) and electrolytes, it is a better conductor of electrical current than fat. Fat is anhydrous and a poor conductor of electrical current. The total body impedance, measured at the constant frequency of 50 kHz, primarily reflects the volumes of the water and muscle compartments composing the FFM and the extracellular water volume (Kushner 1992).

■ **Impedance is a function of resistance and reactance, where $Z = \sqrt{(R^2 + X_c^2)}$. Resistance** (R) is a measure of pure opposition to current flow through the body; **reactance (X_c)** is the opposition to current flow caused by capacitance produced by the cell membrane (Kushner 1992). R is much larger than X_c (at a 50-kHz frequency) when whole-body impedance is measured; therefore, R is a better predictor of FFM and TBW than Z (Lohman 1989). For these reasons, the **resistance index** (ht^2/R), instead of ht^2/Z, is often used in many BIA models to predict FFM or TBW.

Using the Bioelectrical Impedance Analysis Method

The traditional BIA method measures whole-body resistance using a tetrapolar wrist-to-ankle electrode configuration at a single frequency for estimating TBW or FFM (figure 8.11). However, technological advances and changes in theoretical modeling have led to a number of variations in the traditional BIA method. These variations use sophisticated models to assess segmental body composition and fluid subcompartments, thereby improving the clinical usefulness of BIA. Also, user-friendly BIA analyzers designed for home use and individual monitoring of health and fitness use upper- or lower-body impedance measures to estimate body composition (figure 8.12).

Whole-body bioimpedance measures (Z, R, and X_c) are used in BIA prediction equations to estimate TBW and FFM. These prediction equations are based on either population-specific or generalized models. A population-specific equation is valid for only those individuals whose physical characteristics match the sample from which the equation was derived. Researchers have developed equations specific to age (Deurenberg, vanderKooy, Evers, and Hulshof 1990; Lohman 1992), ethnicity (Stolarczyk, Heyward, Hicks, and Baumgartner 1994), body fatness (Gray, Bray, Gemayel, and Kaplan 1989; Segal, VanLoan, Fitzgerald, Hodgdon, and van Itallie 1988), and level of physical activity (Houtkooper, Going, Westfall, and Lohman 1989). Alternatively, generalized BIA equations have been developed for heterogeneous populations varying in age, gender, and body fatness (Deurenberg et al. 1990; Gray et al. 1989; Kyle, Genton, Karsegard,

Slosman, and Pichard 2001; Kushner and Schoeller 1986; Lukaski and Bolonchuk 1988; Van Loan and Mayclin 1987).

Inexpensive lower-body (foot-to-foot) and upper-body (hand-to-hand) BIA devices are available and have been marketed for home use. The Tanita analyzers measure lower-body impedance between the right and left legs as the individual stands on the analyzer's electrode plates (see figure 8.12a). The Omron Body Logic analyzer, which is hand-held, measures upper-body impedance between the right and left arms (see figure 8.12b). The Tanita and Omron analyzers estimate %BF and FFM using proprietary equations developed by the manufacturers. Typically, it is not possible to obtain impedance (resistance and reactance) data from these analyzers. However, they do provide the general public with an inexpensive, simple, and reasonably accurate means of self-assessing body fat.

Table 8.5 presents commonly used population-specific and generalized BIA equations. With these equations, you can accurately estimate the FFM of your clients within the recommended values, ±2.8 kg for women and ±3.5 kg for men (Lohman 1992). To use these equations, obtain R and X_c directly from your BIA analyzer. Estimate the %BF of your client by determining the **fat mass (FM)** (FM =

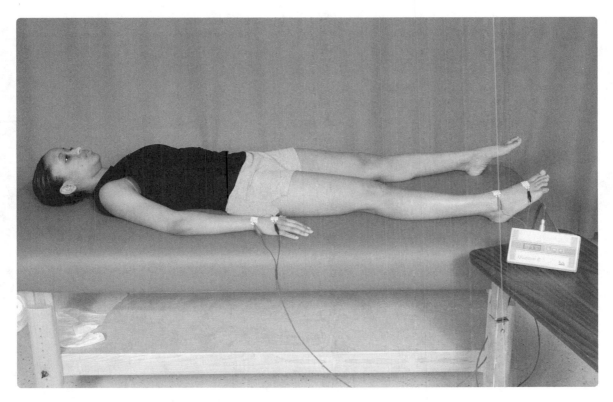

Figure 8.11 Bioelectrical impedance analysis electrode placement and client positioning.

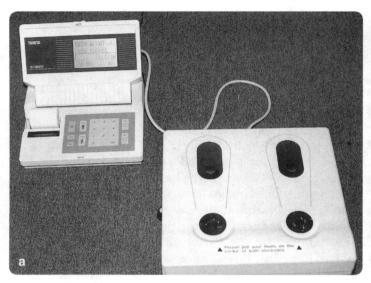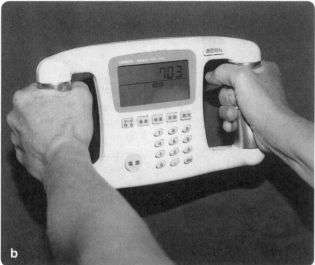

Figure 8.12 *(a)* Tanita and *(b)* Omron bioelectrical impedance analyzers.

TABLE 8.5 Bioelectrical Impedance Analysis Prediction Equations

Population subgroup	%BF level[a]	Equation	Reference
American Indian, Black, Hispanic, or White men, 17-62 years	<20% BF	FFM (kg) = 0.00066360(ht²) − 0.02117(R) + 0.62854(BM) − 0.12380(age) + 9.33285	Segal et al. (1988)
	≥20% BF	FFM (kg) = 0.00088580(ht²) − 0.02999(R) + 0.42688(BM) − 0.07002(age) + 14.52435	Segal et al. (1988)
American Indian, Black, Hispanic, or White women, 17-62 years	<30% BF	FFM (kg) = 0.000646(ht²) − 0.014(R) + 0.421(BM) + 10.4	Segal et al. (1988)
	≥30% BF	FFM (kg) = 0.00091186(ht²) − 0.01466(R) + 0.29990(BM) − 0.07012(age) + 9.37938	Segal et al. (1988)
White boys and girls, 8-15 years	NA	FFM (kg) = 0.62(ht²/R) + 0.21(BM) + 0.10(X_c) + 4.2	Lohman (1992)
White boys and girls, 10-19 years	NA	FFM (kg) = 0.61(ht²/R) + 0.25(BM) + 1.31	Houtkooper et al. (1992)
Female athletes, 18-27 years	NA	FFM (kg) = 0.282(ht) + 0.415(BM) −0.037(R) + 0.096(X_c) − 9.734	Fornetti et al. (1999)
Male athletes, 19-40 years	NA	FFM (kg) = 0.186(ht²/R) + 0.701(BM) + 1.949	Oppliger et al. (1991)

NA = not applicable.

[a]For clients who are obviously lean, use the <20% BF (men) and <30% BF (women) equations. For clients who are obviously obese, use the ≥20% BF (men) and ≥30% BF (women) equations. For clients who are not obviously lean or obese, calculate their FFM using both the lean and obese equations and then average the two FFM estimates.

%BF = percent body fat; FFM = fat-free mass; BM = body mass; R = resistance; X_c = reactance; ht = height.

BM – FFM) and dividing FM by the client's body mass [%BF = (FM/BM) × 100].

Experts recommend not using the FFM and %BF estimates obtained directly from your BIA analyzer (e.g., BMR, Holtain, RJL, or Valhalla) unless you know for sure which equations are programmed in the analyzer's computer software, obtain information from the manufacturer regarding the validity and accuracy of these equations, and determine that these equations are applicable to your clients.

Although the relative predictive accuracy of the BIA method is similar to that of the SKF method, BIA may be preferable in some settings for the following reasons:

- It does not require a high degree of technician skill.

- It is generally more comfortable and does not intrude as much upon the client's privacy.

- It can be used to estimate body composition of obese individuals.

Bioelectrical Impedance Analysis Technique

BIA accuracy highly depends on controlling the factors that may increase measurement error. Regardless of the BIA method (whole, upper, or lower body) being used, your client must adhere to the "BIA Pretesting Client Guidelines", which are designed to control fluctuations in hydration status.

BIA Pretesting Client Guidelines

- No eating or drinking within 4 hr of the test.
- No moderate or vigorous exercise within 12 hr of the test.
- Void completely within 30 min of the test.
- Abstain from alcohol consumption within 48 hr of the test.
- Do not ingest diuretics, including caffeine, before the assessment unless they are prescribed by a physician.
- If you are in a stage of your menstrual cycle during which you perceive you are retaining water, postpone testing (female clients).

Use standardized testing procedures to minimize error in the BIA method (see "Standardized Procedures for the Whole-Body BIA Method").

Standardized Procedures for the Whole-Body BIA Method

- Take bioimpedance measures on the right side of the body with the client lying supine on a nonconductive surface in a room with normal ambient temperature (~25 °C).

- Clean the skin at the electrode sites with an alcohol pad.

- Place the sensor (proximal) electrodes on (a) the dorsal surface of the wrist so that the upper border of the electrode bisects the head of the ulna and (b) the dorsal surface of the ankle so that the upper border of the electrode bisects the medial and lateral malleoli (see figure 8.11). You can use a measuring tape and surgical marking pen to mark these points for electrode placement.

- Place the source (distal) electrodes at the bases of the second or third metacarpophalangeal joints of the hand and foot (see figure 8.11). Make certain there is at least 5 cm between the proximal and distal electrodes.

- Attach the lead wires to the appropriate electrodes. Red leads are attached to the wrist and ankle and black leads are attached to the hand and foot.

- Make certain that the client's legs and arms are comfortably abducted, at about a 30° to 45° angle from the trunk. Ensure that there is no contact between the arms and trunk and between the thighs as contact will short-circuit the electrical path, dramatically affecting the impedance value.

Sources of Measurement Error

The accuracy and precision of the BIA method are affected by instrumentation, client factors, technician skill, environmental factors, and the prediction equation used to estimate FFM. The following questions address sources of BIA measurement error.

- ***Can different types of whole-body BIA analyzers be used interchangeably?***

Research demonstrates significant differences in whole-body resistance when different brands of single-frequency analyzers are used (Graves, Pollock, Colvin, Van Loan, and Lohman 1989; Smye, Sutcliffe, and Pitt 1993). For example, Smye and colleagues (1993) reported lower resistances (6% or 32-36 Ω) for the Holtain device compared to the Bodystat, RJL, and EZcomp analyzers. Graves and colleagues (1989) noted that the correlation between resistance values measured with the Valhalla and Bioelectrical Sciences (BES) analyzers was only $r = 0.59$; the average %BF estimated for men from one BIA equation differed by 6.3% using the resistances from these two instruments. Although there is a high correlation ($r = 0.99$) between resistances measured with the Valhalla and RJL analyzers, the Valhalla analyzer produces significantly higher resistances for men ($\sim 16\ \Omega$) and women ($\sim 19\ \Omega$), corresponding to a systematic underestimation of FFM in men (~ 1.3 kg) and women (~ 1.0 kg) (Graves et al. 1989). Also, differences may exist among the same models of analyzers . The Z values from three RJL (model 101) analyzers differed by 7 to 16 Ω, causing a difference in FFM of 2.1 kg for some individuals (Deurenberg, van der Kooy, and Leenan 1989).

■ Do upper- and lower-body BIA analyzers accurately estimate body composition?

The Tanita Corporation now markets about 20 different models of lower-body analyzers that vary in weight capacity, software and memory, and data output. Compared to two-component model estimates of FFM obtained from underwater weighing, Tanita analyzer estimates of the average FFM of heterogeneous adult samples are reasonably good *(SEE* = 3.5-3.7 kg) (Cable, Nieman, Austin, Hogen, and Utter 2001; Utter, Nieman, Ward, and Butterworth 1999). Estimates by Tanita analyzers also agree well with SKF estimates of %BF in collegiate wrestlers (Utter et al. 2001) and with DXA estimates of FFM in children (Sung, Lau, Yu, Lam, and Nelson 2001; Tyrrel, Richards, Hofman, Gillies, Robinson, and Cutfield 2001).

In the late 1990s, Omron Healthcare developed a low-cost, hand-to-hand BIA analyzer for home use. Omron's proprietary equation was developed and cross-validated on a large heterogeneous sample from three laboratories using HW to obtain two-component model reference measures of %BF and FFM (Loy et al. 1998). The group predictive accuracy *(SEE)* for estimating FFM was 3.9 kg for men and 2.9 kg for women. In an independent cross-validation of the Omron analyzer, Gibson and colleagues (2000) reported slightly smaller prediction errors *(SEE* = 2.9 kg for men and 2.2 kg for women). Loy and colleagues (1998) noted that the average FFM estimates from the Omron device are similar to values obtained with whole-body (RJL and Valhalla) analyzers. Lastly, in a study of Japanese men the accuracy of upper-body (Omron, HBF-300), lower-body (Tanita, TBF-102), and whole-body (Selco, SIF-891) analyzers was compared to two-component model reference measures of %BF obtained from HW. The average difference between reference and predicted %BF values was slightly smaller for the Omron (2.2% BF) than for the whole-body (3.3% BF) and lower-body (3.2% BF) analyzers (Demura, Yamaji, Goshi, Kobayashi, Sato, and Nagasawa 2002). However, estimation errors from the Omron and Tanita devices tended to be greater at the lower and upper extremes of the %BF distribution.

Recently, Omron developed BIA prediction equations to estimate the body composition of physically active adults. These equations are programmed in the new Omron analyzer (model HBF-306) along with prediction equations for nonactive adults and children. The predictor variables in the manufacturer's equation for this unit are upper-body impedance, age, gender, height, weight, and level of physical activity (i.e., athlete or nonathlete). The prediction errors for athletes *(SEE* = 3.8% and 3.6% BF for male and female athletes, respectively) were somewhat less than those for nonathletes *(SEE* = 4.5% BF) (K. Yamanoto, pers. comm.).

The Omron (HBF-306) model has been tested on ethnically diverse samples of European and Asian populations. Generally the group predictive accuracy is good for these subgroups, but individual prediction errors can be high (Deurenberg-Yap, Schmidt, van Staveren, Hautvast, and Deurenberg 2001; Deurenberg and Deurenberg-Yap 2002). Deurenberg-Yap and colleagues (2001) noted that Omron data misclassified (gave false negatives) for 24% of the obese females and 44% of the obese males in their study. In comparing the Omron estimates of %BF to a multicomponent model, the *SEE* was 4.5% BF; the error in estimating %BF using the Omron analyzer was related to the age, body fatness, and arm span-to-height ratio of the subjects (Deurenberg and Deurenberg-Yap 2002).

■ How does my client's hydration level affect the accuracy of bioimpedance measures?

A major source of error with the BIA method is intraindividual variability in whole-body resistance due to factors that alter the client's hydration. Between 3.1% and 3.9% of the variance in resistance may be attributed to day-to-day fluctuations in body water (Jackson, Pollock, Graves, and Mahar 1988). Factors such as eating, drinking, dehydrating, and exercising alter the hydration state, thereby affecting total-body resistance and the estimate of FFM. Measuring resistance 2 to 4 hr after a meal decreases R as much as 13 to

17 Ω and likely overestimates the FFM of your client by almost 1.5 kg (Deurenberg, Weststrate, Paymans, and van der Kooy 1988). Likewise, Gallagher and colleagues (1998) found a significant decrease in impedance 2 hr following breakfast, and this effect lasted for 5 hr after consumption. In contrast to these studies, at only 1 hr postmeal, there appears to be greater individual variability and smaller changes in R (Fogelholm, Sievanan, Kukkonen-Harjula, Oja, and Vuori 1993). Kushner, Gudivaka, and Schoeller (1996) concluded that eating or drinking minimally influences whole-body Z within 1 hr following consumption but is likely to decrease Z (< 3%) at 2 to 4 hr. Dehydration has the opposite effect: R increases (~40 Ω), leading to a 5.0 kg underestimation of FFM (Lukaski 1986).

■ *How does exercise affect bioimpedance measures?*

Kushner and colleagues (1996) suggested three ways in which exercise may influence BIA measurements:

- Increased blood flow and warming of skeletal muscle tissue reduce Z and the specific resistivity (ρ) of muscle.
- Increased cutaneous blood flow, skin temperature, and sweating lower Z.
- Fluid loss due to exercise increases Z.

The effect of aerobic exercise on resistance measurements partially depends on exercise intensity and duration. Jogging and cycling at moderate intensities (~70% $\dot{V}O_2$max) for 90 to 120 min substantially decreased R (by 50-70 Ω), resulting in a large overestimation of FFM (~12 kg) (Khaled et al. 1988; Lukaski 1986). In contrast, cycling at lower intensities (100 and 175 W) for 90 min had a much smaller effect on R (1-9 Ω) (Deurenberg et al. 1988). Liang and Norris (1993) reported a decrease in R of about 3% immediately after 30 min of moderate-intensity exercise, but R returned to normal 1 hr postexercise with water ad libitum. The decrease in R following strenuous exercise most likely reflects a relatively greater loss of body water in the sweat and expired air compared to the loss of electrolytes. This difference leads to a higher electrolyte concentration in the body's fluids, thereby lowering R (Deurenberg et al. 1988).

The BIA method was found to adequately predict changes in TBW after heat-induced dehydration and glycerol-induced hyperhydration but not after exercise-induced dehydration; thus, factors other than just total fluid volume affect BIA measures following exercise (Koulmann et al. 2000). Researchers hypothesized that the redistribution of body fluids to active muscles during exercise, which relatively increases hydration in these segments (legs), might partially conceal the decreased fluid volumes in less active segments (trunk and arms).

■ *Can I measure bioimpedance at any time during my client's menstrual cycle?*

Although the menstrual cycle alters TBW, the ratio of extracellular to intracellular water, and body weight, researchers found only small differences in bioimpedance measures (Z and R) between the follicular and premenstrual stages (~5-8 Ω) and between menses and the follicular stage (~7 Ω) (Deurenberg et al. 1988; Gleichauf and Rose 1989). However, the average body weight of the women studied was stable (< 0.2 kg difference) during the menstrual cycle. In women experiencing relatively large body weight gains (2-4 kg) during the menstrual cycle, a large part of the gain is due to an increase (1.5 kg on average) in TBW (Bunt, Lohman, and Boileau 1989). Until there are more conclusive data on this issue, you should take BIA measurements at a time during the menstrual cycle when the client perceives that she is not experiencing a large weight gain. This practice should minimize error and more accurately estimate FFM for your clients.

■ *Is there high agreement between bioimpedance values measured by two different technicians?*

Technician skill is not a major source of BIA measurement error. There is virtually no difference in R measurements taken by different technicians, provided that standardized procedures for electrode placement and client positioning are closely followed (Jackson et al. 1988). The proximal electrodes in particular need to be correctly positioned at the wrist and ankle, as a 1 cm displacement may result in a 2% error in R (Elsen, Siu, Pineda, and Solomons 1987). Lukaski (1986) reported a 16% increase in R (~79 Ω) due to improper electrode placement.

■ *How does body position affect bioimpedance measures?*

Proper positioning of the client is important for an accurate measurement. As a standard practice, whole-body resistance is measured with the client lying in a supine position. Changes in body position alter Z values as much as 12% (Lozano, Rosell, and Pallas-Areny 1995); moving from a standing to supine position immediately increases Z by about 3% because of fluid shifts (Kushner et al. 1996). Also, the amount of time that the client lies supine before Z is recorded needs to be standardized; in the supine position Z gradually increases over several hours (Kushner et al. 1996). Experts recommend having your client lie supine for at least 10 min before BIA measurement (Ellis et al. 1999). In addition, make sure that your client's arms are abducted (30°-45°) from the trunk and that the thighs are not touching each other. Crossing the limbs short-circuits the electrical path, dramatically affecting bioimpedance values.

■ *Should I measure whole-body bioimpedance on the right or left side of the body?*

The standard practice is to measure whole-body bioimpedance on the right side of the body. The differences between R measurements using ipsilateral (right arm–right leg or left arm–left leg) and contralateral (right arm–left leg or left arm–right leg) electrode placements are generally small (Graves et al. 1989; Lukaski, Johnson, Bolonchuk, and Lykken 1985).

■ *How does temperature affect bioimpedance?*

Bioimpedance measurements should be made with the client lying supine on a nonconductive surface (e.g., stretcher bed or mat) in a room at normal ambient temperature (25 °C [77 °F]). Researchers have demonstrated that ambient temperature affects skin temperature, and R varies inversely with skin temperature (Caton, Mole, Adams, and Heustis 1988; Gudivaka, Schoeller, and Kushner 1996; Liang, Su, and Lee 2000). Cool ambient temperatures ($\sim$14 °C) drop skin temperature (24 °C compared to 33 °C under normal conditions), significantly increasing total body R (by 35 Ω, on average) and decreasing estimated FFM (by $\sim$2.2 kg) (Caton et al. 1988). Liang and colleagues (2000) reported a slightly greater difference in R (46 Ω) between cold (17 °C ambient temperature and 28.7 °C skin temperature) and hot (35 °C ambient and 35.8 °C skin temperature) conditions.

Other Anthropometric Methods

Anthropometry refers to the measurement of the size and proportion of the human body. Body weight and stature (standing height) are measures of body size, whereas ratios of weight to height represent body proportion. Circumferences, skinfold thicknesses, skeletal diameters, and segment lengths may be used to assess the sizes and proportions of body segments. A circumference (C) is a measure of the girth of a body segment such as

the arm, thigh, waist, or hip. A skeletal diameter (D) is a measure of bony width or breadth (e.g., of the knee, ankle, or wrist).

Anthropometric measures such as circumferences, skinfolds, and skeletal diameters have been used to assess total and regional body composition. Also, anthropometric indices such as body mass index (BMI), waist-to-hip circumference ratio (WHR), waist circumference, and sagittal abdominal diameter (SAD) are used to identify individuals at risk for disease. Compared to skinfolds, other anthropometric measures are relatively simple and inexpensive, and they do not require a high degree of technical skill and training. They are well suited for large epidemiological surveys and for clinical purposes.

The basic principles underlying the use of anthropometric measures such as circumference, skeletal diameter, and BMI to estimate body composition are as follows:

■ **Circumferences are affected by fat mass, muscle mass, and skeletal size; therefore, they are related to fat mass and lean body mass.** Jackson and Pollock (1976) reported that circumference and bony diameter are markers of lean body mass (muscle mass and skeletal size); however, some circumferences are also highly associated with body fat. These findings confirm that circumferences reflect both fat and fat-free components of body composition.

■ **Skeletal size directly relates to lean body mass.** Behnke (1961) proposed that lean body mass could be accurately estimated from skeletal diameters and developed equations for doing so. Cross-validation of these equations yielded a moderately high ($r = 0.80$) relationship and closely estimated average lean body mass values obtained from hydrodensitometry (Wilmore and Behnke 1969, 1970). Behnke's hypothesis was also supported by the observation that skeletal diameters, along with circumferences, are strong markers of lean body mass (Jackson and Pollock 1976).

■ **To estimate total body fat from weight-to-height indices, the index should be highly related to body fat but independent of height.** Based on data from two large-scale epidemiological surveys (National Health and Nutrition Examination Surveys I and II), Micozzi, Albanes, Jones, and Chumlea (1986) reported that BMI (body weight divided by height squared) is not significantly related to the height of men ($r = -0.06$) and women ($r = -0.16$). However, BMI is not totally independent of height, especially in younger children (< 15 yr). Although BMI was directly related to skinfold thickness and the estimated fat area of the arm (r = 0.72 to 0.80) (Micozzi et al. 1986), the relationship of BMI to body fat varied with age, gender, and ethnicity (Deurenberg and Deurenberg-Yap 2001; Deurenberg, Yap, and van Staveren 1998; Gallagher, Walker, and O'Dea 1996; Rush, Plank, Laulu, and Robinson 1997; Wang, Thornton, Russell, Burastero, Heymsfield, and Pierson 1994).

Using the Anthropometric Method to Estimate Body Composition

Although some anthropometric prediction models use skinfolds, circumferences, and skeletal diameters to estimate body composition, only those equations using circumferences and diameters are addressed in this chapter for the following reasons:

- The predictive accuracy of anthropometric (circumference and diameter) equations is not greatly improved by adding SKF measures.

- Anthropometric equations using only circumferences estimate the body fatness of obese individuals more accurately than SKF prediction equations (Seip and Weltman 1991).

- Compared to SKFs, circumferences and skeletal diameters can be measured with less error (Bray and Gray 1988a).

- Some practitioners may not have access to SKF calipers.

Anthropometric prediction equations estimate total body density (Db), relative body fat (%BF), and fat-free mass (FFM) from combinations of body weight, height, skeletal diameters, and circumferences. Generally, equations using only skeletal measures have larger prediction errors than those using both circumferences and bony diameters. Like SKF and bioelectrical impedance (BIA) equations, anthropometric equations are based on either population-specific or generalized models.

Population-specific anthropometric equations are valid only for individuals whose physical characteristics (age, gender, ethnicity, and level of body fatness) are similar to those of the specific population. For example, anthropometric equations developed to estimate the body composition of obese individuals (Weltman, Levine, Seip, and Tran 1988; Weltman, Seip, and Tran 1987) should not be applied to nonobese individuals.

On the other hand, generalized equations, applicable to individuals of various age and body fatness, have been developed for heterogeneous populations of women (15-79 yr; 13%-63% BF) and men (20-78 yr; 2%-49% BF) (Tran and Weltman 1988, 1989). The predictive accuracy of these generalized equations for estimating the %BF of obese men and women was similar to that of fatness-specific (obese) equations (Seip and Weltman 1991). Typically, generalized equations include body weight or height, along with two or three circumferences, as predictors of Db or %BF. Like in generalized SKF models, the relationship between some circumference measures and Db is curvilinear (Tran and Weltman 1988, 1989). Also, age was an independent predictor of Db for women (Tran and Weltman 1989). Table 8.6 provides anthropometric prediction equations for various population subgroups.

TABLE 8.6 Circumference Prediction Equations

Population subgroup	Equation	Reference
White women, 15-79 years	Db (g · cc^{-1})^a = 1.168297 − 0.002824(abdom C^b) + 0.0000122098(abdom C^b)^2 − 0.000733128(hip C) + 0.000510477(ht) − 0.00021616(age)	Tran and Weltman (1989)
White men, 15-78 years	% BF = −47.371817 + 0.57914807 (abdom C^b) + 0.025189114 (hipC) + 0.21366088 (iliacC) − 0.35595404 (BM)	Tran and Weltman (1988)
White, obese women, 20-60 years	%BF = 0.11077(abdom C^b) − 0.17666(ht) + 0.14354(BM) + 51.033	Weltman et al. (1988)
White, obese men, 24-68 years	%BF = 0.31457(abdom C^b) − 0.10969(BM) + 10.834	Weltman et al. (1987)

^{a}Use population-specific conversion formula to calculate %BF from Db.

^{b}abdom C (cm) is the average abdominal circumference measured at two sites: (1) anteriorly midway between the xiphoid process of sternum and the umbilicus and laterally between the lower end of the rib cage and iliac crests; (2) at the umbilicus level.

Db = body density; %BF = percent body fat; BM = body mass.

Using Anthropometric Indices to Classify Disease Risk

Anthropometric measures have other uses besides estimating body composition. In large-scale epidemiological surveys and clinical settings, indirect anthropometric indices such as BMI, WHR, waist circumference, and SAD are used to assess regional fat distribution (upper- and lower-body fat) and to identify at-risk individuals.

Body Mass Index

The body mass index (BMI) is used to classify individuals as obese, overweight, and underweight; to identify individuals at risk for obesity-related diseases; and to monitor changes in the body fatness of clinical populations (U.S. Department of Health and Human Services 2000; World Health Organization 1998). BMI is a significant predictor of cardiovascular disease and type 2 diabetes (Janssen, Heymsfield, Allison, Kotler, and Ross 2002). Because of this association and the fact that BMI is easily calculated (BMI = body weight/height squared), BMI is widely used in population-based and prospective studies to identify at-risk individuals.

BMI, however, is limited as an index of obesity (body fatness) because it does not account for the composition of body weight. In addition, factors such as age, ethnicity, body build, and frame size affect the relationship between BMI and %BF. Thus, using BMI as an index of obesity may result in misclassifications of underweight, overweight, and obese. Also, because BMI is a better measure of nonabdominal and abdominal subcutaneous fat than of visceral fat (Janssen et al. 2002), other anthropometric indices need to be used to assess fat distribution.

Body mass index (BMI) is the ratio of body weight to height squared: BMI (in kg/m^2) = wt (in kg)/ht^2 (in m). To calculate BMI, measure the body weight in kilograms and convert the height from centimeters to meters (m = cm/100). Alternatively, you can use a nomogram (see figure 8.13) to calculate your client's BMI (Bray 1978). To use this nomogram, plot your client's height and body weight in the appropriate columns and connect the two points with a ruler. Read the corresponding BMI at the point where the connecting line intersects the BMI column.

Table 8.7 describes standards for classifying BMI values. The World Health Organization (1998) defines *obesity* as a BMI of 30 kg/m^2 or more, *overweight* as a BMI between 25 and 29.9 kg/m^2, and *underweight* as a BMI of less than 18.5 kg/m^2. These suggested cutoffs are based on the relationship between BMI and morbidity and mortality reported in observational studies in Europe and the United States. The use of BMI in health risk appraisals assumes that people who are disproportionately heavy are so because of excess fat mass. However, controversy exists concerning the most appropriate cutoff for designating obesity (Deurenberg 2001).

The relationship between BMI and %BF is affected by age, gender, ethnicity, and body build (Deurenberg et al. 1998; Snijder, Kuyf, and Deurenberg 1999). For a given BMI value, older individuals have a greater %BF compared to their younger counterparts and young adult males have a lesser %BF than young adult females. Also, for a given %BF, age- and gender-matched Whites have a higher BMI (1.3-4.6 kg/m^2) compared to other ethnic groups (e.g., African Americans, Chinese, Indonesians, Ethiopians, and Polynesians) (Deurenberg et al. 1998). These findings suggest that using a universal BMI cutoff to define obesity ($\geq$30 kg/m^2) may not be appropriate. Ethnic-specific cutoff values need to be established that account for the relationship between BMI and %BF and for the morbidity and mortality risks in relation to BMI for specific ethnic groups (Deurenberg 2001).

Waist Circumference

Waist circumference is gaining support as a measure of regional adiposity (i.e., abdominal obesity) and as a predictor of obesity-related health risk. Waist circumference coupled with BMI predicts health risk better than BMI alone, especially for White men (Ardern, Katzmarzyk, and Ross 2003; Zhu et al. 2004). However, recent studies showed that waist circumference alone predicts obesity-related health risk even better than the combination of BMI and waist circumference (Janssen, Katzmarzyk, and Ross 2004; Zhu, Heymsfield, Toyoshima, Wang, Petrobelli, and Heshka 2005). The National Cholesterol Education Program (NCEP 2001) recommends using waist circumference cutoffs of >102 cm for men and >88 cm for women to evaluate obesity as a risk factor for cardiovascular and metabolic diseases. Recently, however, Zhu and colleagues (2005) proposed using waist circumference cutoffs of >100 cm for men and >95 cm for women to identify individuals with a high risk for cardiovascular disease. These cutoffs apply to Black, Mexican American, and White adults (Zhu et al. 2005).

Waist-to-Hip Ratio

The waist-to-hip ratio (WHR) is as an indirect measure of lower- and upper-body fat distribution.

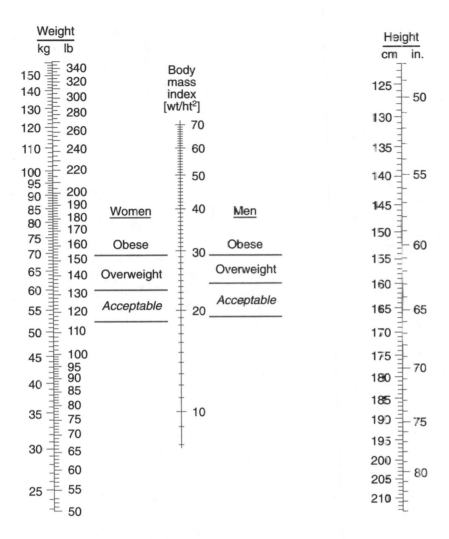

Figure 8.13 Nomogram for body mass index.

Reprinted, by permission, from G.A. Bray, 1978, "Definitions, measurements, and classifications of the syndromes of obesity," *International Journal of Obesity* 2(2): 99-112.

TABLE 8.7 Classification of Overweight and Obesity Based on Body Mass Index (BMI)

Classification	BMI value
Underweight	<18.5
Normal weight	18.5-24.9
Overweight	25.0-29.9
Obesity	
Class I	30.0-34.9
Class II	35.0-39.9
Class III	≥40.0

Data from WHO Report. 1998. *Obesity: Preventing and managing the global epidemic.* Report of a WHO Consultation on Obesity. Geneva: World Health Organization.

Upper-body obesity, or central adiposity, measured by the WHR moderately relates (r = 0.48 to 0.61) to risk factors associated with cardiovascular and metabolic diseases in men and women (Ohrvall, Berglund, and Vessby 2000). Young adults with WHR values in excess of 0.94 for men and 0.82 for women are at high risk for adverse health consequences (Bray and Gray 1988b).

Although the WHR has been used as an anthropometric measure of central adiposity and visceral fat, it has certain limitations:

- The WHR of women is affected by menopausal status (Svendsen, Hassager, Bergmann, and Christiansen 1992; Weits, Van der Beek, Wedel, and Ter Haar Romeny 1988). Postmenopausal women show more of a male pattern of fat distribution than do premenopausal women (Ferland et al. 1989).

- The WHR is not valid for evaluating fat distribution in prepubertal children (Peters, Fox, Armstrong, Sharpe, and Bell 1992).

- The accuracy of the WHR in assessing visceral fat decreases with increasing fatness.

- Hip circumference is influenced only by subcutaneous fat deposition; waist circumference is affected by both visceral fat and subcutaneous fat depositions. Thus, the WHR may not accurately detect changes in visceral fat accumulation (Goran, Allison, and Poehlman 1995; van der Kooy et al. 1993).

The **waist-to-hip ratio (WHR)** is calculated by dividing waist circumference (in cm) by hip circumference (in cm). The measurement site for waist circumference, however, has not been universally standardized. The World Health Organization (1998) recommends measuring waist circumference midway between the lower rib margin and the iliac crest and measuring hip circumference at the widest point over the greater trochanters. In contrast, the *Anthropometric Standardization Reference Manual* (Callaway et al. 1988) recommends measuring the waist circumference at the narrowest part of the torso and the hip circumference at the level of the maximum extension of the buttocks. The WHR norms (table 8.8) were established using the measurement procedures described in the *Anthropometric Standardization Reference Manual*. Instead of calculating the WHR by hand, you can use the WHR nomogram (figure 8.14) to obtain values for your clients. Plot the client's waist and hip circumferences in the corresponding columns

of the nomogram and connect these points with a straight line. Read the WHR at the point where this line intersects the WHR column.

Sagittal Abdominal Diameter

The **sagittal abdominal diameter (SAD)** is a measure of the anteroposterior thickness of the abdomen at the umbilical level. Research suggests that the SAD is an excellent indirect measure of visceral fat (Ohrvall et al. 2000; Zamboni et al. 1998). SAD is strongly related to visceral adipose tissue in men ($r = 0.82$) and women ($r = 0.76$), even after adjusting for BMI ($r = 0.66$ and 0.63, respectively, for men and women) (Zamboni et al. 1998). However, this relationship is stronger in lean or moderately overweight individuals than in obese individuals. Compared to waist circumference, WHR, and BMI, SAD is more strongly related to risk factors for cardiovascular and metabolic diseases in women and men (Ohrvall et al. 2000). SAD is also associated with cardiovascular disease risk factors in older women (67-78 yr) (Turcato et al. 2000).

The procedures for measuring SAD have not been standardized. In most studies, SAD was measured while the client was lying supine, legs extended, on an examination table. A sliding-beam anthropometer is used to measure the vertical distance (to the nearest 0.1 cm) between the top of the table and the abdomen at the level of the umbilicus or iliac crests. In some studies, SAD was measured with the hips and legs flexed or with the client standing instead of lying supine.

TABLE 8.8   Waist-to-Hip Circumference Ratio Norms for Men and Women

| | Age | RISK | | | |
		Low	Moderate	High	Very high
Men	20-29	<0.83	0.83-0.88	0.89-0.94	>0.94
	30-39	<0.84	0.84-0.91	0.92-0.96	>0.96
	40-49	<0.88	0.88-0.95	0.96-1.00	>1.00
	50-59	<0.90	0.90-0.96	0.97-1.02	>1.02
	60-69	<0.91	0.91-0.98	0.99-1.03	>1.03
Women	20-29	<0.71	0.71-0.77	0.78-0.82	>0.82
	30-39	<0.72	0.72-0.78	0.79-0.84	>0.84
	40-49	<0.73	0.73-0.79	0.80-0.87	>0.87
	50-59	<0.74	0.74-0.81	0.82-0.88	>0.88
	60-69	<0.76	0.76-0.83	0.84-0.90	>0.90

Adapted from Bray and Gray, 1988b, "Obesity – Part I – Pathogensis," *Western Journal of Medicine* 149: 432.

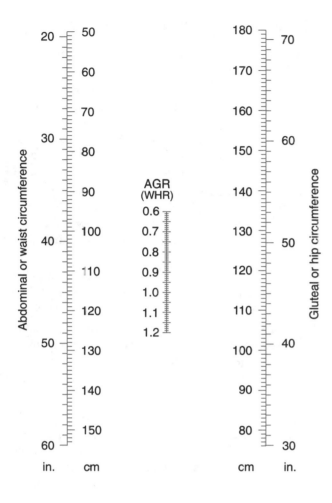

Figure 8.14 Nomogram for waist-to-hip ratio (WHR).

Reprinted, by permission of *The Western Journal of Medicine*, G.A. Bray and D.S. Gray, "Obesity: Part I—Pathogenesis," 1988, 149: 432. ©BMJ Publishing Group.

Using Anthropometric Measures to Classify Frame Size

Skeletal diameters are used to classify frame size in order to improve the validity of height–weight tables for evaluating body weight. The rationale for including frame size is that skeletal breadths are important estimators of the bone and muscle components of fat-free mass. Estimating frame size allows you to differentiate between those who weigh more because of a large musculoskeletal mass and those who weigh more because of a large fat mass (Himes and Frisancho 1988). Since there are health implications for individuals who are overweight, a critical evaluation of body weight is important. You can classify frame size by using reference data for elbow breadth (see table 8.9). The anatomical landmarks for measurement are described in appendix D.5, "Standardized Sites for Bony Breadth Measurements," page 338.

Anthropometric Techniques

You must practice in order to become proficient in measuring skeletal diameters and circumferences. Following the standardized procedures (see p. 204) will increase the accuracy and reliability of your measurements (Callaway et al. 1988; Wilmore et al. 1988).

Sources of Measurement Error

The accuracy and reliability of anthropometric measures are potentially affected by equipment, technician skill, and client factors (Bray 1978;

TABLE 8.9 Elbow Breadth Norms (in cm) for Men and Women in the United States

| | Age (yr) | FRAME SIZE | | |
		Small	Medium	Large
Men	18-24	≤6.6	>6.6 and <7.7	≥7.7
	25-34	≤6.7	>6.7 and <7.9	≥7.9
	35-44	≤6.7	>6.7 and <8.0	≥8.0
	45-54	≤6.7	>6.7 and <8.1	≥8.1
	55-64	≤6.7	>6.7 and <8.1	≥8.1
	65-74	≤6.7	>6.7 and <8.1	≥8.1
Women	18-24	≤5.6	>5.6 and <6.5	≥6.5
	25-34	≤5.7	>5.7 and <6.8	≥6.8
	35-44	≤5.7	>5.7 and <7.1	≥7.1
	45-54	≤5.7	>5.7 and <7.2	≥7.2
	55-64	≤5.8	>5.8 and <7.2	≥7.2
	65-74	≤5.8	>5.8 and <7.2	≥7.2

From A.R. Frisancho, 1984, "New Standards for Weight and Body Composition by Frame Size and Height for Assessment of Nutritional Status of Adults and the Elderly." *American Journal of Clinical Nutrition* 40: 808-819. Reproduced with permission by the American Journal of Clinical Nutrition. © Am J Clin Nutr. American Society for Clinical Nutrition.

STANDARDIZED PROCEDURES FOR ANTHROPOMETRIC MEASUREMENTS

1. Take all circumference and bony diameter measurements of the limbs on the right side of the body.

2. Carefully identify and measure the anthropometric site. Be meticulous about locating anatomical landmarks used to identify the measurement site (see appendix D.4, "Standardized Sites for Circumference Measurements," p. 337; and appendix D.5, "Standardized Sites for Bony Breadth Measurements," p. 338), and instruct your clients to relax their muscles during the measurement.

3. Take a minimum of three measurements at each site in rotational order.

4. To measure the breadth of smaller segments, like the elbow or wrist, use small sliding calipers (range of 30 cm or 11.8 in.) with greater scale precision instead of larger skeletal anthropometers (range of 60 to 80 cm or 23.6 to 31.5 in.).

5. Hold the skeletal anthropometer or caliper in both hands so the tips of the index fingers are adjacent to the tips of the caliper.

6. Place the caliper on the bony landmarks and apply firm pressure to compress the underlying muscle, fat, and skin. Apply pressure to a point where the measurement no longer continues to decrease.

7. Use an anthropometric tape to measure circumferences. Hold the zero end of the tape in your left hand, positioned below the other part of the tape that is held in your right hand.

8. Apply tension to the tape so that it fits snugly around the body part but does not indent the skin or compress the subcutaneous tissue.

9. For some circumferences (e.g., waist, hip, and thigh), you should align the tape in a horizontal plane, parallel to the floor.

Callaway et al. 1988). The following questions and responses concern these sources of measurement error.

■ *What equipment will I need to measure bony widths?*

Use skeletal anthropometers and sliding or spreading calipers to measure bony widths and body breadths (see figure 8.15). The precision characteristics (0.05 to 0.50 cm) and range of measure-

ment (0 to 210 cm) depend on the type of skeletal anthropometer or caliper you are using (Wilmore et al. 1988). The instruments must be carefully maintained and must be calibrated periodically so that their accuracy can be checked and restored.

■ *Can I use any type of tape measure to measure body circumferences?*

Use an anthropometric tape measure to measure circumferences (see figure 8.15). The tape measure

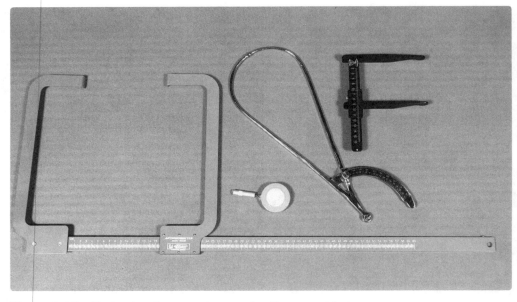

Figure 8.15   Skeletal anthropometers and anthropometric tape measure.

should be made from a flexible material that does not stretch with use. You can use a plastic-coated tape measure if an anthropometric tape measure is not available. Some anthropometric tapes have a spring-loaded handle (i.e., Gulick handle) that allows a constant tension to be applied to the end of the tape during the measurement.

■ *How much skill and practice are required to ensure accurate circumference and skeletal diameter measurements?*

Compared to the SKF method, technician skill is not a major source of measurement error. However, you need to practice in order to perfect the identification of the measurement sites and your measurement technique. Experts recommend practicing on at least 50 people and taking a minimum of three measurements for each site in rotational order (Callaway et al. 1988). Closely follow standardized testing procedures for locating measurement sites, positioning the anthropometer or tape measure, and applying tension during the measurement. Appendix D.4 ("Standardized Sites for Circumference Measurements," p. 337) and appendix D.5 ("Standardized Sites for Bony Breadth Measurements," p. 338) describe some of the most commonly used circumference and skeletal diameter sites.

■ *Is there good agreement in circumference and skeletal diameter values when the measurements are taken by two different technicians?*

Variability in circumference measurements taken by different technicians is relatively small (0.2 to 1.0 cm), with some sites differing more than others (Callaway et al. 1988). Skilled technicians can obtain similar values even when measuring circumferences of obese individuals (Bray and Gray 1988a).

■ *Are the circumferences of obese clients more easily measured than SKFs?*

As with the SKF method, it is more difficult to obtain consistent measurements of circumference for obese compared to lean individuals (Bray and Gray 1988a). However, circumferences are preferable to SKFs for measuring obese clients, for several reasons:

■ You can measure circumferences of obese individuals regardless of their size, whereas the maximum aperture of the SKF caliper may not be large enough to allow measurement.

■ Measurement of circumferences requires less technician skill.

■ Differences between technicians are smaller for circumferences compared to SKF measurements (Bray and Gray 1988a).

■ *Is it possible to accurately measure bony widths of heavily muscled and obese clients?*

Accurate measurement of bony diameters in heavily muscled or obese individuals may be difficult because the underlying muscle and fat tissues must be firmly compressed. It may be difficult to identify and palpate bony anatomical landmarks, leading to error in locating the measurement site.

Near-Infrared Interactance Method

Near-infrared interactance (NIR) is a method that indirectly assesses tissue composition (fat and water) by measuring optical density, or the amount of light absorbed and reflected at a specific body site (typically the biceps site). NIR has been commercially available for years as an alternative method for assessing body composition. Futrex, Inc. is the only manufacturer of a commercial NIR device that measures optical density values for estimating %BF. In the late 1990s, Futrex developed a new line of NIR analyzers (the 1100, 5000/XL, and 6100/XL to replace the 1000, 5000, and 6000, respectively). Most of the upgrades in the Futrex models were designed to make the product more user friendly (e.g., ability to print in color and to download data to computers) rather than to change the way it measures optical density. All of the Futrex analyzers except the Futrex-6100/XL measure NIR light at two wavelengths. The Futrex-6100/XL measures NIR light at up to six wavelengths.

There are over 20 cross-validation studies of the manufacturer's equations for the Futrex NIR analyzers. With few exceptions, the prediction errors have been large (*SEE* > 3.5% BF). In most cases, the Futrex-5000 equation underestimates %BF by 2% to 10% BF. The degree of underestimation appears to be directly related to the level of body fatness (Elia, Parkinson, and Diaz 1990; Heyward, Cook, Hicks, Jenkins, Quatrochi, and Wilson 1992). Some studies noted large underestimations of average %BF when the Futrex-5000 equation was compared to multicomponent model estimates of %BF for obese women (Fuller, Sawyer, and Elia 1994) and for overweight arthritic patients (Heitmann et al. 1994). Thus, the Futrex-5000 manufacturer's equation is likely to grossly underestimate the %BF of fatter clients compared to %BF estimates for leaner clients.

The vast majority of NIR research has been done on the Futrex-5000 analyzer; however, a few studies have used other models. The Futrex-1000 is a handheld, battery-operated device designed for home use. Studies including both the Futrex-5000 and the Futrex-1000 have reported lower validity coefficients and higher prediction errors for the Futrex-1000 (Smith, Johnson, Stout, Housh, Housh, and Evetovich 1997; Stout, Eckerson, Housh, and Johnson 1994; Stout, Eckerson, Housh, Johnson, and Betts 1994; Stout, Housh, Eckerson, Johnson, and Betts 1996). Even though the Futrex-5000A is marketed for use with children, Smith and colleagues (1997) observed that the Futrex-5000 more accurately estimates %BF for female gymnasts (13-17 yr) than the 5000A does. Likewise, Cassady and colleagues (1993) reported unacceptable %BF prediction errors when using the Futrex-5000A

manufacturer's equation to assess the body composition of children. One study compared %BF estimates from the Futrex-6000 and from DXA. In this study of obese females, the mean difference between %BF$_{Futrex-6000}$ and %BF$_{DXA}$ was small (1.4% BF); however, the individual predictive accuracy for the Futrex-6000 was poor (–8.0% to 10.7% BF) (Panotopoulos, Ruiz, Guy-Grand, and Basdevant 2001). From these limited data, it appears that these models (Futrex-5000A and Futrex-6000) of analyzers are no better than the Futrex-5000 at estimating %BF and, in some cases, that they are even worse. Because many research studies have reported unacceptable prediction errors, the Futrex manufacturer's equations should not be used to assess the body fatness of your clients.

Sources for Equipment

Product	Supplier's address
Air displacement plethysmograph	
Bod Pod Body Composition System	LMI, Inc.
	1980 Oliveri Rd., Ste. C
	Concord, CA 94520
	(800) 426-3763
	www.bodpod.com
Anthropometers	
Spreading calipers	Pfister Import-Export, Inc.
Sliding calipers	450 Barell Ave.
Standard skeletal anthropometer	Carlstadt, NJ 07072
	(202) 939-4606
	Rosscraft Industries
	14732 16A Ave.
	Surrey, BC Canada V4A 5M7
	(604) 531-5049
	tep2000.com/Rosscraft.htm
Anthropometric tape measure	Country Technology, Inc.
	P.O. Box 87
	Gays Mills, WI 54631
	(608) 735-4718
	www.fitnessmart.com
Bioimpedance analyzers	
American Weights & Measures (formerly Valhalla Scientific)	American Weights & Measures, Inc.
	16501 Zumaque St.
	Rancho Santa Fe, CA 92067
	(800) 395-4565
	www.americanweightsandmeasures.com
Bio-Analogics	Bio-Analogics
	7909 SW Cirrus Dr.
	Beaverton, OR 97008
	(800) 327-7953
	www.bioanalogics.com

Biodynamics	Biodynamics Corp. 3511 NE 45th St. #2 Seattle, WA 98105 (800) 869-6987 www.biodyncorp.com
Biospace	Biospace, Inc. 8820 Wilshire Blvd., Suite 310 Beverly Hills, CA 90211 (310) 358-0360 www.biospaceamerica.com
Bodystat	Bodystat (USA), Inc. 2 Adalia Ave., Ste. 401 Tampa, FL 33606 (813) 258-3570 www.bodystat.com
Data-Input	Data-Input GmbH Trakehner St. 5 60487 Frankfurt Germany +49 69-970 840-0 www.b-i-a.de
Holtain	Holtain, Ltd. Crosswell, Crymych Pembrokeshire, SA41 3UF United Kingdom +44 (0) 1239-891656 www.fullbore.co.uk/holtain/medical
Impedimed (distributors of SEAC BIA analyzers)	Impedimed Pty., Ltd. P.O. Box 2121 Mansfield, Queensland 4122 Australia +61 (0) 7 3849-3444
Maltron	Maltron International, Ltd. P.O. Box 15 Rayleigh, Essex, SS6 9SN United Kingdom +44 (0) 1268-778251 www.maltronint.com
OMRON	OMRON Healthcare, Inc. 300 Lakeview Pkwy. Vernon Hills, IL 60061 (847) 680-6200 www.omronhealthcare.com
RJL	RJL Systems 33955 Harper Ave. Clinton TWP, MI 48035 (800) 528-4513 www.rjlsystems.com

Tanita

Tanita Corp.
2625 S. Clearbrook Dr.
Arlington Heights, IL 60005
(800) TANITA-8
www.tanita.com

Valhalla

See American Weights & Measures

Xitron Hydra ECF/ICF

Xitron Technologies, Inc.
9770-A Carroll Centre Rd.
San Diego, CA 92126
(858) 530-8099
www.xitron-tech.com

Calibration instruments and supplies

Skinfold calibration blocks (15 mm)

Creative Health Products
7621 E. Joy Rd.
Ann Arbor, MI 48105
(800) 742-4478
www.chponline.com

Standard calibration weights

Ohaus Scale Corp.
29 Hanover Rd.
Florham, NJ 07932
(800) 672-7722
www.ohaus.com

Vernier caliper

L.S. Starrett Co.
121 Cresent St.
Athol, MA 01331
(978) 249-3551
www.lsstarrett.com

Dual-energy X-ray absorptiometers

Hologic

Hologic, Inc.
35 Crosby Dr.
Bedford, MA 01730
(781) 999-7300
www.hologic.com

Norland

Norland Medical Systems, Inc.
W6340 Hackbarth Rd.
Fort Atkinson, WI 53538
(800) 563-9504
www.norland.com

Lunar

GE Lunar Medical Systems
P.O. Box 414
Milwaukee, WI 53201
(608) 274-2663
www.gemedicalsystems.com

Near-infrared interactance

Futrex NIR analyzers

Zelcore, Inc.
130 Western Maryland Pkwy.
Hagerstown, MD 21740
(800) 576-0295
www.futrex.com

Scales

Chatillon underwater weighing scale	Creative Health Products
Detecto balance beam scale	7621 E. Joy Rd.
Health-O-Meter balance beam scale	Ann Arbor, MI 48105
Health-O-Meter digital scale	(800) 742-4478
Seca digital scale	www.chponline.com

Skinfold calipers

AccuMeasure	AccuMeasure
	P.O. Box 4411
	Greenwood, CO 80155
	(800) 866-2727
	www.accumeasurefitness.com
Adipometer (plastic)	Ross Products Division
	Abbott Laboratories
	625 Cleveland Ave.
	Columbus, OH 43216
	(800) 344-9739
	www.ross.com
Body Caliper	The Caliper Company
	7 Millside Ln.
	Mill Valley, CA 94941
	(800) 655-4960
	www.bodycaliper.com
Fat-Control (plastic)	Creative Health Products
Fat-o-Meter	7621 E. Joy Rd.
Lafayette	Ann Arbor, MI 48105
Skyndex	(800) 742-4478
Slim-Guide	www.chponline.com
Harpenden	Quinton Instruments
	3303 Monte Villa Pkwy.
	Bothell, WA 98021
	(800) 426-0347
	www.quinton.com
Holtain	Pfister Import-Export, Inc.
	450 Barell Ave.
	Carlstadt, NJ 07072
	(201) 939-4606
Lange	Cambridge Scientific Products
	26 New St.
	Cambridge, MA 21613
	(888) 354-8908
	www.cambridgescientific.com
McGaw (plastic)	McGaw, Inc.
	P.O. Box 19791
	Irvine, CA 92713
	(714) 660-2055
	www.mcgaw.com

Stadiometers

Harpenden	Pfister Import-Export, Inc.
Holtain	450 Barell Ave.
	Carlstadt, NJ 07072
	(201) 939-4606

KEY POINTS

- Body composition is a key component of health and physical fitness; total body fat and fat distribution are related to disease risk.

- Standards for percent body fat can be used to classify body composition.

- Average %BF and standards for obesity vary according to age, gender, and physical activity levels.

- Hydrostatic weighing is a valid and reliable reference method for assessing body composition.

- Air displacement plethsymography is used to measure body volume and body density.

- Dual-energy X-ray absorptiometry is gaining recognition as a reference method for assessing body composition.

- Population-specific conversion formulas, based on multicomponent models of body composition, should be used to convert Db into percent body fat.

- The SKF method is widely used in field and clinical settings.

- Generalized SKF equations for the prediction of Db are reliable and valid for a wide range of individuals.

- Bioelectrical impedance analysis is a viable alternative for assessing body composition of diverse population subgroups.

- Circumferences and skeletal diameters can be used to estimate body composition.

- Body mass index is a crude index of total body fatness.

- Waist-to-hip ratio, waist circumference, and sagittal abdominal diameter are acceptable indices for identifying at-risk clients.

KEY TERMS

Learn the definition for each of the following key terms. Definitions of terms can be found in the glossary on page 379.

air displacement plethysmography (ADP)

anthropometry

Archimedes' principle

attenuation

bioelectrical impedance analysis (BIA)

body density (Db)

body mass index (BMI)

body surface area

body volume (BV)

Boyle's law

circumference (C)

densitometry

dual-energy X-ray absorptiometry (DXA)

fat-free body (FFB)

fat-free mass (FFM)

fat mass (FM)

hydrodensitometry

hydrostatic weighing (HW)

impedance (Z)

multicomponent model

near-infrared interactance (NIR)

optical density

percent body fat (%BF)

reactance (X_c)

relative body fat (%BF)

residual volume (RV)

resistance (R)

resistance index (ht^2/R)

sagittal abdominal diameter (SAD)

skeletal diameter (D)

skinfold (SKF)

tare weight

thoracic gas volume (TGV)

two-component model

underwater weight (UWW)

waist-to-hip ratio (WHR)

REVIEW QUESTIONS

In addition to being able to define each of the key terms, test your knowledge and understanding of the material by answering the following review questions.

1. Why is it important to assess the body composition of your clients?

2. What are the standards for classifying obesity and minimal levels of body fat for men and women?

3. What are the assumptions of the two-component model of body composition? Identify two commonly used two-component model equations for converting Db into %BF.

4. Explain how gender, ethnicity, and age affect FFB density and therefore two-component model estimates of %BF.

5. Name three methods that can be used to obtain reference measures of body composition. Which method is best? Explain your choice.

6. Identify two ways to measure (not estimate) your client's Db.

7. Distinguish between total Db and FFB density.

8. Describe how the HW method could be modified to test clients who are unable to be weighed underwater at RV.

9. Identify potential sources of measurement error for the SKF method.

10. In lay terms, explain the basic theory underlying the use of BIA.

11. To obtain accurate estimates of body composition using the BIA method, your client must adhere to pretesting guidelines. Identify these client guidelines.

12. Explain how BMI, WHR, and waist circumference may be used to identify clients at risk due to obesity.

13. Identify suitable field methods and prediction equations (i.e., SKF, BIA, or other anthropometric methods) to estimate body composition for each of the following subgroups of the population: older adults, children, obese individuals, and athletes.

chapter 9

Designing Weight Management and Body Composition Programs

Key Questions

- What is obesity and how prevalent is it worldwide?
- What are the health risks associated with having high or low levels of body fat?
- What are the primary causes of overweight and obesity?
- How is healthy body weight determined?
- What are the guidelines for a well-balanced diet? Are vitamin and mineral supplements necessary for most clients?
- What steps should I follow in planning a weight management program?
- What are the recommended guidelines for weight-loss and weight-gain programs?
- Why is exercise important for weight management?
- What types of exercise are best for weight loss?
- Does exercising without dieting improve body composition?

Health and longevity are threatened when a person is either overweight or underweight. Overweight and obesity increase one's risk of developing serious cardiovascular, pulmonary, and metabolic diseases and disorders. Likewise, individuals who are underweight may have a higher risk than others of cardiac, musculoskeletal, and reproductive disorders. Thus, healthy weight is key to a healthy and longer life.

As a health/fitness professional, you have an enormous challenge and responsibility to help determine a healthy body weight for your clients and to provide scientifically sound weight management programs for them. This chapter presents guidelines and techniques for determining healthy body weight. You will learn about weight control principles and practices, as well as guidelines for designing exercise programs for weight loss, weight gain, and body composition change.

OBESITY, OVERWEIGHT, AND UNDERWEIGHT: DEFINITIONS AND TRENDS

Individuals with body fat levels falling at or near the extremes of the body fat continuum are likely to have serious health problems that reduce life expectancy and threaten their quality of life. Obese individuals have a higher risk of cardiovascular disease, dyslipidemia, hypertension, glucose intolerance, insulin resistance, diabetes mellitus, obstructive pulmonary disease, gallbladder disease, osteoarthritis, and certain types of cancer (U.S. Department of Health and Human Services 2000b). The prevalences of hypercholesterolemia, hypertension, and type 2 diabetes are, respectively, 2.9, 2.1, and 2.9 times greater in overweight than non-overweight persons (National Institutes of

Health Consensus Development Panel 1985). Obesity is independently associated with coronary heart disease (CHD), heart failure, cardiac arrhythmia, stroke, and menstrual irregularities (Pi-Sunyer 1999).

At the opposite extreme, underweight individuals with too little body fat tend to be malnourished. These people have a relatively higher risk of fluid-electrolyte imbalances, osteoporosis and osteopenia, bone fractures, muscle wasting, cardiac arrhythmias and sudden death, peripheral edema, and renal and reproductive disorders (Fohlin 1977; Mazess, Barden, and Ohlrich 1990; Vaisman, Corey, Rossi, Goldberg, and Pencharz 1988). One disease associated with extremely low body fat levels is anorexia nervosa. Anorexia nervosa, an eating disorder found primarily in females, is characterized by excessive weight loss. Anorexia nervosa is estimated to afflict 1% of the female population (American Psychiatric Association 1994). Compared to normal women, those with anorexia have extremely low body fat (8% to 13% body fat), signs of muscle wasting, and less bone mineral content and bone density (Mazess et al. 1990; Vaisman, Rossi, Goldberg, Dibden, Wykes, and Pencharz 1988).

Definitions of Obesity, Overweight, and Underweight

Obesity is an excessive amount of body fat relative to body weight and is not synonymous with overweight. In many epidemiological studies, overweight is defined as a body mass index (BMI) between 25 and 29.9 kg/m^2; obesity is defined as a BMI of 30 kg/m^2 or more; and underweight is defined by a BMI of less than 18.5 kg/m^2 (U.S. Department of Health and Human Services 2000b). To identify children and adolescents who are overweight, the 85th and 95th percentile cutoffs for age and sex developed from the Centers for Disease Control and Prevention growth charts are commonly used in the United States. Children with a BMI greater than the 95th percentile for their age and sex are categorized as overweight; those with BMI values between the 85th and 94th percentiles are categorized as at risk for overweight. However, these definitions are not universally accepted. Pooled international data for BMI have been used to develop international standards for evaluating childhood overweight and obesity. These standards are based on growth curves that relate the cutoff points for BMI of different age-gender groups (2-18 yr) to the adult categories for overweight (BMI ≥25 kg/m^2) and obesity (BMI ≥30

kg/m^2) (see Cole, Bellizzi, Flegal, and Dietz 2000). Because these criteria do not take into account the composition of the individual's body weight, they are limited as indexes of obesity and may result in misclassifications of underweight, overweight, and obesity. There is considerable variability in body composition for any given BMI. Some individuals with low BMIs may have as much relative body fat as those with higher BMIs. Older people have more relative body fat at any given BMI than younger people (Baumgartner, Heymsfield, and Roche 1995). Thus, the prevalence of obesity could be worse than currently thought.

Trends in Overweight and Obesity

Globally, the prevalence of overweight and obesity has reached epidemic proportions. The World Health Organization (2004b) reported that more than 1 billion adults are overweight and over 300 million are obese. The prevalence of overweight and obesity in children and adults varies among countries, depending in part on the nation's level of industrialization (see table 9.1). In the European Union, Greece has the highest prevalence of overweight and obesity; over 3 out of 4 adults (>75%) are either overweight or obese (International Obesity Task Force 2005). In Western Samoa, 57% of men and 74% of women are obese, and the prevalence rises to 75% for adults in urban areas. In the United States, over 30% of adults are obese (BMI ≥30 kg/m^2), and 2 out of 3 adults are overweight (BMI = 25-29.9 kg/m^2). On average, the prevalence of obesity is low for men (3%-5%) and women (4%-13%) from less-developed countries (Brazil and Australia), Asia (China and Japan), and Scandinavia (Denmark and Sweden).

Childhood obesity is also a global problem. The prevalence of children and adolescents (6-19 yr) at risk for overweight (BMI = 85th-95th percentile) in Canada and the United States ranges from 29% to 35% (Hedley, Ogden, Johnson, Carroll, Curtin, and Flegal 2004; Tremblay and Willms 2000). In comparison, children in Australia (~20%) and Mexico (10.8%-19.1%) have a relatively lower prevalence of being at risk for overweight (del Rio-Navarro et al. 2004; Magarey, Daniels, and Boulton 2001). Since 1980 the number of overweight American children has doubled and the number of overweight American adolescents has tripled (World Health Organization 2004b). Also, it is alarming that even for preschool children (2-5 yr), the prevalence of overweight and obesity ranges from 18% in

TABLE 9.1   Prevalence of Overweight and Obesity in Selected Countries

Country	Obesity[a]	Overweight[b] or obesity	Source
ADULTS			
Australia, Brazil, China, Denmark, Japan, Sweden	Men: 3%-5% Women: 4%-13%		Flegal 1999
Canada		Men: 57% Women: 35%	Tremblay et al. 2002
England, Cyprus, Czech Republic, Finland, Germany, Greece, Ireland, Malta, Slovakia	Men: 19%-27.5% Women: 19%-38%	Men: 65.4%-78.6% Women: 51%-74.7%	International Obesity Task Force 2005
United States	30.4%[c]	65.1%[c]	Hedley et al. 2004
Western Samoa	Men: 57% Women: 74%		Flegal 1999

Country	Overweight[d]	At risk for overweight[e]	Source
CHILDREN AND ADOLESCENTS			
Australia (7-15 yr)		Boys: 20% Girls: 21.5%	Magarey et al. 2001
Canada (6-19 yr)		Boys: 35.4% Girls: 29.2%	Tremblay and Willms 2000
Crete, Gibraltar, Italy, Malta, Portugal, Sicily, Spain (7-11 yr)	7%-12%[c,f]	31%-35%[c,g]	International Obesity Task Force 2005
Crete, England, Italy, Cyprus, Ireland, Greece, Bulgaria, Spain (13-17 yr)	5%-10%[c,f]	21%-34%[c,g]	International Obesity Task Force 2005
Mexico (10-17 yr)	Boys: 9.2%-14.7% Girls: 6.8%-10.6%	Boys: 10.8%-16.1% Girls: 14.3%-19.1%	del Rio-Navarro et al. 2004
Thailand (5-12 yr)	15.6%		World Health Organization 2004b
United States (6-19 yr)	16.5%[c]	31%[c]	Hedley et al. 2004

Country	Overweight[d]	At risk for overweight[e]	Source
PRESCHOOL CHILDREN			
Australia (2-6 yr)		18%	Canning et al. 2004
Canada (3-5 yr)		25.6%	Canning et al. 2004
United Kingdom (3-4 yr)		23.6%	Bundred et al. 2001
United States (2-5 yr)	10.4%		Ogden et al. 2002

[a]Obesity defined as BMI ≥ 30 kg/m^2.

[b]Overweight defined as BMI between 25.0 and 29.9 kg/m^2.

[c]Males and females combined.

[d]Overweight defined as sex-specific BMI for age in 95th percentile or above.

[e]At risk for overweight defined as sex-specific BMI for age in 85th to 94th percentile.

[f]Percentage of children who are obese, defined by age- and gender-specific BMI cutoffs corresponding to adult cutoff for obesity (BMI ≥ 30 kg/m^2).

[g]Percentage of children who are obese or overweight, defined by age- and gender-specific BMI cutoffs corresponding to adult cutoff for overweight (BMI ≥ 25 kg/m^2).

Australia to 25.6% in Canada (Canning, Courage, and Frizzell 2004).

Because of the health risks and medical costs associated with obesity, the goal of the U.S. Surgeon General is to reduce the prevalence of overweight in children and obesity in adults to no more than 5% and 15%, respectively, by the year 2010 (U.S. Department of Health and Human Services 2000b).

OBESITY: TYPES AND CAUSES

Combating obesity is not an easy task. Many overweight and obese individuals have incorporated patterns of overeating and physical inactivity into their lifestyles, while others have developed eating disorders, exercise addictions, or both. In an effort to lose weight quickly and to prevent weight gain, many are lured by fad diets and exercise gimmicks; and some resort to extreme behaviors, such as avoiding food, bingeing and purging, and exercising compulsively. In a survey of weight control practices of adults in the United States, Serdula et al. (1994) reported that 38% of women and 24% of men were trying to lose weight by counting calories, participating in organized weight-loss programs, taking special supplements or diet pills, or fasting. Only 50% of those trying to lose weight reported using the recommended method of restricting caloric intake and increasing physical activity.

In a report of leisure-time physical activity among overweight adults in the United States ("Prevalence of Leisure-Time Physical Activity" 2000), two-thirds of overweight adults reported that they engaged in physical activity to try to lose weight; however, only 20% met the national recommendation for physical activity (at least 30 min of moderate-intensity activity, most days of the week, preferably daily). Most of these individuals exercised 30 min or longer per session; but only a minority exercised at least five times per week. Therefore, low frequency of physical activity was the main reason that the physical activity recommendation was not met.

Types of Obesity

The way in which fat is distributed in the body may be more important than total body fat for determining one's risk of disease. The waist-to-hip ratio (WHR) is strongly associated with visceral fat, and the impact of regional fat distribution on health is related to the amount of visceral fat located in the abdominal cavity. Abdominal fat is strongly associated with diseases such as CHD, diabetes, hypertension, and hyperlipidemia (Bjorntorp 1988; Blair, Habricht, Sims, Sylwester, and Abraham 1984; Ducimetier, Richard, and Cambien 1989).

The terms **android obesity** and **gynoid obesity** refer to the localization of excess body fat mainly in the upper body (android) or lower body (gynoid). Android obesity (apple shaped) is more typical of males; gynoid obesity (pear shaped) is more characteristic of females. However, some men may have gynoid obesity, and some women may have android obesity. Other terms are also used to describe types of obesity and regional fat distribution. Android obesity is frequently simply called **upper-body obesity**, and gynoid obesity is often described as **lower-body obesity**.

In field settings, you can assess regional fat distribution using the WHR. Chapter 8 presents measurement procedures (see p. 202) and WHR norms (see table 8.8, p. 202). Generally, young adults with WHR values in excess of 0.94 for men and 0.82 for women are at very high risk for adverse health consequences (Bray and Gray 1988b).

Causes of Overweight and Obesity

Many questions may arise in regard to overweight and obesity. This section addresses common questions relating to the causes of overweight and obesity.

■ *Why do people gain or lose weight?*

An energy imbalance in the body results in a weight gain or loss. There is an energy balance when the caloric intake equals the caloric expenditure. A **positive energy balance** is created when the input (food intake) exceeds the expenditure (resting metabolism plus activity level). For every 3500 kcal of excess energy accumulated, 1 lb (0.45 kg) of fat is stored in the body. A **negative energy balance** is produced when the energy expenditure exceeds the energy input. This can be accomplished by reducing the food intake or increasing the physical activity level. A caloric deficit of approximately 3500 kcal produces a loss of 1 lb of fat.

■ *How are energy needs and energy expenditure measured?*

Energy need and expenditure are measured in kilocalories (kcal). A **kilocalorie** is defined as the amount of heat needed to raise the temperature of 1 kg (2.2 lb) of water 1° C. Direct calorimetry is used to measure the energy yield and caloric equivalent of various foods. These foods are burned in a closed chamber in the presence of oxygen, and the amount of heat liberated is measured precisely in kilocalories. Table 9.2 gives the energy yield and caloric equivalents for carbohydrate, protein, and fat.

The energy or caloric need is a function of an individual's metabolic rate and physical activity level. The **basal metabolic rate (BMR)** is a measure of the minimal amount of energy (kcal) needed to maintain basic and essential physiological functions such as breathing, blood circulation, and temperature regulation. Basal metabolic rate varies according to age, gender, body size, and body composition. For assessment of BMR, the individual needs to be rested and fasted and should be in a controlled environment. Since this is not always practical, we use the term *resting metabolic rate (RMR)*, or *resting energy expenditure (REE)*, to indicate the energy required to maintain essential physiological processes in a relaxed, awake, and reclined state. The RMR is approximately 10% higher than the BMR.

Total energy expenditure (TEE) is the sum of the energy expended for BMR or RMR, **dietary thermogenesis** (i.e., energy needed for digesting, absorbing, transporting, and metabolizing foods), and physical activity. The gold standard for measuring TEE is the doubly labeled water (with deuterium and oxygen-18) method. This method is expensive and requires considerable expertise as well as specialized equipment. Therefore, age- and gender-specific prediction equations have been developed to estimate TEE (see table 9.3).

Alternatively, energy expenditure during basal, resting, or activity states can be measured in laboratory settings through indirect calorimetry. In this case, the body's energy expenditure is estimated from oxygen utilization. Every liter of oxygen consumed per minute yields approximately 5 kcal (see table 9.2). For specific physical activities, energy

expenditure is typically expressed in METs (see chapter 4 and appendix E.4) as a multiple of the RMR. One MET equals the relative rate of oxygen consumption of 3.5 ml · min^{-1} for each kilogram of body weight (3.5 · ml · kg^{-1} · min^{-1}) or the relative rate of energy expenditure of 1 kcal · hr^{-1} for each kilogram of body weight (1 kcal · hr^{-1} · kg^{-1}).

Recently, the Western Human Nutrition Research Center of the U.S. Department of Agriculture developed a **digital activity log.** The digital activity log allows the client to record in a handheld computer the type and duration of physical activity performed during the day. The hours spent in various MET-level activities are calculated and used, along with RMR, number of waking hours, and estimated energy expenditure during sleep, to measure TEE. Recent validation studies reported that in women of normal weight this method yields TEE values that are within 10% of reference measures (Kretsch, Blanton, Baer, Staples, Horn, and Keim 2004).

■ *How is RMR regulated?*

Thyroxine is extremely important in regulating RMR. Inadequate levels of this hormone can be produced by thyroid tumors or lack of iodine in the diet. Underproduction of thyroxine can reduce RMR 30% to 50%. If energy input and expenditure are not adjusted accordingly, the positive energy balance that is created results in a weight gain.

Growth hormone, epinephrine, norepinephrine, and various sex hormones may elevate RMR as much as 15% to 20%. These hormones increase during exercise and may be responsible for the elevation in RMR after cessation of exercise.

■ *Does weight gain increase both the number and size of fat cells?*

Obesity is associated with increases in the both the number and size of fat cells. A normal-weight individual has 25 to 30 billion fat cells, whereas an obese person may have as many as 42 to 106 billion fat cells. Also, the adipose cell size of obese individuals is on the average 40% larger than that of non-obese persons (Hirsh 1971). An increase in fat cell number (hyperplasia) occurs rapidly during the first year of life and again during adolescence but remains fairly stable in adulthood, except in cases of morbid obesity. Fat cells increase in size (hypertrophy) during the adolescent growth spurt and continue to grow when excess fat is stored in the cells as triglycerides. Weight gain in adults is typically characterized by the enlargement of existing fat cells, rather than the creation of new fat cells. Also, caloric restriction and exercise are effective in

TABLE 9.2 Energy Yield and Caloric Equivalents for Macronutrients

Nutrient	Energy yield (kcal/g)	Caloric equivalents (kcal/L O$_2$)
Carbohydrate	4.1	5.1
Protein	4.3	4.4
Fat	9.3	4.7

TABLE 9.3 Prediction Equations for Estimating TEE (kcal/day) of Children and Adults

Gender and age	Equation	Physical activity coefficient (PA)
Male 3-18 yr	TEE = 88.5 − (61.9 × age) + PA [(26.7 × wt) + (903 × ht)]	1.00, if PAL ≥ 1.0 and < 1.4 (sedentary)
		1.13, if PAL ≥ 1.4 and < 1.6 (low)
		1.26, if PAL ≥ 1.6 and < 1.9 (active)
		1.42, if PAL ≥ 1.9 and < 2.5 (very active)
Male ≥19 yr	TEE = 662 − (9.53 × age) + PA [(15.9 × wt) + (540 × ht)]	1.00, if PAL ≥ 1.0 and < 1.4 (sedentary)
		1.11, if PAL ≥ 1.4 and < 1.6 (low)
		1.25, if PAL ≥ 1.6 and < 1.9 (active)
		1.48, if PAL ≥ 1.9 and < 2.5 (very active)
Female 3-18 yr	TEE = 135.3 − (30.8 × age) + PA [(10.0 × wt) + (934 × ht)]	1.00, if PAL ≥ 1.0 and < 1.4 (sedentary)
		1.16, if PAL ≥ 1.4 and < 1.6 (low)
		1.31, if PAL ≥ 1.6 and < 1.9 (active)
		1.56, if PAL ≥ 1.9 and < 2.5 (very active)
Female ≥19 yr	TEE = 354 − (6.91 × age) + PA [(9.36 × wt) + (726 × ht)]	1.00, if PAL ≥ 1.0 and < 1.4 (sedentary)
		1.12, if PAL ≥ 1.4 and < 1.6 (low)
		1.27, if PAL ≥ 1.6 and < 1.9 (active)
		1.45, if PAL ≥ 1.9 and < 2.5 (very active)

TEE = total energy expenditure in kcal/day; PA = physical activity coefficient; wt = body weight in kg; ht = height in m; PAL = physical activity level.

Institute of Medicine 2002

reducing fat cell size but not the number of fat cells in adults (Hirsh 1971). Perhaps the key to preventing obesity is to closely monitor the dietary intake and energy expenditure, especially during the adolescent growth spurt and puberty. This could potentially retard the development of new fat cells and control the size of existing fat cells.

■ *What is the relative importance of genetics and environment in developing obesity?*

Scientists have debated the relative contributions of genetics and environment to obesity. Mayer (1968) observed that only 10% of children who had normal-weight parents were obese. The probability of being obese is increased to 40% and 80%, respectively, if one parent or both parents are obese. Although these data suggest a strong genetic influence, they do not rule out environmental influences such as eating and exercise habits.

In a controlled study of long-term (100 days) overfeeding in identical twins, Bouchard et al. (1990) observed large individual differences in the tendency toward obesity and distribution of body fat, even within each pair of twins. Changes in body weight due to overfeeding of twins were moderately correlated ($r = 0.55$). Overall, increases in body weight, fat mass, trunk fat, and visceral fat were three times greater in high-weight gainers compared to low-weight gainers. These data suggest that genotype explains some, but not all, of a person's adaptation to a sustained energy surplus. Approximately 25% of the variability among individuals in absolute and relative body fat is attributed to genetic factors and 30% is associated with cultural (environmental) factors (Bouchard, Perusse, Leblanc, Tremblay, and Theriault 1988).

Hill and Melanson (1999) suggested that the major cause of obesity in the United States is our environment. Over the past 30 years, the U.S. population has been exposed to an environment that strongly promotes the consumption of high-fat, energy-dense foods (increased energy intake) and reliance on technology that discourages physical activity and reduces the amount of physical activity (decreased energy expenditure) needed for daily living.

WEIGHT MANAGEMENT PRINCIPLES AND PRACTICES

Proper nutrition (eating a well-balanced diet) and daily physical activity are key components of a weight management program. In weight management programs, most clients are interested in losing body weight and body fat, but some need to gain body weight. The basic principle underlying safe and effective weight-loss programs is that weight can be lost only through a negative energy balance, which is produced when the caloric expenditure exceeds the caloric intake. The most effective way of creating a caloric deficit is through a combination of diet (restricting caloric intake) and exercise (increasing caloric expenditure). On the other hand, for weight-gain programs, the caloric intake must exceed the caloric expenditure in order to create a positive energy balance. "Weight Management Principles" (p. 220) summarizes principles and practices underlying the design of weight management programs.

People can win the battle of controlling body weight and obesity by not only understanding why they eat and monitoring their food intake closely, but also by incorporating more physical activity into their lifestyles. The physically active lifestyle is characterized by

- daily aerobic exercise;
- strength and flexibility exercises;
- increased participation in recreational activities such as bowling, golf, tennis, and dancing; and
- increased physical activity in the daily routine at home and work through restricting use of labor-saving devices such as escalators, power tools, automobiles, and home and garden appliances.

In addition to these suggestions, you should encourage your clients to follow the *Dietary Guidelines for Americans* (U.S. Department of Health and Human Services 2005a):

Adequate Nutrients Within Calorie Needs

- Consume a variety of nutrient-dense foods within and among the basic food groups; choose foods that limit intake of saturated and trans fats, cholesterol, added sugars, salt, and alcohol.
- Meet recommended intakes within energy needs by adopting a balanced eating pattern.

Weight Management

- To maintain body weight in a healthy range, balance calories from foods and beverages with calories expended.
- To prevent gradual weight gain over time, make small decreases in food and beverage calories and increase physical activity.

Physical Activity

- To reduce risk of chronic disease in adulthood, engage in at least 30 min of moderate-intensity physical activity, above usual activity, at work or home on most days of the week.
- For most people, greater health benefits can be obtained by engaging in physical activity of more vigorous intensity or longer duration.
- To help manage body weight and prevent gradual, unhealthy body weight gain in adulthood, engage in approximately 60 min of moderate-to-vigorous-intensity exercise on most days of the week while not exceeding caloric intake requirements.
- To sustain weight loss in adulthood, participate in at least 60 to 90 min of daily moderate-intensity physical activity while not exceeding caloric intake requirements. Some people may need to consult with a health care provider before participating in this level of activity.
- Achieve physical fitness by including cardiovascular conditioning, stretching exercises for flexibility, and resistance exercises or calisthenics for muscle strength and endurance.

Food Groups to Encourage

- Consume a sufficient amount of fruits and vegetables while staying within energy needs. Two cups of fruit and 2½ cups of vegetables per day are recommended for a reference 2000-calorie intake, with higher or lower amounts depending on the calorie level.
- Choose a variety of fruits and vegetables each day. In particular, select from all five vegetable subgroups (dark green, orange, legumes, starchy vegetables, and other vegetables) several times a week.

Weight Management Principles

Weight loss	Weight gain	Exercise
• A well-balanced diet for good nutrition contains carbohydrate, protein, fat, vitamin, minerals, and water.	• The dietary protein intake should be increased to 1.2–1.6 g · kg^{-1} body weight.	• A major cause of obesity is lack of physical activity.
• The weight loss should be gradual—no more than 2 lb a week.	• The weight gain should be gradual—no more than 2 lb a week.	• For fat-weight loss, aerobic exercise should be performed daily or twice daily.
• The caloric intake should be at least 1200 kcal/day, and the caloric deficit should not exceed 1000 kcal/day.	• The daily caloric intake should exceed caloric needs by 400 to 500 kcal/day.	• Resistance exercise training is excellent for maintaining FFM (for weight loss) and increasing FFM (for weight gain).
• A caloric deficit of 3500 kcal is needed to lose 1 lb of fat.	• A positive energy balance of 2800 to 3500 is needed to gain 1 lb of muscle tissue.	• For weight loss, exercise helps create a caloric deficit by increasing caloric expenditure.
• Weight loss should be due to loss of fat rather than lean body tissue.	• Weight gain should be due to increased FFM rather than fat mass.	• Exercise is better than dieting for maximizing fat loss and minimizing lean tissue loss.
• On the same diet, a taller, heavier person will lose weight at a faster rate than a shorter, lighter person due to a higher RMR.	• The individual should eat 3 meals and 2 to 3 healthy snacks per day (e.g., dried fruits, nuts, seeds, and some liquid meals).	• Compared to fat, muscle tissue is more metabolically active and uses more calories at rest.
• Weight loss rate decreases over time, because the difference between the caloric intake and caloric needs gets smaller as one loses weight.	• Protein powders are no more effective than natural protein sources (e.g., lean meats, skim milk, and egg whites).	• Low-intensity, longer-duration exercise maximizes total energy expenditure better than high-intensity, shorter-duration exercise.
• Men lose weight faster than women due to a higher RMR.	• Amino acid supplements may promote muscle growth if taken immediately before or after exercise.	• RMR remains elevated 30 min or longer after vigorous exercise.
• The individual should eat at least 3 meals a day.	• Vitamin B12, boron, and chromium supplementation does not increase FFM.	• At a given heart rate, the more physically fit individual expends calories at a faster rate than the less fit individual.
• Quick weight-loss diets, diet pills, and appetite suppressants should be avoided.		• Exercise does not increase appetite.
• Carnitine supplementation does not promote body fat loss.		• Passive exercise devices (e.g., vibrators and sauna belts) do not massage away excess fat.
• Compulsive eating behaviors should be identified and modified.		• Spot-reduction exercises do not preferentially mobilize subcutaneous fat stored near the exercising muscles.
		• To increase caloric expenditure, avoid using labor-saving devices at home and work.

■ Consume 3 or more ounce-equivalents of whole-grain products per day, with the rest of the recommended grains coming from enriched or whole-grain products. In general, at least half the grains should come from whole grains.

■ Consume 3 cups per day of fat-free or low-fat milk or equivalent milk products.

Carbohydrates

■ Choose fiber-rich fruits, vegetables, and whole grains often.

■ Choose and prepare foods and beverages with little added sugars or caloric sweeteners.

■ Reduce the incidence of dental caries by practicing good oral hygiene and consuming sugar- and starch-containing foods and beverages less frequently.

Sodium and Potassium

■ Consume less than 2300 mg (approximately 1 tsp of salt) of sodium per day.

■ Choose and prepare foods with little salt. At the same time, consume potassium-rich foods such as fruits and vegetables.

Alcoholic Beverages

- Those who drink alcoholic beverages should do so sensibly and in moderation—defined as the consumption of up to one drink per day for women and up to two drinks per day for men.

- Alcoholic beverages should not be consumed by individuals who cannot restrict their alcohol intake, women of childbearing age who may become pregnant, pregnant and lactating women, children and adolescents, individuals taking medications that can interact with alcohol, and those with specific medical conditions.

- Alcoholic beverages should be avoided by individuals engaging in activities that require attention, skill, or coordination such as driving or operating machinery.

WELL-BALANCED NUTRITION

Before you can help your clients with their weight management, you must understand good nutrition. A well-balanced diet should contain adequate amounts of protein, fat, carbohydrate, vitamins, minerals, and water. The Institute of Medicine (2002) recommends that adults seeking well-balanced nutrition get 45% to 65% of their calories from carbohydrates, 20% to 35% of their calories from fat, and 10% to 25% of their calories from protein.

Recently, trends in the dietary intake of energy and macronutrients by U.S. adults (Wright, Kennedy-Stephenson, Wang, McDowell, and Johnson 2004) were evaluated by studying National Health and Nutrition Examination Survey (NHANES) data from 1971 (NHANES I) to 2000 (NHANES IV). Analysis showed that the average daily energy intake increased ~7% for men and 21% for women. This increase in calorie intake was attributed primarily to increases in the relative and absolute carbohydrate intake. The relative carbohydrate intake increased from 42% to 49% in men and from 45% to 51.6% in women. On average, the absolute carbohydrate intake of men and women increased by 68 g and 62 g, respectively. In comparison, the relative intake of total fat decreased (from ~37% to ~33% for men and from 36% to ~33% for women). However, this relative decrease was attributed to the increase in total calorie intake. In fact, the average absolute amount of fat intake increased by 6.5 g for women but decreased by 5.3 g for men. The percentage of kilocalories obtained from protein slightly decreased for both men (from 16.5% to 15.5%) and women (from 16.9% to 15.1%).

Carbohydrates

Carbohydrates are grouped into two major categories—simple and complex. Simple carbohydrates consist of simple sugars (e.g., glucose and fructose) found in fruits, berries, some vegetables, table sugar, and honey. Complex carbohydrates are found in many plant-based foods, whole grains, and low-fat dairy products. The Institute of Medicine (2002) recommends that the largest proportion (45%-65%) of the daily calorie intake be in the form of carbohydrates. Experts recommend consuming a wide range of carbohydrates and to emphasize fruits, vegetables, whole grains, and low-fat dairy products. Foods with added sugars should be limited to no more than 25% of the total calories consumed; overweight people need much less. Carbohydrates provide an efficient source of energy (i.e., glucose) that the muscles and brain can directly use. The Institute of Medicine (2002) recommends a minimum daily intake of 130 g of carbohydrate to maintain proper brain function for children and adults. Also, many carbohydrates contain fiber; a high-fiber diet lowers the risk of heart disease, diabetes, and colon cancer (Harvard School of Public Health 2004).

Since 1981, the glycemic index (GI) has been used to classify carbohydrate-containing foods. The GI is a measure of the body's glycemic response (i.e., increase in blood glucose and insulin following consumption) to various foods. The GI rates the immediate effect of a specific food on blood glucose levels and is obtained by comparing the glycemic response of that food with the glycemic response of glucose (GI = 100). The glycemic response of simple and complex carbohydrates varies greatly. Some complex carbohydrates are metabolized as rapidly as simple sugars. Generally, refined grain products and potatoes have a high GI (>60), legumes and unprocessed grains have a moderate GI (40-60), and nonstarchy fruits and vegetables have a low GI (<40). Lists of GI values for various foods may be found in nutrition books and journals and on Web sites (see Clark 1997; Foster-Powell and Miller 1995; Miller 2001).

Several popular diet books (e.g., *Sugar Busters*, *The Zone*, and *South Beach Diet*) advocate the consumption of low-GI foods. Although some international health organizations have endorsed the GI, its relevance to health and nutrition is controversial. For example, the American Heart Association, American Diabetes Association, and American Dietetic Association do not endorse using the GI for disease prevention and treatment (Ludwig and Eckel 2002). In fact, Pi-Sunyer (2002) concluded that there is insufficient evidence to justify basing public health recommendations on the GI. Additional research is needed to assess the long-term effects of low-GI diets on the prevention and treatment of disease and obesity.

Recommendations for the dietary carbohydrate intake of athletes and physically active individuals depend on the intensity and duration of exercise. As intensity increases, the use of carbohydrates for energy increases and the proportion of energy coming from fat decreases. During extended exercise (lasting 1-2 hr), muscle glycogen is depleted, and the body must use blood glucose as a carbohydrate source for energy. Generally, a daily carbohydrate intake of 5 to 7 g · kg^{-1} of body weight is recommended for individuals engaging in low-intensity, moderate-duration physical activity. For those performing high-intensity or long-duration exercise, an intake of 7 to 12 g · kg^{-1} of body weight is recommended (Burke, Kiens, and Ivy 2004).

Protein

Approximately 10% to 25% of the daily caloric intake should be protein. The diet should include sources of the essential amino acids needed for protein synthesis. Lack of these essential amino acids may produce a loss of muscle tissue or prevent the synthesis of hormones, enzymes, and cellular structures. The amount of protein that the average individual needs to meet the daily protein requirements of the body is 0.8 g·kg^{-1} of body weight. Experts agree that exercise increases the need for protein (American Dietetic Association 2000; Lemon 2000; Tipton and Wolfe 2004). The additional protein requirement depends on the type (resistance training or aerobic), intensity, and duration of exercise. The recommended daily protein intake for endurance athletes is 1.2 to 1.4 g · kg^{-1} of body weight, whereas strength-trained athletes may need as much as 1.6 to 1.8 g · kg^{-1} of body weight (American Dietetic Association 2000; Lemon 2000). The diets of most athletes adequately meet these protein requirements, especially when the daily calorie intake is sufficient and the diet contains complete sources of protein such as meats, eggs, and fish (Campbell and Geik 2004; Manore 2004).

Amino acids are the building blocks of protein. Nine essential amino acids must be obtained through the diet because the body lacks the ability to synthesize them. Three essential amino acids—leucine, isoleucine, and valine—share a structural similarity and are known as *branched-chain amino acids*. Approximately 99% of the body's amino acids are incorporated into protein structures, and the remaining 1%, known as the free pool, can be found in the plasma and the intracellular and extracellular spaces. Amino acids enter the free pool through absorption of dietary protein, breakdown of tissue protein, and synthesis from carbohydrates or fat (Armsey and Grime 2002). Recent research suggests that muscle protein synthesis is regulated by levels of essential amino acids in the plasma rather than levels of intramuscular amino acids (Bohe, Low, Wolfe, and Rennie 2003). Leucine is one of the most important stimulators of skeletal muscle protein synthesis (Kimball and Jefferson 2002).

Excess protein cannot be stored in the body and is broken down into amino acids. Amino acids also cannot be stored and therefore will be used as fuel for energy. Too much protein in the diet causes dehydration due to excessive production of urea, which must be eliminated in the urine.

Fats

Fats and oils are part of a healthy diet and well-balanced nutrition. Some dietary fat is needed to supply fatty acids and to absorb fat-soluble vitamins. The omega-3 fatty acids (eicosapentaenoic acid [EPA] and docosahexanoic acid [DHA]) have a cardioprotective effect, reducing the risk of cardiovascular disease. In addition, free fatty acids are an important source of energy during aerobic exercise. Approximately 20% to 35% of the daily energy intake should come from fat; however, fats must be chosen wisely. To decrease their risk of elevated LDL-cholesterol, most Americans need to decrease their intake of saturated fat, trans-fatty acid, and cholesterol (U.S. Department of Health and Human Services 2004). Saturated fat should account for less than 10% of the daily calorie intake, and trans-fatty acid consumption should be as low as possible, contributing to no more than 1% of the daily calorie intake. Dietary intake of cholesterol should be less than 300 mg per day for adults whose LDL-C is less than 130 mg · dl^{-1}. For adults with elevated LDL-C (>130 mg · dl^{-1}), dietary cholesterol should be limited to no more than 200 mg per day and saturated fat intake should not exceed 7% of total calorie intake. Also, consuming two servings of fish rich in EPA and DHA (e.g., salmon, trout, and light tuna) each week is recommended (U.S. Department of Health and Human Services 2004).

The National Cholesterol Education Program (2001) recommends a "Therapeutic Lifestyle Changes Diet" (table 9.4) to promote weight loss in those who are overweight and to reduce serum

TABLE 9.4   Nutrient Composition of the Therapeutic Lifestyle Changes Diet

Nutrient	Recommended intake
Saturated fat[a]	<7% of total calories
Polyunsaturated fat	Up to 10% of total calories
Monounsaturated fat	Up to 20% of total calories
Total fat	25-35% of total calories
Carbohydrate[b]	50-60% of total calories
Fiber	20-30 g/day
Protein	Approximately 15% of total calories
Cholesterol	<200 mg/day
Total calories[c]	Balance energy intake and expenditure to maintain desirable body weight/prevent weight gain

[a]Trans fatty acids are another low-density lipoprotein-raising fat that should be kept to a low intake.

[b]Carbohydrates should be derived predominantly from foods rich in complex carbohydrates including grains, especially whole grains, fruits, and vegetables.

[c]Daily energy expenditure should include at least moderate physical activity (contributing approximately 200 kcal/day).

Data from National Cholesterol Education Program, 2001, "Executive Summary of the Third Report of the National Cholesterol Education Program Expert Panel on Detection, Evaluation and Treatment of High Blood Cholesterol in Adults (Adult Treatment Panel I I)," *Journal of the American Medical Association* 285 (19): 2490.

cholesterol levels. This diet limits dietary intakes of saturated fat and trans fatty acids (< 7% of total calories), total fat (25% to 35% of total calories), and cholesterol (< 200 mg per day).

Vitamins, Minerals, and Water

A well-balanced diet usually does not need to be supplemented to meet the minimum daily vitamin and mineral requirements of the body. Table 9.5 gives recommended dietary allowances (RDAs), adequate intakes (AIs), and upper intake levels (ULs) for vitamins and minerals.

Vitamins

Eating a well-balanced diet typically provides an individual's vitamin requirements. The body does not store the water-soluble vitamins (B complex and C); and in the case of most of these vitamins, an excess amount is excreted in the urine. The excess accumulation of fat-soluble vitamins (A, D, E, and K) may produce decalcification of bones, headaches, nausea, diarrhea, and other toxic effects (Williams 1992).

According to the 2005 Dietary Guidelines Advisory Committee Report (U.S. Department of Health and Human Services 2004), many Americans need to increase their intake of vitamins A, C, and E. Also, individuals older than 50 yr should eat foods fortified with vitamin B_{12} or take a vitamin B_{12} supplement daily. Elderly individuals and persons with dark skin may need more than the adequate intake recommen-

dation (see table 9.5) for vitamin D (U.S. Department of Health and Human Services 2004).

Vitamin deficiencies are uncommon in athletes and physically active individuals. However, athletes who restrict their food intake to maintain a low body weight or who engage in severe weight-loss practices (e.g., wrestlers, dancers, and gymnasts) have a greater risk of vitamin deficiency (Manore 2004). Also, athletes who eat diets rich in fast foods or who do not eat a well-balanced diet may suffer from vitamin deficiencies, especially in B complex (B_6 and folate) and antioxidant (C, E, and beta-carotene) vitamins (Benardot, Clarkson, Coleman, and Manore 2001). To be on the safe side, athletes and physically active individuals can take a multivitamin and mineral supplement daily or every other day. Vitamin supplementation improves sport performance *only* in athletes who are vitamin deficient (Benardot et al. 2001).

Minerals

The most common mineral deficiencies are of iron, zinc, and calcium. Physically active individuals, particularly those who choose to exclude meat from their diets, need to plan their diets carefully so that adequate amounts of iron and zinc are available. In some cases, it may be appropriate for you to recommend daily supplementation of iron, zinc, and calcium at 100% RDA in order to ensure adequate intake of these nutrients.

TABLE 9.5 Guidelines for Vitamin and Mineral Intakes: RDAs, AIs, and ULs* for Adults

	MEN AGE (YR)				WOMEN AGE (YR)				UL BOTH SEXES
	19-30	31-50	51-70	70+	19-30	31-50	51-70	70+	19-70+
VITAMINS									
A (μg RE)[a]	1000	1000	1000	1000	800	800	800	800	NA[c]
D (μg/day)	**5**	**5**	**10**	**15**	**5**	**5**	**10**	**15**	50
E (mg/day)	15	15	15	15	15	15	15	15	1000
K (μg)	70	80	80	80	60	65	65	65	NA
C (mg/day)	90	90	90	90	75	75	75	75	NA
Thiamin (mg/day)	1.2	1.2	1.2	1.2	1.1	1.1	1.1	1.1	NA
Riboflavin (mg/day)	1.3	1.3	1.3	1.3	1.1	1.1	1.1	1.1	NA
Niacin (mg/day)	1.6	1.6	1.6	1.6	1.4	1.4	1.4	1.4	35
B_6 (mg/day)	1.3	1.3	1.7	1.7	1.3	1.3	1.5	1.5	100
Folate (μg/day)	400	400	400	400	400	400	400	400	1000
B_{12} (μg/day)	2.4	2.4	2.4	2.4	2.4	2.4	2.4	2.4	NA
Pantothenic acid (mg/day)	**5**	**5**	**5**	**5**	**5**	**5**	**5**	**5**	NA
Biotin (μg/day)	**30**	**30**	**30**	**30**	**30**	**30**	**30**	**30**	NA
Choline (mg/day)	**550**	**550**	**550**	**550**	**425**	**425**	**425**	**425**	3500
MINERALS									
Calcium (mg/d⁻¹)	**1000**	**1000**	**1200**	**1200**	**1000**	**1000**	**1200**	**1200**	2500
Phosphorous (mg/d⁻¹)[b]	700	700	700	700	700	700	700	700	3000-4000
Magnesium (mg/d⁻¹)	400	420	420	420	310	320	320	320	350[d]
Fluoride (mg/d⁻¹)	**4**	**4**	**4**	**4**	**3**	**3**	**3**	**3**	10
Iron (mg)	10	10	10	10	15	15	10	10	NA
Zinc (mg)	15	15	15	15	12	12	12	12	NA
Iodine (μg)	150	150	150	150	150	150	150	150	NA
Selenium (μg/d⁻¹)	55	55	55	55	55	55	55	55	400

[a]Retinol equivalents: 1 RE = 1 μg retinol or 6 μg beta-carotene.

[b]3000 mg/day for >70 years; 4000 mg/day for 19-70 years.

[c]Not available.

[d]UL is for supplemental magnesium only.

*Recommended dietary allowances (RDAs) are in ordinary type, and adequate intakes (AIs) are in bold type. The RDA is the intake that meets the needs of almost all (97-98%) individuals in a group. The AI is believed to cover needs of all individuals in the group; however, sufficient scientific evidence is not available to estimate the RDA for this nutrient. The AI can be used to set goals for individuals. The tolerable upper intake level (UL) is the maximum amount of the nutrient that is unlikely to have adverse health effects in most healthy individuals.

Based on data from the National Academy of Sciences. National Academy Press, Washington, D.C., 2000.

Iron is found in hemoglobin (in the red blood cells), which transports oxygen to exercising muscles. Iron deficiency has been frequently reported for both male and female athletes but is more common among women (Clarkson 1990). Thus, iron supplementation may be warranted for some exercising individuals (Rajaram et al. 1995).

Zinc plays an important role in energy metabolism (as a cofactor for enzymes), hormonal function, and the immune system. The average zinc intake of sedentary and athletic women in the United States is below the RDA (12 mg per day); for men, it typically exceeds the RDA (Clarkson and Haymes 1994). Zinc deficiency may result in decreased strength and endurance (Krotkiewski, Gudmundsson, Backstrom, and Mandroukas 1982).

The recommended adequate intake (AI) for calcium is 1000 mg per day for men and women less than 51 years of age and 1200 mg per day for older (51-70 + yr) adults. Most individuals can meet their calcium requirements by eating a well-balanced diet that contains milk products. When this is not possible, they should use calcium supplements.

Adequate dietary calcium intake and exercise are essential for bone mineralization and skeletal growth. Inadequate bone mineralization or excessive bone resorption results in bone loss and osteoporosis (Sanborn 1990). In early-menopausal women, a high calcium intake (1500 mg per day), in combination with estrogen therapy, deterred bone loss. Calcium supplementation alone did not prevent bone loss in this group (Ettinger, Genault, and Cann 1987).

The typical American diet contains more sodium than the recommended daily amount. The *Dietary Guidelines for Americans* (U.S. Department of Health and Human Services 2005a) recommends limiting salt intake to less than 2300 mg per day (approximately 1 level teaspoon of salt). Excess salt (sodium chloride) intake may disrupt the electrolyte balance of the body and lead to increased fluid retention, hypertension, and calcium excretion. Thus, the amount of sodium in the diet should be restricted, especially for hypertensive or coronary-prone individuals. To counteract the effect of salt on blood pressure, foods rich in potassium are recommended; potassium lowers blood pressure.

Fraudulent claims sway many physically active individuals, particularly bodybuilders and strength-trained athletes, into believing that multivitamin and mineral supplements enhance muscle growth and exercise performance. Research suggests that long-term use of vitamin–mineral supplements does not increase strength or sport performance (Telford, Catchpole, Deakin, Hahn, and Plank 1992). Scientific studies (Williams 1993) demonstrate that

- vitamin B_{12} supplementation does not increase muscle growth or strength;
- carnitine (a vitamin-like compound) supplementation does not facilitate loss of body fat;
- chromium supplementation does not increase fat-free mass or decrease body fat;
- boron supplementation does not increase serum testosterone or fat-free mass; and
- magnesium supplementation does not improve muscle strength.

Water

The major sources of water for the body are fluid intake, food intake, and oxidation of foodstuffs by the body. Water is lost in urine, feces, perspiration, and expired air. During strenuous exercise, as much as 3 L of water may be lost through sweating. To prevent dehydration and electrolyte imbalances, athletes and physically active individuals need to hydrate before exercise, drink fluids during exercise, and rehydrate immediately after exercise. Although plain water is effective much of the time, carbohydrate sport drinks may also be used to maintain blood glucose levels and to replace fluids lost during exercise. The ideal fluid-replacement beverage contains some sodium to help maintain plasma osmolality and some glucose or sucrose to provide energy during exercise and to replenish muscle glycogen stores after exercise. Guidelines for maintaining hydration before, during, and after exercise have been developed by the ACSM (American College of Sports Medicine 1996) and the National Athletic Trainers' Association (Casa et al. 2002):

- Consume generous amounts of fluids 24 hr before exercise.
- Consume 400 to 600 ml of fluid 2 hr before exercise.
- Do not restrict fluid intake during exercise; drink at least 150 to 350 ml (6-12 oz) of fluid every 15 to 20 min.
- Consume sport drinks containing carbohydrate and sodium when engaging in intense, long-duration (>1 hr) activity or when exercising in the heat.

DESIGNING WEIGHT-MANAGEMENT PROGRAMS: PRELIMINARY STEPS

In designing weight-management programs for weight loss or weight gain, you need to set body weight goals and assess the calorie intake and expenditure for your clients.

Setting Body Weight Goals

To set healthy body weight goals for your clients, you must first assess their present body weight, BMI, or body fat levels. You can easily measure the client's body weight by using a calibrated bathroom or doctor's scale. Clients should wear indoor clothing but not shoes.

When you are evaluating your client's body weight, you should not use height–weight tables established by the Metropolitan Life Insurance Company (Society of Actuaries and Association of Life Insurance Medical Directors of America 1980). These tables are limited for two reasons:

- The values represent height and weight with shoes and clothing. Whether individuals were measured with shoes and clothing was not standardized.

- Data were obtained from individuals who could afford life insurance; the data represent predominantly young to middle-aged White males and females and therefore are not representative of other population groups.

The *Dietary Guidelines for Americans* (U.S. Department of Health and Human Services 2005a) recommends using BMI to determine a healthy body weight range. Use table 9.6 to determine if your client's BMI value falls within the healthy range. Individuals with a BMI from 18.5 up to 25 are considered to be at a **healthy body weight**.

Determining a healthy body weight from either BMI or any height–weight table alone may lead to invalid conclusions regarding your client's level of body fatness and health risk. These methods do not take into account the body composition of the individual. For example, with the use of BMI or height–weight tables, many mesomorphs having a large fat-free mass are classified as overweight, yet

TABLE 9.6 Body Mass Index Chart

BMI[a]	NORMAL (HEALTHY) WEIGHT						OVERWEIGHT					OBESE					
	19	20	21	22	23	24	25	26	27	28	29	30	31	32	33	34	35
HT (in.)	BODY WEIGHT (LB)																
58	91	96	100	105	110	115	119	124	129	134	138	143	148	153	158	162	167
59	94	99	104	109	114	119	124	128	133	138	143	148	153	158	163	168	173
60	97	102	107	112	118	123	128	133	138	143	148	153	158	163	168	174	179
61	100	106	111	116	122	127	132	137	143	148	153	158	164	169	174	180	185
62	104	109	115	120	126	131	136	142	147	153	158	164	169	175	180	186	191
63	107	113	118	124	130	135	141	146	152	158	163	169	175	180	186	191	197
64	110	116	122	128	134	140	145	151	157	163	169	174	180	186	192	197	204
65	114	120	126	132	138	144	150	156	162	168	174	180	186	192	198	204	210
66	118	124	130	136	142	148	155	161	167	173	179	186	192	198	204	210	216
67	121	127	134	140	146	153	159	166	172	178	185	191	198	204	211	217	223
68	125	131	138	144	151	158	164	171	177	184	190	197	203	210	216	223	230
69	128	135	142	149	155	162	169	176	182	189	196	203	209	216	223	230	236
70	132	139	146	153	160	167	174	181	188	195	202	209	216	222	229	236	243
71	136	143	150	157	165	172	179	186	193	200	208	215	222	229	236	243	250
72	140	147	154	162	169	177	184	191	199	206	213	221	228	235	242	250	258
73	144	151	159	166	174	182	189	197	204	212	219	227	235	242	250	257	265
74	148	155	164	171	179	186	194	202	210	218	225	233	241	249	256	264	272
75	152	160	168	176	184	192	200	208	216	224	232	240	248	256	264	272	279
76	156	164	172	180	189	197	205	213	221	230	238	246	254	263	271	279	287

[a]BMI in kg/m^2; BMI <18.5 kg/m^2 is classified as underweight. To convert body weight in lb to kg, divide body weight by 2.2; to convert height in in. to cm, multiply height by 2.54.

Instructions: Find your client's height (HT in in.) and body weight (in lb). Read up the chart to find the corresponding BMI. If your client's BMI is classified as overweight or obese, use this chart to determine a healthy body weight for the client (i.e., a body weight corresponding to a BMI <25 kg/m^2).

their body fat content may be lower than average. Similarly, individuals may be overfat or obese even though they are underweight according to the BMI and height–weight tables. Therefore, you should use the body composition technique to estimate a healthy body weight and body fat level for your clients.

When you use the body composition technique for estimating healthy body weight and body fat levels, assess the fat-free mass (FFM) and percent fat (%BF) using one of the methods described in chapter 8. A healthy body weight is based on the client's present FFM and %BF goal. Because some fat is needed for good health and nutrition, individuals should attempt to achieve a %BF somewhere between the low and upper values recommended in table 8.1 (see p. 172). Remember, minimal %BF depends on age and is estimated to be 5% to 10% for males and 12% to 15% for females. Cutoff values for obesity are also age dependent, ranging from >22% to >31% BF for males and >35% to >38% BF for females. Figure 9.1 illustrates a sample calculation of healthy body weight using the body composition technique.

With aging, there is a tendency to accumulate body weight and excess fat. Typically, adults may expect to gain 15 lb (9 kg) of fat weight and lose 5 lb (2.3 kg) of lean body mass per decade of life (Evans and Rosenberg 1992; Forbes 1976; Paffenbarger and Olsen 1996). This weight gain is primarily characterized by an increase in body fat and a decrease in muscle mass and is associated with declining physical activity levels with age. Each individual should attempt to maintain body weight and fatness at healthy levels.

Assessing Calorie Intake and Energy Expenditure

The second step in planning weight management programs is to assess the client's energy (calorie) intake and expenditure. You will use these baseline data to estimate the rate of weight loss or weight gain and the amount of time needed to achieve long-term goals of body composition and body weight.

Energy Intake

A food record (see appendix E.1, "Food Record and RDA Profile," p. 340) is used to determine an individual's daily caloric intake. The client keeps a record of the type and quantity of foods eaten each day for 3 to 7 days. Make certain that your client records all foods consumed; under reporting of food intake ranges from 10% to 45%. Use computer software to assess the average daily caloric intake and to compare average nutrient intakes to recommended amounts for each nutrient (see appendix E.2, "Sample Computerized Analysis of Food Intake," p. 342, for sample output). The food record also can help you analyze dietary patterns

---

Demographic Data

Client: 31-year-old male

Current body composition:

Body weight = 185 lb (84.1 kg)
Body fat = 20% BF
Fat-free mass (FFM) = 148 lb (67.3 kg)

Goals: 12% BF and 88% FFM

Steps:

1. Determine the client's present %BF using one of the body composition methods (see chapter 8).

2. Calculate the client's present FFM (in lb): 185 lb × 0.80 (current %FFM) = 148 lb.

3. Set reasonable body composition goals for client: 12% BF and 88% FFM.

4. Divide the present FFM (in lb) by the %FFM goal to obtain target body weight: 148 lb/0.88 = 168 lb (76.4 kg).

5. Calculate weight loss by subtracting target body weight from present body weight: 185 − 168 = 17 lb (7.7 kg). Assuming that FFM is maintained, this client must lose 17 lb of fat to achieve his target body weight and body fat level.

Figure 9.1 Sample calculation of healthy body weight using body composition method.

such as types of foods consumed, frequency of eating, and the caloric content of each meal.

Energy Expenditure

You can use either the factorial method or the total energy expenditure (TEE) method to assess the energy needs of your clients. For the **factorial method**, RMR or REE and the additional calories expended during work, household chores, personal daily activities, and exercise are estimated. Various methods used to estimate RMR and the additional energy requirements for occupational and physical activities are presented in this section. Although the factorial approach may reasonably estimate your client's energy expenditure, it is limited in that the equations used to estimate RMR have prediction errors and it is neither feasible nor practical to measure the wide range of activities performed throughout a normal day. Therefore, the TEE method for estimating total energy expenditure has been endorsed by the Institute of Medicine (2002). For the **total energy expenditure (TEE) method**, the individual's TEE is predicted using equations derived from doubly-labeled water measures of TEE in free-living individuals (see table 9.3, p. 218).

Factorial Method: Estimation of Resting Metabolic Rate

Indirect calorimetry can be used to obtain reference measures of RMR or REE. Prediction equations are an inexpensive alternative to indirect calorimetry (see "Methods of Estimating Resting Metabolic Rate," below). You can estimate body surface area (BSA) from height and weight using the nomogram in figure 9.2.

The average male or female between 20 and 40 years of age burns 38 kcal $\cdot$ hr^{-1} and 35 kcal $\cdot$ hr^{-1}, respectively, for each square meter of BSA. For example, according to method I for estimating RMR, a 5 ft 2 in. (157.5 cm), 120-lb (54.5 kg) female has a body surface area of 1.54 m^2 and a daily resting metabolic need of 1294 kcal (1.54 m^2 × 35 kcal $\cdot$ hr^{-1} × 24 hr).

You can obtain a quicker but less accurate estimate of RMR by multiplying the body weight by a factor of 10 (for BW measured in lb) or 22 (for BW measured in kg) for women and a factor of 11 (for BW in lb) or 24.2 (for BW in kg) for men (see method IV). With this method, the RMR for the woman in our example is 1200 kcal (120 lb × 10).

Resting metabolic rate gradually decreases with age because the number of metabolically active

Methods of Estimating Resting Metabolic Rate (RMR)	
Method	**Equation**
I. Body surface area (BSA)[a]	
Men	RMR = BSA × 38 kcal $\cdot$ hr^{-1} × 24 hr
Women	RMR = BSA × 35 kcal $\cdot$ hr^{-1} × 24 hr
II.A. Harris-Benedict equations[b]	
Men	RMR = 66.473 + 13.751 (BM) + 5.0033 (HT) − 6.755 (AGE)
Women	RMR = 655.0955 + 9.463 (BM) + 1.8496 (HT) − 4.6756 (AGE)
II.B. Mifflin et al. equations[b]	
Men	RMR = [9.99 (BM) + 6.25 (HT) − 4.92 (AGE)] + 5.0
Women	RMR = [9.99 (BM) + 6.25 (HT) − 4.92 (AGE)] − 161
III. Fat-free mass (FFM)	
Men and women	RMR = 500 + 22 (FFM in kg)
IV. Quick estimate (from body mass)	
Men	RMR = BM (in lb) × 11 kcal $\cdot$ lb^{-1}
	RMR = BM (in kg) × 24.2 kcal $\cdot$ kg^{-1}
Women	RMR = BM (in lb) × 10 kcal $\cdot$ lb^{-1}
	RMR = BM (in kg) × 22.0 kcal $\cdot$ kg^{-1}

[a]Adjust RMR for age. RMR decreases 2% to 5% per decade after age 40.

[b]BM in kg; HT in cm; AGE in yr.

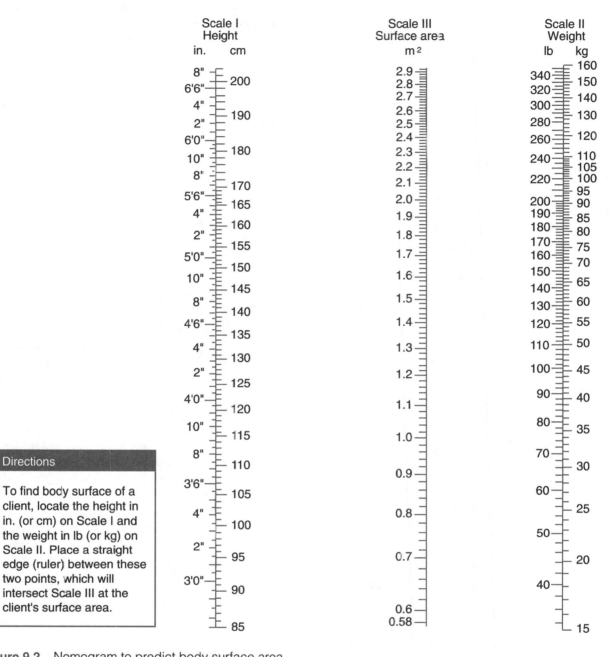

Figure 9.2 Nomogram to predict body surface area.

Reprinted, by permission, from W.E. Collins, 1967, *Clinical Spirometry*, Braintree, MA: Warren E. Collins. Copyright 1967 by Warren E. Collins. 33.

cells is reduced. The RMR declines 2% to 5% during each decade of life after age 25 (Sharkey 1990). To prevent gradual weight gain with aging, people must reduce caloric intake or increase physical activity level. In the past, the Harris-Benedict (1919) equations (method IIA) were widely used to estimate RMR. However, the American Dietetic Association (2003) recommends using the equations of Mifflin and colleagues (1990) to estimate the RMR of healthy individuals (see method IIB). Both equations (Harris-Benedict and Mifflin) are gender specific and take into account not only

height and weight but also age. Roza and Shizgal (1984) cross-validated the original Harris-Benedict equations, developed new equations using data from a large number of subjects, and concluded that the original equations published in 1919 yielded identical estimates of RMR. Also, the Harris-Benedict equations accurately estimated the REE of a large sample ($N = 2528$) of normal weight, overweight, and obese individuals, but these equations tended to overestimate REE in underweight persons (Muller et al. 2004). In contrast, the American Dietetic Association (2003) reported that the Harris-Benedict equations generally overestimated RMR but that the Mifflin et al. equations accurately estimated (within ±10%) the RMR for 80% of their sample. Compared to indirect calorimetry, both the Harris-Benedict and the Mifflin et al. equations are more practical in terms of effort and expense, and their accuracy is adequate for planning weight management programs.

In addition to body size and age, RMR is influenced by body composition. Muscular individuals have a higher RMR than fatter individuals of the same body weight because fat tissue is less metabolically active than muscle tissue. The RMRs of women are 5% to 10% lower than those of men (McArdle, Katch, and Katch 1996). This lower rate may be attributable to a greater relative fat content and lower FFM for women. To use method III (p. 228), you must measure the fat-free mass of your client using one of the body composition methods suggested in chapter 8.

Factorial Method: Estimation of Additional Caloric Requirements

Resting metabolic rate accounts for 50% to 70% of total daily caloric needs, but this value depends on the activity level and occupation of the person. The percentage is greater for less active individuals, who require fewer calories above the resting level. For example, if a sedentary male office worker has a resting metabolic need of 1680 kcal, the additional caloric need as a consequence of the nature of his work is approximately 40% above resting level, or 672 kcal. Provided he performs no additional physical activities, his total daily caloric need is 2352 kcal. In this case, RMR accounts for 71% of his total daily caloric requirements. Table 9.7 presents additional caloric requirements for selected occupational activity levels.

After determining the daily energy needs of your clients from their RMR and occupation, you can estimate their additional calorie expenditure due to physical activity and exercise by using a physical activity log (appendix E.3, "Physical Activity Log," p. 347). The individual records every activity performed and the total amount of time spent in each activity. The estimated energy expenditure for a variety of activities is listed in appendix E.4, "Gross Energy Expenditure for Conditioning Exercises, Sports, and Recreational Activities," page 348. You can calculate the total caloric expenditure for each activity by converting the METs to kcal · kg^{-1} · hr^{-1} (1 MET = 1 kcal · kg^{-1} · hr^{-1}) and multiplying this value by the client's body weight (kg). This yields the total amount of kilocalories that the client

TABLE 9.7 Additional Energy Requirements for Selected Activity Levels

Occupational activity level*	PERCENTAGE ABOVE BASAL METABOLISM	
	Men	Women
Sedentary	15	15
Lightly active	40	35
Moderately active	50	45
Very active	85	70
Exceptionally active	110	100

*Examples for each occupational activity level are as follows:

Sedentary = inactive.

Lightly active = most professionals, office workers, shop workers, teachers, homemakers.

Moderately active = workers in light industry, most farm workers, active students, department store workers, soldiers not in active service, commercial fishing workers.

Very active = full-time athletes and dancers, unskilled laborers, forestry workers, military recruits and soldiers in active service, mine workers, steel workers.

Exceptionally active = lumberjacks, blacksmiths, female construction workers.

expends per hour of that activity. You can determine the kcal · min^{-1} expenditure by dividing the kcal · hr^{-1} by 60 min. Calculate the total energy expenditure by multiplying the kcal · min^{-1} by the duration of the activity.

Keeping a physical activity log is a very time-consuming process for both you and your client; and it may not increase the accuracy of your estimate of additional caloric expenditure because many clients tend to overestimate the actual duration of their physical activity. It may be best to just ask your clients to list the frequency, intensity, and average time for the physical activities and sports that they perform on a regular basis; you can then determine their calorie expenditure for each activity as just described. Add these values to the daily caloric need estimated for the individual's RMR and occupation, and advise clients that on days they are active they can increase their calorie intake accordingly.

TEE Method

For this method, the age- and gender-specific equations in table 9.3, page 218, are used to estimate your client's TEE. These equations predict TEE from your client's age, body weight, height, and physical activity coefficient. The physical activity coefficient depends on your client's **physical** activity level (PAL); given that energy expenditure is highly dependent on physical activity, PAL is commonly described as the ratio of TEE to BMR (PAL = TEE/BMR). The PAL categories were developed from doubly labeled water measures of TEE and BMR in normal, healthy individuals. Data from elite athletes and extremely active individuals (i.e., military personnel and astronauts) were not included (Brooks, Butte, Rand, Flatt, and Caballero 2004). PALs are classified as sedentary (1.0 to < 1.4), low (1.4 to < 1.6), active (1.6 to 1.9), and very active (1.9 to < 2.5). To obtain a fairly good estimate of your client's PAL, you can use various tools such as self-reported physical activity questionnaires, physical activity diaries, pedometers, accelerometers, heart rate monitors, and digital activity logs (Keim, Blanton, and Kretsch 2004). The "Steps for Estimating TEE" illustrates how you can use the TEE equations to estimate your client's daily energy expenditure.

Steps for Estimating TEE

To estimate your client's total energy expenditure (TEE) from age- and gender-specific TEE equations, follow these steps:

Step 1: Determine the client's gender and age (50-year-old male).

Step 2: Measure the client's body weight and height (BW = 180 lb; HT = 70 in.). Convert body weight in pounds to body weight in kilograms: 180 lb/2.204 = 81.7 kg. Convert height in inches to height in meters: 70 in. × 0.0254 = 1.78 m.

Step 3: Estimate your client's PAL (1.70, or active, from physical activity log).

Step 4: Select the appropriate age- and gender-specific TEE prediction equation from table 9.3: for males ≥19 yr.

$$\text{TEE (kcal/day)} = 662 - (9.53 \times \text{age}) + \text{PA} [(15.9 \times \text{wt}) + (540 \times \text{ht})].$$

Step 5: Determine the physical activity coefficient corresponding to your client's PAL (1.25 for PAL = 1.70).

Step 6: Substitute the values for age, body weight, physical activity, and height into the equation:

$$\text{TEE (kcal/day)} = 662 - (9.53 \times 50 \text{ yr}) + 1.25 [(15.9 \times 81.7 \text{ kg}) + (540 \times 1.78 \text{ m})].$$

Step 7: Calculate the estimated TEE (kcal/day):

$$\begin{aligned}
\text{TEE (kcal/day)} &= 662 - (9.53 \times 50 \text{ yr}) + 1.25 [(15.9 \times 81.7 \text{ kg}) + (540 \times 1.78 \text{ m})] \\
&= 662 - (476.5) + [1.25 \times (1{,}299 + 961)] \\
&= 185.5 + 2{,}260.
\end{aligned}$$

$$\text{TEE} = 2445.7, \text{ or } 2446 \text{ kcal/day.}$$

DESIGNING WEIGHT-LOSS PROGRAMS

When the caloric expenditure exceeds the caloric intake, a negative energy balance or caloric deficit is created. The most effective way of producing this deficit is to use a combination of caloric restriction and exercise. Because a deficit of 3500 kcal is needed to lose 1 lb (0.45 kg) of fat, you can easily calculate the daily caloric deficit that is needed to result in the target weekly weight loss you set for your client. An average deficit of 500 kcal will produce a weekly weight loss of approximately 1 lb (0.45 kg), given that 500 kcal × 7 days = 3500 calories. An average deficit of 1000 will produce a weight loss of 2 lb (0.90 kg) a week (1000 kcal × 7 days, or 2 lb). The daily caloric deficit should not exceed 1000 kcal per day.

To ensure that the weight loss is a result of the loss of body fat rather than lean body tissue, you should

- use the body composition method to estimate the client's healthy body weight and fat loss;

- encourage daily participation in aerobic exercise and resistance training programs to enhance the loss of fat and to conserve FFM; and

- plan a diet that restricts calorie intake but contains adequate amounts of good sources of carbohydrate, protein and fat. The diet should contain at least 130 g of carbohydrate per day and 0.8 g of protein per kilogram of body weight per day. Table 9.8 lists good sources of carbohydrate, protein, and fat recommended by the Harvard School of Public Health (2004).

When you design the weight-loss program of diet and exercise, use descriptive data to help you set reasonable goals for your clients. These data include age, gender, height, body weight, relative body fat (%BF), %BF goal, average calorie intake, cardiorespiratory fitness level and occupation. Figure 9.3 illustrates the steps to follow in designing a weight-loss program.

Weight-Loss Diets

You may be overwhelmed by the vast amount of information about popular weight-loss diets in magazines, newspapers, news shows, and scientific and professional journals. There is much controversy and hype about the effectiveness of low-carbohydrate, high-protein, or low-fat diets for weight loss.

TABLE 9.8 Good Sources of Carbohydrate, Protein, and Fat

Macronutrient	Food sources
Carbohydrate	Whole grains, whole wheat bread, oatmeal, brown rice, fruits, vegetables
Protein	Fish, poultry, eggs, nuts, legumes, black beans, navy beans, garbanzo beans, nonfat or low-fat milk
Fat	Unsaturated plant oils such as olive, canola, soy, corn, sunflower, and peanut

Also, in scientific journals it is possible to find arguments for or against any particular diet. According to a recent survey (Partnership for Essential Nutrition 2004), almost 50% of American adults believe that people can lose weight by cutting back on carbohydrates without cutting back on calories (a major premise of the popular Atkins diet). Studies show that high-protein or low-carbohydrate diets result in greater weight losses ($\sim$2.5-4.0 kg) over 3 to 6 mo than do low-fat diets (Foster et al. 2003; Samaha et al. 2003). These findings have led some researchers to question whether a *calorie* is a *calorie* or whether a calorie depends on the macronutrient composition of the diet (Buchholz and Schoeller 2004). Buchholz and Schoeller (2004) noted that increasing protein intake from 15% to 30%-35% increases resting and sleeping energy expenditure; however, these changes account for only one-third of the difference in average weight loss between high protein-low-carbohydrate diets and high carbohydrate-low-fat diets. Also, the greater weight loss for high-protein diets cannot be explained by a greater loss of glycogen and water. Some evidence suggests that individuals on high-protein diets eat less (i.e., reduce their energy intake) over the long term and may be more compliant because protein increases satiety. In fact, comprehensive review articles and meta-analyses on this issue conclude that weight loss depends on calorie intake and not on the macronutrient composition (i.e., low carbohydrate, low fat, or high protein) of the diet (Bravata et al. 2003; Buchholz and Schoeller 2004; Ornish 2004; Seshadri 2004).

In addition to efficacy for weight loss, the long-term health benefits and risks of any diet that limits the intake of specific macronutrients should be assessed. Weight-loss programs should help individuals lose weight in ways that promote health. Foster and colleagues (2003) conducted a 1 yr, multicenter, randomized control trial to compare the weight-loss and health effects of a low-carbohydrate, high-protein, high-fat diet (i.e., Atkins diet) to those of a conventional high-carbohydrate, low-fat, energy-deficit diet. Results indicated that in the short term (up to 6 mo), the Atkins diet pro-

duces greater weight loss ($\sim$4%) in obese men and women (BMI $\sim$34 kg/m^2); however, after 1 yr there was no statistically significant difference in the amount of weight loss between the groups. During the first 6 mo, the Atkins dieters had a greater energy deficit even though their protein and fat intake was not limited, and the energy intake of the conventional dieters was restricted. Thus, a greater calorie deficit, not the macronutrient composition of the diet, was most likely responsible for the greater weight loss seen in the Atkins diet group. In terms of the overall long-term (1 yr) effect on CHD risk, the low-carbohydrate diet group showed greater relative improvements in some risk factors: triglycerides decreased 28% with the Atkins diet and increased 1.4% with the conventional diet, while HDL-cholesterol increased 18% with the Atkins diet but only 3.1% with the conventional diet. Changes in the other risk factors (blood pressure, insulin sensitivity, and LDL-cholesterol) were not statistically significant in either group. Given that the large amounts of saturated fats and small amounts of fruits, vegetables, and fiber in low-carbohydrate diets can independently increase the risk of CHD (Schaefer 2002), the authors concluded that there is insufficient information to determine if the beneficial health effects of the Atkins diet (i.e., improvements in triglycerides and HDL-cholesterol levels) outweigh the potential adverse effects on CHD risk in obese individuals. Additional long-term studies are needed to evaluate the potential benefits and risks of low-carbohydrate and high-protein diets.

In the meantime, the optimal diet for health and long-term maintenance of weight loss may be one that not only restricts calorie intake but also contains adequate amounts of *good* sources of carbohydrate, protein, and fat (see table 9.8). An effective strategy for reducing energy intake is to eat less refined, processed food as well as less saturated and trans fat. The Healthy Eating Pyramid (see figure 9.4), a product of the Harvard School of Public Health, summarizes the best dietary information presently available. This pyramid has a foundation of daily physical activity and weight

Summary of Client's Demographic Data

1. Client's age and gender (35 yr female)
2. Height (62 in. or 157.5 cm)
3. Body weight (131 lb or 59.55 kg)
4. Percent fat (26% BF); relative FFM (74%)
5. Percent fat goal (20% BF); relative FFM goal (80%)
6. Average daily calorie intake (2000 kcal)
7. Cardiorespiratory fitness level (below average)
8. Occupation (secretary)

Steps

1. Assess the body weight and body composition of the client.

2. Assess the daily calorie intake of the subject (use 3- or 7-day food records).

3. Estimate a healthy target body weight based on the client's percent fat goal.
   Present FFM = 96.9 lb (131 lb × 0.74) (relative FFM)
   Target body weight = 121 lb (96.9 lb/0.80) (relative FFM goal)

4. Calculate the weight loss and total calorie deficit needed to achieve that weight loss.
   a. Weight loss = 10 lb (131 lb − 121 lb)
   b. Caloric deficit = 35,000 kcal (10 lb × 3500 kcal $\cdot$ lb^{-1})

5. Estimate the daily energy expenditure of the client from the equation: Energy expenditure = RMR + daily activity level.
   a. RMR = 655.0955 + 9.463 (59.55 kg) + 1.8496 (157.5 cm) − 4.6756 (35 yr) = 1346 kcal
   b. Daily occupational activity level: lightly active 35% above basal level (see table 9.7).
      Additional kcal = 1346 × 0.35 = 471 kcal
   c. Total energy expenditure = 1346 + 471 = 1817 kcal

6. Plan to produce a calorie deficit of 700 to 800 kcal per day by reducing the calorie intake by 500 kcal per day and increasing the calorie expenditure by 200 to 300 kcal per day through exercise. To calculate caloric expenditure during exercise refer to appendix E.4. Multiply the calories burned per minute per kilogram of body weight by the duration of the activity and the client's body weight. Continue this program until the total calorie deficit of 35,000 kcal is reached.

Week 1	exercise = 100 kcal $\cdot$ day^{-1} × 7 days	=	700 kcal
	diet = 500 kcal $\cdot$ day^{-1} × 7 days	=	3500 kcal
	Total	=	4200 kcal
Week 2	exercise = 150 kcal $\cdot$ day^{-1} × 7 days	=	1050 kcal
	diet = 500 kcal $\cdot$ day^{-1} × 7 days	=	3500 kcal
	Total	=	4550 kcal
Weeks 3-4	exercise = 200 kcal $\cdot$ day^{-1} × 14 days	=	2800 kcal
	diet = 500 kcal $\cdot$ day^{-1} × 14 days	=	7000 kcal
	Total	=	9800 kcal
Weeks 5-6	exercise = 250 kcal $\cdot$ day^{-1} × 14 days	=	3500 kcal
	diet = 500 kcal $\cdot$ day^{-1} × 14 days	=	7000 kca
	Total	=	10,500 kca.
Week 7	exercise = 300 kcal $\cdot$ day^{-1} × 7 days	=	2100 kcal
	diet = 500 kcal $\cdot$ day^{-1} × 7 days	=	3500 kcal
	Total	=	5600 kcal
	Total Weeks 1-7	=	34,650 kcal

   In a little over 7 weeks the client will lose approximately 10 lb (4.5 kg). This is a gradual average weight loss of 1 1/2 lb (0.7 kg) per week. Reassess the body composition to see if the percent fat goal was reached.

7. Put the client on a maintenance diet and exercise program.
   a. Calculate the total energy expenditure using an estimate of RMR based on the new body weight.
      RMR + activity level + exercise = total energy expenditure where:
      RMR = 1303 kcal (use Harris-Benedict formula substituting a body weight of 55 kg)
      Occupational activity level = 456 kcal (1303 × 0.35)
      Exercise = 300 kcal
      Total energy expenditure = 1303 + 456 + 300 = 2059 kcal
   b. Advise the client that if she continues to exercise daily, expending approximately 300 kcal per workout, she may increase her calorie intake to 2060 kcal per day. However, for days in which she cannot exercise, the calorie intake must be restricted to 1760 kcal.

Figure 9.3 Steps for designing a weight-loss program. FFM = fat-free mass; BF = body fat; RMR = resting metabolic rate.

control and includes the following recommendations for food choices that promote health and weight control:

■ **Whole grains.** The body needs carbohydrates for energy. Compared to highly processed carbohydrates such as white flour, whole grains have a lower glycemic index, allowing better control of blood glucose and insulin and reducing the risk of type 2 diabetes.

■ **Plant oils.** When healthy unsaturated fats are eaten in place of highly processed carbohydrates, cholesterol levels improve and the risk of cardiac arrhythmias decreases.

■ **Vegetables and fruits.** Diets rich in vegetables and fruits lower blood pressure and decrease the risk of heart attack, stroke, and certain cancers.

■ **Fish, poultry, and eggs.** These are good sources of protein. Chicken and turkey can be low in saturated fat. Eating fish can reduce the risk of CHD.

■ **Nuts and legumes.** These are excellent sources of protein, fiber, vitamins, and minerals, and many kinds of nuts contain healthy fats.

■ **Dairy products.** Nonfat or low-fat dairy products (e.g., milk, yogurt, and cheese) are an excellent source of calcium, which helps prevent osteopenia and osteoporosis. Two glasses of whole milk, however, contain as much saturated fat as 8 slices of cooked bacon.

The apex of the pyramid lists foods that should be eaten sparingly. Red meats and butter contain saturated fat, which can increase total cholesterol and LDL-cholesterol levels. White rice, white bread, potatoes, pasta, and sweets should also be eaten sparingly because they are high-glycemic foods that can cause rapid increases in blood glucose levels and insulin resistance (which increases risk of type 2 diabetes), weight gain, and increased risk of developing CHD, and other chronic disorders.

Recently, the *Dietary Guidelines for Americans* (U.S. Department of Health and Human Services 2005a) and a revised U.S. food guide pyramid (see figure 9.5) were released. The *Dietary Guidelines for Americans* describes a healthy diet as one that

■ emphasizes fruits, vegetables, whole grains, and fat-free or low-fat milk and milk products;

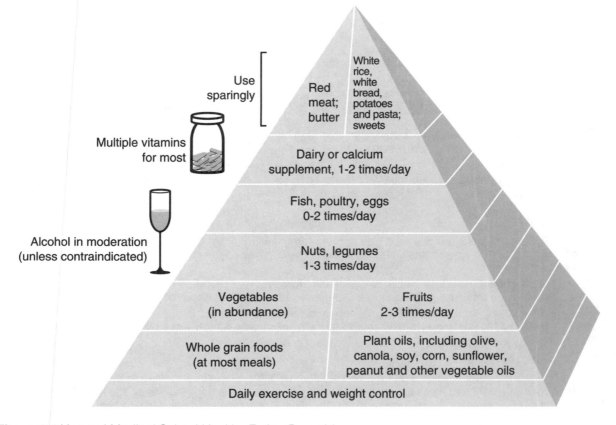

Figure 9.4 Harvard Medical School Healthy Eating Pyramid.

- includes lean meats, poultry, fish, beans, eggs, and nuts; and

- is low in saturated fats, trans fats, cholesterol, salt (sodium), and added sugars.

The revised U.S. food guide pyramid contains rainbow bands running from the tip to the base of the pyramid (U.S. Department of Health and Human Services 2005b). The color and width of the bands differ to indicate various food groups and the relative amount of servings that should be eaten from each food group. Daily physical activity is represented by the figure of a person climbing steps. This new pyramid, called *MyPyramid*, encourages Americans to use 1 of 12 models to customize their diet and exercise. The model selected varies with the client's age, gender, and level of daily physical activity. Figure 9.5 illustrates the recommended model for a moderately active 58-year-old female. To generate food guide pyramids for your clients, see www.MyPyramid.com.

Other evidence-based food guides that depict healthy eating are the Asian, Latin American, Mediterranean, and Vegetarian pyramids (see appendix E.5, "Food Guide Pyramids," pp. 353-356). Each of these food guides has a foundation of daily physical activity and reflects traditional but healthy foods indigenous to its culture. For an overview and comparison of food guides from 12 different countries, see Painter, Rah, and Lee (2002).

It is strongly recommended that you work closely with a licensed nutritionist or registered dietitian when planning diets for your clients. Food guides are useful tools for determining the recommended number of servings from each food group for healthy eating. When comparing your client's typical nutrient intake to recommended intakes, ask the following questions:

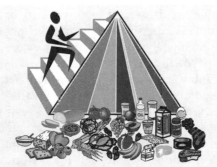

MyPyramid
STEPS TO A HEALTHIER YOU

Based on the information you provided, this is your daily recommended amount from each food group.

Grains 6 ounces	Vegetables 2 1/2 cups	Fruits 1 1/2 cups	Milk 3 cups	Meat & Beans 5 ounces
Make half your grains whole Aim for at least **3 ounces** of whole grains a day	**Vary your veggies** aim for these amounts each week: **Dark green veggies** = 3 cups **Orange veggies** = 2 cups **Dry beans & peas** = 3 cups **Starchy veggies** = 3 cups **Other veggies** = 6 1/2 cups	**Focus on fruits** Eat a variety of fruit Go easy on fruit juices	**Get your calcium-rich foods** Go low-fat or fat-free when you choose milk, yogurt, or cheese	**Go lean with protein** Choose low-fat or lean meats and poultry Vary your protein routine— choose more fish, beans, peas, nuts, and seeds

Find your balance between food and physical activity

Be physically active for at least **30 minutes** most days of the week.

Know your limits on fats, sugars, and sodium

Your allowance for oil is **5 teaspoons a day.**

Limit extras—solid fats and sugars—to **195 calories a day.**

Your results are based on a 1800 calorie pattern.   Name: _____

This calorie level is only an estimate of your needs. Monitor your body weight to see if you need to adjust your calorie intake.

From www.mypyramid.gov

Figure 9.5   U.S. food guide pyramid for a moderately active 58-year-old female.

- How does the average caloric intake compare with the caloric needs and expenditure of the individual?

- What is the relative percentage of carbohydrate, protein, and fat in the diet?

- How much of the total fat intake is saturated fat and trans fat?

- Is the minimum daily protein requirement being met?

- What is the dietary cholesterol level?

- What is the sodium intake?

- Are the vitamin and mineral requirements being met through the food intake?

- How many meals per day does the person eat? What is the average caloric content of each meal? At what meal are most of the kilocalories consumed?

- What types of snack foods does the person eat? (If the diet contains a lot of junk food, suggest more nutritious snack foods.)

- At what time of day does eating appear to be a problem?

Exercise Prescription for Weight Loss

Exercise alone—without dieting—has only a modest effect on weight loss. The most successful weight-loss programs, therefore, use a combination of dieting and exercising to optimize the energy deficit and to maintain weight loss (ACSM 2001). The exercise portion of the weight-loss regimen is designed to produce a weight loss by increasing the calorie expenditure. Generally, aerobic activities (Group I or II) are recommended for weight management programs.

The amount of physical activity and exercise needed to benefit health, prevent overweight and obesity, or maintain weight loss differs (see table 9.9). For health benefits, the CDC and ACSM recommend at least 30 min of moderate-intensity physical activity on most, preferably all, days of the week (Pate et al. 1995). However, the International Association for the Study of Obesity (IASO) consensus statement suggests that 30 min of daily physical activity may be insufficient to prevent gaining weight or regaining weight after weight loss (Saris et al. 2003). To maintain weight and to prevent unhealthy weight gain and transition to overweight or obesity in adults, 45 to 60 min of moderate-to-vigorous activity (PAL = 1.7) on most, preferably all, days are recommended (Institute

of Medicine 2002; U.S. Department of Health and Human Services 2005a; Saris et al. 2003). For children and adolescents, at least 60 min of moderate-to-vigorous physical activity on most days is recommended to maintain healthy body weight as well as good health and fitness (U.S. Department of Health and Human Services 2004).

The optimal physical activity level (PAL) for preventing weight gain differs from that for creating a negative energy balance for weight loss and maintenance of weight loss. For weight loss, the ACSM (2001) recommends moderate-intensity exercise beginning at 150 min/wk and progressing to more than 200 min/wk. The ACSM (2001) also acknowledges that to prevent regaining weight after weight loss, energy expenditure may need to exceed 2000 kcal/wk. To maintain weight loss and to prevent weight regain in formerly obese adults, the IASO consensus statement (see Saris et al. 2003) recommends a minimum of 60 min, but preferably 80 to 90 min, of moderate-intensity (2.8 to 4.3 METs) physical activity and exercise (e.g., walking or cycling) per day. This intensity and duration of physical activity approximately equals 35 min of vigorous activity (6 to 10 METs or PAL = 1.9 to 2.5).

Table 9.9 summarizes physical activity recommendations for health benefit, healthy weight loss, and weight management. The exercise prescription for weight loss and weight management will differ depending on your client's goal. You can use the information in table 9.9 to develop exercise prescriptions for weight loss, weight maintenance, and prevention of weight gain or regain.

Benefits of Exercise

This section highlights some common questions about the benefits of exercise in a weight-loss program.

- *Why is exercise an essential part of weight-loss programs?*

In addition to increasing energy expenditure and helping to create a negative energy balance for weight loss, adding exercise to dieting increases the amount of fat lost. Exercise also maintains or slows down the loss of FFM that occurs with dieting only and is important for maintaining weight loss after dieting.

Pavlou, Steffee, Lerman, and Burrows (1985) studied the contribution of exercise to the preservation of FFM in mildly obese males on a rapid weight-loss diet. The exercise group dieted and participated in an 8 wk walking-jogging program, 3 days/wk. The nonexercising group dieted only.

TABLE 9.9   Physical Activity and Exercise Recommendations for Health Benefit, Healthy Weight Loss, and Weight Management

Goal	Intensity	Duration (min)	Frequency (days/wk)	Source*
Health benefit	Moderate[a]	At least 30	5-7	CDC and ACSM
	Moderate to vigorous[b]	30	5-7	USDHHS
Weight loss	Moderate	At least 30, progressing to 40-60[c]	5-7	ACSM
Weight maintenance and prevention of weight gain	Moderate (PAL ≅ 1.7) to vigorous (PAL ≅ 1.9-2.5)	45-60	5-7	IASO, IOM, and USDHHS
Prevention of weight regain	Moderate	60-90	7	USDHHS
	Moderate	At least 60 but preferably 80-90	7	IASO
	Vigorous	At least 35	7	IASO

*ACSM = American College of Sports Medicine; CDC = Centers for Disease Control (U.S.); IASO = International Association for the Study of Obesity; IOM = Institute of Medicine (U.S.); USDHHS = U.S. Department of Health and Human Services; PAL = physical activity level.

[a]Moderate intensity ≅ 2.8 to 4.3 METs; PAL ≅ 1.7.

[b]Vigorous intensity ≅ 6 to 10 METs; PAL ≅ 1.9 to 2.5.

[c]Accumulate a total duration of activity of 150 min/wk, progressing to 200 to 300 min/wk; total weekly exercise energy expenditure ≥ 2,000 kcal/wk.

Although the total weight loss of the exercise (–11.8 kg) and nonexercise (–9.2 kg) groups was similar, the composition of the weight loss differed significantly. The exercise group maintained FFM (–0.6 kg) while the nonexercise group lost a significant amount of FFM (–3.3 kg). Also, the exercise group lost more fat (11.2 kg) than the nonexercise group (5.9 kg). In other words, for the nonexercising subjects, only 64% of the total weight loss was fat weight compared to 95% for the exercising subjects. The researchers concluded that the addition of aerobic exercise to the dietary regimen preserves existing FFM, increases fat utilization for energy production, and is more effective in reducing fat stores than diet alone.

Similarly, Kraemer, Volek, et al. (1999) compared the effects of a weight-loss dietary regimen with and without exercise in overweight men. The diet-only group did not exercise; the exercise groups participated in either an aerobic exercise program or a combined aerobic and resistance training exercise program, 3 days/wk for 12 wk. By the end of the program, all three groups lost a similar amount of body weight (~9 to 10 kg), but the composition of the weight loss differed significantly. For the diet-only group, only 69% of the total weight loss was fat weight compared to 78% for the diet plus aerobic exercise group and

97% for the diet and exercise (aerobic + resistance training) group. These results suggest that using a combination of aerobic and resistance training exercises in conjunction with dieting is more effective than dieting alone for preserving FFM and maximizing fat loss.

■ *How does exercise promote fat loss and the preservation of lean body mass?*

In response to aerobic and resistance training exercise, levels of growth hormone, epinephrine, and norepinephrine increase. These hormones stimulate the mobilization of fat from storage and activate the enzyme lipase, which breaks down triglycerides into free fatty acids. Free fatty acids are then metabolized and serve as an important energy source, especially during aerobic exercise. Heavy resistance training exercise also stimulates the release of anabolic hormones such as testosterone and growth hormone, resulting in increased protein synthesis, muscle growth, and FFM (Kraemer et al. 1991).

■ *How does improved cardiorespiratory fitness help control body weight?*

As the individual's cardiorespiratory fitness level increases through training, the amount of work that the person can accomplish at a given submaximal heart rate increases. Thus, the more fit individual expends calories at a faster rate than the less fit individual at a given exercise heart rate. For example, at a heart rate of 150 bpm, the rate of energy expenditure is approximately 10 and 15 kcal·min^{-1} for fair and superior fitness levels, respectively (Sharkey 1990).

During high-intensity aerobic exercise, lactate production increases and inhibits fatty acid metabolism. However, endurance training increases the lactate threshold (point at which lactate accumulates significantly in the blood). In aerobically trained individuals, the percentage of the energy derived from the oxidation of free fatty acids during submaximal exercise is greater than that derived from glucose oxidation (Coyle 1995; Mole, Oscai, and Holloszy 1971). The reduction in muscle glycogen utilization is also associated with a greater rate of oxidation of intramuscular triglyceride (Coyle 1995).

In order to expend the amount of energy (2000 kcal/wk) recommended to prevent weight regain after weight loss, cardiorespiratory fitness ($\dot{V}O_2$max) needs to increase. Therefore, weight reduction programs should increase cardiorespiratory fitness so that participants are able to reach this physical activity goal within a reasonable amount of time (Saris et al. 2003).

■ *What effect does exercise have on the RMR?*

Another reason for including exercise in the weight-loss program is its positive effect on RMR. Research indicates that exercise may counter the reduction in RMR that usually occurs as a result of dieting (Thompson, Manore, and Thomas 1996). It is well known that the rate of weight loss declines in the later stages of dieting due to a decrease in RMR. The lowered RMR is an energy-conserving metabolic adaptation to prolonged periods of caloric restriction (Donahue, Lin, Kirschenbaum, and Keesey 1984). In a study of 12 overweight females, Donahue et al. (1984) reported that diet alone caused a 4.4% reduction in the relative RMR (RMR/BW). After the addition of 8 wk of aerobic exercise to the program, the relative RMR increased by 5%. The net effect of exercise was to offset the diet-induced metabolic adaptation and return the RMR to the normal, pre-diet level.

Exercise may also facilitate weight loss by causing an increase in postexercise RMR. Moderate- to high-intensity aerobic exercise increases the postexercise RMR by 5% to 16%, and the elevated RMR may persist for 12 to 39 hr postexercise

(Bahr et al 1987; Bielinski, Schultz, and Jequier 1985; Sjodin et al. 1996). The postexercise elevation in RMR appears to be related to the exercise intensity and duration (Brehm 1988). Cycling at 70% $\dot{V}O_2$max for 20 min produced a 5% to 14% elevation in RMR for 12 hr in young, healthy men (Bahr et al. 1987). Although it is tempting to apply these findings to clients who are elderly or obese, it is not known whether the postexercise metabolic response of these individuals is similar to that of young men.

Types of Exercise

This section addresses common concerns regarding the types of exercise suitable for weight-loss programs.

■ *Is aerobic exercise better than resistance exercise for weight loss?*

One study evaluated the effects of aerobic and/or resistance training, in combination with dieting (i.e., moderate caloric restriction), in moderately overweight women (Marks, Ward, Morris, Castellani, and Rippe 1995). All the exercise intervention groups (cycling only, resistance training only, and combination of cycling and resistance training) maintained FFM. The diet-only group lost only a minimal amount of FFM; this result suggests that FFM can be maintained provided that the daily caloric intake is at least 1200 kcal a day. Compared to a control group, all diet and exercise intervention groups lost greater amounts of body weight (–3.7 to –5.4 kg) and fat mass, but there were no differences in weight loss and fat loss among the intervention groups. These data suggest that resistance training may be as effective as aerobic training in weight-loss programs.

Another study (Bryner et al. 1999) compared the effects of 12 wk of resistance or aerobic training on the FFM and RMR of individuals on a very low calorie diet (800 kcal/day liquid diet). One group exercised aerobically (walking, biking, or stair-climbing) for 1 hr, four days per week; the other group performed resistance training exercises (2 to 4 sets, 8- to 15-RM for 10 exercises). The body weight of the aerobic exercise group decreased more than that of the resistance-trained group; however, the FFM and RMR of the aerobic exercise group also decreased significantly. The resistance-trained group, on the other hand, maintained FFM and significantly increased RMR. These findings suggest that resistance training may be superior to aerobic training in preserving FFM and RMR of individuals on a very low calorie diet.

■ *Is high-intensity exercise better than light- to moderate-intensity exercise for weight loss?*

An important reason for including exercise as part of a weight-loss program is to maximize energy expenditure, thereby creating a larger negative energy balance. Weight loss and loss of fat mass are positively related to weekly energy expenditure (Ross and Janssen 2001). When the same amount of energy is expended, total fat oxidation is higher during low-intensity exercise than during high-intensity exercise. Close examination of energy expenditure during selected physical activities (appendix E.4, "Gross Energy Expenditure for Conditioning Exercises, Sports, and Recreational Activities," p. 348) reveals that increases in speed (intensity) of exercise produce only small increases in the rate of energy expenditure (METs). For example, if a 123-lb woman increases the speed of running from a slow (5.0 mph or 12 min/mile) to a faster speed (7.0 mph or 8.5 min/mile), the rate of expenditure increases only 3.2 kcal·min^{-1}. At the 8.5 min/mile pace, the woman expends 11.5 METs (11.5 kcal·kg^{-1}·min^{-1} or 10.7 kcal·min^{-1}) and is able to run a maximum distance of 3 miles (4.8 km). The duration of the workout is 25.5 min (8.5 min·mile^{-1} × 3 miles), and the total caloric expenditure is 274 kcal (25.5 min × 10.7 kcal·min^{-1}). When she reduces the exercise intensity by decreasing her speed to a 12 min/mile pace, her relative energy expenditure decreases (8 METs or 8 kcal·kg^{-1}·min^{-1} or 7.5 kcal·min^{-1}), but she is able to run a distance of 4 miles (6.4 km). The duration of the workout increases to 48 min (12 min·mile^{-1} × 4 miles), and the total caloric expenditure is increased (48 min × 7.5 kcal·min^{-1} = 360 kcal). Thus, the duration of the exercise and total distance may be somewhat more important than the speed (intensity) of exercise for maximizing the energy expenditure.

■ *Which aerobic exercise mode is best to maximize fat loss?*

In a meta-analysis of 53 studies dealing with the effects of exercise on body weight and composition, Ballor and Keesey (1991) reported that fat loss for males participating in aerobic exercise training was, on average, 1.9 kg for cycling (0.11 kg/wk) and 1.6 kg for running and walking (0.12 kg/wk). For resistance training, body weight increased an average of 1.2 kg, but fat mass was reduced by 1.0 kg. For females, fat mass decreased significantly (1.3 kg) for running and walking but not cycling. These studies suggest that in terms of fat loss, aerobic exercise modes are equally effective for men, but running and walking may be better than cycling for women.

■ *Are spot reduction exercises effective for decreasing body fat in localized regions of the body?*

Specific spot reduction exercises are no more effective than general aerobic exercise for changing limb and body girth measurements or for altering total body composition (Carns, Schade, Liba, Hellebrandt, and Harris 1960; Noland and Kearney 1978; Roby 1962; Schade, Hellebrandt, Waterland, and Carns 1962). Katch, Clarkson, Kroll, McBride, and Wilcox (1984) assessed changes in the diameter of adipose cells from the abdomen, gluteal, and subscapular sites resulting from a 27-day training program in which each subject performed 5004 sit-ups. Although the training significantly reduced fat cell diameter, the effect was similar at all three sites: abdomen, −6.4%; gluteal, −5.0%; and subscapular, −3.7%. It appears that a sit-up exercise program does not preferentially reduce the fat in the abdominal region.

Despres, Bouchard, Tremblay, Savard, and Marcotte (1985) reported that a 20-wk cycling program significantly reduced %BF and body weight. Cycling affected trunk skinfolds (SKFs) (−22%) more than extremity SKFs (−12.5%). If fat was mobilized preferentially from subcutaneous stores near the exercising muscle mass, one would expect the lower-extremity SKFs to be more affected by cycling than the trunk SKFs. Yet Despres et al. (1985) noted an 18% reduction in the suprailiac SKF compared to a 13% reduction in the thigh SKF. This suggests that subcutaneous fat cells in the abdomen are more sensitive to the lipolytic effect of catecholamines than subcutaneous fat cells in the thighs (Smith, Hammerstein, Bjorntorp, and Kral 1979).

The enzyme lipoprotein-lipase is responsible for lipid accumulation. In women, lipoprotein-lipase activity is higher in the gluteofemoral region than in the abdominal region (Litchell and Boberg 1978). Estrogen and progesterone appear to enhance lipoprotein-lipase activity in women. Also, the lipolytic response to catecholamines is lower in the femoral than in the abdominal depots for both men and women (Rebuffe-Scrive 1985).

Thus, the regional distribution and mobilization of adipose tissue appear to follow a biologically selective pattern regardless of type of exercise. Even with weight reduction, the relative fat distribution remains stable as measured by the WHR; however, the waist-to-thigh ratio decreases, suggesting that the thigh region is slightly more resistant to fat mobilization in women (Ashwell, McCall, Cole, and Dixon 1985).

DESIGNING WEIGHT-GAIN PROGRAMS

Because genetics plays an important role in weight gain, some clients may have difficulty gaining weight, especially if they have inherited a high RMR. Before prescribing weight-gain programs, you should rule out the possibility that diseases and psychological disorders associated with malnutrition (e.g., anorexia nervosa) are not causing your client to be underweight.

The number of additional calories needed in order for a person to gain 1 lb (0.45 kg) of muscle tissue has not yet been firmly established. However, research suggests that an excess of 2800 to 3500 kcal is required. Thus, adding 400 to 500 kcal to the estimated daily caloric needs (RMR + occupational activity level) of the individual should produce a gradual weight gain of 1 lb per week (Williams 1992). The caloric intake must also be adjusted for additional calories expended during exercise.

Weight-Gain Diets

Again, it is highly recommended that you consult with a trained nutrition professional when planning weight-gain diets. When comparing your client's typical nutrient intakes to recommended dietary intakes, you should focus on the same questions as outlined for weight-loss programs (see p. 236).

To ensure that your client's weight gain is due to increases in lean tissues rather than body fat, you should

- use the body composition method to estimate a healthy target body weight and gain in FFM;
- plan a high-calorie, well-balanced diet in which 60% to 65% of the total kilocalorie intake is derived from carbohydrate, 12% to 15% from protein, and 23% to 25% from fat;
- increase daily protein intake to 1.2 to 1.6 g per kilogram of body weight to increase muscle size; and
- monitor body composition regularly throughout the weight gain program using methods described in chapter 8.

Exercise Prescription for Weight Gain

As part of the weight-gain program, you should prescribe resistance training to increase muscle size. A high-volume resistance training program is the best approach to maximize the development of muscle size. Because some clients may not be able to tolerate this volume of training at first, novice weightlifters should start slowly by performing only three sets of each exercise at the prescribed intensity and by reducing the number of exercises for each muscle group. Depending on your client's goal, this may be sufficient to increase FFM. For some clients, however, you may need to progressively increase the training volume in order to elicit further improvements in muscle size and FFM. Recommended guidelines for developing an exercise prescription for weight gain are as follows:

GUIDELINES FOR EXERCISE PRESCRIPTION FOR WEIGHT GAIN

- **Mode:** Resistance training
- **Intensity:** 70% to 75% 1-RM or 10- to 12-RM
- **Sets:** Three for novices; more than three for advanced weightlifters
- **Number of exercises:** One to two per muscle group for novices; three to four per muscle group for advanced weightlifters
- **Duration:** 60 min or longer
- **Frequency:** 3 days/wk for novices; 5 to 6 days/wk for advanced weightlifters
- **Length of program:** Dependent on desired weight gain

DESIGNING PROGRAMS TO IMPROVE BODY COMPOSITION

Some clients may wish to improve their body composition without changing their body weight. For these individuals, you can design exercise programs to either decrease body fat, increase FFM, or both. Research has shown that regular participation in an exercise program may alter an individual's body composition. Aerobic exercise and resistance training are effective modes for decreasing SKF thicknesses, fat weight, and %BF of both women and men.

Questions About Exercise and Body Composition Changes

- *What is the effect of aerobic exercise training on body fat?*

Numerous studies have been conducted to determine the effect of aerobic exercise training on body composition. The modes of exercise include cycling, walking, jogging, running, and swimming. Wilmore, Royce, Girandola, Katch, and Katch (1970) reported that a 10-wk jogging program (3 days/wk) produced a significant increase in body density of sedentary men. Because total body weight decreased and FFM remained stable, the increase in body density was attributed almost entirely to fat loss. Pollock et al. (1971) also noted that a 20-wk (4 days/wk) walking program produced a decrease in %BF and total body weight of men.

■ *Which aerobic exercise mode is best for maximizing fat loss?*

One study compared cycling, running, and walking of equal frequency, duration, and intensity (Pollock, Dimmick, Miller, Kendrick, and Linnerud 1975). All three programs produced significant reductions in %BF and body weight. Also, Despres et al. (1985) reported that a 20-wk cycling program (4 to 5 times a week) resulted in significant reductions in body weight, %BF, and fat cell weight in a group of sedentary men. On the basis of these studies it appears that aerobic exercise modes are equally effective in altering body composition.

■ *How many times a week should I exercise to maximize the loss of body fat?*

The frequency of the training program may affect the magnitude of the changes in body composition. Pollock, Miller, Linnerud, and Cooper (1975) compared aerobic exercise programs consisting of 2, 3, or 4 days/wk. Even though the total mileage and caloric expenditure were the same, exercising 2 days/wk was not sufficient to produce significant alterations in body composition. The authors concluded that a 3 or 4 day a week program produces significant body composition changes, with 4 days/wk being superior to 3 days/wk.

■ *What effect does resistance training have on body fat and FFM?*

Although resistance training may increase body weight, it positively affects fat mass, %BF, and FFM (Ballor and Keesey 1991). Cullinen and Caldwell (1998) found that normal-weight women (19 to 44 yr) participating in a moderate-intensity resistance training program (2 days/wk for 12 wk) significantly increased FFM (~4.5%) and decreased %BF (~8.7%). In Wilmore's

study (1974), subjects trained 2 days/wk for 10 wk. At each training session, they performed 2 sets of 7- to 9-RM for 8 different weight training exercises. Men and women exhibited similar alterations in body composition. Although the total body weight remained stable, the FFM increased significantly for both sexes. As a result of resistance training, the relative body fat decreased 9.6% and 10.0% for women and men, respectively.

■ *How does exercise promote body composition changes?*

The significant loss of fat weight and %BF with aerobic exercise and resistance training is a function of hormonal responses to the exercise. Exercise increases the circulatory levels of growth hormone (GH), and the levels remain elevated for 1 to 2 hr after exercise (Hartley et al. 1972; Hartley 1975). Exercise also stimulates the release of catecholamines from the adrenal medulla. Both GH and catecholamines increase the mobilization of free fatty acids from storage (Hartley 1975). Eventually, the muscle may metabolize these free fatty acids during rest and low-intensity exercise.

The increase in FFM with resistance training may be due to muscle hypertrophy, increased protein content in the muscle, or increased bone density. Muscle hypertrophy and increased protein are mediated by changes in serum testosterone and GH levels in response to weightlifting. Immediately following heavy resistance weightlifting, serum testosterone levels are significantly elevated for men but not for women (Fahey, Rolph, Moungmee, Nagel, and Mortara 1976; Weiss, Cureton, and Thompson 1983). Growth hormone levels in men are increased significantly for 15 min following a 21-min bout of high-intensity (85% of 1-RM) leg press exercises. However, low-intensity, high-repetition (28% of 1-RM, 21 reps per set) leg presses produced no significant change in GH even though the total amount of work and duration of exercise were equal. Thus, the intensity and number of repetitions play a role in GH release in response to weightlifting exercise (Vanhelder, Radomski, and Goode 1984).

In addition, resistance training has an effect on the hormonal profiles of younger (30 yr) and older (62 yr) men (Kraemer, Hakkinen, et al. 1999). Following a 10-wk, periodized strength-power training program, young men had significant increases in free testosterone at rest and in response to weightlifting exercise. Younger men also showed increases in resting levels of insulin-like growth factor-binding protein-3 after training. For the older men, training produced a significant increase in total testosterone in response to weightlifting exercise, as well as a significant reduction in resting cortisol levels.

Exercise Prescription for Body Composition Change

While light- to moderate-intensity aerobic exercise may be more beneficial for fat loss, high-intensity resistance training is better for FFM gain. Thus, combining aerobic and resistance training exercises may be the most effective way to alter body composition of non-dieting individuals (Dolezal and Potteiger 1998). When designing exercise programs to promote changes in body composition, adhere to the following guidelines. Prescribe aerobic exercise to reduce body fat and resistance training exercise to increase FFM.

GUIDELINES FOR EXERCISE PRESCRIPTION FOR FAT LOSS

- **Goal:** Fat loss
- **Mode:** Group I or II aerobic activities (see p. 95)
- **Intensity:** Light to moderate (50% to 75% $\dot{V}O_2$ reserve)
- **Duration:** 30 to 45 min
- **Frequency:** Minimum of 3 days/wk
- **Length:** Minimum of 8 wk

GUIDELINES FOR EXERCISE PRESCRIPTION FOR FAT-FREE MASS GAIN

- **Goal:** Increase FFM and reduce body fat
- **Mode:** Dynamic resistance training
- **Intensity:** 70% to 85% 1-RM
- **Repetitions:** 6 to 12 reps
- **Sets:** 3 sets
- **Frequency:** Minimum of 3 days/wk
- **Length:** Minimum of 8 wk

KEY POINTS

- Obesity is an excess of body fat that increases health risks.
- Two types of obesity are upper-body (android) and lower-body (gynoid) obesity.
- The number of fat cells in the body is determined primarily during childhood and adolescence.
- Weight gain in adults is associated with an increase in the size of existing fat cells (hypertrophy), rather than an increase in the number of fat cells (hyperplasia).
- Physical inactivity is a common cause of obesity.
- The body composition method provides a useful estimate of a healthy body weight.
- Well-balanced nutrition includes adequate amounts of carbohydrate, protein, fat, minerals, vitamins, and water.
- Weight loss depends on calorie intake, not on the macronutrient composition of the diet.
- Effective weight-loss programs create a negative energy balance by restricting caloric intake

and increasing physical activity and exercise; weight-gain programs create a positive energy balance by increasing caloric intake.
- For weight-loss programs, the combined daily caloric deficit due to calorie restriction and extra exercise should not exceed 1000 kcal; for weight-gain programs, the daily caloric intake should exceed the energy need by no more than 400 to 500 kcal.
- Adding a combination of aerobic and resistance training exercises to the dieting regimen is an effective way to maximize fat loss and preserve FFM during weight loss.
- The optimal amount of physical activity for preventing weight gain differs from that needed to create a negative energy balance for weight loss and for maintenance of weight loss.
- For weight-gain programs, resistance training will ensure that most of the weight gain is due to increases in lean body tissues.
- Aerobic exercise and resistance training are effective ways to improve body composition without changing body weight.

KEY TERMS

Learn the definition for each of the following key terms. Definitions of terms can be found in the glossary on page 379.

android obesity
anorexia nervosa
at risk of overweight
basal metabolic rate (BMR)
complex carbohydrates
dietary thermogenesis
digital activity log
factorial method
glycemic index (GI)
gynoid obesity
healthy body weight
hyperplasia
hypertrophy

kilocalorie
lower-body obesity
negative energy balance
obesity
overweight
physical activity level (PAL)
positive energy balance
resting energy expenditure (REE)
resting metabolic rate (RMR)
simple carbohydrates
total energy expenditure (TEE)
underweight
upper-body obesity

REVIEW QUESTIONS

In addition to being able to define each of the key terms, test your knowledge and understanding of the material by answering the following review questions.

1. Using BMI, what are the cutoff values for classification of obesity, overweight, healthy body weight, and underweight?

2. Describe how you can determine a healthy body weight for your client.

3. For typical weight-loss programs, identify the minimal caloric intake per day and maximal caloric deficit (i.e., negative energy balance) per day. What is the best way to create this daily caloric deficit?

4. Explain why a taller, heavier person will lose weight at a faster rate than a shorter, lighter person when both individuals are on the same diet.

5. For well-balanced nutrition, what are the recommended proportions of carbohydrate, fat, and protein in the diet?

6. Explain why exercise is an important component of weight-loss and weight-gain programs.

7. Describe two methods that you can use to estimate the energy needs of your clients.

8. Describe the optimal amount of physical activity (intensity, duration, and frequency) for health benefits, weight loss, weight maintenance, and prevention of weight regain.

9. Estimate the daily caloric intake for a 50-year-old, 150-lb (68-kg) female professor who is 5 ft 5 in. and who bikes a total of 60 min, 5 days/wk, to and from the university.

10. Describe the basic exercise prescriptions for weight-loss and weight-gain programs.

chapter 10

Assessing Flexibility

Key Questions

- What is the difference between static and dynamic flexibility?
- What factors affect flexibility?
- How is flexibility assessed?
- Are indirect measures of flexibility valid and reliable?
- What are the general guidelines for flexibility testing?
- What test can I use to assess the flexibility of older adults?

Flexibility is an important, yet often neglected, component of health-related fitness. Adequate levels of flexibility are needed for maintenance of functional independence and performance of activities of daily living such as bending to pick up a newspaper or getting out of the back seat of a two-door car. Over the years, flexibility tests have been included in most health-related fitness test batteries, since it has been long thought that lack of flexibility is associated with musculoskeletal injuries and low back pain. However, compared to research on other physical fitness components, there are not many studies substantiating the importance of flexibility to health-related fitness.

Research suggests that individuals with too little (ankylosis) or too much (hypermobility) flexibility are at higher risk than others for musculoskeletal injuries (Jones and Knapik 1999), but there is limited evidence that a greater-than-normal amount of flexibility actually decreases injury risk (Knudson, Magnusson, and McHugh 2000). Also, research fails to support an association between lumbar/hamstring flexibility and the occurrence of low back pain (Jackson, Morrow, Brill, Kohl, Gordon, and Blair 1998; Plowman 1992). Still, flexibility should be included in health-related fitness test batteries to identify individuals at the extremes who may have a higher risk of musculotendinous injury.

This chapter describes direct and indirect methods for assessing flexibility. It presents guidelines for flexibility testing as well as norms for commonly used flexibility tests.

BASICS OF FLEXIBILITY

Flexibility and joint stability are highly dependent on the joint structure, as well as the strength and number of ligaments and muscles spanning the joint. To fully appreciate the complexity of flexibility, you should review the anatomy of joints and muscles. This section deals with the definitions and nature of flexibility and also presents factors influencing joint mobility.

Definitions and Nature of Flexibility

Flexibility is the ability of a joint, or series of joints, to move through a full range of motion (ROM) without injury. Static flexibility is a measure of the total ROM at the joint and is limited by the extensibility of the musculotendinous unit. Dynamic flexibility is a measure of the rate of torque or resistance developed during stretching throughout the ROM. Although dynamic flexibility accounts for 44% to 66% of the variance in static flexibility (Magnusson et al. 1997; McHugh, Kremenic, Fox, and Gleim 1998), more research is needed to firmly establish the relationship between static and dynamic flexibility and to determine whether these two types of flexibility are distinct entities or two aspects of the same flexibility component (Knudson et al. 2000).

The ROM is highly specific to the joint (i.e., specificity principle) and depends on morphological factors such as the joint geometry and the joint capsule, ligaments, tendons, and muscles spanning the joint. The joint structure determines the planes of motion and may limit the ROM at a given joint. **Triaxial joints** (e.g., ball-and-socket joints of the hip and shoulder) afford a greater degree of movement in more directions than either the **uniaxial** or **biaxial joints** (see table 10.1).

The tightness of soft-tissue structures such as muscle, tendons, and ligaments is a major limitation to both static and dynamic flexibility. Johns and Wright (1962) determined the relative contribution of soft tissues to the total resistance encountered by the joint during movement:

- Joint capsule—47%
- Muscle and its fascia—41%
- Tendons and ligaments—10%
- Skin—2%

The joint capsule and ligaments consist predominantly of collagen, a nonelastic connective tissue. The muscle and its fascia, however, have elastic connective tissue; therefore, they are the most important structures in terms of reducing resistance to movement and increasing dynamic flexibility.

The tension within the muscle-tendon unit affects both static flexibility (ROM) and dynamic flexibility (stiffness or resistance to movement). The tension within this unit is attributed to the **viscoelastic properties** of connective tissues, as well as to the degree of muscular contraction resulting from the stretch reflex (McHugh, Magnusson, Gleim, and Nicholas 1992). Individuals with less flexibility and tighter muscles and tendons have a greater contractile response during stretching exercises and a greater resistance to stretching. The **elastic deformation** of the muscle-tendon unit during stretching is proportional to the load or tension applied, whereas the **viscous deformation** is proportional to the speed at which the tension is applied. When the muscle and tendon are stretched and held at a fixed length (e.g., during **static stretching**), the tension within the unit, or tensile stress, decreases over time (McHugh et al. 1992). This is called **stress relaxation**. A single static stretch sustained for 90 sec produces a 30% increase in viscoelastic stress relaxation and decreases muscle stiffness for up to 1 hr (Magnusson 1998). Thus, static stretching exercise is an excellent way to induce viscoelastic stress relaxation.

Factors Affecting Flexibility

Flexibility is related to body type, age, gender, and physical activity level. This section addresses some commonly asked questions about flexibility.

- *Does body type limit flexibility?*

Individuals with large hypertrophied muscles or excessive amounts of subcutaneous fat may score poorly on ROM tests because adjacent body segments in these people contact each other sooner than in those with smaller limb and trunk girths. However, this does not necessarily mean that all heavily muscled or obese individuals have poor flexibility. Many bodybuilders and obese individuals who routinely stretch their muscles have adequate levels of flexibility.

TABLE 10.1   Joint Classification by Structure and Function

Type of joint	Axes of rotation	Movements	Examples
Gliding	Nonaxial	Gliding, sliding, twisting	Intercarpal, intertarsal, tarsometatarsal
Hinge	Uniaxial	Flexion, extension	Knee, elbow, ankle, interphalangeal
Pivot	Uniaxial	Medial and lateral rotation	Proximal radioulnar, atlantoaxial
Condyloid and saddle	Biaxial	Flexion, extension, abduction, adduction, circumduction	Wrist, atlanto-occipital, metacarpophalangeal, first carpometacarpal
Ball and socket	Triaxial	Flexion, extension, abduction, adduction, circumduction, rotation	Hip, shoulder

■ *Why do older individuals tend to be less flexible than younger people?*

Inflexible and older individuals have increased muscle stiffness and a lower stretch tolerance compared to younger individuals with normal flexibility (Magnusson 1998). As muscle stiffness increases, static flexibility progressively decreases with aging (Brown and Miller 1998; Gajdosik, Vander Linden, and Williams 1999). A decline in physical activity and development of arthritic conditions, rather than a specific effect of aging, are the primary causes for the loss of flexibility as one grows older. Still, flexibility training can help to counteract age-related decreases in ROM. Girouard and Hurley (1995) reported significant improvements in shoulder and hip ROM of older men (50 to 69 years) following 10 wk of flexibility training. Thus, older persons can benefit from flexibility training and should be encouraged to perform stretching exercises at least three times a week to counteract age-related decreases in ROM.

■ *Are females more flexible than males?*

Some evidence suggests that females generally are more flexible than males at all ages (Alter 1996; Payne, Gledhill, Katzmarzyk, Jamnik, and Keir 2000). The greater flexibility of women is usually attributed to gender differences in pelvic structure and hormones that may affect connective tissue laxity (Alter 1996). However, the effect of gender on ROM appears to be joint and motion specific. Females tend to have more hip flexion and spinal lateral flexion than males of the same age. On the other hand, males have greater ROM in hip extension and spinal flexion and extension in the thoracolumbar region (Norkin and White 1995).

■ *How do physical activity and inactivity affect flexibility?*

Habitual movement patterns and physical activity levels apparently are more important determinants of flexibility than gender, age, and body type (Harris 1969; Kirby, Simms, Symington, and Garner 1981). Lack of physical activity is a major cause of inflexibility. It is well documented that inactive persons tend to be less flexible than active persons (McCue 1953) and that exercise increases flexibility (deVries 1962; Chapman, deVries, and Swezey 1972; Hartley-O'Brien 1980). Disuse, due to lack of physical activity or immobilization, produces shortening of the muscles (i.e., contracture) and connective tissues, which in turn restricts joint mobility.

Moving the joints and muscles in a repetitive pattern or maintaining habitual body postures may restrict ROM because of the tightening and shortening of the muscle tissue. For example, joggers and people who sit behind a desk for long periods need to stretch the hamstrings and low back muscles to counteract the tautness developed in these muscle groups.

■ *Does warming up affect flexibility?*

Although active warm-up exercises such as walking, jogging, and stair-climbing increase muscle temperature and decrease muscle stiffness, warming up alone does not increase range of motion (deWeijer, Gorniak, and Shamus 2003; Shrier and Gossal 2000). Studies have reported that active warm-up combined with static stretching is more effective than static stretching alone in increasing the length of the hamstring muscles (deWeijer et al. 2003) and in improving range of motion (Shrier and Gossal 2000). Therefore, when you administer flexibility (ROM) tests, make certain that your clients warm up and statically stretch the muscle groups before you measure them, and administer multiple trials for each test item.

■ *Can you develop too much flexibility?*

It is important to recognize that excessive amounts of stretching and flexibility training may result in hypermobility, or an increased ROM of joints beyond normal, acceptable values. Hypermobility leads to joint laxity (looseness or instability) and may increase one's risk of musculoskeletal injuries. For example, it is not uncommon for gymnasts and swimmers to experience shoulder dislocations because of joint laxity and hypermobility. As an exercise specialist, you need to be able to accurately assess ROM and to design stretching programs that improve your clients' flexibility without compromising joint stability.

ASSESSMENT OF FLEXIBILITY

Field and clinical tests are available for assessing static flexibility. Although ROM data are important, measures of dynamic flexibility (i.e., joint stiffness and resistance to movement) may be more meaningful in terms of physical performance. Dynamic flexibility tests measure the increase in resistance during muscle elongation; several studies have shown that less stiff muscles are more effective in using the elastic energy during movements involving the stretch-shortening cycle (Kubo, Kawakami, and Fukunaga 1999; Kubo, Kaneshisa, Takeshita, Kawakami, Fukashiro, and Fukunaga 2000). However, dynamic flexibility testing is limited to the research setting because the equipment is expensive. Typically, static flexibility is assessed in field and clinical settings by direct or indirect measurement of the ROM.

GENERAL GUIDELINES FOR FLEXIBILITY TESTING

To assess a client's flexibility, you should select a number of test items because of the highly specific nature of flexibility (Dickinson 1968; Harris 1969). Direct tests that measure the range of joint rotation in degrees are usually more useful than indirect tests that measure static flexibility in linear units. When administering these tests,

- have the client perform a general warm-up followed by static stretching prior to the test and avoid fast, jerky movements and stretching beyond the pain-free range of joint motion;

- administer three trials of each test item;

- compare the client's best score to norms in order to obtain a flexibility rating for each test item; and

- use the test results to identify joints and muscle groups in need of improvement.

Direct Methods of Measuring Static Flexibility

To assess static flexibility directly, measure the amount of joint rotation in degrees using a goniometer, flexometer, or inclinometer. The following sections describe the procedures for these tests.

Universal Goniometer Test Procedures

The universal **goniometer** is a protractor-like device with two steel or plastic arms that measure the joint angle at the extremes of the ROM (see figure 10.1). The stationary arm of the goniometer is attached at the zero line of the protractor, and the other arm is movable. To use the goniometer, place the center of the instrument so it coincides with the fulcrum, or axis of rotation, of the joint. Align the arms of the goniometer with bony landmarks along the longitudinal axis of each moving body segment. Measure the ROM as the difference between the joint angles (degrees) at the extremes of the movement.

Table 10.2 summarizes procedures for measuring ROM for various joints using a universal goniometer. For more detailed descriptions of these procedures, see Greene and Heckman (1994) and Norkin and White (1995). Table 10.3 presents average ROM values for healthy adults.

Flexometer Test Procedures

Another tool you can use to measure ROM is the Leighton **flexometer** (see figure 10.2). This device

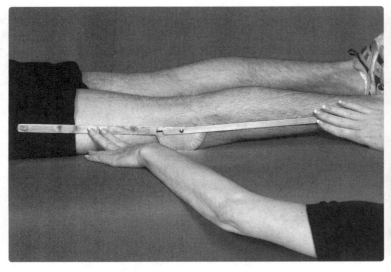
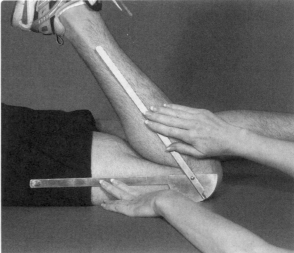

Figure 10.1 Measuring range of motion at knee joint using universal goniometer.

TABLE 10.2 Universal Goniometer Measurement Procedures

GONIOMETER POSITION

Joint	Body position	Axis of rotation	Stationary arm	Moving arm	Stabilization	Special considerations
Shoulder						
Extension	Prone	Acromion process	Midaxillary line	Lateral epicondyle of humerus	Scapula and thorax	Elbow is slightly flexed and palm of hand faces body.
Flexion	Supine	Same as extension	Same as extension	Same as extension	Scapula and thorax	Palm of hand faces body.
Abduction	Supine	Anterior axis of acromion process	Midline of anterior aspect of sternum	Medial midline of humerus	Scapula and thorax	Palm of hand faces anteriorly; humerus is laterally rotated; elbow is extended.
Medial/lateral rotation	Supine	Olecranon process	Perpendicular to floor	Styloid process of ulna	Distal end of humerus and scapula	Arm is abducted 90°; forearm is perpendicular to supporting surface in mid-pronated-supinated position; humerus rests on pad so that it is level with acromion process.
Elbow						
Flexion	Supine	Lateral epicondyle of humerus	Lateral midline of humerus	Lateral midline of radial head and styloid process	Distal end of humerus	Arm is close to body; pad is placed under distal end of humerus; forearm is fully supinated.
Forearm						
Pronation	Sitting	Lateral to ulna styloid process	Parallel to anterior midline of humerus	Lies across dorsal aspect of forearm, just proximal to styloid processes of radius and ulna	Distal end of humerus	Arm is close to body, elbow flexed 90°; forearm is midway between supination and pronation (thumb toward ceiling).
Supination	Sitting	Medial to ulna styloid process	Parallel to anterior midline of humerus	Lies across ventral aspect of forearm, just proximal to styloid processes of radius and ulna	Distal end of humerus	Testing position is same as for pronation of forearm.

(continued)

TABLE 10.2 *(continued)*

GONIOMETER POSITION

Joint	Body position	Axis of rotation	Stationary arm	Moving arm	Stabilization	Special considerations
Wrist						
Flexion and extension	Sitting	Lateral aspect of wrist over the triquetrum	Lateral midline of ulna, using olecranon and ulnar styloid processes for reference	Lateral midline of fifth metacarpal	Radius and ulna	Client sits next to supporting surface, abducts shoulder 90°, and flexes elbow 90°; forearm is in mid-supinated-pronated position; palm of hand faces ground; forearm rests on supporting surface; hand is free to move.
Radial or ulnar deviation	Sitting	Middle of dorsal aspect of wrist over capitate	Dorsal midline of forearm, using lateral humeral epicondyle as reference	Dorsal midline of third metacarpal	Distal ends of radius and ulna	Same as for wrist flexion.
Hip						
Flexion and extension	Supine Prone	Lateral aspect of hip joint, using greater trochanter as reference	Lateral midline of pelvis	Lateral midline of femur, using lateral epicondyle for reference	Pelvis	Knee is allowed to flex as range of hip flexion is completed; knee is flexed during hip extension.
Abduction and adduction	Supine	Centered over anterior superior iliac spine	Horizontally align arm with imaginary line between anterior superior iliac spines	Anterior midline of femur, using midline of patella for reference	Pelvis	Knee is extended during abduction.
Medial/lateral rotation	Sitting	Centered over anterior aspect of patella	Perpendicular to floor	Anterior midline of lower leg, using crest of tibia and point midway between malleoli for reference	Distal end of femur; avoid rotation and lateral tilt of pelvis	Client sits on supporting surface, knees flexed 90°; place towel roll under distal end of femur; contralateral knee may need to be flexed so that hip being measured can complete full range of lateral rotation.

	Position	Axis	Stationary arm	Moving arm	Stabilization	Comments
Knee						
Flexion	Supine	Over the lateral epicondyle of femur	Lateral midline of femur, using greater trochanter for reference	Lateral midline of fibula, using lateral malleolus and fibular head for reference	Femur to prevent rotation, abduction, and adduction	As knee flexes, the hip also flexes.
Ankle						
Dorsiflexion and plantar flexion	Sitting	Over the lateral aspect of lateral malleolus	Lateral midline of fibula, using head of fibula for reference	Parallel to lateral aspect of fifth metatarsal	Tibia and fibula	Client sits on end of table with knee flexed and ankle positioned at 90°.
Subtalar						
Inversion and eversion	Sitting	Centered over anterior aspect of ankle mid way between malleoli	Anterior midline of lower leg, using the tibial tuberosity for reference	Anterior midline of second metatarsal	Tibia and fibula	Client sits with knee flexed 90° and lower leg over edge of supporting surface.
Lumbar spine						
Lateral flexion	Standing	Centered over posterior aspect of spinous process of S1	Perpendicular to ground	Posterior aspect of spinous process of C7	Pelvis to prevent lateral tilt	Client stands erect with 0° of spinal flexion, extension, and rotation.
Rotation	Sitting	Centered over superior aspect of client's head	Parallel to imaginary line between tubercles of iliac crests	Imaginary line between two acromion processes	Pelvis to prevent rotation	Keep feet flat on floor to stabilize pelvis,

TABLE 10.3 Average Range of Motion (ROM) Values for Healthy Adults

Joint	ROM (degrees)	Joint	ROM
Shoulder		Thoracic-lumbar spine	
Flexion	150-180	Flexion	60-80
Extension	50-60	Extension	20-30
Abduction	180	Lateral flexion	25-35
Medial rotation	70-90	Rotation	30-45
Lateral rotation	90	Hip	
Elbow		Flexion	100-120
Flexion	140-150	Extension	30
Extension	0	Abduction	40-45
Radioulnar		Adduction	20-30
Pronation	80	Medial rotation	40-45
Supination	80	Lateral rotation	45-50
Wrist		Knee	
Flexion	60-80	Flexion	135-150
Extension	60-70	Extension	0-10
Radial deviation	20	Ankle	
Ulnar deviation	30	Dorsiflexion	20
Cervical spine		Plantar flexion	40-50
Flexion	45-60	Subtalar	
Extension	45-75	Inversion	30-35
Lateral flexion	45	Eversion	15-20
Rotation	60-80		

Data from the American Academy of Orthopaedic Surgeons (Greene and Heckman 1994) and the American Medical Association (1988).

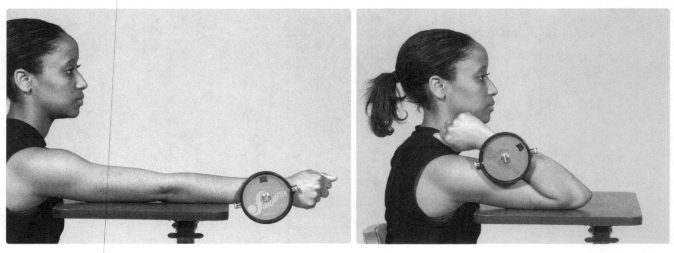

Figure 10.2 Measuring range of motion at elbow joint using Leighton flexometer.

consists of a weighted 360° dial and weighted pointer. The ROM is measured in relation to the downward pull of gravity on the dial and pointer. To use this device, strap the instrument to the body segment, and lock the dial at 0° at one extreme of the ROM. After the client executes the movement, lock the pointer at the other extreme of the ROM. The degree of arc through which the movement takes place is read directly from the dial. Tests have been devised to measure the ROM at the neck, trunk, shoulder, elbow, radioulnar, wrist, hip, knee, and ankle joints using the Leighton flexometer (Hubley-Kozey 1991; Leighton 1955).

Inclinometer Test Procedures

The **inclinometer** is another type of gravity-dependent goniometer (see figure 10.3). To use this device, hold it on the distal end of the body segment. The inclinometer measures the angle between the long axis of the moving segment and the line of gravity. This device is easier to use than the flexometer and universal goniometer because it is held by hand on the moving body segment during the measurement and does not have to be aligned with specific bony landmarks. Also, the American Medical Association (1988) recommends the double-inclinometer technique, using two inclinometers, to measure spinal mobility (see figure 10.3).

Validity and Reliability of Direct Measures

The validity and reliability of these devices for directly measuring ROM are highly dependent on the joint being measured and technician skill. Radiography is considered to be the best reference method for establishing validity of goniometric measurements. Research shows high agreement between ROM measured by radiographs and universal goniometers for the hip and knee joints (Ahlback and Lindahl 1964; Enwemeka 1986). Mayer, Tencer, and Kristoferson (1984) reported no difference between radiography and the double-inclinometer technique for assessing spinal ROM of patients with low back pain.

The intratester and intertester reliability of goniometric measurements is affected by difficulty in identifying the axis of rotation and palpating bony landmarks. Measurements of upper-extremity joints are generally more reliable than ROM measurements of the lower-extremity joints (Norkin and White 1995). Generally, the inclinometer reliably measures ROM at most joints; however, the intertester reliability of inclinometer measurements is variable and joint specific. Studies have reported reliability coefficients ranging from 0.48 for lumbar extension (Williams, Binkley, Bloch, Goldsmith, and Minuk 1993) to 0.96 for subtalar joint position (Sell, Verity, Worrell, Pease, and Wigglesworth 1994). Also, the intrarater reliabilities for inclinometer measurements of the flexibility of the iliotibial band (hip adduction), and for ROM measurements of the lumbar spine and lordosis generally exceed 0.90 (Ng, Kippers, Richardson, and Parnianpour 2001; Reese and Bandy 2003). In order to obtain accurate and reliable ROM measurements, you need a thorough knowledge of anatomy and of standardized testing procedures, as well as training and practice to develop your measurement techniques.

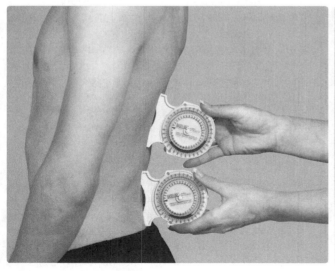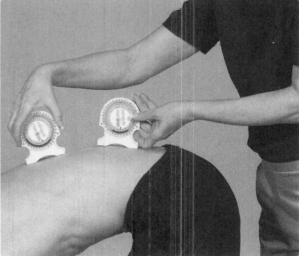

Figure 10.3 Measuring lumbosacral flexion using the double-inclinometer technique.

Indirect Methods of Measuring Static Flexibility

Because of the belief that lack of flexibility is associated with low back pain and musculoskeletal injuries, most health-related fitness test batteries include a sit-and-reach test to evaluate the static flexibility of the lower back and hamstring muscles (Payne et al. 2000). The sit-and-reach test provides an indirect, linear measurement of the ROM. Several sit-and-reach protocols have been developed using either a yardstick (meter stick) or a box, or both, to measure flexibility in inches or centimeters.

Although some fitness professionals assume the sit-and-reach to be a valid measure of low back and hamstring flexibility, research has shown that these tests are moderately related to hamstring flexibility ($r = 0.39$ to 0.89), but poorly related to low back flexibility ($r = 0.10$ to 0.59) in children (Patterson, Wiksten, Ray, Flanders, and Sanphy 1996), adults (Jackson and Langford 1989; Hui, Yuen, Morrow, and Jackson 1999; Hui and Yuen 2000; Martin, Jackson, Morrow, and Liemohn 1998; Minkler and Patterson 1994), and older adults (Jones, Rikli, Max, and Noffal 1998). Moreover, in a prospective study of adults, Jackson et al. (1998) reported that the sit-and-reach test has poor criterion-related validity and is unrelated to self-reported low back pain. Likewise, Grenier, Russell, and McGill (2003) noted that sit-and-reach test scores do not relate to a history of low back pain or discomfort in industrial workers. Although sit-and-reach scores were moderately related ($r = 0.42$) to lumbar ROM in the sagittal plane, the sit-and-reach test could not distinguish between workers who had low back discomfort and workers who did not. The researchers concluded that standard fitness test batteries should include measures of lumbar ROM instead of the sit-and-reach test to assess low back fitness. Lumbar ROM in the sagittal plane can be measured directly with an inclinometer (double-inclinometer technique, see figure 10.3) or indirectly with the skin distraction test (see "Skin Distraction Test," page 257). Sit-and-reach tests should be limited to identifying individuals at the extremes who may have a higher risk of muscle injury because of hypermobility or lack of flexibility in the hamstring muscles.

The following sections describe the protocols for various types of sit-and-reach tests, as well as the skin distraction test. Before clients take any of these tests, have them perform a general warm-up to increase muscle temperature, as well as stretching exercises for the muscle groups to be tested. Unless otherwise stated, have your clients remove their shoes for all sit-and-reach test protocols.

Standard Sit-and-Reach Test

The ACSM (2006) and CSEP (2003) recommend using the standard sit-and-reach test to assess low back and hamstring flexibility. This test uses a sit-and-reach box with a zero point at 26 cm. Have the client sit on the floor with his knees extended and the soles of his feet against the edge of the box. The inner edges of the soles of the feet must be 6 in. (15.2 cm) apart. Instruct the client to keep his knees fully extended, arms evenly stretched, and hands parallel with the palms down (fingertips may overlap) as he slowly reaches forward as far as possible along the top of the box. Have the client hold this position for ~2 sec. Advise your client that lowering the head maximizes the distance reached. The client's score is the most distant point along the top of the box that the fingertips contact. If the client's knees are flexed or motion is jerky or bouncing, do not count the score. Administer 2 trials and record the maximum score to the nearest 0.5 cm. Table 10.4 presents age-gender norms for this test.

V Sit-and-Reach Test

The V sit-and-reach, also known as the YMCA sit-and-reach test, uses a yardstick instead of a box. Secure the yardstick to the floor by placing tape (12 in. long) at a right angle to the 15-in. (38 cm) mark on the yardstick. The client sits, straddling the yardstick, with the knees extended (but not locked) and legs spread 12 in. (30.5 cm) apart. The heels of the feet touch the tape at the 15-in. mark. Instruct the client to reach forward slowly and as far as possible along the yardstick while keeping the two hands parallel (fingertips may overlap) and to hold this position momentarily (~2 sec). Make certain that the knees do not flex and that the client avoids leading with one hand. The score (in centimeters or inches) is the most distant point on the yardstick contacted by the fingertips. Table 10.5 presents norms for the V sit-and-reach test.

Modified Sit-and-Reach Test

To account for a potential bias due to limb-length differences (i.e., individuals who have short legs relative to the trunk and arms may have an advantage when performing the standard sit-and-reach test), Hoeger (1989) developed a modified sit-and-reach test that takes into account the distance between the end of the fingers and the sit-and-

TABLE 10.4 Age-Gender Norms for Standard Sit-and-Reach Test[a]

	AGE (YR)					
	15-19	20-29	30-39	40-49	50-59	60-69
MEN						
Excellent	≥39	≥40	≥38	≥35	≥35	≥33
Very good	34-38	34-39	33-37	29-34	28-34	25-32
Good	29-33	30-33	28-32	24-28	24-27	20-24
Fair	24-28	25-29	23-27	18-23	16-23	15-19
Needs improvement	≤23	≤24	≤22	≤17	≤15	≤14
WOMEN						
Excellent	≥43	≥41	≥41	≥38	≥39	≥35
Very good	38-42	37-40	36-40	34-37	33-38	31-34
Good	34-37	33-36	32-35	30-33	30-32	27-30
Fair	29-33	28-32	27-31	25-29	25-29	23-26
Needs improvement	≤28	≤27	≤26	≤24	≤24	≤22

[a]Distance measured in cm using a sit-and-reach box with the zero point at 26 cm. If using a box with the zero point at 23 cm, subtract 3 cm from each value in this table.

The Canadian Physical Activity, Fitness & Lifestyle Approach: CSEP-Health & Fitness Program's Health-Related Appraisal and Counselling Strategy, 3rd edition. © 2003. Reprinted with permission of the Canadian Society for Exercise Physiology.

TABLE 10.5 Percentile Ranks for the V Sit-and-Reach Test*

Rank	AGE (YR)											
	18-25		26-35		36-45		46-55		56-65		>65	
	M	F	M	F	M	F	M	F	M	F	M	F
90	22	24	21	23	21	22	19	21	17	20	17	20
80	20	22	19	21	19	21	17	20	15	19	15	18
70	19	21	17	20	17	19	15	18	13	17	13	17
60	18	20	17	20	16	18	14	17	13	16	12	17
50	17	19	15	19	15	17	13	16	11	15	10	15
40	15	18	14	17	13	16	11	14	9	14	9	14
30	14	17	13	16	13	15	10	14	9	13	8	13
20	13	16	11	15	11	14	9	12	7	11	7	11
10	11	14	9	13	7	12	6	10	5	9	4	9

*Sit-and-reach scores measured in inches.

Data from YMCA of the USA, 2000, *YMCA Fitness Testing and Assessment Manual* 4th ed., (Champaign, IL: Human Kinetics).

reach box and uses the finger-to-box distance as the relative zero point. This test uses a 12-in. (30.5 cm) sit-and-reach box (see figure 10.4). The client sits on the floor with buttocks, shoulders, and head in contact with the wall; extends the knees; and places the soles of the feet against the box. A yardstick is placed on top of the box with the zero end toward the client. Keeping the head and shoulders in contact with the wall, the client reaches forward with one hand on top of the other, and the yardstick is positioned so that it touches the fingertips. This procedure establishes the relative zero point for each client. As you firmly hold the yardstick in place, the client reaches forward slowly, sliding the fingers along the top of the yardstick. The score (in inches) is the most distant point on the yardstick contacted by the fingertips. Table 10.6 provides age-gender percentile norms for the modified sit-and-reach test.

Research comparing the standard and modified sit-and-reach test scores indicated that individuals with proportionally longer arms than legs (lower finger-to-box distance) had significantly better scores on the standard sit-and-reach test than those with moderate or high finger-to-box distances; in contrast, the modified sit-and-reach test scores did not differ significantly among the three groups (Hoeger, Hopkins, Button, and Palmer 1990; Hoeger and Hopkins 1992). However, Minkler and Patterson (1994) reported that the modified sit-and-reach test was only moderately related to criterion measures of hamstring flexibility for women ($r = 0.66$) and men ($r = 0.75$) and poorly related to low back flexibility of women ($r = 0.25$) and men ($r =$

0.40). Similarly, Hui, Yuen, Morrow, and Jackson (1999) compared the criterion-related validity of the standard and modified sit-and-reach tests and concluded that both tests were moderately valid measures of hamstring flexibility but poor measures of low back flexibility. Consequently, it appears that the validity of the modified sit-and-reach test is no better than that of the standard sit-and-reach test for assessing flexibility of the low back and hamstring muscle groups.

Back-Saver Sit-and-Reach Test

The standard, modified, and V sit-and-reach tests require the client to stretch the hamstring muscles of both legs simultaneously, causing some discomfort when the anterior portions of the vertebrae are compressed during the stretch. The back-saver sit-and-reach test was devised to relieve some of this discomfort by measuring the flexibility of the hamstring muscles, one leg at a time. Instruct your client to place the sole of the foot of the extended (tested) leg against the edge of the sit-and-reach box and to flex the untested leg, placing the sole of that foot flat on the floor 2 to 3 in. to the side of the extended (tested) knee (see figure 10.5). Then follow the instructions for the standard sit-and-reach test to determine your client's flexibility score for each leg. Research suggests that the validity of this test ($r = 0.39$ to 0.71) is similar to that of the standard sit-and-reach test ($r = 0.46$ to 0.74) for assessing hamstring flexibility of men and women (Hui and Yuen 2000; Jones et al. 1998). Norms for this test are available elsewhere (see Cooper Institute for Aerobics Research 1992).

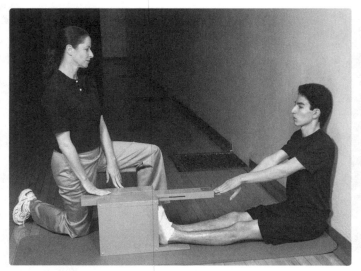 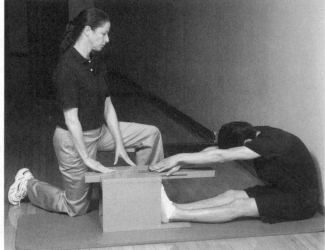

Figure 10.4 Modified sit-and-reach test.

TABLE 10.6	Percentile Ranks for the Modified Sit-and-Reach Test*					
PERCENTILE RANK	**WOMEN**			**MEN**		
	≤35 yr	36-49 yr	≥50 yr	≤35 yr	36-49 yr	≥50 yr
99	19.8	19.8	17.2	24.7	18.9	16.2
95	18.7	19.2	15.7	19.5	18.2	15.8
90	17.9	17.4	15.0	17.9	16.1	15.0
80	16.7	16.2	14.2	17.0	14.6	13.3
70	16.2	15.2	13.6	15.8	13.9	12.3
60	15.8	14.5	12.3	15.0	13.4	11.5
50	14.8	13.5	11.1	14.4	12.6	10.2
40	14.5	12.8	10.1	13.5	11.6	9.7
30	13.7	12.2	9.2	13.0	10.8	9.3
20	12.6	11.0	8.3	11.6	9.9	8.8
10	10.1	9.7	7.5	9.2	8.3	7.8
5	8.1	8.5	3.7	7.9	7.0	7.2
1	2.6	2.0	1.5	7.0	5.1	4.0

*Sit-and-reach scores measured to the nearest 0.25 in.

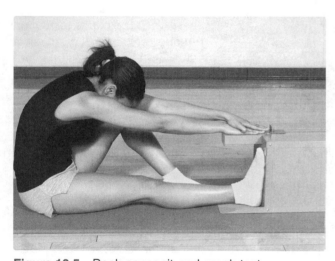

Figure 10.5 Back-saver sit-and-reach test.

Modified Back-Saver Sit-and-Reach Test

While performing the back-saver sit-and-reach test, some participants may complain about the uncomfortable position of the untested leg. Hui and Yuen (2000), therefore, modified this test by having the client perform a single-leg sit-and-reach on a 12-in. (30.5 cm) bench (see figure 10.6). Instruct the client to place the untested leg on the floor with the knee flexed at a 90° angle.

Align the sole of the foot of the tested leg with the 50-cm mark on the meter rule. Then follow the instructions for the standard sit-and-reach test to determine your client's hamstring flexibility for each leg. Hui and Yuen (2000) reported that the validity of this test (r = 0.50 to 0.67) for assessing hamstring flexibility was similar to that of the standard (r = 0.46 to 0.53) and V (r = 0.44 to 0.63) sit-and-reach tests. The modified back-saver test, however, was rated as the most comfortable compared to the other test protocols. Norms for this test have not yet been established.

Skin Distraction Test

The modified Schober test (Mcrae and Wright 1969) or the simplified skin distraction test (Van Adrichem and van der Korst 1973) is useful in assessing low back flexibility. These field tests are reliable and have good agreement with radiographic measurements of spinal flexion and extension (Williams et al. 1993). For the simplified skin distraction test, place a 0-cm mark on the midline of the lumbar spine at the intersection of a horizontal line connecting the left and right posterior superior iliac spines while the client is standing erect. Place a second mark 15 cm (5.9 in.) superior to the 0-cm mark (see figure 10.7). As the client flexes the lumbar spine, these marks move away

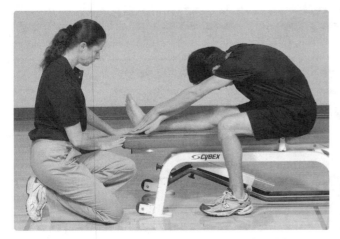

Figure 10.6   Modified back-saver sit-and-reach test.

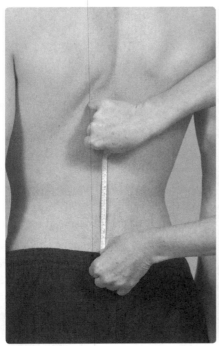
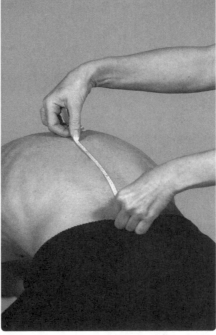

Figure 10.7   Measuring lumbosacral flexion using the simplified skin distraction test.

from each other; use an anthropometric tape measure to measure the new distance between the two marks. The lumbar flexion score is the difference between this measurement and the initial length between the skin markings (15 cm). In a group of 15- to 18-year-old subjects, the simplified skin distraction scores averaged 6.7 ± 1.0 cm in males and 5.8 ± 0.9 cm in females. However, normal values for other age groups are not yet available. You can also use this technique to measure lumbar spinal extension (simplified skin attraction test) by having the client extend backward and measuring the difference between the initial length and the new distance between the superior and inferior skin markings.

Lumbar Stability Tests

Lumbar instability increases the risk of developing low back pain. The primary muscle groups responsible for stabilizing the lumbar spine are the trunk extensors (erector spinae), trunk flexors (rectus abdominis and abdominal oblique muscles), and lateral flexors (quadratus lumborum). Research indicates that muscle endurance is more protective than muscle strength for reducing low back injury (McGill 2001). To evaluate the balance in the isometric endurance capabilities of these muscle groups in healthy individuals, McGill, Childs, and Liebenson (1999) used three tests: trunk extension, trunk flexion, and side bridge.

To measure the isometric endurance of the trunk extensors, have your client lie prone with the lower body secured (use straps) to the test bed at the ankles, knees, and hips and with the upper body extended over the edge of the bed. The test bed should be approximately 25 cm (10 in.) above the surface of the floor. During the test, the client holds the upper arms across the chest, with the hands resting on the opposite shoulders. Instruct your client to assume and maintain a horizontal position above the floor for as long as possible. Use a stopwatch to record in seconds the time from which the client assumes the horizontal position until the time at which the upper body contacts the floor.

To measure the isometric endurance of the trunk flexors, have your client sit on a test bench with a moveable back support set at a 60° angle. The client flexes the knees and hips to 90° and folds the arms across the chest. Use toe straps to secure the client's feet to the test bench. Instruct your client to maintain this body position for as long as possible after you lower or remove the back support. End the test when the client's trunk falls below the 60° angle. Use a stopwatch to record in seconds the elapsed time.

To measure the isometric endurance of the lateral flexors, use the side bridge. Ask your client to assume a side-lying position on a mat, with her legs extended. Place the top foot in front of the lower foot for support. Instruct your client to lift her hips off the mat while supporting her body in a straight line on one elbow and the feet for as long as possible. She should hold the uninvolved arm across the chest. End the test when her hips return to the mat. Use a stopwatch to record in seconds the elapsed time. Administer this test for both the right and left sides of the body.

Table 10.7 contains gender-specific reference data for the isometric endurance of the trunk extensor, trunk flexor, and lateral flexor muscle groups. You can use these reference values to evaluate lumbar stability and to set training goals for your clients.

FLEXIBILITY TESTING OF OLDER ADULTS

Flexibility is an important component of the functional fitness of older individuals. Older adults need to perform activities of daily living (ADL) safely in order to maintain their functional independence as they age. Flexibility facilitates ADL such as getting in and out of a car or chair, dressing, and bathing. The Senior Fitness Test, developed by Rikli and Jones (2001), includes 2 measures of flexibility for older adults—the chair sit-and-reach and the back scratch tests.

Chair Sit-and-Reach Test (Rikli and Jones 2001)

Many older individuals have difficulty performing sit-and-reach tests because functional limitations (e.g., low back pain and poor ROM) prevent them from getting down to and up from the floor. Jones and colleagues (1998) devised a chair sit-and-reach test that is similar to the back-saver protocol (see

figure 10.6, page 258) in that it tests only one leg, thereby reducing stress on the spine and lower back. Compared to standard (r = 0.71 to 0.74) and back-saver (r = 0.70 to 0.71) sit-and-reach protocols, the chair test yielded similar criterion-related validity coefficients (r = 0.76 to 0.81) as a measure of hamstring flexibility in older (>60 yr) men and women. Table 10.8 presents age-gender norms for the chair sit-and-reach test.

Purpose: Assess lower-body (hamstring) flexibility.

Application: A measure of the ability to perform ADL such as climbing stairs and getting in and out of a car, chair, or bathtub.

Equipment: You will need a folding chair that has a seat height of 17 in. (43 cm) and that will not tip forward, as well as an 18 in. (46 cm or half a yardstick) ruler.

Test Procedures: Place the folding chair against a wall for stability and have your client sit on the front edge of the seat. The client extends the leg being tested in front of the hip, with the heel on the floor and the ankle dorsiflexed approximately 90°. The client flexes the untested leg so that the sole of the foot is flat on the floor about 6 to 12 in. (15-30.5 cm) to side of the body's midline. With the extended leg as straight as possible and the hands on top of each other (palms down), the client slowly bends forward at the hip joint, keeping the spine as straight as possible and the head in normal alignment (not tucked) with the spine (see figure 10.8). The client reaches down the extended leg, trying to touch the toes, and holds this position for 2 sec. Place the ruler parallel to your client's lower leg and administer 2 practice trials followed by 2 test trials.

Scoring: The middle of the big toe (medial aspect) at the end of the shoe represents a zero score.

TABLE 10.7 Reference Values for Isometric Lumbar Stabilization Tests in Healthy Adults

Test item	MEN		WOMEN	
	Endurance time (sec)	Ratio*	Endurance time (sec)	Ratio*
Trunk extension	146	1.00	189	1.00
Trunk flexion	144	0.99	149	0.79
Side bridge (right)	94	0.64	72	0.38
Side bridge (left)	97	0.66	77	0.40

*Ratio is calculated by dividing endurance time of each item by trunk extension endurance time.

Data from S.M. McGill, A. Childs, and D.C. Liebenson, 1999, "Endurance times for low back stabilization exercises: Clinical targets for testing and training from a normal database," *Archives of Physical Medicine and Rehabilitation* 80: 941-944.

TABLE 10.8   Chair Sit-and-Reach Test Norms*

Percentile rank	60-64 YR F	60-64 YR M	65-69 YR F	65-69 YR M	70-74 YR F	70-74 YR M	75-79 YR F	75-79 YR M	80-84 YR F	80-84 YR M	85-89 YR F	85-89 YR M	90-94 YR F	90-94 YR M
95	8.7	8.5	7.9	7.5	7.5	7.5	7.4	6.6	6.6	6.2	6.0	4.5	4.9	3.5
90	7.2	6.7	6.6	5.9	6.1	5.8	6.1	4.9	5.2	4.4	4.6	3.0	3.4	1.9
85	6.3	5.6	5.7	4.8	5.2	4.7	5.2	3.8	4.3	3.2	3.7	2.0	2.5	0.9
80	5.5	4.6	5.0	3.9	4.5	3.8	4.4	2.8	3.6	2.2	3.0	1.1	1.7	0.0
75	4.8	3.8	4.4	3.1	3.9	3.0	3.7	2.0	3.0	1.4	2.4	0.4	1.0	−0.7
70	4.2	3.1	3.9	2.4	3.3	2.4	3.2	1.3	2.4	0.6	1.8	−0.2	0.4	−1.4
65	3.7	2.5	3.4	1.8	2.8	1.8	2.7	0.7	1.9	0.0	1.3	−0.8	−0.1	−1.9
60	3.1	1.8	2.9	1.1	2.3	1.1	2.1	0.1	1.4	−0.8	0.8	−1.3	−0.7	−2.5
55	2.6	1.2	2.5	0.6	1.9	0.6	1.7	−0.5	1.0	−1.4	0.4	−1.9	−1.2	−3.0
50	2.1	0.6	2.0	0.0	1.4	0.0	1.2	−1.1	0.5	−2.0	−0.1	−2.4	−1.7	−3.6
45	1.6	0.0	1.5	−0.6	0.9	−0.6	0.7	−1.7	0.0	−2.6	−0.6	−2.9	−2.2	−4.2
40	1.1	−0.6	1.1	−1.1	0.5	−1.2	0.2	−2.3	−0.4	−3.2	−1.0	−3.5	−2.7	−4.7
35	0.5	−1.3	0.6	−1.8	0.0	−1.8	−0.3	−2.9	−0.9	−4.0	−1.5	−4.0	−3.3	−5.3
30	0.0	−1.9	0.1	−2.4	−0.5	−2.4	−0.8	−3.5	−1.4	−4.6	−2.0	−4.6	−3.8	−5.8
25	−0.6	−2.6	−0.4	−3.1	−1.1	−3.1	−1.3	−4.2	−2.0	−5.3	−2.6	−5.3	−4.4	−6.5
20	−1.3	−3.4	−1.0	−3.9	−1.7	−3.9	−2.0	−5.0	−2.6	−6.2	−3.2	−5.9	−5.1	−7.2
15	−2.1	−4.4	−1.7	−4.8	−2.4	−4.8	−2.8	−6.0	−3.3	−7.2	−3.9	−6.8	−5.9	−8.1
10	−3.0	−5.5	−2.6	−5.9	−3.3	−5.9	−3.7	−7.1	−4.2	−8.4	−4.8	−7.8	−6.8	−9.1
5	−4.0	−7.3	−3.9	−7.5	−4.7	−7.6	−5.0	−8.8	−5.0	−10.2	−6.3	−9.3	−7.9	−10.7

*Score is measured in inches.

F = females; M = males.

To convert in. to cm, multiply value in table by 2.54.

Adapted, by permission, from R. Rikli and C. Jones, 2001, *Senior fitness test manual* (Champaign, IL: Human Kinetics).

Reaches short of the toes are recorded as minus scores; reaches beyond the toes are recorded as plus scores. Record the best score to the nearest half inch and compare it to the norms in table 10.8.

Back Scratch Test (Rikli and Jones 2001)

Limited ROM in the upper body, especially in the shoulder joints, may cause painful movement and increase the chance of injury while performing common tasks such as putting on and taking off clothes. The back scratch test appears to have good construct validity, as evidenced by its ability to detect declines in shoulder flexibility across age groups (60-90 yr) (Rikli and Jones 1999). Table 10.9 presents age-gender norms for the back scratch test.

Purpose: Assess upper-body (shoulder joint) flexibility.

Application: A measure of the ability to perform ADLs such as combing hair, dressing, and reaching for a seat belt.

Equipment: You will need an 18 in. (46 cm) ruler.

Test Procedures: Ask your client to reach, with the preferred hand (palm down and fingers

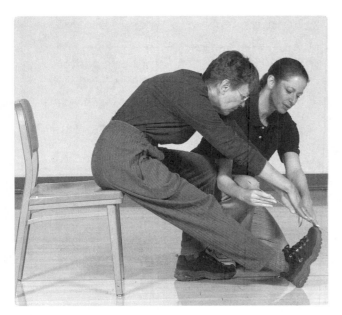

Figure 10.8 Chair sit-and-reach test.

extended), over the shoulder and down the back while reaching around and up the middle of the back with the other hand (palm up and fingers extended) (see figure 10.9). Allow the client to choose the best, or preferred, hand through trial and error. Administer 2 practice trials followed by 2 test trials.

Scoring: Use the ruler to measure the overlap (plus score) or gap (minus score) between the middle fingers of each hand. If the fingers just touch each other, record a zero. Record the best score to the nearest half inch and compare this value to the norms in table 10.9.

TABLE 10.9 Back Scratch Test Norms*

Percentile rank	60-64 YR		65-69 YR		70-74 YR		75-79 YR		80-84 YR		85-89 YR		90-94 YR	
	F	M	F	M	F	M	F	M	F	M	F	M	F	M
95	5.0	4.5	4.9	3.9	4.5	3.5	4.5	2.8	4.3	3.2	3.5	1.7	3.9	0.7
90	3.8	2.7	3.5	2.2	3.2	1.8	3.1	0.9	2.8	1.2	1.9	−0.1	2.2	−1.1
85	2.9	1.6	2.6	1.0	2.3	0.6	2.2	−0.3	1.8	−0.1	0.8	−1.2	0.9	−2.2
80	2.2	0.6	1.9	0.0	1.5	−0.4	1.3	−1.3	0.9	−1.2	−0.1	−2.2	−0.1	−3.2
75	1.6	−0.2	1.3	−0.8	0.8	−1.2	0.6	−2.2	0.2	−2.1	−0.9	−3.0	−1.0	−4.0
70	1.1	−0.9	0.7	−1.6	0.3	−2.0	0.0	−2.9	−0.4	−2.9	−1.6	−3.7	−1.8	−4.7
65	0.7	−1.5	0.2	−2.2	−0.2	−2.6	−0.5	−3.6	−1.0	−3.6	−2.1	−4.3	−2.5	−5.3
60	0.2	−2.2	−0.3	−2.9	−0.8	−3.3	−1.1	−4.3	−1.6	−4.3	−2.8	−5.0	−3.2	−6.0
55	−0.2	−2.8	−0.7	−3.5	−1.2	−3.9	−1.6	−4.9	−2.1	−5.0	−3.3	−5.6	−3.8	−6.6
50	−0.7	−3.4	−1.2	−4.1	−1.7	−4.5	−2.1	−5.6	−2.6	−5.7	−3.9	−6.2	−4.5	−7.2
45	−1.2	−4.0	−1.7	−4.7	−2.2	−5.1	−2.6	−6.3	−3.1	−6.4	−4.5	−6.8	−5.2	−7.8
40	−1.6	−4.6	−2.1	−5.3	−2.6	−5.7	−3.1	−6.9	−3.7	−7.1	−5.0	−7.4	−5.8	−8.4
35	−2.1	−5.3	−2.6	−6.0	−3.2	−6.4	−3.7	−7.6	−4.2	−7.8	−5.7	−8.1	−6.5	−9.1
30	−2.5	−5.9	−3.1	−6.6	−3.7	−7.0	−4.2	−8.3	−4.8	−8.5	−6.2	−8.7	−7.2	−9.7
25	−3.0	−6.6	−3.7	−7.4	−4.2	−7.8	−4.8	−9.0	−5.4	−9.3	−6.9	−9.4	−8.0	−10.4
20	−3.6	−7.4	−4.3	−8.2	−4.9	−8.6	−5.5	−9.9	−6.1	−10.2	−7.7	−10.2	−8.9	−11.2
15	−4.3	−8.4	−5.0	−9.2	−5.7	−9.6	−6.4	−10.9	−7.0	−11.3	−8.6	−11.2	−9.9	−12.2
10	−5.2	−9.5	−5.9	−10.4	−6.6	−10.8	−7.3	−12.1	−8.0	−12.5	−9.7	−12.3	−11.2	−13.3
5	−6.4	−11.3	−7.3	−12.1	−7.9	−12.5	−8.8	−14.0	−9.5	−14.6	−11.3	−14.1	−13.0	−15.1

*Score is measured in inches.

F = females; M = males.

To convert in. to cm, multiply value in table by 2.54.

Adapted, by permission, from R. Rikli and C. Jones, 2001, *Senior fitness test manual* (Champaign, IL: Human Kinetics)

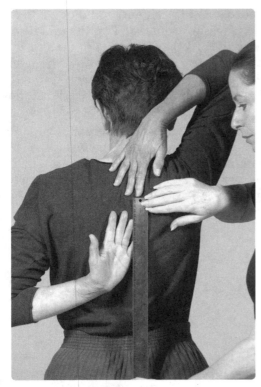

Figure 10.9   Back scratch test.

Sources for Equipment

Product	Supplier's address
Flexometer Inclinometer Sit-and-reach box Universal goniometer	Country Technology Inc. P.O. Box 87 Gay Mills, WI 54631 Phone: (608) 735-4718 www.fitnessmart.com
Pilates equipment	Balanced Body Inc. 8220 Ferguson Ave. Sacramento, CA 95828 Phone: (800) 745-2837 www.pilates.com

KEY POINTS

- Static flexibility is a measure of the total ROM at the joint.
- Dynamic flexibility is a measure of the rate of torque or resistance developed during movement through the ROM.
- Flexibility is highly joint specific, and the ROM depends, in part, on the structure of the joint.
- Lack of physical activity is a major cause of inflexibility.
- A universal goniometer, flexometer, or inclinometer can be used to obtain direct measures of ROM.

- A yardstick and anthropometric tape measure can be used to obtain indirect measures of ROM.
- Sit-and-reach tests measure flexibility of the hamstrings but not low back flexibility.
- The chair sit-and-reach and the back scratch tests can be used to assess flexibility of older adults.
- Lumbar instability increases risk of developing low back pain.
- Muscle endurance is more protective than muscle strength for reducing low back injury.

KEY TERMS

Learn the definition for each of the following key terms. Definitions of terms can be found in the glossary on page 379.

ankylosis
biaxial joints
contracture
dynamic flexibility
elastic deformation
flexibility
flexometer
goniometer
hypermobility
inclinometer

joint laxity
range of motion (ROM)
static flexibility
static stretching
stress relaxation
triaxial joints
uniaxial joints
viscoelastic properties
viscous deformation

REVIEW QUESTIONS

In addition to being able to define each of the key terms, test your knowledge and understanding of the material by answering the following review questions.

1. Why are flexibility tests included in most health-related fitness test batteries?

2. Identify and explain how morphological factors affect range of joint motion.

3. How do age, gender, and physical activity (or lack thereof) affect flexibility?

4. Identify and briefly describe three direct methods for measuring static flexibility.

5. Do sit-and-reach tests yield valid measures of hamstring and low back flexibility? Explain.

6. Is the modified standard sit-and-reach test more valid than the standard sit-and-reach test for assessing hamstring and low back flexibility?

7. Describe three tests that can be used to evaluate lumbar stability.

8. Describe two tests that indirectly measure the flexibility of older adults.

chapter 11

Designing Programs for Flexibility and Low Back Care

Key Questions

- How do training principles apply to the design of flexibility training programs?

- Are all methods of stretching safe and effective for improving flexibility?

- What are the recommended guidelines for designing a stretching program?

- How do you individualize flexibility programs to meet the goals and abilities of each client?

- How often does a client need to exercise to improve flexibility?

- Is there an optimal combination of stretch duration and repetitions for improving range of motion?

- Can low back syndrome be prevented?

- What exercises are recommended for low back care?

Flexibility training is a systematic program of stretching exercises designed to progressively increase the range of motion (ROM) of joints over time. It is well documented that stretching improves flexibility and ROM. Generic exercise prescriptions for improving flexibility are not recommended; flexibility programs should be individualized to address the needs, abilities, and physical activity interests of each client. Your client's flexibility assessment (see chapter 10) can help you focus on joints and muscle groups needing improvement. Lifestyle assessments (see appendix A.5, p. 288) can help identify muscle groups and body parts with limited joint mobility caused by habitual body postures (e.g., sitting at a desk for long times at work) or repetitive movement patterns during exercise (e.g., jogging).

This chapter presents guidelines for designing flexibility programs. Basic training principles are applied to developing flexibility programs. It compares various methods of stretching and addresses questions about the flexibility exercise prescription. In addition, it presents approaches and recommendations for designing low back care programs.

TRAINING PRINCIPLES

The principles of overload, specificity, progression, and interindividual variability (see chapter 3, pp. 44) apply to flexibility programs. Flexibility is joint specific (Cotten 1972; Harris 1969; Munroe and Romance 1975); to increase the ROM of a particular joint, select exercises that stretch the appropriate muscle groups (i.e., apply the specificity principle). Review your anatomy and kinesiology, particularly muscle origins and insertions, joint structures and functions, and agonist–antagonist muscle pairs. To improve ROM at a joint, your client must overload the muscle group by stretching the muscles beyond their normal resting length but not beyond the pain-free ROM. The pain-free ROM varies among individuals (interindividual variability principle), depending on their **stretch tolerance** (the amount of resistive force to stretch within target muscles that a person can tolerate before experiencing pain) and their perception of stretch and pain (Magnusson 1998; Shrier and Gossal 2000). Periodically your client will need to increase the total time of stretching by increasing the duration or number of repetitions of each stretch in order to ensure the overload required for further ROM improvements (progression principle).

STRETCHING METHODS

Traditionally, three stretching methods have been used to improve ROM: ballistic, slow static, and proprioceptive neuromuscular facilitation. **Ballistic stretching** uses jerky, bouncing movements to lengthen the target muscle, whereas **static stretching** uses slow, sustained muscle lengthening to increase ROM. Commonly used **proprioceptive neuromuscular facilitation (PNF)** stretching techniques involve maximal or submaximal contractions (isometric or dynamic) of target (agonist) and opposing (antagonist) muscle groups followed by passive stretching of the target muscles (Chalmers 2004). Stretching techniques are classified as active, passive, or active-assisted. In **active stretching**, the client moves the body part without external assistance (i.e., voluntarily contracts the muscle). In **passive stretching**, the client relaxes the target muscle group as the body part is moved by an assistant (e.g., partner, personal trainer, physical therapist, or athletic trainer). In **active-assisted stretching**, the client moves the body part to the end of its active ROM and the

assistant then moves the body part beyond its active ROM. Table 11.1 summarizes the advantages and disadvantages of stretching methods. The following questions address issues that you should consider when selecting a stretching method for your client's flexibility program.

■ *Which method of stretching is best for improving ROM?*

All three stretching methods (ballistic, slow static, and PNF) produce acute and chronic gains in flexibility and ROM at the knee, hip, trunk, shoulder, and ankle joints (Thacker, Gilchrist, Stroup, and Kimsey 2004). Although slow static stretching is considered safer than ballistic or PNF stretching and is easier to perform because it does not require special equipment or an assistant, each stretching method has its proponents. Studies generally indicate that PNF stretching improves ROM more effectively than either slow static or ballistic stretching (Anderson and Burke 1991; Etnyre and Abraham 1986; Holt, Travis, and Okita 1970; Shrier and Gossal 2000; Wallin, Ekblom, Grahn, and Nordenburg 1985), but this finding has not been consistent (Thacker et al. 2004). Choose a method, therefore, that meets your client's specific abilities (e.g., stretch tolerance and pain threshold), needs, and long-term goals. PNF stretching is frequently used in sport and rehabilitation settings.

■ *What are some of the commonly used PNF stretching techniques and how are they performed?*

There are various PNF techniques that use different combinations of dynamic (concentric and eccentric) and isometric contraction of target and opposing muscle groups. The **contract-relax**

TABLE 11.1   Comparison of Stretching Techniques

Factor	Ballistic	Slow static	PNF[a]
Risk of injury	High	Low	Medium
Degree of pain	Medium	Low	High
Resistance to stretch	High	Low	Medium
Practicality (time and assistance needed)	Good	Excellent	Poor
Efficiency (energy consumption)	Poor	Excellent	Poor
Effective for increasing ROM[b]	Good	Good	Excellent

[a]Proprioceptive neuromuscular facilitation.
[b]Range of motion.

(CR) and **contract-relax agonist contract (CRAC)** techniques are common PNF procedures. In the CR technique, your client first isometrically contracts the target muscle group; this is immediately followed by slow, passive stretching of the target muscle group. The first two steps of the CRAC and CR techniques are identical except that the client assists the CRAC stretching phase by actively contracting the opposing muscle group. For example, to stretch the pectoral muscles, the client sits on the floor and extends the arms horizontally. The client isometrically contracts the pectoral muscles as the partner offers resistance to horizontal flexion. Following the isometric contraction, the partner slowly stretches the pectorals as the client actively contracts the horizontal extensors in the upper back (see figure 11.1). For detailed explanations and illustrations of nine PNF stretching techniques, see Alter (1996).

■ *What are the general recommendations for performing PNF stretches?*

The following steps are recommended for performing PNF stretches to increase ROM:

- Stretch the target muscle group by moving the joint to the end of its ROM.
- Isometrically contract the stretched muscle group against an immovable resistance (such as a partner or wall) for 5 to 10 sec.
- Relax the target muscle group as you stretch it actively or passively (with a partner) to a new point of limitation.
- For the CRAC technique, contract the opposing muscle group submaximally for 5 to 6 sec to facilitate further stretching of the target muscle group.

■ *Which is best—the CR or CRAC procedure?*

It has been reported that the CRAC technique improves ROM more effectively (Alter 1996; Moore and Hutton 1980). Moore and Hutton compared the relative levels of muscle relaxation during CR and CRAC stretching. CRAC produced larger gains in hip flexion, but it also produced greater electromyographic activity in the hamstring muscle group and was ranked as more uncomfortable than CR

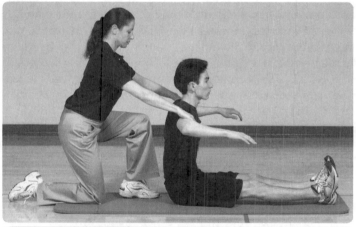

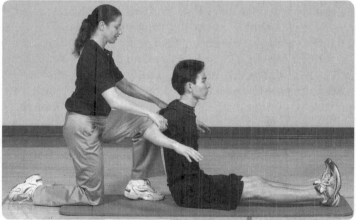

Figure 11.1 Contract-relax agonist contract (CRAC) proprioceptive neuromuscular facilitation stretching technique for the shoulder horizontal flexors.

in terms of perceived pain. Therefore, you need to consider your client's stretch tolerance when selecting a PNF stretching technique.

■ Is PNF stretching always superior to slow static stretching?

A major disadvantage of the PNF technique is that most of the exercises cannot be performed alone. An assistant is needed to resist movement during the isometric contraction phase and to apply external force during the stretching phase. Overstretching may cause injury, especially if the assistant has not been carefully trained in the correct PNF procedures. Assisted stretching procedures such as PNF should be carefully performed by trained clients or exercise professionals who understand the correct procedures and the risks of incorrect stretching (Knudson, Magnusson, and McHugh 2000).

■ Why is slow static stretching safer than ballistic stretching?

Many exercise professionals recommend slow static stretching over ballistic stretching because there is less chance of injury and muscle soreness resulting from jerky, rapid movements. Ballistic stretching uses relatively fast bouncing motions to produce stretch. The momentum of the moving body segment rather than external force pushes the joint beyond its present ROM. This technique appears counterproductive for increasing muscle relaxation and stretch. During the movement, the muscle spindles signal changes in both muscle length and contraction speed. The spindle responds more (due to a lower threshold) to the speed of the movement than to the length or position of the muscle. In fact, muscle spindle activity is directly proportional to the speed of movement. Thus, ballistic stretching evokes the stretch reflex, producing more contraction and resistance to stretch in the target muscle group. Also, the muscle has viscous properties. The viscous material resists elongation more when the stretch is applied rapidly (Taylor, Dalton, Seaber, and Garrett, 1990). Therefore, ballistic stretching places greater strain on the muscle and may cause microscopic tearing of muscle fibers and connective tissues.

In slow static stretching, your client stretches the target muscle group when the joint is at the end of its ROM. While maintaining this lengthened position, the client slowly applies torque to the target muscle group to stretch it further. Because the dynamic portion of the muscle spindle rapidly adapts to the lengthened position, spindle discharge decreases. This decrease lessens the reflex contraction of the target muscle group and allows the muscle to relax and be stretched even further. The force needed to lengthen a muscle is affected by the rate of stretching and by the duration the target muscle group is held at a specific length (Taylor et al. 1990). Resistance to elongation is greater for rapid (e.g., ballistic) stretching than for slow static stretching. Also, the resistance produced by the viscous properties of the muscle decreases over time as the target muscle is held at its stretched length. The resulting **stress relaxation** allows further elongation of the target muscle group (Chalmers 2004).

■ What are the physiological mechanisms underlying the increased ROM produced by the PNF method?

The mechanisms responsible for gains in ROM from PNF stretching are controversial. Two suggested hypotheses are the neurophysiological and the viscoelastic (Burke, Culligan, and Holt 2000). Traditionally in the PNF literature, increases in ROM were explained by neurophysiological modifications such as inhibition of the spinal reflexes (e.g., stretch reflex and Golgi tendon organ, or GTO, reflex) in target muscles. These modifications are caused by decreased muscle spindle discharge during slow static stretching (i.e., less spindle activity leads to less reflex contraction and more muscle relaxation) and by increased GTO activity during isometric contraction (i.e., greater GTO activation leads to reflex relaxation). Also, voluntary contraction of opposing muscle groups during CRAC stretching was simply explained by **reciprocal inhibition** (as the opposing muscle group is voluntarily contracted, the target muscle group is reflexively inhibited).

The neuromuscular mechanisms underlying muscle stretch are extremely complicated and not fully understood. Simple explanations of the role of reciprocal inhibition during muscle stretching are inadequate. For example, recurrent collateral pathways from motor neurons of the opposing muscle group inhibit interneurons that reduce the excitation of alpha motor neurons of the target muscle group, thereby blocking inhibitory input to target muscle groups (Hultborn, Illert, and Santini 1974). In addition, presynaptic inhibition can modify transmission from sensory neurons, and interneurons can receive input from more than one sensory receptor as well as from multiple descending tracts in the central nervous system. For example, the interneuron activated by the sensory signals of GTOs in a target muscle group also receives input from many sensory and descending tracts. This input potentially modifies the simple spinal reflex pathway (Chalmers 2004).

Obviously, neurophysiological mechanisms such as muscle spindle and GTO reflexes do not singularly explain how PNF stretching improves ROM. Therefore, other mechanisms such as changes in the viscoelastic properties of stretched muscle (viscoelastic hypothesis) and the ability to tolerate stretch have been suggested. In light of the viscoelastic changes accompanying slow static stretching, ROM improvements from PNF stretching may also be partly explained by greater elastic deformation (proportional to the tension applied during stretching) and viscous deformation (proportional to the speed at which the tension is applied during stretching) as well as enhanced viscoelastic stress relaxation over time (Burke et al. 2000; Chalmers 2004). In addition, long-term PNF stretching enhances **stretch tolerance** because of the analgesic effect of stretching. As a result, more force can be applied to the muscle before the individual feels pain (Shrier and Gossal 2000).

■ *During PNF stretches, what is the recommended duration of the isometric contraction phase to maximize long-term gains in ROM?*

Traditionally, isometric contractions of 5 to 10 sec are recommended for PNF stretching programs; however, there is a lack of research justifying these durations or documenting their continued effectiveness for improving ROM during training. One study (Rowlands, Marginson, and Lee 2003) compared chronic gains in passive flexibility between two CRAC stretching programs with different durations of isometric contraction (5 sec vs. 10 sec). Training consisted of performing 3 repetitions of 2 different passive stretching exercises twice per week over 6 wk. Compared to a control group that did not stretch, both training groups experienced significant increases in hip flexion. However, greater gains in hip flexion resulted from 10 sec isometric contraction compared to 5 sec contraction. The authors concluded that the 10 sec isometric contraction allowed more time for changes in viscoelastic properties and therefore allowed greater relaxation of the target muscle group. They suggested that more research is needed comparing different PNF training programs and quantifying the roles of the neurophysiological and viscoelastic mechanisms underlying chronic gains in both active and passive flexibility.

DESIGNING FLEXIBILITY PROGRAMS: EXERCISE PRESCRIPTION

After assessing your client's flexibility, you must identify the joints and muscle groups needing improvement and select an appropriate stretching method and the specific exercises for the exercise prescription. Appendix F.1, "Selected Flexibility Exercises," on page 358 illustrates flexibility exercises for various regions of the body. For additional stretching exercises, see Anderson (1980) and Alter (1996). Follow the guidelines (see "Guidelines for Designing Flexibility Programs" on page 272 and "Client Guidelines for Stretching Programs" on page 272) and be sure to address the following questions regarding your client's exercise prescription.

■ *How many exercises should be included in a flexibility program?*

A well-rounded program includes at least one exercise for each of the major muscle groups of the body. It is important to select exercises for problem areas such as the lower back, hips, and posterior thighs and legs. Use the results of the flexibility tests to identify specific muscle groups with relatively poor flexibility, and include more than one exercise for these muscle groups. The workout should take 15 to 30 min depending on the number of exercises to be performed.

■ *Are some stretching exercises safer than others?*

Some stretching exercises are not recommended for flexibility programs because they create excessive stress, thereby increasing your client's chance of musculoskeletal injuries—especially to the knee joints and low back region. Appendix F.2, "Exercise Do's and Don'ts," page 367, illustrates exercises that are contraindicated for flexibility programs and suggests alternative exercises that you can prescribe to increase the flexibility of specific muscle groups. For detailed analysis of risk factors and options for minimizing risk for certain stretching exercises, see Alter (1996).

■ *What is a safe intensity for stretching exercises?*

The intensity of the exercise for the slow static stretching and PNF stretching exercises should always be below the pain threshold of the individual. Some mild discomfort will occur, especially during the PNF exercises when the target muscle is contracted isometrically. However, the joint should not be stretched beyond its pain-free ROM (ACSM 2006).

■ *How long does each stretch need to be held?*

To date there is a limited amount of research concerning the optimal time that a static stretch should be sustained to improve ROM. In the past, some experts have suggested varying lengths of static stretch, ranging from 10 to 60 sec (Beaulieu 1980). The ACSM (2006) recommends holding the stretched position 15 to 30 sec.

Borms, Van Roy, Santens, and Haentjens (1987) compared the effects of 10, 20, and 30 sec of static stretching on hip flexibility of women engaging in a 10-wk (two sessions a week) static flexibility training program. They reported similar improvements in hip flexibility for all three groups, suggesting that a duration of 10 sec of static stretching is sufficient for improving hip flexibility.

Another study compared the effect of three static stretching durations (15, 30, and 60 sec) on the hip flexibility of men and women with "tight" hamstring muscles (Bandy and Irion 1994). The subjects participated in a 6 wk static flexibility training program, stretching five times a week. The authors noted that 30 and 60 sec of static stretching were more effective than stretching 15 sec for increasing hip flexibility. They observed no significant difference between stretching for 30 sec and for 60 sec, indicating that a 30-sec stretch of the hamstring muscles was as effective as the longer-duration stretch.

Some research suggests that the total stretching time in a workout may be more important than the duration of each stretch (Cipriani, Abel, and Pirrwitz 2003; Roberts and Wilson 1999). Roberts and Wilson (1999) compared the effects of stretching 5 or 15 sec on active and passive ROM in the lower extremity. The treatment groups participated in a static stretching program three times a week for a 5-wk period. The investigators controlled the total amount of time spent stretching (45 sec) by having the 5-sec group perform 9 repetitions and the 15-sec group 3 repetitions for each exercise. The improvement in passive ROM was similar for the 5- and 15-sec groups; however, the 15-sec group showed significantly greater improvement in active ROM.

Similarly, Cipriani and colleagues (2003) compared two stretching protocols that controlled for total stretch time (10 sec × 6 reps vs. 30 sec × 2 reps). Stretching was performed twice daily for a

total workout duration of 2 min/day for 6 wk. The resulting gains in passive ROM at the hip joint were equal for these two protocols. The findings from these two studies have implications for designing flexibility programs. For clients with a low stretch tolerance, you can prescribe shorter stretch duration (e.g., 10 sec) and more repetitions; for those who can tolerate longer stretch durations (30 sec or more), you can prescribe less repetitions.

In light of these findings, you should consider having your clients perform each stretching exercise for a total of 45 sec to 2 min. The combination of duration and repetitions used to reach this recommended total should be individualized to your client's tolerance for the sensation of stretching. For short durations, the stretch should be sustained at least 10 to 15 sec. As flexibility improves, you can progressively overload the target muscle groups by changing either the stretch duration (10-30 sec) or the number of repetitions so that the total time that the stretched position is held gradually increases. As your client's stretch tolerance improves, consider increasing the duration and decreasing the number of repetitions of each stretch. Remember that you must gradually increase the total stretching time for each exercise in order to ensure overload and further improvements in ROM.

■ *How many repetitions of each exercise should be performed?*

Beginners should start with 2 to 4 repetitions of each exercise (ACSM 2006). As flexibility improves during the training program, the number of repetitions of each flexibility exercise may be gradually increased to 5 repetitions to progressively overload the muscle group.

■ *How often should flexibility exercises be performed?*

Flexibility exercises should be performed a minimum of 2 to 3 days a week (ACSM 2006) but preferably daily (Knudson et al. 2000). Flexibility exercises should be performed after moderate or vigorous physical activity and are often an integral part of the cool-down segments of aerobic exercise and resistance training workouts.

■ *Does stretching prevent injury and improve physical performance?*

For years clinicians, coaches, and exercise practitioners have recommended stretching as part of the warm-up. Because an active warm-up prevents injury and because stretching is commonly included in the warm-up, one could easily but mistakenly conclude that stretching prevents injury. However, there is a lack of scientific evidence supporting the long-held belief that stretching before physical activity prevents injury (Pope, Herbert, Kirwan, and Graham 2000; Shrier 1999; Thacker et al. 2004; Weldon and Hill 2003). Theories based on research data and clinical observations have been proposed to explain why stretching does not reduce the risk of injury:

- The ability of muscles to absorb energy is not related to flexibility. No scientific evidence supports the idea that more compliant (i.e., more flexible) muscles and connective tissues have a greater ability to absorb energy and are thus less likely to sustain injury (Shrier 1999).

- Stretching, even mild stretching, can cause damage at the cellular level (Shrier 2000).

- The analgesic effect of stretching increases pain tolerance (Shrier and Gossal 2000).

Experts agree that there is insufficient evidence to either endorse or decry routine preevent stretching for preventing injuries among competitive and recreational athletes (Herbert and Gabriel 2002; Thacker et al. 2004). To resolve this issue additional research, particularly well-controlled randomized trials, is needed.

Also, some evidence suggests that stretching may be detrimental to performance (Knudson et al. 2000). Intense, prolonged stretching may create a strength deficit for up to 1 hr afterward (Fowles, Sales, and MacDougall 2000). To reach peak tension during contraction, stretched muscles need time to take up the slack in the musculotendinous unit produced by stretching. Therefore, stretching immediately before performance may impair strength and performance, especially when the muscle is not allowed enough time to take up slack (Bracko 2002). Knudson (1999) recommended stretching during the warm-up only for those engaging in activities that require extreme ROM, such as dancing, diving, and gymnastics.

■ Does the flexibility exercise prescription need to be adapted for older individuals?

Range of motion decreases with age due to disuse, changes in tissue viscoelasticity, and diseases such as arthritis. However, stretching improves ROM in older adults (Feland, Myrer, Schulthies, Fellingham, and Measom 2001; Ferber, Osternig, and Gravelle 2002). There is a lack of research addressing optimal stretching

methods and durations for older adults. Ferber and colleagues (2002) compared the effects of three stretching methods—static stretching, contract-relax (CR) PNF stretching, and agonist contract-relax (ACR) PNF stretching—on knee joint ROM in older adults (50-75 yr). The ACR technique produced greater gains in ROM (29% and 34%) than did the static stretching and CR methods, even though the ACR technique produced more electromyographic activity in the target muscles.

Feland and colleagues (2001) studied the effects of 15, 30, and 60 sec of static stretching on the rate of ROM improvement in older adults (65-97 yr) with tight hamstrings. The subjects trained 5 times/wk for 6 wk, and knee extension ROM was measured weekly. The group that stretched for 60 sec had a greater rate of improvement (2.4°/wk) than that of those stretching for 30 sec (1.3°/wk) and 15 sec (0.6°/wk). Although these findings suggest that 60 sec is optimal for improving flexibility in older adults, the total time of stretching was not controlled in this study (i.e., the total time of stretching was 30 min for the 60 sec group and only 15 min and 7.5 min for the 30 sec and 15 sec groups, respectively). The difference in total time most likely explains why the 60 sec stretch duration was superior.

Swank, Funk, Durham, and Roberts (2003) assessed the effectiveness of adding light wrist and ankle weights to a low-intensity, rhythmic movement program (the Body Recall Program) designed to improve and maintain the strength and flexibility of older adults. Compared to a control group and a group that participated only in the Body Recall Program, the group that added weights to the Body Recall Program showed significantly greater improvements in ROM at the neck (cervical rotation), hip (extension), and ankle (plantar flexion). Thus, adding weights may enhance the effectiveness of rhythmic movement and stretching programs designed to improve the flexibility of older adults.

Given the limited number of studies dealing with flexibility in older adults, at this time it is not possible to firmly recommend how to change program guidelines when designing flexibility programs for older adults. However, if you use the PNF method with older adults, take care that you do not exceed the stretch tolerance of your clients. The stretch tolerance of older adults is reduced due to age-related changes in the viscoelastic properties of muscle and connective tissue.

You can use the general guidelines presented in this section as a starting point for designing flexibility programs. You should individualize programs to take into account client factors such as tolerance to stretch and pain, needs, and long-range goals. For example, shorter duration–higher repetitions static stretching may be more appropriate for clients with low stretch tolerance, whereas longer duration PNF stretching may be more suitable for athletes or for clients in injury rehabilitation programs. Also, the optimal duration, frequency, and total time of stretching may vary among muscle groups because their viscoelastic properties and response to the stretch stimulus may differ (Shrier and Gossal 2000). Table 11.2 presents a sample program for a 35-year-old woman who wants to improve her overall flexibility. Note that this program includes more than one exercise for muscle groups with poor-to-fair flexibility ratings.

GUIDELINES FOR DESIGNING FLEXIBILITY PROGRAMS

- **Mode:** Static or PNF stretching
- **Number of exercises:** 10 to 12
- **Frequency:** Minimum of 2 to 3 days a week, preferably daily
- **Intensity:** Slowly stretch the muscle to a position of mild discomfort
- **Duration of stretch:** 10 to 30 sec for static stretching; 5-10 sec contraction, followed by 10 to 30 sec of assisted stretching for PNF
- **Repetitions:** 2 to 6 for each exercise so that the total duration of each stretching exercise is 45-120 sec.
- **Time:** 15 to 30 min per session

Instruct clients who are engaging in stretching programs to adhere to the following guidelines (Kravitz and Heyward 1995):

CLIENT GUIDELINES FOR STRETCHING PROGRAMS

- Perform a general warm-up before stretching to increase body temperature and to warm the muscles to be stretched.
- Stretch all major muscle groups, as well as opposing muscle groups.
- Focus on the target muscles involved in the stretch, relax the target muscle, and minimize the movement of other body parts.

- Hold the stretch for 10 to 30 sec.
- Stretch to the limit (end point) of the movement, not to the point of pain.
- Keep breathing slowly and rhythmically while holding the stretch.
- Stretch the target muscle groups in different planes to improve overall ROM at the joint.

DESIGNING LOW BACK CARE EXERCISE PROGRAMS

Low back pain frequently causes activity restrictions for middle-aged and older adults, disabling 3 to 4 million people each year. Chronic low back pain is the number-one cause of disability in the working population (Carpenter and Nelson 1999). The safest and most effective way to prevent and rehabilitate low back injuries remains controversial. This section describes two approaches for low back care programs. The approach you select depends on your client's needs, health/fitness status, and training objective (e.g., reducing low back pain, lowering the risk of low back injury, or maximizing athletic performance).

Traditional Approach

Traditionally, low back care programs have been designed to correct improper alignment and support of the spinal column and pelvis. Generally, a combination of stretching and strengthening exercises is prescribed to increase (a) the ROM of the hip flexors, hamstrings, and low back extensor muscles and (b) the strength of the abdominal muscles.

Exercise professionals have focused primarily on strengthening the abdominal muscles in order to prevent low back pain and injury, giving little or no attention to the low back muscles. Recent research, however, suggests that low back-strengthening programs are effective for relieving and preventing low back pain and injury (Carpenter and Nelson 1999). A current practice in some low back care programs is to include exercises to increase the strength and endurance of both the abdominal and low back extensor muscles.

To strengthen the low back (lumbar extensor) muscles, **pelvic stabilization** is a key requirement. If the pelvis is not stabilized during extension of the trunk, the hip extensor muscles rotate the pelvis ($\sim 110°$), and the lumbar vertebrae maintain their relative position to each other (do not extend). On the

TABLE 11.2 Sample Flexibility Program

Client data

Age	35 yr
Gender	Female
Body weight	140 lb (63.6 kg)
Program goal	Improve overall flexibility
Time commitment	20-30 min/workout
Number of exercises	12
Method	Static stretching
Intensity	Just below pain threshold
Duration of stretch	10 sec
Repetitions	4-6 per exercise
Total stretch time	50-120 sec per exercise
Frequency	Daily
Overload	Gradually increase stretch duration or repetitions up to a maximum of 2 min per exercise

Exercise[a]	Week	Duration (sec)	Reps	Total time (sec)	Muscle groups
Quad stretch (side lying)	1-3	10	5	50	Quadriceps femoris
	4-6	12	5	60	
	7-9	15	6	90	
Half-straddle stretch*	1-3	10	5	50	Hamstrings; trunk extensors (low back)
	4-6	12	5	60	
	7-9	15	6	90	
Double knee to chest (supine)*	1-3	10	6	60	Hamstrings; trunk extensors (low back)
	4-6	15	6	90	
	7-9	20	6	120	
Butterfly stretch (seated)	1-3	10	5	50	Hip adductors
	4-6	10	6	60	
	7-9	12	6	72	
Trunk flex (hands and knees)*	1-3	15	5	75	Trunk extensors (low back)
	4-6	20	5	100	
	7-9	20	6	120	
Crossed-leg trunk rotation	1-3	10	5	50	Hip abductors; trunk rotators
	4-6	15	5	75	
	7-9	15	6	90	
Achilles (calf) stretch	1-3	10	5	50	Ankle plantar flexors
	4-6	12	5	60	
	7-9	15	5	75	
Pelvic tilt	1-3	15	5	75	Abdominals
	4-6	20	5	100	
	7-9	30	4	120	
Towel stretch (standing)	1-3	10	5	50	Shoulder extensors
	4-6	12	5	60	
	7-9	15	5	75	
Towel stretch (kneeling prone)	1-3	12	5	60	Shoulder flexors
	4-6	15	5	75	
	7-9	20	5	100	
Triceps stretch	1-3	10	5	50	Elbow extensors
	4-6	12	5	60	
	7-9	15	5	75	
Neck rotation	1-3	12	5	60	Neck flexors; neck lateral flexors; neck rotators
	4-6	12	6	72	
	7-9	15	5	75	

[a]For descriptions of exercises, see appendixes F.1 and F.3, pages 352 and 372.

*Two or more exercises are included for the muscle groups with poor flexibility—the hamstrings and trunk extensors (low back).

other hand, when the pelvis is immobilized, the lumbar vertebrae extend ($\sim 72°$) as the low back extensor muscles contract (Carpenter and Nelson 1999). Most calisthenic-type floor exercises do not isolate the low back muscles because the pelvis is free to move. Using a lumbar extension machine, with thigh and femur restraints to stabilize the pelvis, prevents hip extension and isolates the low back muscles during the movement. Exercising on a lumbar extension machine with a minimal training volume (one set of 8 to 15 repetitions of lumbar extension exercise to fatigue per week) significantly improves lumbar muscle strength and bone mineral density (Graves et al. 1994; Pollock, Garzarella, and Graves 1992) and reduces the incidence of back injuries (Mooney, Kron, Rummerfield, and Holmes 1995). Individuals with chronic low back pain who participate in this type of low back-strengthening program can expect significant improvements in joint mobility and muscular strength and endurance, as well as relief from pain (Carpenter and Nelson 1999).

To strengthen the abdominal muscles, select exercises that maximize the activation of the abdominal muscles but minimize the compression (load) of the lumbar vertebrae (i.e., a high challenge : compression ratio). Since the psoas muscle (prime mover for hip flexion) is a major source of spinal loading, choose exercises that minimize the activation of this muscle, such as bent-knee curl-ups (feet free or anchored), dynamic cross-knee curl-ups (curl-ups with a twist), isometric side support (side bridge), and dynamic sideward curl exercises (Axler and McGill 1997; Juker, McGill, Kropf, and Steffen 1998; Knudson 1999). The bent-knee curl-up exercise emphasizes the rectus abdominis, while the isometric side support emphasizes the abdominal oblique and quadratus lumborum muscles. Because of their low challenge to compression ratios, the following abdominal exercises are not recommended: straight-leg or bent-knee sit-ups, supine straight-leg raises, and hanging bent-knee raises (Axler and McGill 1997).

Using the traditional approach, the following exercises are recommended for low back care. Some of these exercises are described and illustrated in appendix F.3, "Exercises for Low Back Care," page 372.

- Pelvic tilt (supine-lying position) to stretch the abdominal muscles
- Knee-to-chest (supine-lying position) to stretch the hamstring, buttock, and low back muscles

- Trunk flex (on hands and knees) to stretch the back, abdominal, and hamstring muscles
- Lumbar extension exercises with pelvic stabilization (on machine) to strengthen the low back extensors
- Curl-ups, dynamic cross-knee curl-ups, and isometric side-support exercises to strengthen the abdominal and quadratus lumborum muscles
- Single-leg extension (prone-lying position) to strengthen the hamstring and buttock muscles and to stretch the hip flexor muscles

A New Approach

Studies suggest that the major cause of low back injury during exercise or performance of activities of daily living is lumbar instability, rather than improper alignment of the spinal column and pelvis per se (McGill 2001). Research also indicates that muscle *endurance* is more protective than muscle *strength* for reducing low back injury and that greater lumbar mobility (ROM) actually increases one's risk of low back injury (McGill 1998, 2001). Thus, sufficient stability of the lumbar spine (i.e., **lumbar stabilization**) is the major emphasis in this new approach to low back care. To measure lumbar stability, see "Lumbar Stability Tests," in chapter 10, page 258. For detailed discussion and suggestions for applying the concept of lumbar stabilization to low back care programs, see Bracko (2004) and Norris (2000).

To develop and maintain lumbar stability, experts (McGill 2001) recommend:

- "Bracing" the lumbar spine during activity by isometrically co-contracting the abdominal wall and low back muscles
- Maintaining a "neutral" spine (i.e., the natural lordotic curve in the lumbar spine while standing upright) during activity
- Avoiding end ROM positions (fully flexed or extended) of the trunk while lifting or exercising
- Performing exercises that emphasize the development of muscle endurance rather than strength

The following sequence of exercises is specifically recommended for beginners who are starting a low back care program. These exercises are illustrated in appendix F.3, "Exercises for Low Back Care," page 372.

- Cat-camel exercise to slowly and dynamically move through the full range of spinal flexion and extension, with emphasis on spinal mobility rather than pressing and holding the trunk position at the ends of the ROM (usually five to six cycles of this exercise are sufficient)
- Stretching exercises to increase mobility at the hip and knee joints
- Curl-ups with one leg flexed and hands placed underneath the lumbar spine to help in maintaining a neutral spine

- Isometric side support (side bridge) exercises for the quadratus lumborum and abdominal oblique muscles
- Single-leg extension holds (modified bird dog exercises) while on hands and knees for the low back and hip extensor muscles
- Isometric stabilization exercises requiring simultaneous contraction of the abdominal muscles to generate an abdominal "brace" during performance of other exercises
- Dynamic "hollowing" or drawing of the navel toward the spine for the deeper abdominal wall muscles (i.e., transverse abdominis and internal obliques)

KEY POINTS

- The specificity, overload, progression, and interindividual variability principles should be applied to designing flexibility programs.
- Three methods of stretching are static, ballistic, and proprioceptive neuromuscular facilitation.
- Typically, larger gains in ROM result from PNF stretching than from ballistic or static stretching.
- The contract-relax (CR) and contract-relax agonist contract (CRAC) are common PNF stretching techniques.
- Ballistic stretching is not recommended because of its high risk for injury and muscle soreness.
- For static stretching programs, gains in ROM are related to the total time the stretch is sustained; total time of stretching is a function of stretch duration and the number of repetitions of the exercise.
- A well-rounded flexibility program includes at least one exercise for each major muscle group.
- Muscle groups should not be stretched beyond the pain-free ROM.

- Typically, the duration of the stretch should be 10 to 15 sec for beginners and no more than 30 sec for more advanced clients.
- Beginners should start with 5 to 6 repetitions of each exercise.
- Flexibility exercises should be performed a minimum of 2 to 3 days/wk, but preferably daily.
- To progressively overload the target muscle group, gradually increase the total time of the stretch (45-120 sec) by increasing the duration of stretch (10-30 sec) and the number of repetitions (3-6 repetitions).
- Stretching does not prevent injury or improve physical performance.
- Lumbar instability is a major cause of low back problems.
- Exercises that develop and maintain lumbar stability are recommended for low back care programs.
- Exercises developing muscle endurance may be more effective than exercises developing muscle strength for the prevention and treatment of low back injuries.

KEY TERMS

Learn the definition of each of the following key terms. Definition of terms can be found in the glossary on page 379.

active stretching

active-assisted stretching

ballistic stretching

contract-relax agonist contract (CRAC) technique

contract-relax (CR) technique

flexibility training

lumbar stabilization

passive stretching

pelvic stabilization

proprioceptive neuromuscular facilitation (PNF)

reciprocal inhibition

static stretching

stress relaxation

stretch tolerance

REVIEW QUESTIONS

In addition to being able to define each of the key terms, test your knowledge and understanding of material by answering the following review questions.

1. Explain why ballistic stretching is not recommended for flexibility programs.

2. Identify two sensory receptors of the musculotendinous unit and explain how each receptor is affected by slow static stretching.

3. What are the physiological mechanisms responsible for gains in ROM from PNF stretching?

4. Identify three high-risk flexibility exercises and suggest safe alternatives.

5. What are the advantages and disadvantages of slow static and PNF stretching?

6. Describe the basic guidelines for designing flexibility programs. Explain how the specificity and overload training principles apply.

7. Explain why stretching does not prevent injury.

8. Describe three abdominal exercises that have high challenge-to-compression ratios.

9. What are the similarities and differences between the traditional and new approaches to low back care programs?

10. Describe the recommended sequence of exercises for beginners starting a low back care program.

Health and Fitness Appraisal

This appendix includes questionnaires and forms that you can duplicate and use for the pretest health screening of your clients. The PAR-Q (appendix A.1) is used to identify individuals who need medical clearance from their physicians before taking any physical fitness tests or starting an exercise program. The Medical History Questionnaire (appendix A.2) is used to obtain a personal and family health history for your client. As part of the pretest health screening, ask your clients if they have any of the conditions or symptoms listed in the Checklist for Signs and Symptoms of Disease (appendix A.3). The PARmed-X (appendix A.4) may be used by physicians to assess and convey medical clearance for physical activity participation of your clients.

You can obtain a lifestyle profile for your clients by using either the Lifestyle Evaluation form or the Fantastic Lifestyle Checklist provided in appendix A.5. Be sure that each participant signs the Informed Consent (appendix A.6) before conducting any physical fitness tests or allowing your client to engage in an exercise program.

You can use the Sample ECG Tracings (appendix A.7) to practice measuring heart rates. Appendix A.8 provides the answers to the questions posed in the sample case study presented in chapter 5 (see p. 111). Appendix A.9 includes Web sites for selected professional organizations and institutes.

Physical Activity Readiness
Questionnaire - PAR-Q
(revised 2002)

PAR-Q & YOU

(A Questionnaire for People Aged 15 to 69)

Regular physical activity is fun and healthy, and increasingly more people are starting to become more active every day. Being more active is very safe for most people. However, some people should check with their doctor before they start becoming much more physically active.

If you are planning to become much more physically active than you are now, start by answering the seven questions in the box below. If you are between the ages of 15 and 69, the PAR-Q will tell you if you should check with your doctor before you start. If you are over 69 years of age, and you are not used to being very active, check with your doctor.

Common sense is your best guide when you answer these questions. Please read the questions carefully and answer each one honestly: check YES or NO.

YES	NO		
☐	☐	1.	**Has your doctor ever said that you have a heart condition <u>and</u> that you should only do physical activity recommended by a doctor?**
☐	☐	2.	**Do you feel pain in your chest when you do physical activity?**
☐	☐	3.	**In the past month, have you had chest pain when you were not doing physical activity?**
☐	☐	4.	**Do you lose your balance because of dizziness or do you ever lose consciousness?**
☐	☐	5.	**Do you have a bone or joint problem (for example, back, knee or hip) that could be made worse by a change in your physical activity?**
☐	☐	6.	**Is your doctor currently prescribing drugs (for example, water pills) for your blood pressure or heart condition?**
☐	☐	7.	**Do you know of <u>any other reason</u> why you should not do physical activity?**

If

you

answered

YES to one or more questions

Talk with your doctor by phone or in person BEFORE you start becoming much more physically active or BEFORE you have a fitness appraisal. Tell your doctor about the PAR-Q and which questions you answered YES.

- You may be able to do any activity you want — as long as you start slowly and build up gradually. Or, you may need to restrict your activities to those which are safe for you. Talk with your doctor about the kinds of activities you wish to participate in and follow his/her advice.
- Find out which community programs are safe and helpful for you.

NO to all questions

If you answered NO honestly to <u>all</u> PAR-Q questions, you can be reasonably sure that you can:

- start becoming much more physically active — begin slowly and build up gradually. This is the safest and easiest way to go.
- take part in a fitness appraisal — this is an excellent way to determine your basic fitness so that you can plan the best way for you to live actively. It is also highly recommended that you have your blood pressure evaluated. If your reading is over 144/94, talk with your doctor before you start becoming much more physically active.

DELAY BECOMING MUCH MORE ACTIVE:

- if you are not feeling well because of a temporary illness such as a cold or a fever — wait until you feel better; or
- if you are or may be pregnant — talk to your doctor before you start becoming more active.

PLEASE NOTE: If your health changes so that you then answer YES to any of the above questions, tell your fitness or health professional. Ask whether you should change your physical activity plan.

<u>Informed Use of the PAR-Q</u>: The Canadian Society for Exercise Physiology, Health Canada, and their agents assume no liability for persons who undertake physical activity, and if in doubt after completing this questionnaire, consult your doctor prior to physical activity.

No changes permitted. You are encouraged to photocopy the PAR-Q but only if you use the entire form.

NOTE: If the PAR-Q is being given to a person before he or she participates in a physical activity program or a fitness appraisal, this section may be used for legal or administrative purposes.

"I have read, understood and completed this questionnaire. Any questions I had were answered to my full satisfaction."

NAME _____

SIGNATURE _____ DATE _____

SIGNATURE OF PARENT _____ WITNESS _____
or GUARDIAN (for participants under the age of majority)

Note: This physical activity clearance is valid for a maximum of 12 months from the date it is completed and becomes invalid if your condition changes so that you would answer YES to any of the seven questions.

CSEP
SCPE © Canadian Society for Exercise Physiology   Supported by: ▪◆▪ Health   Santé   continued on other side...
                                                                  Canada   Canada

...continued from other side

PAR-Q & YOU

Physical Activity Readiness
Questionnaire - PAR-Q
(revised 2002)

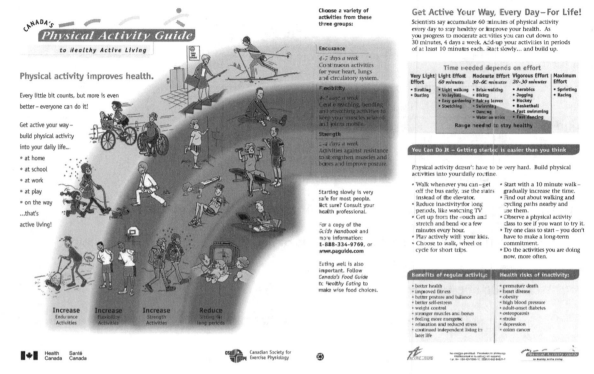

Source: *Canada's Physical Activity Guide to Healthy Active Living,* Health Canada, 1998 *http://www.hc-sc.gc.ca/hppb/paguide/pdf/guideEng.pdf*

© Reproduced with permission from the Minister of Public Works and Government Services Canada, 2002.

FITNESS AND HEALTH PROFESSIONALS MAY BE INTERESTED IN THE INFORMATION BELOW:

The following companion forms are available for doctors' use by contacting the Canadian Society for Exercise Physiology (address below):

The **Physical Activity Readiness Medical Examination (PARmed-X)** – to be used by doctors with people who answer YES to one or more questions on the PAR-Q.

The **Physical Activity Readiness Medical Examination for Pregnancy (PARmed-X for Pregnancy)** – to be used by doctors with pregnant patients who wish to become more active.

References:

Arraix, G.A., Wigle, D.T., Mao, Y. (1992). Risk Assessment of Physical Activity and Physical Fitness in the Canada Health Survey
Follow-Up Study. **J. Clin. Epidemiol.** 45:4 419-428.

Mottola, M., Wolfe, L.A. (1994). Active Living and Pregnancy, In: A. Quinney, L. Gauvin, T. Wall (eds.), **Toward Active Living: Proceedings of the International Conference on Physical Activity, Fitness and Health**. Champaign, IL: Human Kinetics.

PAR-Q Validation Report, British Columbia Ministry of Health, 1978.

Thomas, S., Reading, J., Shephard, R.J. (1992). Revision of the Physical Activity Readiness Questionnaire (PAR-Q). **Can. J. Spt. Sci.** 17:4 338-345.

To order multiple printed copies of the PAR-Q, please contact the:

Canadian Society for Exercise Physiology
202-185 Somerset Street West
Ottawa, ON K2P 0J2
Tel. 1-877-651-3755 • FAX (613) 234-3565
Online: www.csep.ca

The original PAR-Q was developed by the British Columbia Ministry of Health. It has been revised by an Expert Advisory Committee of the Canadian Society for Exercise Physiology chaired by Dr. N. Gledhill (2002).

Disponible en français sous le titre «Questionnaire sur l'aptitude à l'activité physique - Q-AAP (revisé 2002)».

 © Canadian Society for Exercise Physiology

Supported by: Health Canada Santé Canada

Medical History Questionnaire

Demographic Information

Last name	First name	Middle initial
Date of birth	Sex	Home phone
Address	City, State	Zip code
Work phone	Family physician	

Section A

1. When was the last time you had a physical examination?

2. If you are allergic to any medications, foods, or other substances, please name them.

3. If you have been told that you have any chronic or serious illnesses, please list them.

4. Give the following information pertaining to the last 3 times you have been hospitalized. *Note*: Women, do not list normal pregnancies.

	Hospitalization 1	Hospitalization 2	Hospitalization 3
Reason for hospitalization	_____	_____	_____
Month and year of hospitalization	_____	_____	_____
Hospital	_____	_____	_____
City and state	_____	_____	_____

Section B

During the past 12 months

1. Has a physician prescribed any form of medication for you?	Yes	No
2. Has your weight fluctuated more than a few pounds?	Yes	No
3. Did you attempt to bring about this weight change through diet or exercise?	Yes	No
4. Have you experienced any faintness, light-headedness, or blackouts?	Yes	No
5. Have you occasionally had trouble sleeping?	Yes	No
6. Have you experienced any blurred vision?	Yes	No
7. Have you had any severe headaches?	Yes	No
8. Have you experienced chronic morning cough?	Yes	No
9. Have you experienced any temporary change in your speech pattern, such as slurring or loss of speech?	Yes	No
10. Have you felt unusually nervous or anxious for no apparent reason?	Yes	No
11. Have you experienced unusual heartbeats such as skipped beats or palpitations?	Yes	No
12. Have you experienced periods in which your heart felt as though it were racing for no apparent reason?	Yes	No

At present

1. Do you experience shortness or loss of breath while walking with others your own age?   Yes   No

2. Do you experience sudden tingling, numbness, or loss of feeling in your arms, hands, legs, feet, or face?   Yes   No

3. Have you ever noticed that your hands or feet sometimes feel cooler than other parts of your body?   Yes   No

4. Do you experience swelling of your feet and ankles?   Yes   No

5. Do you get pains or cramps in your legs?   Yes   No

6. Do you experience any pain or discomfort in your chest?   Yes   No

7. Do you experience any pressure or heaviness in your chest?   Yes   No

8. Have you ever been told that your blood pressure was abnormal?   Yes   No

9. Have you ever been told that your serum cholesterol or triglyceride level was high?   Yes   No

10. Do you have diabetes?   Yes   No

     If yes, how is it controlled?

     ❏ Dietary means   ❏ Insulin injection

     ❏ Oral medication   ❏ Uncontrolled

11. How often would you characterize your stress level as being high?   Yes   No

     ❏ Occasionally   ❏ Frequently   ❏ Constantly

12. Have you ever been told that you have any of the following illnesses?   Yes   No

     ❏ Myocardial infarction   ❏ Arteriosclerosis   ❏ Heart disease   ❏ Thyroid disease

     ❏ Coronary thrombosis   ❏ Rheumatic heart   ❏ Heart attack   ❏ Heart valve disease

     ❏ Coronary occlusion   ❏ Heart failure   ❏ Heart murmer

     ❏ Heart block   ❏ Aneurysm   ❏ Angina

13. Have you ever had any of the following medical procedures?   Yes   No

     ❏ Heart surgery   ❏ Pacemaker implant

     ❏ Cardiac catheterization   ❏ Defibrilator

     ❏ Coronary angioplasty   ❏ Heart transplantation

Section C

Has any member of your immediate family been treated for or suspected to have had any of these conditions? Please identify their relationship to you (father, mother, sister, brother, etc.).

A. Diabetes

B. Heart disease

C. Stroke

D. High blood pressure

From Vivian H. Heyward, 2006, *Advanced Fitness Assessment and Exercise Prescription*, 5th ed. (Champaign, IL: Human Kinetics).

Checklist for Signs and Symptoms
of Disease

Instructions: Ask your clients if they have any of the following conditions and risk factors. If so, refer them to their physicians to obtain a signed medical clearance prior to any exercise testing or participation. See the glossary on p. 379 for definitions of terms.

Client's name _____ Date _____

Condition	Yes	No	Comments
Cardiovascular			
Hypertension			
Hypercholesterolemia			
Heart murmurs			
Myocardial infarction (heart attack)			
Fainting/dizziness			
Claudication			
Chest pain			
Palpitations			
Ischemia			
Tachycardia (rhythm disturbances)			
Ankle edema			
Stroke			
Pulmonary			
Asthma			
Bronchitis			
Emphysema			
Nocturnal dyspnea			
Coughing up blood			
Exercise-induced asthma			
Breathlessness during or after mild exertion			
Metabolic			
Diabetes			
Obesity			
Glucose intolerance			
McArdle's syndrome			

From Vivian H. Heyward, 2006, *Advanced Fitness Assessment and Exercise Prescription*, 5th ed. (Champaign, IL: Human Kinetics).

APPENDIX A.3

Condition	Yes	No	Comments
Metabolic *(continued)*			
Hypoglycemia			
Thyroid disease			
Cirrhosis			
Musculoskeletal			
Osteoporosis			
Osteoarthritis			
Low back pain			
Prosthesis			
Muscular atrophy			
Swollen joints			
Orthopedic pain			
Artificial joints			
Risk factors*			
Male older than 45 yr			
Female older than 55 yr, or had hysterectomy, or are postmenopausal			
Smoking or quit smoking within previous 6 mo			
Blood pressure > 140/90 mmHg			
Don't know blood pressure			
Taking blood pressure medication			
Blood cholesterol > 200 mg · dl^{-1}			
Do not know cholesterol level			
Have close relative who had heart attack or heart surgery before age 55 (father or brother) or age 65 (mother or sister)			
Physically inactive (<30 min of physical activity more than 4 days/wk)			
Overweight by more than 20 lb (9 kg)			

*If you have two or more risk factors, you should consult your physician before engaging in exercise.

From Vivian H. Heyward, 2006, *Advanced Fitness Assessment and Exercise Prescription*, 5th ed. (Champaign, IL: Human Kinetics).

Physical Activity Readiness
Medical Examination
(revised 2002)

PARmed-X PHYSICAL ACTIVITY READINESS
MEDICAL EXAMINATION

The PARmed-X is a physical activity-specific checklist to be used by a physician with patients
who have had positive responses to the Physical Activity Readiness Questionnaire (PAR-Q). In addition, the
Conveyance/Referral Form in the PARmed-X can be used to convey clearance for physical activity participation,
or to make a referral to a medically-supervised exercise program.

Regular physical activity is fun and healthy, and increasingly more people are starting to become more active every day. Being more active is very safe for most people. The PAR-Q by itself provides adequate screening for the majority of people. However, some individuals may require a medical evaluation and specific advice (exercise prescription) due to one or more positive responses to the PAR-Q.

Following the participant's evaluation by a physician, a physical activity plan should be devised in consultation with a physical activity professional (CSEP-Professional Fitness & Lifestyle Consultant or CSEP-Exercise Therapist™). To assist in this, the following instructions are provided:

PAGE 1: • Sections A, B, C, and D should be completed by the participant BEFORE the examination by the physician. The bottom section is to be completed by the examining physician.

PAGES 2 & 3: • A checklist of medical conditions requiring special consideration and management.

PAGE 4: • Physical Activity & Lifestyle Advice for people who do not require specific instructions or prescribed exercise.

• Physical Activity Readiness Conveyance/Referral Form - an optional tear-off tab for the physician to convey clearance for physical activity participation, or to make a referral to a medically-supervised exercise program.

This section to be completed by the participant

A PERSONAL INFORMATION:

NAME _____

ADDRESS _____

_____

TELEPHONE _____

BIRTHDATE _____ GENDER _____

MEDICAL No. _____

B PAR-Q: Please indicate the PAR-Q questions to which you answered YES

❑	Q 1	Heart condition
❑	Q 2	Chest pain during activity
❑	Q 3	Chest pain at rest
❑	Q 4	Loss of balance, dizziness
❑	Q 5	Bone or joint problem
❑	Q 6	Blood pressure or heart drugs
❑	Q 7	Other reason:

_____

C RISK FACTORS FOR CARDIOVASCULAR DISEASE:
Check all that apply

❑ Less than 30 minutes of moderate physical activity most days of the week.

❑ Currently smoker (tobacco smoking 1 or more times per week).

❑ High blood pressure reported by physician after repeated measurements.

❑ High cholesterol level reported by physician.

❑ Excessive accumulation of fat around waist.

❑ Family history of heart disease.

Please note: Many of these risk factors are modifiable. Please refer to page 4 and discuss with your physician.

D PHYSICAL ACTIVITY INTENTIONS:

What physical activity do you intend to do?

_____

_____

_____

This section to be completed by the examining physician

Physical Exam:

Ht	Wt	BP	i)	/
		BP	ii)	/

Conditions limiting physical activity:

❑ Cardiovascular ❑ Respiratory ❑ Other
❑ Musculoskeletal ❑ Abdominal

Tests required:

❑ ECG ❑ Exercise Test ❑ X-Ray
❑ Blood ❑ Urinalysis ❑ Other

Physical Activity Readiness Conveyance/Referral:

Based upon a current review of health status, I recommend:

Further Information:
❑ Attached
❑ To be forwarded
❑ Available on request

❑ No physical activity

❑ Only a medically-supervised exercise program until further medical clearance

❑ Progressive physical activity:

  ❑ with avoidance of: _____

  ❑ with inclusion of: _____

  ❑ under the supervision of a CSEP-Professional Fitness & Lifestyle Consultant or CSEP-Exercise Therapist™

❑ Unrestricted physical activity–start slowly and build up gradually

CSEP
SCPE © Canadian Society for Exercise Physiology

Supported by: Health Santé
Canada Canada

1

PARmed-X
PHYSICAL ACTIVITY READINESS MEDICAL EXAMINATION

Following is a checklist of medical conditions for which a degree of precaution and/or special advice should be considered for those who answered "YES" to one or more questions on the PAR-Q, and people over the age of 69. Conditions are grouped by system. Three categories of precautions are provided. Comments under Advice are general, since details and alternatives require clinical judgement in each individual instance.

	Absolute Contraindications	Relative Contraindications	Special Prescriptive Conditions	ADVICE
	Permanent restriction or temporary restriction until condition is treated, stable, and/or past acute phase.	Highly variable. Value of exercise testing and/or program may exceed risk. Activity may be restricted. Desirable to maximize control of condition. Direct or indirect medical supervision of exercise program may be desirable.	Individualized prescriptive advice generally appropriate: • limitations imposed; and/or • special exercises prescribed. May require medical monitoring and/or initial supervision in exercise program.	

Cardiovascular	❑ aortic aneurysm (dissecting)
	❑ aortic stenosis (severe)
	❑ congestive heart failure
	❑ crescendo angina
	❑ myocardial infarction (acute)
	❑ myocarditis (active or recent)
	❑ pulmonary or systemic embolism—acute
	❑ thrombophlebitis
	❑ ventricular tachycardia and other dangerous dysrhythmias (e.g., multi-focal ventricular activity)
		❑ aortic stenosis (moderate)
		❑ subaortic stenosis (severe)
		❑ marked cardiac enlargement
		❑ supraventricular dysrhythmias (uncontrolled or high rate)
		❑ ventricular ectopic activity (repetitive or frequent)
		❑ ventricular aneurysm
		❑ hypertension—untreated or uncontrolled severe (systemic or pulmonary)
		❑ hypertrophic cardiomyopathy
		❑ compensated congestive heart failure
			❑ aortic (or pulmonary) stenosis—mild angina pectoris and other manifestations of coronary insufficiency (e.g., post-acute infarct)
			❑ cyanotic heart disease
			❑ shunts (intermittent or fixed)
			❑ conduction disturbances
			  • complete AV block
			  • left BBB
			  • Wolff-Parkinson-White syndrome
			❑ dysrhythmias—controlled
			❑ fixed rate pacemakers
				• clinical exercise test may be warranted in selected cases, for specific determination of functional capacity and limitations and precautions (if any).
				• slow progression of exercise to levels based on test performance and individual tolerance.
				• consider individual need for initial conditioning program under medical supervision (indirect or direct).

			❑ intermittent claudication	progressive exercise to tolerance
			❑ hypertension: systolic 160-180; diastolic 105+	progressive exercise; care with medications (serum electrolytes; post-exercise syncope; etc.)
Infections	❑ acute infectious disease (regardless of etiology)	❑ subacute/chronic/recurrent infectious diseases (e.g. malaria, others)	❑ chronic infections ❑ HIV	variable as to condition
Metabolic		❑ uncontrolled metabolic disorders (diabetes mellitus, thyrotoxicosis, myxedema)	❑ renal, hepatic & other metabolic insufficiency	variable as to status
			❑ obesity ❑ single kidney	dietary moderation, and initial light exercises with slow progression (walking, swimming, cycling)
Pregnancy		❑ complicated pregnancy (e.g., toxemia, hemorrhage, incompetent cervix, etc.)	❑ advanced pregnancy (late 3rd trimester)	refer to the "PARmed-X for PREGNANCY"

References:

Arraix, G.A., Wigle, D.T., Mao, Y. (1992). Risk Assessment of Physical Activity and Physical Fitness in the Canada Health Survey Follow-Up Study. **J. Clin. Epidemiol.** 45:4 419-428.

Mottola, M., Wolfe, L.A. (1994). Active Living and Pregnancy, In: A. Quinney, L. Gauvin, T. Wall (eds.), **Toward Active Living: Proceedings of the International Conference on Physical Activity, Fitness and Health.** Champaign, IL: Human Kinetics.

PAR-Q Validation Report. British Columbia Ministry of Health, 1978.

Thomas, S., Reading, J., Shephard, R.J. (1992). Revision of the Physical Activity Readiness Questionnaire (PAR-Q). **Can. J. Spt. Sci.** 17: 4 338-345.

The PAR-Q and PARmed-X were developed by the British Columbia Ministry of Health. They have been revised by an Expert Advisory Committee of the Canadian Society for Exercise Physiology chaired by Dr. N. Gledhill (2002).

No changes permitted. You are encouraged to photocopy the PARmed-X, but only if you use the entire form

Disponible en français sous le titre
«Évaluation médicale de l'aptitude à l'activité physique (X-AAP)»

Continued on page 3...

2

	Special Prescriptive Conditions	**ADVICE**
Lung	❏ chronic pulmonary disorders	special relaxation and breathing exercises
	❏ obstructive lung disease	breath control during endurance exercises to tolerance; avoid polluted air
	❏ asthma	
	❏ exercise-induced bronchospasm	avoid hyperventilation during exercise; avoid extremely cold conditions; warm up adequately; utilize appropriate medication.
Musculoskeletal	❏ low back conditions (pathological, functional)	avoid or minimize exercise that precipitates or exasperates e.g., forced extreme flexion, extension, and violent twisting; correct posture, proper back exercises
	❏ arthritis—acute (infective, rheumatoid; gout)	treatment, plus judicious blend of rest, splinting and gentle movement
	❏ arthritis—subacute	progressive increase of active exercise therapy
	❏ arthritis—chronic (osteoarthritis and above conditions)	maintenance of mobility and strength; non-weightbearing exercises to minimize joint trauma (e.g., cycling, aquatic activity, etc.)
	❏ orthopaedic	highly variable and individualized
	❏ hernia	minimize straining and isometrics; stregthen abdominal muscles
	❏ osteoporosis or low bone density	avoid exercise with high risk for fracture such as push-ups, curl-ups, vertical jump and trunk forward flexion; engage in low-impact weight-bearing activities and resistance training
CNS	❏ convulsive disorder not completely controlled by medication	minimize or avoid exercise in hazardous environments and/or exercising alone (e.g., swimming, mountainclimbing, etc.)
	❏ recent concussion	thorough examination if history of two concussions; review for discontinuation of contact sport if three concussions, depending on duration of unconsciousness, retrograde amnesia, persistent headaches, and other objective evidence of cerebral damage
Blood	❏ anemia—severe (< 10 Gm/dl)	control preferred; exercise as tolerated
	❏ electrolyte disturbances	
Medications	❏ antianginal ❏ antiarrhythmic ❏ antihypertensive ❏ anticonvulsant ❏ beta-blockers ❏ digitalis preparations ❏ diuretics ❏ ganglionic blockers ❏ others	NOTE: consider underlying condition. Potential for: exertional syncope, electrolyte imbalance, bradycardia, dysrhythmias, impaired coordination and reaction time, heat intolerance. May alter resting and exercise ECG's and exercise test performance.
Other	❏ post-exercise syncope	moderate program
	❏ heat intolerance	prolong cool-down with light activities; avoid exercise in extreme heat
	❏ temporary minor illness	postpone until recovered
	❏ cancer	if potential metastases, test by cycle ergometry, consider non-weight bearing exercises; exercise at lower end of prescriptive range (40-65% of heart rate reserve), depending on condition and recent treatment (radiation, chemotherapy); monitor hemoglobin and lymphocyte counts; add dynamic lifting exercise to strengthen muscles, using machines rather than weights.

*Refer to special publications for elaboration as required

The following companion forms are available online: http://www.csep.ca/forms.asp

The **Physical Activity Readiness Questionnaire (PAR-Q)** - a questionnaire for people aged 15-69 to complete before becoming much more physically active.

The **Physical Activity Readiness Medical Examination for Pregnancy (PARmed-X for PREGNANCY)** - to be used by physicians with pregnant patients who wish to become more physically active.

For more information, please contact the:

Canadian Society for Exercise Physiology
202 - 185 Somerset St. West
Ottawa, ON K2P 0J2
Tel. 1-877-651-3755 • FAX (613) 234-3565 • Online: www.csep.ca

Note to physical activity professionals...

It is a prudent practice to retain the completed Physical Activity Readiness Conveyance/Referral Form in the participant's file.

 © Canadian Society for Exercise Physiology

Supported by: Health Santé
Canada Canada

Continued on page 4...

3

PARmed-X PHYSICAL ACTIVITY READINESS MEDICAL EXAMINATION

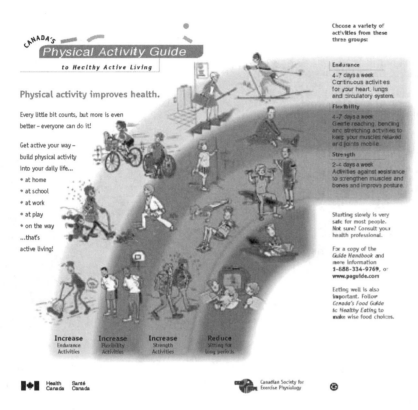

Choose a variety of activities from these three groups:

Endurance
4-7 days a week
Continuous activities for your heart, lungs and circulatory system.

Flexibility
4-7 days a week
Gentle reaching, bending and stretching activities to keep your muscles relaxed and joints mobile.

Strength
2-4 days a week
Activities against resistance to strengthen muscles and bones and improve posture.

Starting slowly is very safe for most people. Not sure? Consult your health professional.

For a copy of the *Guide Handbook* and more information
1-888-334-9769, or
www.paguide.com

Eating well is also important. Follow *Canada's Food Guide to Healthy Eating* to make wise food choices.

Physical activity improves health.

Every little bit counts, but more is even better – everyone can do it!

Get active your way – build physical activity into your daily life...
* at home
* at school
* at work
* at play
* on the way
...that's active living!

Increase Endurance Activities   **Increase** Flexibility Activities   **Increase** Strength Activities   **Reduce** Sitting for long periods.

Get Active Your Way, Every Day–For Life!

Scientists say accumulate 60 minutes of physical activity every day to stay healthy or improve your health. As you progress to moderate activities you can cut down to 30 minutes, 4 days a week. Add-up your activities in periods of at least 10 minutes each. Start slowly... and build up.

Time needed depends on effort

Very Light Effort	Light Effort 60 minutes	Moderate Effort 30-60 minutes	Vigorous Effort 20-30 minutes	Maximum Effort
• Strolling • Dusting	• Light walking • Volleyball • Easy gardening • Stretching	• Brisk walking • Biking • Raking leaves • Swimming • Dancing • Water aerobics	• Aerobics • Jogging • Hockey • Basketball • Fast swimming • Fast dancing	• Sprinting • Racing

Range needed to stay healthy

You Can Do It – Getting started is easier than you think

Physical activity doesn't have to be very hard. Build physical activities into your daily routine.

* Walk whenever you can – get off the bus early, use the stairs instead of the elevator.
* Reduce inactivity for long periods, like watching TV.
* Get up from the couch and stretch and bend for a few minutes every hour.
* Play actively with your kids.
* Choose to walk, wheel or cycle for short trips.

* Start with a 10 minute walk – gradually increase the time.
* Find out about walking and cycling paths nearby and use them.
* Observe a physical activity class to see if you want to try it.
* Try one class to start – you don't have to make a long-term commitment.
* Do the activities you are doing now, more often.

Benefits of regular activity:	Health risks of inactivity:
• better health • improved fitness • better posture and balance • better self-esteem • weight control • stronger muscles and bones • feeling more energetic • relaxation and reduced stress • continued independent living in later life	• premature death • heart disease • obesity • high blood pressure • adult-onset diabetes • osteoporosis • stroke • depression • colon cancer

 Health Canada / Santé Canada   Canadian Society for Exercise Physiology

Source: Canada's Physical Activity Guide to Healthy Active Living, Health Canada, 1998 http://www.hc-sc.gc.ca/hppb/paguide/pdf/guideEng.pdf
© Reproduced with permission from the Minister of Public Works and Government Services Canada, 2002.

PARmed-X Physical Activity Readiness Conveyance/Referral Form

Based upon a current review of the health status of _____ I recommend:

❑ No physical activity

❑ Only a medically-supervised exercise program until further medical clearance

❑ Progressive physical activity

    ❑ with avoidance of: _____

    ❑ with inclusion of: _____

    ❑ under the supervision of a CSEP-Professional Fitness & Lifestyle Consultant or CSEP-Exercise Therapist™

❑ Unrestricted physical activity — start slowly and build up gradually

Further Information:
❑ Attached
❑ To be forwarded
❑ Available on request

Physician/clinic stamp:

_____ M.D.

_____ 20_____
        (date)

NOTE: This physical activity clearance is valid for a maximum of six months from the date it is completed and becomes invalid if your medical condition becomes worse.

4

Source: Physical Activity Readiness Medical Examination (PARmed-X), ©2002. Reprinted with permission from the Canadian Society for Exercise Physiology.
http://www.csep.ca/forms.asp

Lifestyle Evaluation

Smoking habits

   1. Have you ever smoked cigarettes, cigars, or a pipe?   Yes   No

   2. Do you smoke presently?   Yes   No

            Cigarettes _____ a day

            Cigars _____ a day

            Pipefuls _____ a day

   3. At what age did you start smoking? _____ years

   4. If you have quit smoking, when did you quit? _____

Drinking habits

   1. During the past month, how many days did you drink alcoholic beverages? _____

   2. During the past month, how many times did you have 5 or more drinks per occasion? _____

   3. On average, how many glasses of beer, wine, or highballs do you consume a week?

            Beer _____ glasses or cans

            Wine _____ glasses

            Highballs _____ glasses

            Other _____ glasses

Exercise habits

   1. Do you exercise vigorously on a regular basis?   Yes   No

   2. What activities do you engage in on a regular basis?

   3. If you walk, run, or jog, what is the average number of miles you cover each workout? _____ miles

   4. How many minutes on the average is each of your exercise workouts? _____ minutes

   5. How many workouts a week do you participate in on average? _____ workouts

   6. Is your occupation?

            _____ Inactive (e.g., desk job)

            _____ Light work (e.g., housework, light carpentry)

            _____ Heavy work (e.g., heavy carpentry, lifting)

   7. Check those activities that you would prefer in a regular exercise program for yourself:

_____ Walking, running, or jogging	_____ Handball, racquetball, or squash
_____ Stationary running	_____ Basketball
_____ Jumping rope	_____ Swimming
_____ Bicycling	_____ Tennis
_____ Stationary cycling	_____ Aerobic dance
_____ Step aerobics	_____ Stair-climbing
	_____ Other (specify)

From Vivian H. Heyward, 2006, *Advanced Fitness Assessment and Exercise Prescription*, 5th ed. (Champaign, IL: Human Kinetics).

                                                        APPENDIX A.5

Dietary habits

1. What is your current weight? ____ lb ____ kg height? ____ in. ____ cm
2. What would you like to weigh? ____ lb ____ kg
3. What is the most you ever weighed as an adult? ____ lb ____ kg
4. What is the least you ever weighed as an adult? ____ lb ____ kg
5. What weight-loss methods have you tried? _____

_____

6. Which do you eat regularly?

❑ Breakfast ❑ Midafternoon snack

❑ Midmorning snack ❑ Dinner

❑ Lunch ❑ After-dinner snack

7. How often do you eat out each week? _____ times
8. What size portions do you normally have?

❑ Small ❑ Moderate ❑ Large ❑ Extra large ❑ Uncertain

9. How often do you eat more than one serving?

❑ Always ❑ Usually ❑ Sometimes ❑ Never

10. How long does it usually take you to eat a meal? _____ minutes
11. Do you eat while doing other activities (e.g., watching TV, reading, working)? _____
12. When you snack, how many times a week do you eat the following?

Cookies, cake, pie ____ Candy ____ Diet soda ____

Soft drinks ____ Doughnuts ____ Fruit ____

Milk or milk beverage ____ Potato chips, pretzels, etc. ____

Peanuts or other nuts ____ Ice cream ____

Cheese and crackers ____ Other _____

13. How often do you eat dessert? _____ times a day _____ times a week
14. What dessert do you eat most often? _____
15. How often do you eat fried foods? _____ times a week
16. Do you salt your food at the table? ❑ Yes ❑ No

❑ Before tasting it ❑ After tasting it

From Vivian H. Heyward, 2006, *Advanced Fitness Assessment and Exercise Prescription*, 5th ed. (Champaign, IL: Human Kinetics).

Fantastic Lifestyle Checklist

INSTRUCTIONS: Unless otherwise specified, place an 'X' beside the box which best describes your behaviour or situation in the past month. Explanations of questions and scoring are provided on the next page.

FAMILY FRIENDS	I have someone to talk to about things that are important to me	almost never	seldom	some of the time	fairly often	almost always
	I give and receive affection	almost never	seldom	some of the time	fairly often	almost always
ACTIVITY	I am vigorously active for at least 30 minutes per day e.g., running, cycling, etc.	less than once/week	1-2 times/week	3 times/week	4 times/week	5 or more times/week
	I am moderately active (gardening, climbing stairs, walking, housework)	less than once/week	1-2 times/week	3 times/week	4 times/week	5 or more times/week
NUTRITION	I eat a balanced diet (see explanation)	almost never	seldom	some of the time	fairly often	almost always
	I often eat excess 1) sugar, or 2) salt, or 3) animal fats, or 4) junk foods.	four of these	three of these	two of these	one of these	none of these
	I am within ____ kg of my healthy weight	not within 8 kg	8 kg (20 lbs)	6 kg (15 lbs)	4 kg (10 lbs)	2 kg (5 lbs)
TOBACCO TOXICS	I smoke tobacco	more than 10 times/week	1 - 10 times/week	none in the past 6 months	none in the past year	none in the past 5 years
	I use drugs such as marijuana, cocaine	sometimes				never
	I overuse prescribed or 'over the counter' drugs	almost daily	fairly often	only occasionally	almost never	never
	I drink caffeine-containing coffee, tea, or cola	more than 10/day	7-10/day	3-6/day	1-2/day	never
ALCOHOL	My average alcohol intake per week is ____ (see explanation)	more than 20 drinks	13-20 drinks	11-12 drinks	8-10 drinks	0-7 drinks
	I drink more than four drinks on an occasion	almost daily	fairly often	only occasionally	almost never	never
	I drive after drinking	sometimes				never
SLEEP SEATBELTS STRESS SAFE SEX	I sleep well and feel rested	almost never	seldom	some of the time	fairly often	almost always
	I use seatbelts	never	seldom	some of the time	most of the time	always
	I am able to cope with the stresses in my life	almost never	seldom	some of the time	fairly often	almost always
	I relax and enjoy leisure time	almost never	seldom	some of the time	fairly often	almost always
	I practice safe sex (see explanation)	almost never	seldom	some of the time	fairly often	always
TYPE of behaviour	I seem to be in a hurry	almost always	fairly often	some of the time	seldom	almost never
	I feel angry or hostile	almost always	fairly often	some of the time	seldom	almost never
INSIGHT	I am a postive or optimistic thinker	almost never	seldom	some of the time	fairly often	almost always
	I feel tense or uptight	almost always	fairly often	some of the time	seldom	almost never
	I feel sad or depressed	almost always	fairly often	some of the time	seldom	almost never
CAREER	I am satisfied with my job or role	almost never	seldom	some of the time	fairly often	almost always

STEP 1 Total the X's in each column → [ ] [ ] [ ] [ ] [ ]

STEP 2 Multiply the totals by the numbers indicated (write your answer in the box below) → 0   x 1   x 2   x 3   x 4

STEP 3 Add your scores across the bottom for your grand total → [ ] + [ ] + [ ] + [ ] = [ ]

Grand total (see explantion)

APPENDIX A.5

▼ A BALANCED DIET:

According to Canada's Food Guide to Healthy Eating (for people four years and over):

Different People Need Different Amounts of Food

The amount of food you need every day from the 4 food groups and other foods depends on your age, body size, activity level, whether you are male or female and if your are pregnant or breast feeding. That's why the Food Guide gives a lower and higher number of servings for each food group. For example, young children can choose the lower number of servings, while male teenagers can select the higher number. Most other people can choose servings somewhere in between.

Grain Products	Vegetables & Fruit	Milk Products	Meat & Alternatives	Other Foods
Choose whole grain and enriched products more often.	Choose dark green and orange vegetables more often.	Choose lower fat milk products more often.	Choose leaner meats, poultry and fish, as well as dried peas, beans and lentils more often.	Taste and enjoyment can also come from other foods and beverages that are not part of the 4 food groups. Some of these are higher in fat or calories, so use these foods in moderation.

recommended number of servings per day:

5-12	5-10	Children 4-9 years: 2-3 Youth 10-16 years: 3-4 Adults: 2-4 Pregnant and breast-feeding women: 3-4	2-3	

▼ ALCOHOL INTAKE:

1 drink equals:

		Canadian	Metric	U.S.
1 bottle of beer	5% alcohol	12 cz.	340.8 ml	10 oz.
1 glass wine	12% alcohol	5 oz.	142 ml	4.5 oz
1 shot spirits	40% alcohol	1.5 oz	42.6 ml	1.25 oz.

▼ SAFE SEX:

Refers to the use of methods of preventing infection or conception.

WHAT DOES THE SCORE MEAN?

➥	85-100	70-84	55-69	35-54	0-34
	EXCELLENT	VERY GOOD	GOOD	FAIR	NEEDS IMPROVEMENT

NOTE: A low total score does not mean that you have failed. There is always the chance to change your lifestyle — starting now. Look at the areas where you scored a 0 or 1 and decide which areas you want to work on first.

TIPS:

1. Don't try to change all the areas at once. This will be too overwhelming for you.

2. Writing down your proposed changes and your overall goal will help you to succeed.

3. Make changes in small steps towards the overall goal.

4. Enlist the help of a friend to make similar changes and/or to support you in your attempts.

5. Congratulate yourself for achieving each step. Give yourself appropriate rewards.

6. Ask your physical activity professional (CSEP-Professional Fitness and Lifestyle Consultant), family physician, nurse or health department for more information on any of these areas.

From Vivian H. Heyward, 2006, *Advanced Fitness Assessment and Exercise Prescription*, 5th ed. (Champaign, IL: Human Kinetics). Adapted from D. Wilson, 1998, *Fantastic lifestyle assessment, as it appears in CSEP's The Canadian physical activity, fitness, and lifestyle appraisal*, 2nd ed.

Informed Consent

In order to assess cardiovascular function, body composition, and other physical fitness components, the undersigned hereby voluntarily consents to engage in one or more of the following tests (check the appropriate boxes):

❐ Graded exercise stress test
❐ Body composition tests
❐ Muscle fitness tests
❐ Flexibility tests

Explanation of the tests

The graded exercise test is performed on a cycle ergometer or motor-driven treadmill. The workload is increased every few minutes until exhaustion or until other symptoms dictate that we terminate the test. You may stop the test at any time because of fatigue or discomfort.

The underwater weighing procedure involves being completely submerged in a tank or tub after fully exhaling the air from your lungs. You will be submerged for 3 to 5 seconds while we measure your underwater weight. This test provides an accurate assessment of your body composition.

For muscle fitness testing, you lift weights for a number of repetitions using barbells or exercise machines. These tests assess the strength and endurance of the major muscle groups in the body.

For evaluation of flexibility, you perform a number of tests. During these tests, we measure the range of motion in your joints.

Risks and discomforts

During the graded exercise test, certain changes may occur. These changes include abnormal blood pressure responses, fainting, irregularities in heartbeat, and heart attack. Every effort is made to minimize these occurrences. Emergency equipment and trained personnel are available to deal with these situations if they occur.

You may experience some discomfort during the underwater weighing, especially after you expire all the air from your lungs. However, this discomfort is momentary, lasting only 3 to 5 seconds. If this test causes you too much discomfort, an alternative procedure (e.g., skinfold or bioelectrical impedance test) can be used to estimate your body composition.

There is a slight possibility of pulling a muscle or spraining a ligament during the muscle fitness and flexibility testing. In addition, you may experience muscle soreness 24 or 48 hours after testing. These risks can be minimized by performing warm-up exercises prior to taking the tests. If muscle soreness occurs, appropriate stretching exercises to relieve this soreness will be demonstrated.

Expected benefits from testing

These tests allow us to assess your physical working capacity and to appraise your physical fitness status. The results are used to prescribe a safe, sound exercise program for you. Records are kept strictly confidential unless you consent to release this information.

Inquiries

Questions about the procedures used in the physical fitness tests are encouraged. If you have any questions or need additional information, please ask us to explain further.

From Vivian H. Heyward, 2006, *Advanced Fitness Assessment and Exercise Prescription*, 5th ed. (Champaign, IL: Human Kinetics).

APPENDIX A.6

Freedom of Consent

Your permission to perform these physical fitness tests is strictly voluntary. You are free to stop the tests at any point, if you so desire.

_____

I have read this form carefully and I fully understand the test procedures that I will perform and the risks and discomforts. Knowing these risks and having had the opportunity to ask questions that have been answered to my satisfaction, I consent to participate in these tests.

Date	Signature of patient
Date	Signature of witness
Date	Signature of supervisor

From Vivian H. Heyward, 2006 *Advanced Fitness Assessment and Exercise Prescription* 5th ed. (Champaign, IL: Human Kinetics).

Sample ECG Tracings

Directions: Use these ECG tracings to practice techniques described in chapter 2 for measuring heart rate from ECG recordings.

3 Lead
ST Lead V5
Speed   MPH
Filter on

Date 1/27/1995 9:48A
Resting
Level +0.7 Slope +4 HR 65
Grade 0.0%
Gain x1   25 mm/sec

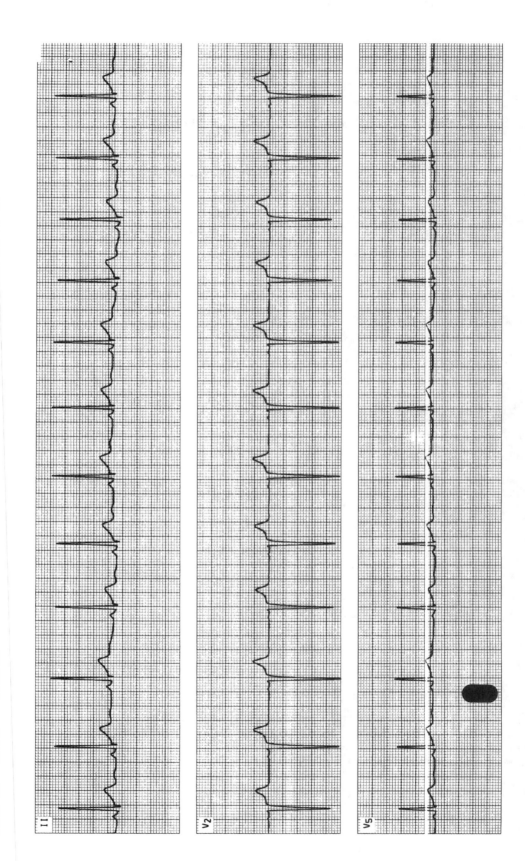

From Vivian H. Heyward, 2006, *Advanced Fitness Assessment and Exercise Prescription*, 5th ed. (Champaign, IL: Human Kinetics).

12 Lead Sml
ST Lead V5
Speed

Date 11/06/1996 11:44A
Resting
Level -0.1 Slope +4 HR 106
MPH Grade 0.0%
Gain x1 25 mm/sec

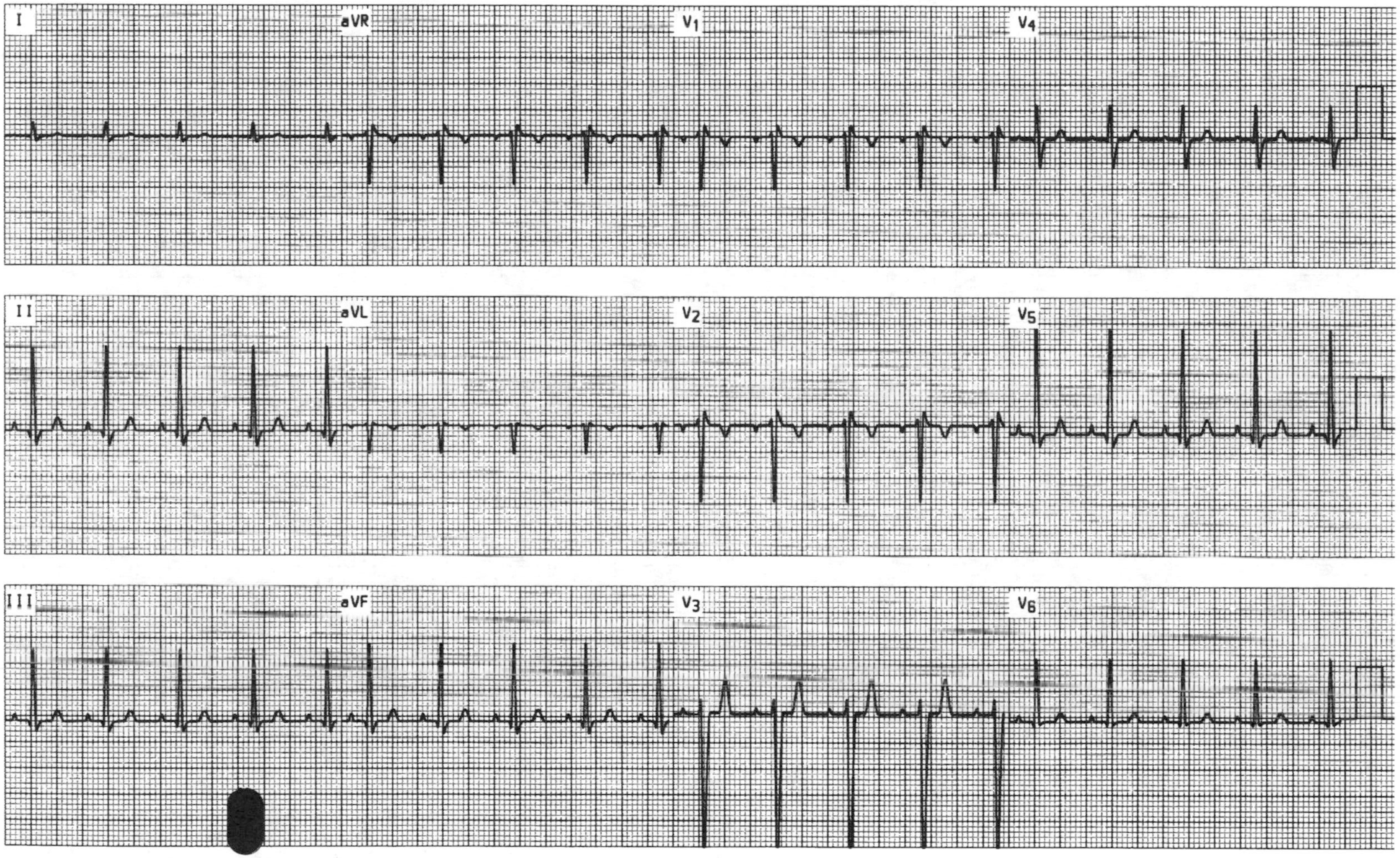

From Vivian H. Heyward, 2006. *Advanced Fitness Assessment and Exercise Prescription*, 5th ed. (Champaign, IL: Human Kinetics).

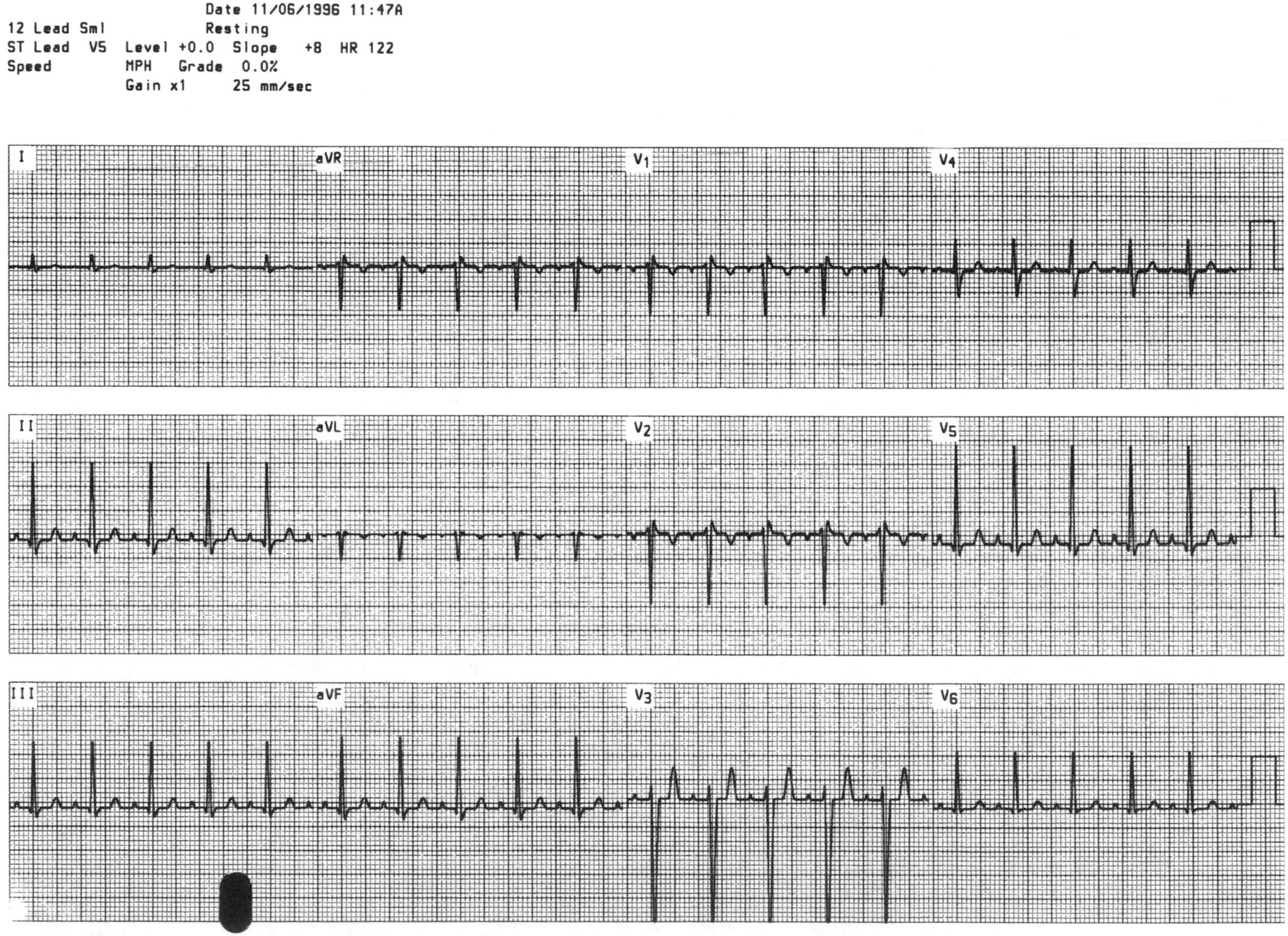

12 Lead Sml   Date 11/06/1996 11:47A
ST Lead   V5   Resting
Speed   Level +0.0 Slope +8   HR 122
                  MPH Grade 0.0%
                  Gain x1   25 mm/sec

I

aVR

V1

V4

II

aVL

V2

V5

III

aVF

V3

V6

From Vivian H. Heyward, 2006, *Advanced Fitness Assessment and Exercise Prescription*, 5th ed. (Champaign, IL: Human Kinetics).

12 Lead Sml   Date 11/06/1996 11:48A
ST Lead V5   Resting
Speed   Level -0.1 Slope +2 HR 134
              MPH Grade 0.0%
              Gain x1   25 mm/sec

From Vivian H. Heyward, 2006, *Advanced Fitness Assessment and Exercise Prescription*, 5th ed. (Champaign, IL: Human Kinetics).

12 Lead Sml
Date 11/06/1996 11:49A
ST Lead V5   Resting
Speed   Level -0.1 Slope +2 HR 147
              MPH Grade 0.0%
              Gain x1   25 mm/sec

From Vivian H. Heyward, 2006, *Advanced Fitness Assessment and Exercise Prescription*, 5th ed. (Champaign, IL: Human Kinetics).

12 Lead Sml   Date 11/06/1996 11:50A
ST Lead V5   Resting
Speed   Level +0.1 Slope +4 HR 155
                     MPH   Grade 0.0%
                     Gain x1   25 mm/sec

From Vivian H. Heyward, 2006, *Advanced Fitness Assessment and Exercise Prescription*, 5th ed. (Champaign, IL: Human Kinetics).

12 Lead Sml   Date 11/06/1996 11:52A
ST Lead   V5   Level -0.2   Slope   +4   HR 170
Speed   MPH   Grade   0.0%
           Gain x1   25 mm/sec

Resting

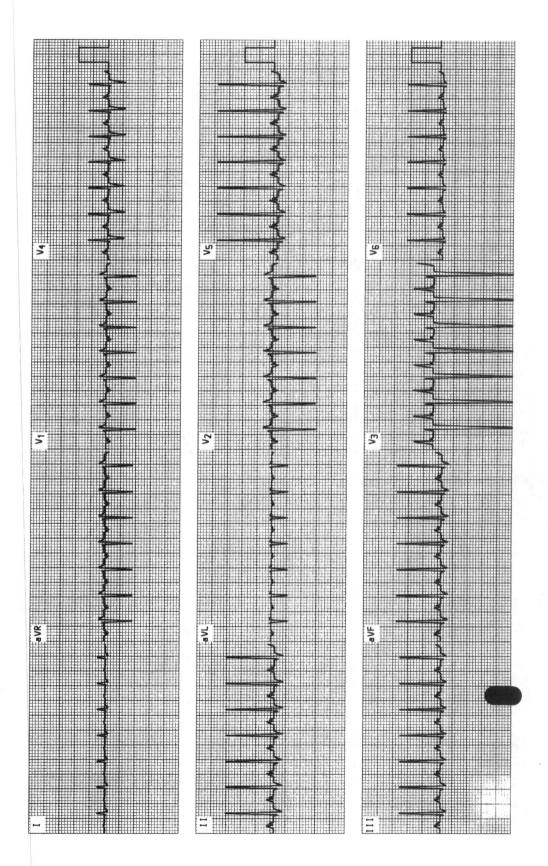

From Vivian H. Heyward, 2006, *Advanced Fitness Assessment and Exercise Prescription*, 5th ed. (Champaign, IL: Human Kinetics).

12 Lead Sml   Date 11/06/1996 11:54A
ST Lead   V5   Resting
Speed   Level -0.1 Slope +4 HR 190
                   MPH   Grade 0.0%
                   Gain x1   25 mm/sec

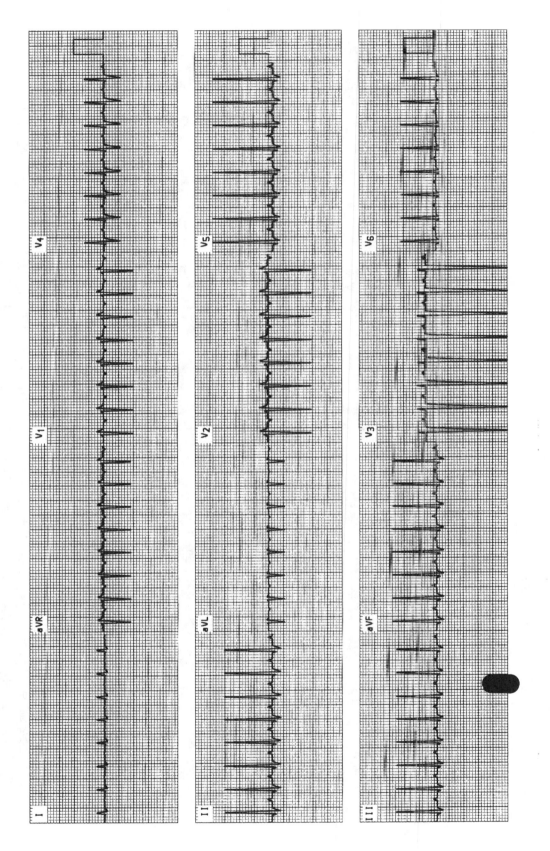

12 Lead Sml
ST Lead V5
Speed

Date 11/06/1996 11:57A
Resting
Level +0.0 Slope +2 HR 217
MPH   Grade 0.0%
Gain x1   25 mm/sec

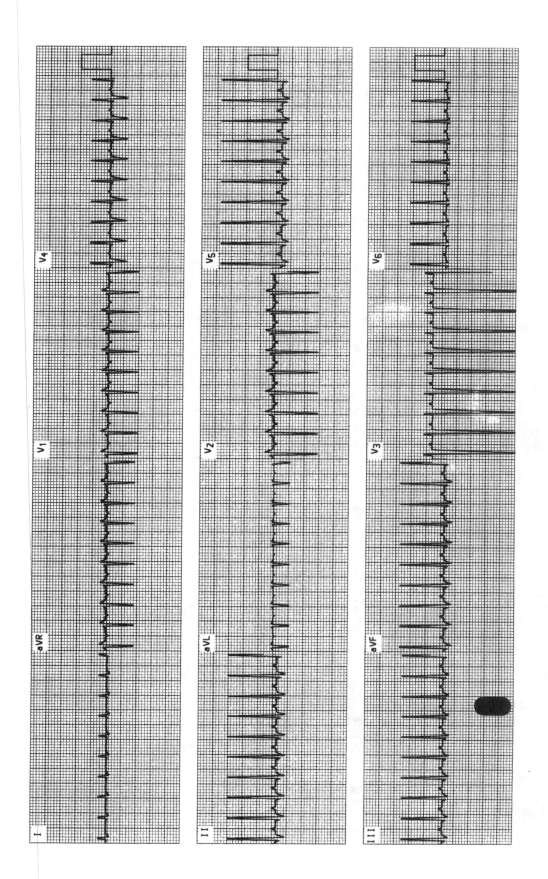

APPENDIX A.7

Analysis of Sample Case Study
in Chapter 5

1. CHD Risk Profile

This client has risk factors for CHD. Her total cholesterol (TC; 220 mg $\cdot$ dl^{-1}) is borderline high (200 to 230 mg $\cdot$ dl^{-1}), and her blood pressure (140/82 mmHg) is categorized as Stage I hypertension (140 to 159 mm Hg). Also, her HDL-C (37 mg $\cdot$ dl^{-1}) and TC/HDL ratio (5.9) place her at higher risk (< 40 mg $\cdot$ dl^{-1} and > 5.0, respectively). She quit smoking cigarettes (one pack a day) three years ago, which is a step in the right direction. Following the National Cholesterol Education Program's recommendation, you should encourage this client to have her LDL-C assessed to determine if she needs a cholesterol treatment program. Engaging in an aerobic exercise program should lower her systolic blood pressure. Her triglycerides and blood glucose levels are normal. She should be encouraged to dine out less frequently and to eat three well-balanced meals a day. When dining out, she should select foods that are low in saturated fat, cholesterol, and sodium. This may help to lower her blood cholesterol and blood pressure.

The client is also at greater risk because of

- the high stress associated with her job (police officer) and lifestyle (divorced parent raising two children),
- family history of cardiovascular disease, and
- physical inactivity (she does not exercise regularly outside of work-related physical activity).

2. Special Considerations

The client has not exercised aerobically for the past six years, and she has gained 15 lb during that time. It is likely that she will experience some discomfort when she starts her aerobic exercise program. Thus, it is important to initially prescribe low-intensity exercise to minimize her physical discomfort.

You also need to consider her busy schedule to find a convenient time for her to exercise. She reports feeling dizzy after eating. The likely reason is that she is eating only one meal a day, and the insulin surge after eating is lowering her blood glucose level. It is important to convince this client to start eating at least three meals a day to avoid this problem.

3. HR, BP, and RPE Responses to Graded Exercise Test

The client's HR response to the graded exercise test was normal. The exercise HR increased during each stage of the exercise test. The maximal heart rate (190 bpm) was very close to her age-predicted maximal HR (220 − 28 = 192 bpm). The client's BP response to the graded exercise test was normal. The diastolic BP remained fairly constant (78 to 82 mmHg), and the systolic BP increased with each stage of the exercise test. The RPEs were normal. The ratings increased linearly with exercise intensity.

4. Functional Aerobic Capacity

The graded exercise test was voluntarily terminated by the client due to fatigue. This was most likely a maximal-effort exercise test as indicated by the RPE (18) and the exercise heart rate (190 bpm) during the last stage of the graded exercise test. The treadmill speed and grade during the last stage of the protocol was 2.5 mph and 12%, respectively. This corresponds to a functional aerobic capacity of 7.0 METs or 24.5 ml $\cdot$ kg^{-1} $\cdot$ min^{-1}. According to the norms, this client's cardiorespiratory fitness level is *poor* for her age.

5. & 6. Training HRs

The graph of the client's HR and RPE responses to the graded exercise test is presented in figure A.8 (see p. 305).

From Vivian H. Heyward, 2006, *Advanced Fitness Assessment and Exercise Prescription*, 5th ed. (Champaign, IL: Human Kinetics).

Given the client's poor cardiorespiratory fitness level and her lack of regular aerobic exercise, the initial minimal training intensity will be 50% $\dot{V}O_2R$ (4.0 METs), gradually increasing to a maximum intensity of 75% $\dot{V}O_2R$ (5.5 METs). The corresponding training HRs, extrapolated from figure A.8, are 152 bpm (50% $\dot{V}O_2R$ or 4.0 METs) and 174 bpm (75% $\dot{V}O_2R$ or 5.5 METs). The HRs and RPEs corresponding to the relative exercise intensities in the following chart were extrapolated from the graph.

%$\dot{V}O_2R$	METs	HR (bpm)	RPE
50%	4.0	152	12
60%	4.6	165	14
70%	5.2	170	15
75%	5.5	174	16

7. Speed Calculations (ACSM Formula for Walking on Level Course)

To calculate walking speed corresponding to 60% of client's $\dot{V}O_2R$ [.60 × (7 – 1) + 1] = 4.6 METs):

a. Convert METs into ml · kg^{-1} · min^{-1}.

$$4.6 \text{ METs} \times 3.5 \text{ ml} \cdot \text{kg}^{-1} \cdot \text{min}^{-1} = 16.1 \text{ ml} \cdot \text{kg}^{-1} \cdot \text{min}^{-1}$$

b. Substitute into ACSM walking equation and solve for speed (m · min^{-1}).

$$\dot{V}O_2 = [\text{speed} \times 0.1] + [1.8 \times \text{speed} \times \text{grade}] + \text{resting } \dot{V}O_2$$

$$16.1 \text{ ml} \cdot \text{kg}^{-1} \cdot \text{min}^{-1} = [\text{speed} \times 0.1] + [1.8 \times \text{speed} \times 0\% \text{ grade}] + 3.5 \text{ ml} \cdot \text{kg}^{-1} \cdot \text{min}^{-1}$$

$$12.6 \text{ ml} \cdot \text{kg}^{-1} \cdot \text{min}^{-1} = \text{m} \cdot \text{min}^{-1} \times 0.1$$

$$126 \text{ m} \cdot \text{min}^{-1} = \text{speed}$$

c. Convert speed (m · min^{-1}) into miles per hour (26.8 m · min^{-1} = 1 mph).

$$126 \text{ m} \cdot \text{min}^{-1}/26.8 \text{ m} \cdot \text{min}^{-1} = 4.7 \text{ mph}$$

d. Convert miles per hour into minutes per mile walking pace.

$$60 \text{ min} \cdot \text{hr}^{-1}/4.7 \text{ mph} = 12.8 \text{ min} \cdot \text{mile}^{-1}, \text{ or } 12:48 \text{ (12 min, 48 sec per mile)}$$

Follow these same steps to calculate the walking speed corresponding to 70% $\dot{V}O_2R$ and 75% $\dot{V}O_2R$.

(Answers: 70% $\dot{V}O_2R$ = 5.5 mph; 75% $\dot{V}O_2R$ = 5.9 mph.)

8. Lifestyle Modifications

- Eat three well-balanced meals a day.
- Avoid fried foods high in saturated fats, cholesterol, and sodium.
- Dine out less frequently and select restaurants offering healthy food choices (e.g., salad bar, grilled skinless chicken, or fish).
- Exercise aerobically at least three days a week.
- Try using relaxation techniques (e.g., stretching, progressive relaxation, mental imagery) to relax in the evening instead of drinking wine.

From Vivian H. Heyward, 2006, *Advanced Fitness Assessment and Exercise Prescription*, 5th ed. (Champaign, IL: Human Kinetics).

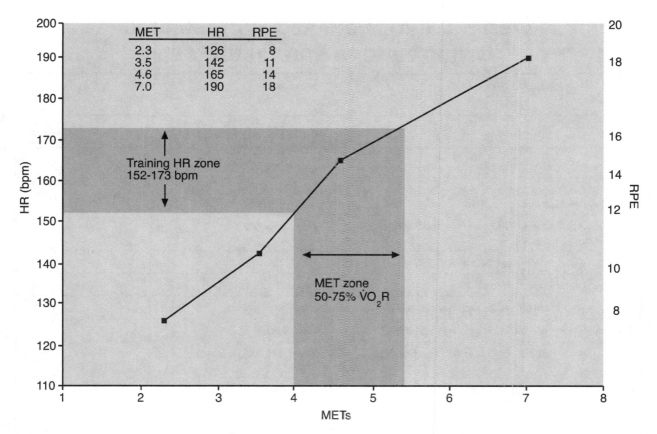

Figure A.8 Plotting heart rate versus METs for graded exercise test.

From Vivian H. Heyward, 2006, *Advanced Fitness Assessment and Exercise Prescription*, 5th ed. (Champaign, IL: Human Kinetics).

Web Sites for Selected Professional Organizations and Institutes[a]

Name	Web site address
Aerobics and Fitness Association of America (AFAA)	www.afaa.com
American Association for Health, Physical Education, Recreation and Dance (AAHPERD)	www.aapherd.org
American Association of Cardiovascular and Pulmonary Rehabilitation (AACPR)	www.aacvpr.org
American College of Sports Medicine (ACSM)	www.acsm.org
American Council on Exercise (ACE)	www.acefitness.org
American Fitness Professionals and Associates (AFPA)	www.afpafitness.org
American Society of Exercise Physiologists (ASEP)	www.asep.org
Australian Association for Exercise and Sport Sciences (AAESS)	www.aaess.com.au
Canadian Academy of Sports Medicine (CASM)	www.casm-acms.org
Canadian Society for Exercise Physiology (CSEP)	www.csep.ca
Cooper Institute for Aerobics Research	www.cooperinst.org
Ethics and Safety Compliance Standards	www.escs.info
Gatorade Sport Science Institute (GSSI)	www.gssiweb.com
IDEA Health and Fitness Association	www.ideafit.com
International Association of Fitness Certifying Agencies	www.iafca.org
International Federation of Sports Medicine (FIMS)	www.fims.org
International Fitness Professionals Association (IFPA)	www.ifpa-fitness.com
International Health, Racquet, & Sportsclub Association	www.ihrsa.org
International Society for Aging and Physical Activity (ISAPA)	www.isapa.org
National Athletic Trainers Association (NATA)	www.nata.org
National Board of Fitness Examiners	www.nbfe.org
National Commission for Certifying Agencies (NCCA)	www.NOCA.org/
National Organization for Competency Assurance (NOCA)	www.NOCA.org
National Strength and Conditioning Association (NSCA)	www.nsca-lift.org
North American Society for Pediatric Exercise Medicine (NASPEM)	www.naspem.org
Sports Medicine Australia	www.sma.org.au
Sports Medicine New Zealand	www.sportsmedicine.co.nz

[a]Organizations and institutes dealing with exercise physiology, sports medicine, and/or physical fitness.

From Vivian H. Heyward, 2006, *Advanced Fitness Assessment and Exercise Prescription*, 5th ed. (Champaign, IL: Human Kinetics).

APPENDIX A.9

Cardiorespiratory Assessments

Appendix B.1 includes a Summary of GXT and Cardiorespiratory Field Test Protocols that are presented in more detail in chapter 4. This appendix summarizes popular maximal and submaximal protocols for treadmill, cycle ergometer, bench stepping, stair-climbing, rowing ergometer, and distance run/walk tests, as well as methods that you can use to obtain an estimate of your client's $\dot{V}O_2$max for each protocol.

Appendix B.2, the Rockport Fitness Charts, provides age-gender norms for the Rockport Walking Test. These charts may be used to classify your client's aerobic capacity.

Appendix B.3 presents a variety of step test protocols. Testing and scoring procedures are included for each protocol. For some protocols, prediction equations are available to estimate your client's $\dot{V}O_2$ max.

Summary of Graded Exercise Test and Cardiorespiratory Field Test Protocols

Test mode/Protocol	Population	Type	Method to estimate $\dot{V}O_2max$	Description (page)
Treadmill				
Balke	Active/sedentary men and women	Max or submax	Prediction equation Multistage equation/graphing	65
Modified Balke	Children	Max or submax	ACSM equations (walk/run) Multistage equations/graphing	85
Bruce	Active/sedentary men and women	Max or submax	Prediction equation Multistage equation/graphing	65
	Elderly	Max or submax	Prediction equation Multistage equation/graphing	
	Cardiac patients	Max or submax	Prediction equation Multistage equation/graphing	
Modified Bruce	High-risk and elderly	Max or submax	ACSM walking equation Multistage equation/graphing	67
Ebbeling (single-stage walking)	Healthy adults (20-59 years)	Submax	Prediction equation	76
George (single-stage jogging)	Healthy adults (18-28 years)	Submax	Prediction equation	76
Latin and Elias (single-stage walking or jogging)	Healthy adults (19-40 years)	Submax	Prediction equation	76
Naughton	Male cardiac patients	Max or submax	Prediction equation Multistage equation/graphing	66
Cycle ergometer				
Åstrand	Healthy adults	Max	ACSM leg ergometry equation	71
Åstrand-Ryhming	Healthy adults	Submax	Nomogram	78
Fox	Healthy adults	Max or submax	ACSM leg ergometry equation Prediction equation	72
YMCA	Healthy adults	Submax	Multistage equation/graphing	77
McMaster	Children	Max or submax	ACSM leg ergometry equation Multistage equation/graphing	85
Swain	Healthy adults	Submax	ACSM leg ergometry equation	77
Bench stepping				
Åstrand-Ryhming	Healthy adults	Submax	Nomogram	80
Nagle	Healthy adults	Max	ACSM stepping equation	73
Queens College	Healthy adults (college age)	Submax	Prediction equation	80

From Vivian H. Heyward, 2006, *Advanced Fitness Assessment and Exercise Prescription*, 5th ed. (Champaign, IL: Human Kinetics).

APPENDIX B.1

Test mode/Protocol	Population	Type	Method to estimate $\dot{V}O_2max$	Description (page)
Stair-climbing				
Howley	Healthy adults	Submax	Multistage equation/graphing	80
Rowing ergometer				
Hagerman	Noncompetitive and unskilled rowers	Submax	Nomogram	81
Distance run/walk				
1.0-mile run/walk	Children (8-17 years)	Submax	Prediction equation	85
1.0-mile steady-state jog	Healthy adults (college age)	Submax	Prediction equation	83
1.5-mile run/walk	Healthy adults	Submax	Prediction equation	83
1.5-mile steady-state run	Healthy adults	Submax	Prediction equation	83
1.0-mile walk	Healthy adults	Submax	Prediction equation	83
12-min run	Healthy adults	Submax	Prediction equation	83
15-min run	Healthy adults	Submax	Prediction equation	81
20-meter shuttle run	Children (8-19 years)	Submax	Prediction equation	85

From Vivian H. Heyward, 2006, Advanced Fitness Assessment and Exercise Prescription, 5th ed. (Champaign, IL: Human Kinetics).

Rockport Fitness Charts

Age-Gender Norms for the Rockport Walking Test

Relative Fitness Level

From Vivian H. Heyward, 2006, *Advanced Fitness Assessment and Exercise Prescription,* 5th ed. (Champaign, IL: Human Kinetics). Reprinted with permission of The Rockport Company, Inc.

Age-Gender Norms for the Rockport Walking Test

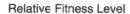

Relative Fitness Level

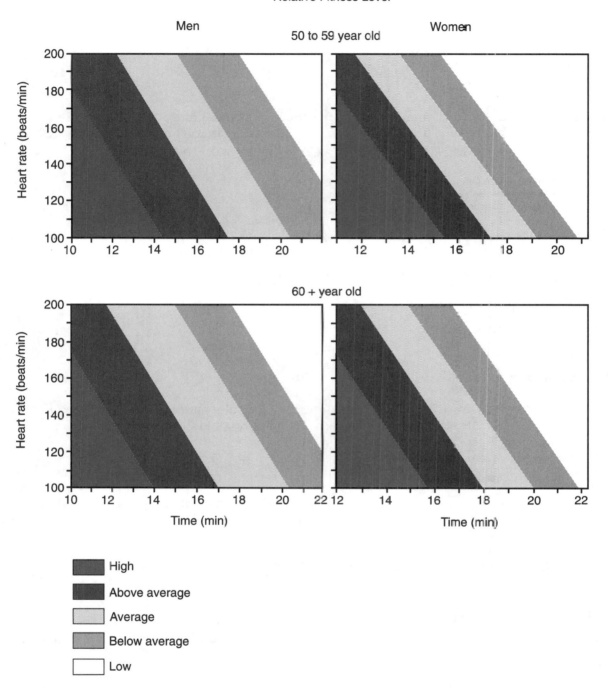

APPENDIX B.2

311

Step Test Protocols

Harvard Step Test (Brouha 1943)

Age and sex: Young men

Stepping rate: 30 steps · min^{-1}

Bench height: 20 in.

Duration of exercise: 5 min

Scoring procedures: Sit down immediately after exercise. The pulse rate is counted in 1/2-min counts, from 1 to 1 1/2, 2 to 2 1/2, and 3 to 3 1/2 min after exercise. The three 1/2-min pulse counts are summed and used in the following equation to determine physical efficiency index (PEI):

$$PEI = \frac{\text{duration of exercise (sec)} \times 100}{2 \times \text{sum of recovery HRs}}$$

You can evaluate the performance of college-age males using the following PEI classifications: < 55 = poor, 55-64 = low average, 65-79 = average, 80-89 = good, and ≥90 = excellent.

Three-Minute Step Test (Hodgkins and Skubic 1963)

Age and sex: High school- and college-age women

Stepping rate: 24 steps · min^{-1}

Bench height: 18 in.

Duration of exercise: 3 min

Scoring procedures: Sit down immediately after exercise. The pulse rate is counted for 30 sec after 1 min of rest (1 to 1 1/2 min after exercise). Use the recovery pulse count in the following equation:

$$CV\ efficiency = \frac{\text{duration of exercise (sec)} \times 100}{\text{recovery pulse} \times 5.6}$$

You can evaluate the performance of college-age women using the following classifications for cardiovascular (CV) efficiency: 0-27 = very poor, 28-38 = poor, 39-48 = fair, 49-59 = good, 60-70 = very good, and 71-100 = excellent.

OSU Step Test (Kurucz, Fox, and Mathews 1969)

Age and sex: Men 19-56 years

Stepping rate: 24 to 30 steps · min^{-1}

Bench height: Split-level bench 15 and 20 in. high with an adjustable hand bar

Duration of exercise: 18 innings, 50 sec each

Phase I: 6 innings, 24 steps · min^{-1}, 15-in. bench

Phase II: 6 innings, 30 steps · min^{-1}, 15-in. bench

Phase III: 6 innings, 30 steps · min^{-1}, 20-in. bench

(Each inning consists of 30 sec of stepping and 20 sec of rest.)

Scoring procedures: Exactly 5 sec into each rest period, take a 10-sec pulse count. Terminate the test when the heart rate reaches 150 bpm (25 counts × 6). The score is the inning during which the heart rate reaches 150 bpm.

From Vivian H. Heyward, 2006, *Advanced Fitness Assessment and Exercise Prescription*, 5th ed. (Champaign, IL: Human Kinetics).

Eastern Michigan University Step Test (Witten 1973)

Age and sex: College-age women

Stepping rate: 24 to 30 steps $\cdot$ min^{-1}

Bench height: Tri-level bench 14 to 20 in.

Duration of exercise: 20 innings, 50 sec each

　Phase I: 5 innings, 24 steps $\cdot$ min^{-1}, 14-in. bench

　Phase II: 5 innings, 30 steps $\cdot$ min^{-1}, 14-in. bench

　Phase III: 5 innings, 30 steps $\cdot$ min^{-1}, 17-in. bench

　Phase IV: 5 innings, 30 steps $\cdot$ min^{-1}, 20-in. bench

　(Each inning consists of 30 sec of stepping and 20 sec of rest.)

Scoring procedures: Exactly 5 sec into each rest period, take a 10-sec pulse count. Terminate the test when the heart rate reaches 168 bpm (28 counts $\times$ 6). The score is the inning during which the heart rate reaches 168 bpm.

Cotten Revision of OSU Step Test (Cotten 1971)

Age and sex: High school- and college-age men

Stepping rate: 24 to 36 steps $\cdot$ min^{-1}

Bench height: 17 in.

Duration of exercise: 18 innings, 50 sec each

　Phase I: 6 innings, 24 steps $\cdot$ min^{-1}, 17-in. bench

　Phase II: 6 innings, 30 steps $\cdot$ min^{-1}, 17-in. bench

　Phase III: 6 innings, 36 steps $\cdot$ min^{-1}, 17-in. bench

　(Each inning consists of 30 sec of stepping and 20 sec of rest.)

Scoring procedures: As with the OSU Step Test, the score is the inning during which the heart rate reaches 150 bpm (25 counts in 10 sec). $\dot{V}O_2$max in ml $\cdot$ kg^{-1} $\cdot$ min^{-1} can be estimated using the following equation:

$\dot{V}O_2$max = (1.69978 $\times$ step test score) $-$ (0.06252 $\times$ body weight in lb) + 47.12525

Queens College Step Test (McArdle et al. 1972)

Age and sex: College-age women and men

Stepping rate: 22 steps $\cdot$ min^{-1} for women; 24 steps $\cdot$ min^{-1} for men

Bench height: 16 1/4 in.

Duration of exercise: 3 min

Scoring procedures: Remain standing after exercise. Beginning 5 sec after the cessation of exercise, take a 15-sec pulse count. Multiply the 15-sec count by 4 to express the score in beats per minute (bpm). $\dot{V}O_2$max in ml $\cdot$ kg^{-1} $\cdot$ min^{-1} can be estimated using the following equations:

　Women: $\dot{V}O_2$max = 65.81 $-$ (0.1847 $\times$ HR)

　Men: $\dot{V}O_2$max = 111.33 $-$ (0.42 $\times$ HR)

From Vivian H. Heyward, 2006, *Advanced Fitness Assessment and Exercise Prescription*, 5th ed. (Champaign, IL: Human Kinetics).

References

Brouha, L. 1943. The step test: A simple method of measuring physical fitness for muscular work in young men. *Research Quarterly* 14: 31–36.

Cotten, D.J. 1971. A modified step test for group cardiovascular testing. *Research Quarterly* 42: 91–95.

Hodgkins, J. and Skubic, V. 1963. Cardiovascular efficiency test scores for college women in the United States. *Research Quarterly* 34: 454–461.

Kurucz, R., Fox, E.L., and Mathews, D.K. 1969. Construction of a submaximal cardiovascular step test. *Research Quarterly* 40: 115–122.

McArdle, W.D., Katch, F.I., Pechar, G.S., Jacobson, L., and Ruck, S. 1972. Reliability and interrelationships between maximal oxygen intake, physical working capacity and step-test scores in college women. *Medicine and Science in Sports* 4: 182–186.

Witten, C. 1973. Construction of a submaximal cardiovascular step test for college females. *Research Quarterly* 44: 46–50.

Muscular Fitness Exercises and Norms

Appendix C.1 includes norms for isokinetic (Omni-Tron) muscular fitness tests. Average strength, endurance, and power values are presented for young adults, older adults, and weight-trained individuals.

Appendix C.2 describes and illustrates some sample basic isometric exercises for a variety of muscle groups.

Appendix C.3 provides an extensive list of dynamic resistance training exercises. Exercises for the upper and lower extremities are organized by body region (e.g., chest, upper arm, thigh, etc.). For each exercise, equipment, body positions, joint actions, prime movers, and exercise variations are presented.

Average Strength, Endurance, and Power Values for Isokinetic (Omni-Tron) Tests

Strength[a]	Young adult[b]	Older adult[c]	Weight trained[d]
Females			
Chest press	88.1	76.7	131.8
Lateral row	82.6	77.4	111.4
Shoulder press	32.9	30.4	60.1
Lateral pull-down	70.8	66.3	101.2
Knee extension	67.7	59.3	82.7
Knee flexion	51.5	43.3	64.3
Males			
Chest press	173.8	154.9	218.6
Lateral row	153.5	143.2	178.6
Shoulder press	69.2	62.4	102.6
Lateral pull-down	134.8	115.3	176.0
Knee extension	110.9	95.5	127.2
Knee flexion	75.9	67.3	89.9

Note: Data courtesy of Hydra-Fitnesss, Belton, TX: 1988.
[a]Values of strength measured in foot-pounds at dial setting 10.
[b]Average age for females = 15.1 ± 2.6 years; for males = 15.8 ± 2.7 years.
[c]Average age for females = 38.2 ± 9.7 years; for males = 37.6 ± 9.6 years.
[d]Average age for females = 21.2 ± 2.0 years; for males = 20.6 ± 2.1 years.

Endurance[a]	Young adult[b]	Older adult[c]	Weight trained[d]
Females			
Chest press	64.3	53.4	125.7
Lateral row	102.4	85.7	143.7
Shoulder press	28.1	25.1	56.3
Lateral pull-down	109.1	91.5	216.3
Knee extension	88.7	86.6	111.6
Knee flexion	114.3	89.2	148.2
Males			
Chest press	211.8	167.3	321.1
Lateral row	266.9	221.2	312.5
Shoulder press	112.4	94.2	170.9
Lateral pull-down	352.2	296.3	501.5
Knee extension	72.9	80.8	98.9
Knee flexion	83.5	84.2	130.9

[a]Values of endurance measured in foot-pounds at dial setting 3.
[b]Average age for females = 15.1 ± 2.6 years; for males = 15.8 ± 2.7 years.
[c]Average age for females = 38.2 ± 9.7 years; for males = 37.6 ± 9.6 years.
[d]Average age for females = 21.2 ± 2.0 years; for males = 20.6 ± 2.1 years.

From Vivian H. Heyward, 2006, *Advanced Fitness Assessment and Exercise Prescription*, 5th ed. (Champaign, IL: Human Kinetics).

Power[a]	Young adult[b]	Older adult[c]	Weight trained[d]
Females			
Chest press	86.3	73.7	163.0
Lateral row	121.3	113.6	156.3
Shoulder press	39.5	32.9	81.9
Lateral pull-down	165.4	128.4	254.1
Knee extension	101.9	73.4	122.5
Knee flexion	103.5	74.6	142.1
Males			
Chest press	264.9	228.4	392.3
Lateral row	302.4	268.4	345.0
Shoulder press	130.7	122.0	224.5
Lateral pull-down	430.9	354.7	550.9
Knee extension	198.4	159.4	233.5
Knee flexion	182.0	155.5	259.5

[a] Values of power measured in foot-pounds at dial setting 6.
[b] Average age for females = 15.1 ± 2.6 years; for males = 15.8 ± 2.7 years.
[c] Average age for females = 38.2 ± 9.7 years; for males = 37.6 ± 9.6 years.
[d] Average age for females = 21.2 ± 2.0 years; for males = 20.6 ± 2.1 years.

From Vivian H. Heyward, 2006, *Advanced Fitness Assessment and Exercise Prescription*, 5th ed. (Champaign, IL: Human Kinetics)

Isometric Exercises

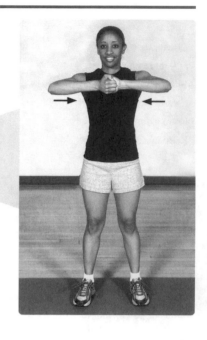

Exercise 1: Chest Push

Muscle groups: Shoulder and elbow flexors

Equipment: None

Description:

1. Lock hands together.
2. Keep forearms parallel to ground and hands close to chest.
3. Push hands together.

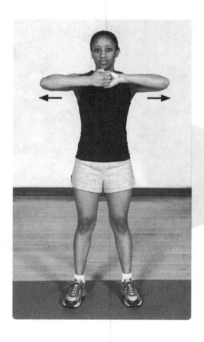

Exercise 2: Shoulder Pull

Muscle groups: Shoulder and elbow flexors

Equipment: None

Description:

1. Using same position as in chest push, attempt to pull hands apart

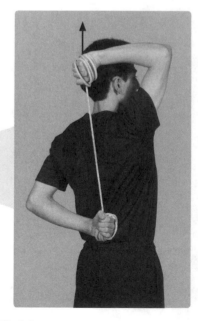

Exercise 3: Triceps Extension

Muscle groups: Elbow extensors

Equipment: Towel or rope

Description:

1. Placing right hand over shoulder and left hand at small of back, grasp rope or towel behind back.
2. Attempt to pull towel or rope upward with right hand.
3. Change position of hands.

From Vivian H. Heyward, 2006, *Advanced Fitness Assessment and Exercise Prescription*, 5th ed. (Champaign, IL: Human Kinetics).

APPENDIX C.2

Exercise 4: Arm Curls

Muscle groups: Elbow flexors

Equipment: Towel or rope

Description:

1. Stand with knees flexed about 45°.
2. Place rope or towel behind thighs and grasp each end with hands shoulder-width apart.
3. Attempt to flex elbows.

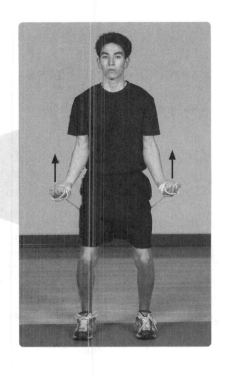

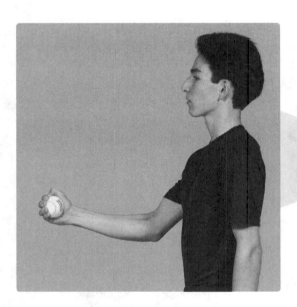

Exercise 5: Ball Squeeze

Muscle groups: Wrist and finger flexors

Equipment: Tennis ball

Description:

1. Hold tennis ball firmly in hand and squeeze maximally.

Exercise 6: Leg and Thigh Extensions

Muscle groups: Hip and knee extensors

Equipment: Rope

Description:

1. Stand on rope with knees flexed.
2. Grasp rope firmly with hands at sides, elbows fully extended.
3. Keeping trunk erect, attempt to extend legs by lifting upward.

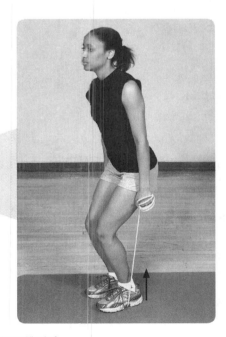

From Vivian H. Heyward, 2006, *Advanced Fitness Assessment and Exercise Prescription*, 5th ed. (Champaign, IL: Human Kinetics).

Exercise 7: Leg Press

Muscle groups: Hip and knee extensors

Equipment: Doorway

Description:

1. Sit in doorway facing side of door frame.
2. Grasp door frame behind head.
3. Attempt to extend legs by pushing feet against door frame.

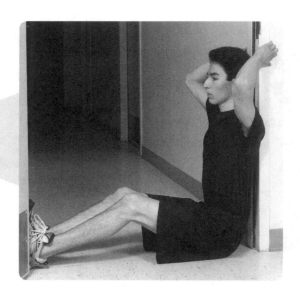

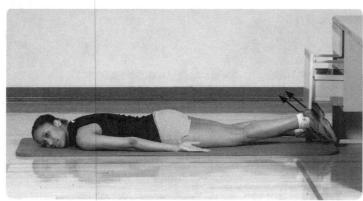

Exercise 8: Leg Curl

Muscle groups: Knee flexors

Equipment: Dresser or desk

Description:

1. Pull out lower dresser drawer slightly.
2. Lying prone, with knees flexed, hook heels under bottom of drawer.
3. Attempt to pull heels toward head.

Exercise 9: Knee Squeeze or Pull

Muscle groups: Hip adductors or abductors

Equipment: Chair

Description:

1. Sitting on chair with forearms crossed and hands on inside of knees, attempt to squeeze knees together (adductors).
2. Same position but place hands on outside of knees; attempt to pull knees apart (abductors).

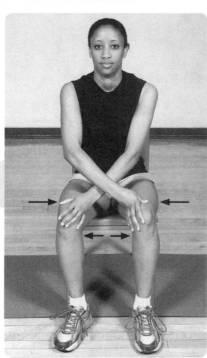

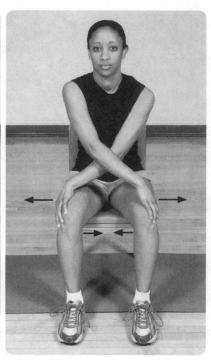

From Vivian H. Heyward, 2006, *Advanced Fitness Assessment and Exercise Prescription*, 5th ed. (Champaign, IL: Human Kinetics).

APPENDIX C.2

Exercise 10: Pelvic Tilt

Muscle groups: Abdominals

Equipment: None

Description:

1. Supine with knees flexed and arms overhead.
2. Tighten abdominal muscles while pressing lower back into floor.

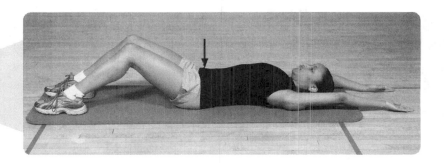

Exercise 11: Gluteal Squeeze

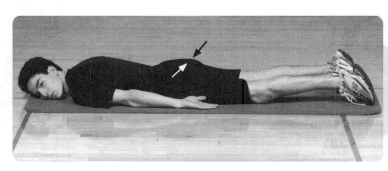

Muscle groups: Hip extensors and abductors

Equipment: None

Description:

1. Lie prone with legs together and fully extended.
2. Tighten and squeeze the buttocks together.

From Vivian H. Heyward, 2006, *Advanced Fitness Assessment and Exercise Prescription*, 5th ed. (Champaign, IL: Human Kinetics).

Dynamic Resistance Training Exercises

Exercise	Type[a]	Variations	Equipment[b]	Body position	Joint actions	Prime movers
Upper extremity						
Chest						
Bench press	M-J	Flat	B, D, M	Supine lying on flat bench	Shoulder horizontal adduction, elbow extension	Pectoralis major (midsternal), triceps brachii
		Incline	B, D, M	Sitting on incline bench	Shoulder flexion, elbow extension	Pectoralis major (clavicular), triceps brachii
		Decline	B, D	Supine lying on decline bench	Shoulder flexion, elbow extension	Pectoralis major (lower sternal), triceps brachii
Push-up	M-J	Hands wider than shoulders	None	Prone; BW supported by hands and feet	Shoulder horizontal adduction, elbow extension	Pectoralis major (midsternal), triceps brachii
		Hands narrower than shoulders	None	Same as above	Shoulder flexion, elbow extension	Pectoralis major (clavicular), ant deltoid, triceps brachii
Bar dip	M-J	Neutral grip	Parallel bars	Vertically supported by bars	Shoulder flexion, elbow extension	Pectoralis major (clavicular), ant deltoid, triceps brachii
		Pronated grip		Same as above	Shoulder adduction, elbow extension	Pectoralis major (midsternal), triceps brachii
Fly	S	Flat	D	Supine lying on flat bench	Shoulder adduction	Pectoralis major (midsternal)
Pullover (bent arm)	S	Flat	B, D	Supine lying on flat bench	Shoulder extension	Pectoralis major (lower sternal), post deltoid, latissimus dorsi

Upper extremity (cont.)

Shoulders

Exercise	Type[a]	Variations	Equipment[b]	Body position	Joint actions	Prime movers
Overhead press	M-J	Military	B, D, M	Sitting or standing	Shoulder flexion, elbow extension	Pectoralis major (clavicular), ant deltoid, triceps brachii
		Behind the head	B	Sitting	Shoulder abduction, elbow extension	Ant/mid deltoid, supraspinatus
Upright row	M-J		B, D	Standing	Shoulder abduction, scapula upward rotation, elbow flexion	Mid deltoid, supraspinatus, trapezius (upper), brachialis
Front arm raise	S		B, C, D	Standing	Shoulder flexion	Pectoralis major (clavicular), ant deltoid
Lateral arm raise	S		C, D, M	Sitting or standing	Shoulder abduction	Mid deltoid, supraspinatus, pectoralis major (clavicular)
Reverse fly	S		C, D	Standing	Shoulder horizontal extension	Post deltoid, infraspinatus, teres minor

Upper arm

Exercise	Type[a]	Variations	Equipment[b]	Body position	Joint actions	Prime movers
Arm curl	S	Supinated grip	B, D, M	Standing or sitting on incline bench or preacher bench	Elbow flexion	Biceps brachii, brachialis
	S	Neutral grip	Same as above		Elbow flexion	Brachioradialis, brachialis, biceps brachii
	S	Pronated grip	Same as above		Elbow flexion	Brachialis
Triceps press-down	M-J		M	Seated	Shoulder flexion, elbow extension	Ant deltoid, pectoralis major (clavicular), triceps brachii

(continued)

From Vivian H. Heyward, 2006, *Advanced Fitness Assessment and Exercise Prescription*, 5th ed. (Champaign, IL: Human Kinetics).

Dynamic Resistance Training Exercises (continued)

Exercise	Type[a]	Variations	Equipment[b]	Body position	Joint actions	Prime movers
Upper extremity (cont.)						
Upper arm (cont.)						
Triceps extension	S		B	Supine lying on flat bench	Elbow extension	Triceps brachii
Triceps push-down	S	V-bar or strength bar	C	Standing	Elbow extension	Triceps brachii
French press	S		D	Standing or sitting	Elbow extension	Triceps brachii (medial head)
Overhead press	S		C, R	Standing with trunk flexed 45°	Elbow extension	Triceps brachii
Triceps kickback	S		D	Standing with one knee/hand on flat bench and trunk horizontal to floor	Elbow extension	Triceps brachii (long head)
Forearm						
Radioulnar rotation	S		D	Forearm/elbow supported on bench; hand free	Supination and pronation	Supinator, pronator teres, biceps brachii, brachioradialis
Wrist curl	S		D	Same as above	Wrist flexion	FCU, FCR
Reverse wrist curl	S		D	Same as above	Wrist extension	ECU, ECR (longus, brevis)
Radioulnar flexion	S		D	Standing with arm at side	Radial flexion, ulna flexion	FCR, ECR, FCU, ECU
Upper-mid back						
Lat pull-down	M-J	Pronated, wide grip	M	Sitting	Shoulder adduction, scapula adduction	Latissimus dorsi (upper), teres major, pectoralis major (upper), trapezius, rhomboids
	M-J	Narrow, neutral grip	M	Sitting	Shoulder extension, elbow flexion	Latissimus dorsi (lower), pectoralis major (lower sternal), biceps brachii

From Vivian H. Heyward, 2006, *Advanced Fitness Assessment and Exercise Prescription*, 5th ed. (Champaign, IL: Human Kinetics).

Exercise	Type[a]	Variations	Equipment[b]	Body position	Joint actions	Prime movers
Upper mid-back (cont.)						
Seated row	M-J	Neutral grip	M	Sitting	Shoulder extension, elbow flexion	Latissimus dorsi (lower), biceps brachii
	M-J	Pronated grip	M	Sitting with elbows horizontal to floor	Shoulder horizontal extension, elbow flexion	Post deltoid, latissimus dorsi (upper), infraspinatus, brachialis
Bent-over row	M-J	Neutral grip	D	Standing with trunk flexed 90°	Shoulder extension, elbow flexion	Latissimus dorsi, biceps brachii
	M-J	Pronated grip	D	Standing with trunk flexed 90° and elbows out	Shoulder horizontal extension, elbow flexion	Post deltoid, infraspinatus, latissimus dorsi, brachialis
Pull-up	M-J	Pronated grip	Pull-up bar	Vertically hanging from bar	Shoulder adduction, elbow flexion	Latissimus dorsi (upper), pectoralis major (sternal), brachialis
Chin-up	M-J	Supinated or neutral grip	Pull-up bar	Vertically hanging from bar	Shoulder extension, elbow flexion	Latissimus dorsi (lower), pectoralis major (sternal), biceps brachii
Shoulder shrug	S	Regular	B, D, M	Standing	Shoulder girdle (scapula and clavicle) elevation	Trapezius (upper), levator scapulae, rhomboids
	S	Elevation with shoulder roll		Standing	Shoulder girdle elevation, scapula adduction	Trapezius (mid), rhomboids
Lower back						
Trunk extension	M-J		M	Sitting with pelvis/thighs stabilized	Spinal extension	Erector spinae
Back raise	M-J		Glut-ham developer	Prone with pelvis supported; trunk flexed	Spinal extension	Erector spinae
Side bends	M-J		D	Standing	Spinal lateral flexion	Quadratus lumborum

(continued)

From Vivian H. Heyward, 2006, *Advanced Fitness Assessment and Exercise Prescription*, 5th ed. (Champaign, IL: Human Kinetics).

Dynamic Resistance Training Exercises *(continued)*

Exercise	Type[a]	Variations	Equipment[b]	Body position	Joint actions	Prime movers
Lower back (cont.)						
Isometric side support (side bridge)	M-J		None	Side-lying with BW supported by forearm and feet	None	Quadratus lumborum, abdominal obliques
Single-leg extension	M-J		None	Hands and knees	Spinal extension, hip extension	Erector spinae, gluteus maximus, hamstrings (upper)
Abdomen						
Curl-up	M-J	Bent knee	None	Supine lying with knees bent	Spinal flexion	Rectus abdominis
	M-J	With twist	None	Same as above	Spinal flexion	Abdominal obliques
Abdominal crunch	M-J		M	Sitting	Spinal flexion	Rectus abdominis
Reverse sit-up	M-J		None	Supine lying on floor on bench	Spinal flexion	Rectus abdominis (lower)
Lower extremity						
Hip						
Half squat	M-J		B, M	Standing	Hip extension, knee extension	Gluteus maximus, hamstrings (upper), quadriceps femoris
Leg press	M-J		M	Sitting	Hip extension, knee extension	Gluteus maximus, hamstrings (upper), quadriceps femoris
Lunge	M-J		B, D	Standing	Hip extension, knee extension	Gluteus maximus hamstrings (upper), quadriceps femoris
Glut-ham raise	M-J		Glut-ham developer	Prone with thighs supported and trunk flexed	Hip extension and knee flexion	Gluteus maximus, hamstrings

From Vivian H. Heyward, 2006, *Advanced Fitness Assessment and Exercise Prescription*, 5th ed. (Champaign, IL: Human Kinetics).

Exercise	Type[a]	Variations	Equipment[b]	Body position	Joint actions	Prime movers
Lower extremity (cont.)						
Hip (cont.)						
Hip flexion	S		C, M	Standing	Hip flexion	Iliopsoas, rectus femoris (upper)
Hip extension	S		C, M	Standing	Hip extension	Gluteus maximus, hamstrings (upper)
Hip adduction	S		M	Sitting or supine lying	Hip adduction	Adductor longus, brevis, and magnus; gracilis
Hip abduction	S		M	Sitting or supine lying	Hip abduction	Gluteus medius
Side leg raise	S		None	Lying on side	Hip abduction	Gluteus medius, hamstrings (upper)
Good morning exercise	S		B, D	Standing	Hip extension	Gluteus maximus, hamstrings (upper)
Thigh						
Leg extension	S		M	Seated	Knee extension	Quadriceps femoris
Leg curl	S	Straight	M	Prone lying, seated, or standing	Knee flexion	Hamstrings (lower)
	S	Knee externally rotated	M	Same as above	Knee flexion	Biceps femoris
	S	Knees internally rotated	M	Same as above	Knee flexion	Semitendinosus, semimembranosus
Lower leg						
Heel raise	S	Standing	D, M	Standing	Ankle plantar flexion	Gastrocnemius
	S	Seated	M	Sitting	Ankle plantar flexion	Soleus
Toe raise	S		Strength bar	Sitting	Ankle dorsiflexion	Tibialis anterior, peroneus tertius, extensor digitorum longus

Note: FCU = flexor carpi ulnaris; ECU = extensor carpi ulnaris; FCR = flexor carpi radialis; ECR = extensor carpi radialis.
[a]Type of exercise: M-J = multijoint exercise; S = single-joint exercise; [b]Equipment codes: B = barbell; C = cables; D = dumbbells; M = exercise machine; R = rope.

From Vivian H. Heyward, 2006, *Advanced Fitness Assessment and Exercise Prescription*, 5th ed. (Champaign, IL: Human Kinetics).

Body Composition Assessments

Appendix D.1 presents prediction equations for estimating residual lung volume. Use these equations only when it is not possible to directly measure your client's residual lung volume.

Appendix D.2 describes and illustrates the standardized sites for skinfold measurements, and appendix D.3 describes the skinfold sites and measurement procedures for Jackson's generalized skinfold prediction equations for men and women.

Standardized sites for circumference (appendix D.4) and bony breadth (appendix D.5) measurements are also provided. Follow these procedures to identify and measure various sites.

Prediction Equations
for Residual Volume

Population	Smoking history[a]	n	Equation[b]
MEN			
Boren, Kory, and Syner (1966)	Mixed	422	RV = 0.0115 (Age) + 0.019 (HT) − 2.24 $r = 0.57$, SEE = 0.53 L
Goldman and Becklake (1959)			RV − 0.017 (Age) + 0.06858 (HT) − 3.477
Berglund et al. (1963)			RV = 0.022 (Age) + 0.0198 (HT) − 0.015 (WT) − 1.54
WOMEN			
O'Brien and Drizd (1983)	Nonsmokers	926	RV = 0.03 (Age) + 0.0387 (HT) − 0.73 (BSA) − 4.78 $r = 0.66$, SEE = 0.49 L
Black, Offord, and Hyatt (1974)	Mixed	110	RV = 0.021 (Age) + 0.023 (HT) − 2.978 $r = 0.70$, SEE = 0.46 L
Goldman and Becklake (1959)			RV = 0.009 (Age) + 0.08128 (HT) − 3.9
Berglund et al. (1963)			RV = 0.007 (Age) + 0.0268 (HT) − 3.42

[a]Mixed indicates that sample included both smokers and nonsmokers.
[b]Age (in yr); HT = height (in cm); BSA = body surface area (in m^2); WT = body mass (in kg).

References

Berglund, E., Birath, G., Bjure, J., Grimby, G., Kjellmar, I., Sandvist, L., and Soderholm, B. 1963. Spirometric studies in normal subjects. I. Forced expirograms in subjects between 7 and 70 years of age. *Acta Medica Scandinavica* 173: 185-192.

Black, L.F., Offord, K., and Hyatt, R.E. 1974. Variability in the maximum expiratory flow volume curve in asymptomatic smokers and nonsmokers. *American Review of Respiratory Diseases* 110: 282–292.

Boren, H.G., Kory, R.C., and Syner, J.C. 1966. The Veteran's Administration-Army cooperative study of pulmonary function: II. The lung volume and its subdivisions in normal men. *American Journal of Medicine* 41: 96–114.

Goldman, H.I., and Beckland, M.R. 1959. Respiratory function tests: Normal values at medium altitudes and the prediction of normal results. *American Review of Tuberculosis and Respiratory Diseases* 79: 457-467.

O'Brien, R.J., and Drizd, T.A. 1983. Roentgenographic determination of total lung capacity: Normal values from a national population survey. *American Review of Respiratory Diseases* 128: 949–952.

From Vivian H. Heyward, 2006, *Advanced Fitness Assessment and Exercise Prescription,* 5th ed. (Champaign, IL: Human Kinetics).

APPENDIX D.1

Standardized Sites
for Skinfold Measurements

Site	Direction of fold	Anatomical reference	Measurement
Chest	Diagonal	Axilla and nipple	Fold is taken between axilla and nipple as high as possible on anterior axillary fold, with measurement taken 1 cm below fingers.
Subscapular	Diagonal	Inferior angle of scapula	Fold is along natural cleavage line of skin just inferior to inferior angle of scapula, with caliper applied 1 cm below fingers.
Midaxillary	Horizontal	Xiphisternal junction (point where costal cartilage of ribs 5-6 articulates with sternum, slightly above inferior tip of xiphoid process)	Fold is taken on midaxillary line at level of xiphisternal junction.
Suprailiac	Oblique	Iliac crest	Fold is grasped posteriorly to midaxillary line and superiorly to iliac crest along natural cleavage of skin with caliper applied 1 cm below fingers.
Abdominal	Horizontal	Umbilicus	Fold is taken 3 cm lateral and 1 cm inferior to center of the umbilicus.
Triceps	Vertical (midline)	Acromial process of scapula and olecranon process of ulna	Using a tape measure, distance between lateral projection of acromial process and inferior margin of olecranon process is measured on lateral aspect of arm with elbow flexed 90°. Midpoint is marked on lateral side of arm. Fold is lifted 1 cm above marked line on posterior aspect of arm. Caliper is applied at marked level.
Biceps	Vertical (midline)	Biceps brachii	Fold is lifted over belly of the biceps brachii at the level marked for the triceps and on line with anterior border of the acromial process and the antecubital fossa. Caliper is applied 1 cm below fingers.
Thigh	Vertical (midline)	Inguinal crease and patella	Fold is lifted on anterior aspect of thigh midway between inguinal crease and proximal border of patella. Body weight is shifted to left foot and caliper is applied 1 cm below fingers.
Calf	Vertical (medial aspect)	Maximal calf circumference	Fold is lifted at level of maximal calf circumference on medial aspect of calf with knee and hip flexed to 90°.

Adapted from Harrison et al. (1988, pp. 55–70).

From Vivian H. Heyward, 2006, *Advanced Fitness Assessment and Exercise Prescription*, 5th ed. (Champaign, IL: Human Kinetics).

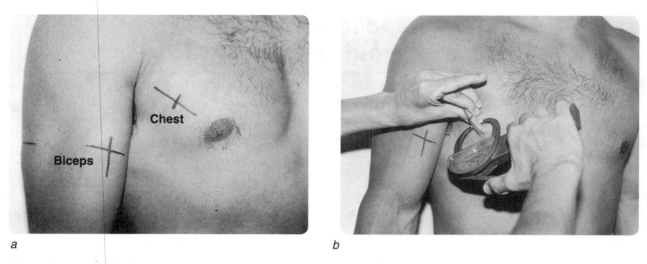

Figure D.2.1 *(a)* Site and *(b)* measurement of the chest skinfold. Photos courtesy of Linda K. Gilkey.

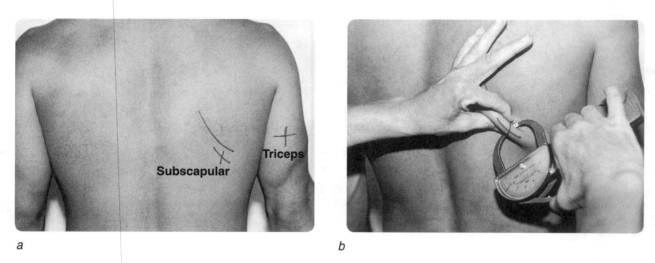

Figure D.2.2 *(a)* Site and *(b)* measurement of the subscapular skinfold. Photos courtesy of Linda K. Gilkey.

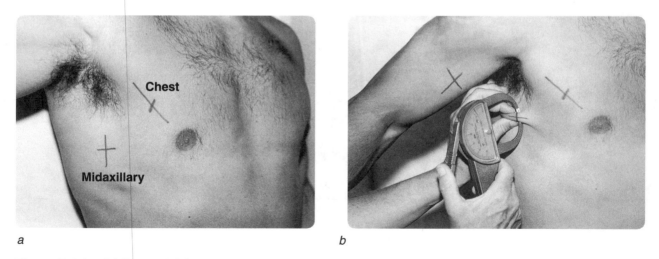

Figure D.2.3 *(a)* Site and *(b)* measurement of the midaxillary skinfold. Photos courtesy of Linda K. Gilkey.

From Vivian H. Heyward, 2006, *Advanced Fitness Assessment and Exercise Prescription*, 5th ed. (Champaign, IL: Human Kinetics).

APPENDIX D.2

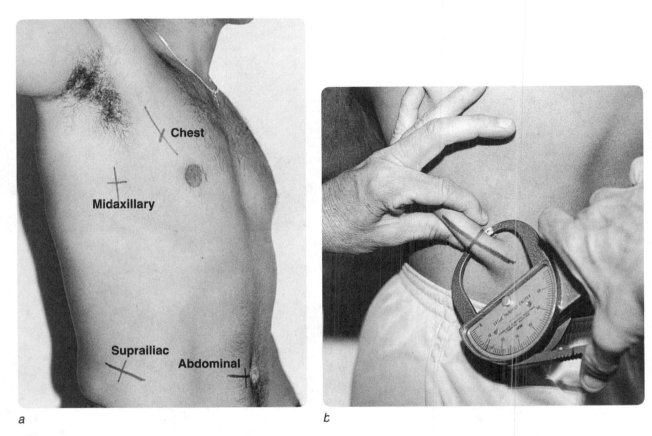

a

b

Figure D.2.4 *(a)* Site and *(b)* measurement of the suprailiac skinfold. Photos courtesy of Linda K. Gilkey.

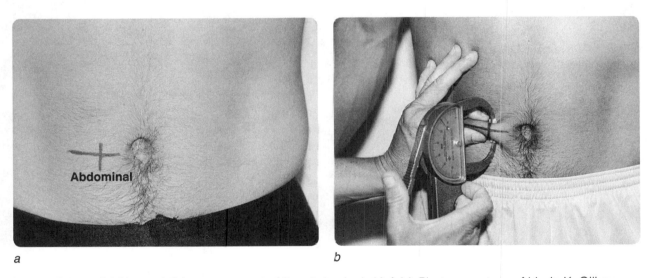

a

b

Figure D.2.5 *(a)* Site and *(b)* measurement of the abdominal skinfold. Photos courtesy of Linda K. Gilkey.

From Vivian H. Heyward, 2006, *Advanced Fitness Assessment and Exercise Prescription*, 5th ed. (Champaign, IL: Human Kinetics).

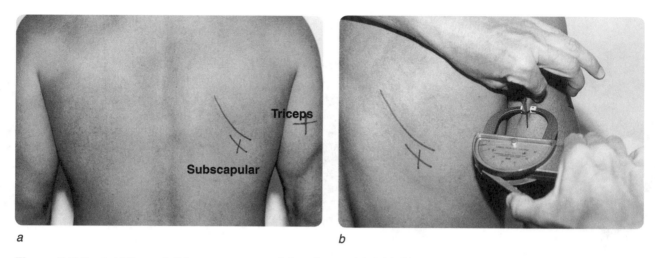

Figure D.2.6 *(a)* Site and *(b)* measurement of the triceps skinfold. Photos courtesy of Linda K. Gilkey.

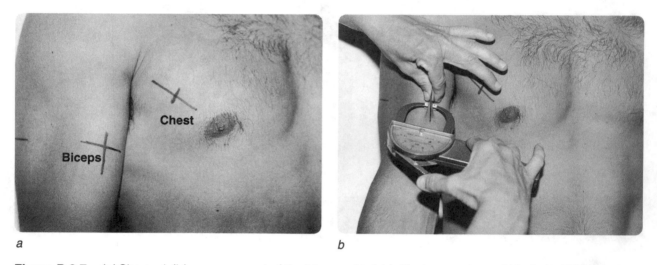

Figure D.2.7 *(a)* Site and *(b)* measurement of the biceps skinfold. Photos courtesy of Linda K. Gilkey.

From Vivian H. Heyward, 2006, *Advanced Fitness Assessment and Exercise Prescription,* 5th ed. (Champaign, IL: Human Kinetics).

APPENDIX D.2

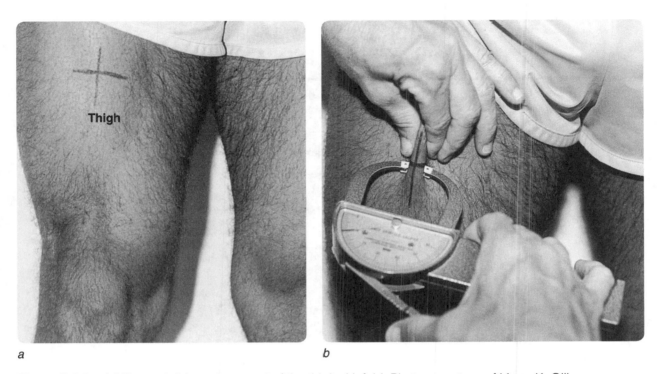

a   b

Figure D.2.8   *(a)* Site and *(b)* measurement of the thigh skinfold. Photos courtesy of Linda K. Gilkey.

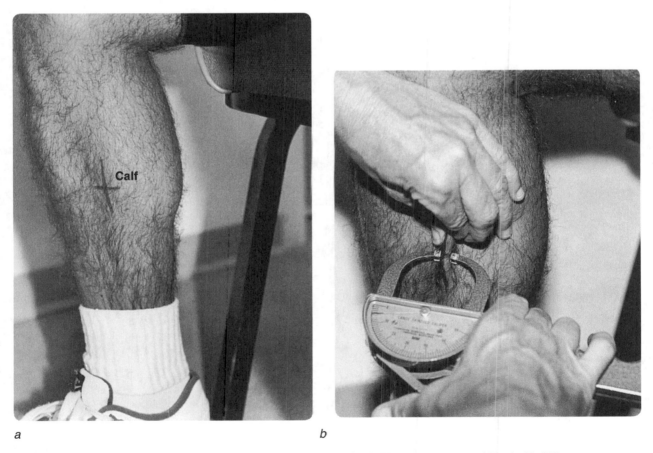

a   b

Figure D.2.9   *(a)* Site and *(b)* measurement of the calf skinfold. Photos courtesy of Linda K. Gilkey.

From Vivian H. Heyward, 2006, *Advanced Fitness Assessment and Exercise Prescription*, 5th ed. (Champaign, IL: Human Kinetics).

Skinfold Sites for Jackson's Generalized Skinfold Equations

Site	Direction of fold	Anatomical reference	Measurement
Chest	Diagonal	Axilla and nipple	Fold is taken 1/2 the distance between the anterior axillary line and nipple for men and 1/3 of this distance for women.
Subscapular	Oblique	Vertebral border and inferior angle of scapula	Fold is taken on diagonal line coming from the vertebral border, 1-2 cm below the inferior angle.
Midaxillary	Vertical	Xiphoid process of sternum	Fold is taken at level of xiphoid process along the midaxillary line.
Suprailiac	Diagonal	Iliac crest	Fold is taken diagonally above the iliac crest along the anterior axillary line.
Abdominal	Vertical	Umbilicus	Fold is taken vertically 2 cm lateral to the umbilicus.

Adapted from Jackson and Pollock (1978) and Jackson, Pollock, and Ward (1980).

From Vivian H. Heyward, 2006, *Advanced Fitness Assessment and Exercise Prescription*, 5th ed. (Champaign, IL: Human Kinetics).

Standardized Sites
for Circumference Measurements

Site	Anatomical reference	Position	Measurement
Neck	Laryngeal prominence ("Adam's apple")	Perpendicular to long axis of neck	Apply tape with minimal pressure just inferior to the Adam's apple.
Shoulder	Deltoid muscles and acromion processes of scapula	Horizontal	Apply tape snugly over maximum bulges of the deltoid muscles, inferior to acromion processes. Record measurement at end of normal expiration.
Chest	Fourth costosternal joints	Horizontal	Apply tape snugly around the torso at level of fourth costosternal joints. Record at end of normal expiration.
Waist	Narrowest part of torso, level of the "natural" waist between ribs and iliac crest	Horizontal	Apply tape snugly around the waist at level of narrowest part of torso. An assistant is needed to position tape behind the client. Take measurement at end of normal expiration.
Abdominal	Maximum anterior protuberance of abdomen, usually at umbilicus	Horizontal	Apply tape snugly around the abdomen at level of greatest anterior protuberance. An assistant is needed to position tape behind the client. Take measurement at end of normal expiration.
Hip (buttocks)	Maximum posterior extension of buttocks	Horizontal	Apply tape snugly around the buttocks. An assistant is needed to position tape on opposite side of body.
Thigh (proximal)	Gluteal fold	Horizontal	Apply tape snugly around thigh, just distal to the gluteal fold.
Thigh (mid)	Inguinal crease and proximal border of patella	Horizontal	With client's knee flexed 90° (right foot on bench), apply tape at level midway between inguinal crease and proximal border of patella.
Thigh (distal)	Femoral epicondyles	Horizontal	Apply tape just proximal to the femoral epicondyles.
Knee	Patella	Horizontal	Apply tape around the knee at midpatellar level with knee relaxed in slight flexion.
Calf	Maximum girth of calf muscle	Perpendicular to long axis of leg	With client sitting on end of table and legs hanging freely, apply tape horizontally around the maximum girth of calf.
Ankle	Malleoli of tibia and fibula	Perpendicular to long axis of leg	Apply tape snugly around minimum circumference of leg, just proximal to the malleoli.
Arm (biceps)	Acromion process of scapula and olecranon process of ulna	Perpendicular to long axis of arm	With client's arms hanging freely at sides and palms facing thighs, apply tape snugly around the arm at level midway between the acromion process of scapula and olecranon process of ulna (as marked for triceps and biceps skinfolds).
Forearm	Maximum girth of forearm	Perpendicular to long axis of forearm	With client's arms hanging down and away from trunk and forearm supinated, apply tape snugly around the maximum girth of the proximal part of the forearm.
Wrist	Styloid processes of radius and ulna	Perpendicular to long axis of forearm	With client's elbow flexed and forearm supinated, apply tape snugly around wrist, just distal to the styloid processes of the radius and ulna.

Adapted from Callaway et al. (1988, pp. 41-53).

From Vivian H. Heyward, 2006, *Advanced Fitness Assessment and Exercise Prescription*, 5th ed. (Champaign, IL: Human Kinetics).

Standardized Sites for Bony Breadth Measurements

Site	Anatomical reference	Position	Measurement
Biacromial (shoulder)	Lateral borders of acromion processes of scapula	Horizontal	With client standing, arms hanging vertically and shoulders relaxed, downward and slightly forward, apply blades of anthropometer to lateral borders of acromion processes. Measurement is taken from the rear.
Chest	Sixth rib on midaxillary line or fourth costosternal joints anteriorly	Horizontal	With client standing, arms slightly abducted, apply the large spreading caliper tips lightly on the sixth ribs on the midaxillary line. Take measurement at end of normal expiration.
Bi-iliac (bicristal)	Iliac crests	45° downward angle	With client standing, arms folded across the chest, apply anthropometer blades firmly at a 45° downward angle, at maximum breadth of iliac crest. Measurement is taken from rear.
Bitrochanteric	Greater trochanter of femur	Horizontal	With client standing, arms folded across the chest, apply anthropometer blade with considerable pressure to compress soft tissues. Measure maximum distance between the trochanters from the rear.
Knee	Femoral epicondyles	Diagonal or horizontal	With client sitting and knee flexed to 90°, apply caliper blades firmly on lateral and medial femoral epicondyles.
Ankle (bimalleolar)	Malleoli of tibia and fibula	Oblique	With client standing and weight evenly distributed, place the caliper blades on the most lateral part of lateral malleolus and most medial part of medial malleolus. Measurement is taken on an oblique plane from the rear.
Elbow	Epicondyles of humerus	Oblique	With client's elbow flexed 90°, arm raised to the horizontal, and forearm supinated, apply the caliper blades firmly to the medial and lateral humeral epicondyles at an angle that bisects the right angle at the elbow.
Wrist	Styloid process of radius and ulna, anatomical "snuff box"	Oblique	With client's elbow flexed 90°, upper arm vertical and close to torso, and forearm pronated, apply caliper tips firmly at an oblique angle to the styloid processes of the radius (at proximal part of anatomical snuff box) and ulna.

Adapted from Wilmore et al. (1988, pp. 28–38).

From Vivian H. Heyward, 2006, *Advanced Fitness Assessment and Exercise Prescription*, 5th ed. (Champaign, IL: Human Kinetics).

Energy Intake and Expenditure

You can use the Food Record and RDA Profile (appendix E.1) to obtain information about your client's energy intake and daily energy needs. Appendix E.2 shows a sample computerized analysis of food intake that summarizes your client's recommended daily nutrients, compares the daily intake to caloric needs, and provides a detailed nutrient analysis for each food item ingested.

Your clients may use the Physical Activity Log (appendix E.3) to record the type and duration of physical activities they engage in on a daily basis. This provides an estimate of the client's daily caloric expenditure due to activity. Appendix E.4 presents MET estimates of gross expenditure for conditioning exercises, sports, and recreational activities. You can use these estimates to calculate your client's energy expenditure (kcal · min^{-1}) for a variety of activities. Appendix E.5 includes illustrations of healthy eating pyramids for Asian, Latin American, Mediterranean, and Vegetarian diets.

Food Record and RDA Profile

Food code	Amount	Description

Food code: This is generally for office use. If you have the food code list, however, use this space to more precisely describe your food item.

Amount: You can use common measures (cup, slice, etc.) or weight for your foods.

Food description: Be specific. For example, bread choices include soft and firm textures; vegetables may be raw or cooked fresh, frozen, or canned; meats should be lean only or lean with some fat; fruit juices are fresh, frozen, or canned; and cheese might be cream or skim, soft, hard, or cottage.

From Vivian H. Heyward, 2006, *Advanced Fitness Assessment and Exercise Prescription*, 5th ed. (Champaign, IL: Human Kinetics).

RDA Profile Information

Name:_____

Age: _____ Height: _____

Sex: Male _____ Weight: _____

    Female _____ Activity level: _____

       Pregnant _____   (enter number from choices below)

       Nursing _____

Most people engage in a variety of activities in a 24-hr period, and each activity can use a different amount of energy. Thus, any table of activity levels must depend on averages. Choose the level that represents your *normal daily average*.

1. Sedentary

   Inactive, sometimes under someone else's care. Energy level is for basal metabolism plus about 15% for minimal activities.

2. Lightly active

   Most professionals (lawyers, doctors, accountants, architects, etc.), office workers, shop workers, teachers, homemakers with mechanical appliances, unemployed persons.

3. Moderately active

   Most persons in light industry, building workers (excluding heavy laborers), many farm workers, active students, department store workers, soldiers not in active service, people engaged in commercial fishing, homemakers without mechanical household appliances.

4. Very active

   Full-time athletes, dancers, unskilled laborers, some agricultural workers (especially in peasant farming), forestry workers, army recruits, soldiers in active service, mine workers, steel workers.

5. Exceptionally active

   Lumberjacks, blacksmiths, women construction workers, rickshaw pullers.

Courtesy of ESHA Research, 606 Juntura Way SE, Salem, OR 97302; phone: (503) 585-6242.

From Vivian H. Heyward, 2006, *Advanced Fitness Assessment and Exercise Prescription*, 5th ed. (Champaign, IL: Human Kinetics).

Sample Computerized Analysis of Food Intake

Jane Doe Personal Profile Report

Gender:	Female
Activity Level:	Lightly Active
Height:	5 ft 3 in
Weight:	132 lbs
Age:	25 yrs
BMI:	23.38

Recommended Daily Nutrients

Basic Components						
Calories	2044		*	Vitamin D mcg	5.00	mcg
Protein	47.9	g		Vit E-Alpha Equiv.	8.00	mg
Carbohydrates	296	g	**	Folate	180.00	mcg
Dietary Fiber	20	g	#	Vitamin K	6.00	mcg
Fat - Total	68	g	**	Pantothenic	7.00	mg **
Saturated Fat	20	g	**	**Minerals**		
Mono Fat	25	g	**	Calcium	800.00	mg
Poly Fat	23	g	**	Chromium	125.00	mcg**
Cholesterol	300	mg		Copper	2.50	mg **
Vitamins				Fluoride	2.75	mg **
Vitamin A IU	4000	IU		Iodine	150	mcg
Vitamin A RE	800	RE		Iron	15	mg
Thiamin-B1	1.02	mg		Magnesium	280	mg
Riboflavin-B2	1.23	mg		Manganese	3.50	mg **
Niacin	13.49	NE		Molybdenum	163	mcg**
Vitamin-B6	1.60	mg		Phosphorus	800	mg
Vitamin-B12	2.00	mcg		Potassium	3750	mg
Biotin	65.00	mcg**		Selenium	55	mcg
Vitamin C	60.00	mg		Sodium	2400	mg
				Zinc	12	mg

* Suggested values within recommended ranges
** Dietary goals   # Fiber = 1 gram/100 kcal

The Food Processor® Nutrition Analysis program from ESHA Research, Salem, Oregon.

From Vivian H. Heyward, 2006, *Advanced Fitness Assessment and Exercise Prescription*, 5th ed. (Champaign, IL: Human Kinetics).

Source of Calories

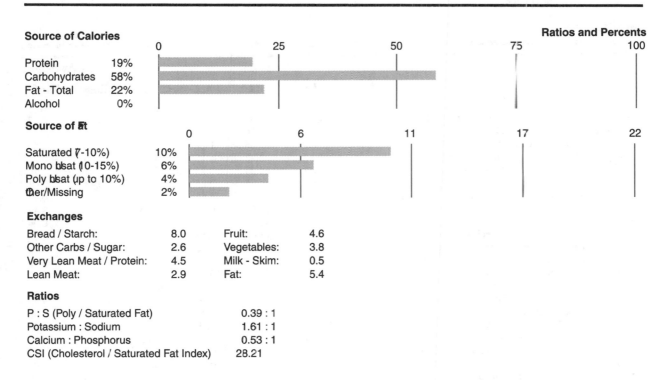

	Ratios and Percents
Protein	19%
Carbohydrates	58%
Fat - Total	22%
Alcohol	0%

Source of Fat

Saturated (7-10%)	10%
Mono bsat (10-15%)	6%
Poly bsat (up to 10%)	4%
Other/Missing	2%

Exchanges

Bread / Starch:	8.0	Fruit:	4.6
Other Carbs / Sugar:	2.6	Vegetables:	3.8
Very Lean Meat / Protein:	4.5	Milk - Skim:	0.5
Lean Meat:	2.9	Fat:	5.4

Ratios

P : S (Poly / Saturated Fat)	0.39 : 1
Potassium : Sodium	1.61 : 1
Calcium : Phosphorus	0.53 : 1
CSI (Cholesterol / Saturated Fat Index)	28.21

% comparison to: Jane Doe

Bar Graph

Nutrient	Value	Goal%
Basic Components		
Calories	1691.39	83%
Protein	84.04 g	175%
Carbohydrates	251.82 g	85%
Dietary fiber	20.71 g	101%
Fat - Total	42.41 g	62%
Saturated fat	19.24 g	94%
Mono fat	11.86 g	47%
Poly fat	7.47 g	33%
Cholesterol	175.49 mg	58%
Vitamins		
Vitamin A RE	1326.90 RE	166%
Thiamin-B1	1.79 mg	176%
Riboflavin-B2	2.11 mg	171%
Niacin-B3	37.54 mg	278%
Vitamin-B6	3.37 mg	211%
Vitamin-B12	2.55 mcg	127%
Vitamin C	266.19 mg	444%
Vitamin D mcg	7.07 mcg	141%
Vit E-Alpha Equiv.	3.79 mg	47%
Folate	440.36 mcg	245%
Pantothenic Acid	4.87 mg	70%
Minerals		
Calcium	665.59 mg	83%
Copper	1.24 mg	49%
Iron	12.83 mg	86%
Magnesium	267.18 mg	95%
Manganese	2.25 mg	64%
Phosphorus	1254.53 mg	157%
Potassium	3187.63 mg	85%
Selenium	144.48 mcg	263%
Sodium	1974.93 mg	82%
Zinc	5.78 mg	48%

From Vivian H. Heyward, 2006, *Advanced Fitness Assessment and Exercise Prescription*, 5th ed. (Champaign, IL: Human Kinetics).

Spreadsheet

Amount	Food Item	Weight (g)	Cals	Prot (g)	Carb (g)	Fiber (g)	Fat-T (g)
1/2 cup	Orange Juice prepared from frozen	124.50	56.03	0.85	13.45	0.25	0.07
2 oz-wt	Kelloggs Corn Flakes Cereal	56.70	220.56	4.59	48.82	1.47	0.17
1 each	Banana--Medium size	118.00	108.56	1.22	27.61	2.83	0.57
1/2 cup	Skim Milk-Vitamin A Added	122.50	42.75	4.18	5.94	0	0.22
1 piece	Whole Wheat Bread-Toasted	25.00	69.25	2.73	12.93	1.85	1.20
2 tsp	Jelly	12.67	34.33	0.05	8.97	0.13	0.01
1 each	White Pita Pocket Bread 6 1/2"diameter	60.00	165.00	5.46	33.42	1.32	0.72
1/2 cup	Tuna Salad	102.50	191.67	16.40	9.65	0	9.49
1/4 cup	Alfalfa Sprouts-Raw	8.25	2.39	0.33	0.31	0.21	0.06
2 piece	Fresh Tomato Wedge(1/4 of Medium Tomato)	62.00	13.02	0.53	2.88	0.68	0.20
8 oz-wt	Diet soda pop - average assorted	226.80	0	0	0	0	0
1 each	Medium Apple w/Peel	138.00	81.42	0.26	21.11	3.73	0.50
4 oz-wt	Chicken light meat - roasted	113.40	173.50	30.73	0	0	4.62
1 each	Baked Potato w/skin - medium	122.00	132.98	2.82	30.74	2.93	0.12
1 oz-wt	Cheddar Cheese-Shredded	28.35	114.25	7.06	0.36	0	9.38
4 oz-wt	Broccoli Pieces-Steamed	113.40	31.75	3.39	5.95	3.40	0.40
1/2 cup	Rich Vanilla Ice Cream	74.00	178.34	2.59	16.58	0	11.99
1/2 cup	Fresh Strawberries-Slices-Cup	83.00	24.90	0.51	5.83	1.91	0.31
2 tbs	Frozen Dessert Topping-Semi Solid	9.38	29.81	0.12	2.17	0	2.37
1 cup	Brewed Coffee	237.00	4.74	0.24	0.95	0	0.01
1 tsp	White Granulated Sugar	4.17	16.13	0	4.16	0	0
	Totals	1841.61	1691.39	84.04	251.82	20.71	42.41

Amount	Food Item	Fat-S (g)	Fat-M (g)	Fat-P (g)	Chol (mg)	A-RE (RE)	B1 (mg)
1/2 cup	Orange Juice prepared from frozen	0.01	0.01	0.01	0	9.96	0.10
2 oz-wt	Kelloggs Corn Flakes Cereal	0.02	0.09	0.03	0	750.71	0.74
1 each	Banana--Medium size	0.22	0.05	0.11	0	9.44	0.05
1/2 cup	Skim Milk-Vitamin A Added	0.14	0.06	0.01	2.21	74.73	0.04
1 piece	Whole Wheat Bread-Toasted	0.26	0.47	0.28	0	0	0.08
2 tsp	Jelly	0.00	0.00	0.01	0	0.25	0.00
1 each	White Pita Pocket Bread 6 1/2"diameter	0.10	0.06	0.32	0	0	0.36
1/2 cup	Tuna Salad	1.58	2.96	4.22	13.32	27.67	0.03
1/4 cup	Alfalfa Sprouts-Raw	0.01	0.00	0.03	0	1.32	0.01
2 piece	Fresh Tomato Wedge(1/4 of Medium Tomato)	0.03	0.03	0.08	0	38.44	0.04
8 oz-wt	Diet soda pop - average assorted	0	0	0	0	0	0
1 each	Medium Apple w/Peel	0.08	0.02	0.14	0	6.90	0.02
4 oz-wt	Chicken light meat - roasted	1.24	1.75	1.05	85.05	9.07	0.07
1 each	Baked Potato w/skin - medium	0.03	0.00	0.05	0	0	0.13
1 oz-wt	Cheddar Cheese-Shredded	6.01	2.66	0.27	29.77	85.90	0.01
4 oz-wt	Broccoli Pieces-Steamed	0.06	0.03	0.19	0	165.79	0.07
1/2 cup	Rich Vanilla Ice Cream	7.39	3.45	0.45	45.14	136.16	0.03
1/2 cup	Fresh Strawberries-Slices-Cup	0.02	0.04	0.15	0	2.49	0.02
2 tbs	Frozen Dessert Topping-Semi Solid	2.05	0.15	0.05	0	8.06	0
1 cup	Brewed Coffee	0.00	0	0.00	0	0	0
1 tsp	White Granulated Sugar	0	0	0	0	0	0
	Totals	19.24	11.86	7.47	175.49	1326.90	1.79

The Food Processor® Nutrition Analysis program from ESHA Research, Salem, Oregon.

From Vivian H. Heyward, 2006, *Advanced Fitness Assessment and Exercise Prescription*, 5th ed. (Champaign, IL: Human Kinetics).

Spreadsheet

Amount	Food Item	B2 (mg)	B3 (mg)	B6 (mg)	B12 (mcg)	Vit C (mg)	D-mcg (mcg)
1/2 cup	Orange Juice prepared from frozen	0.02	0.25	0.05	0	48.43	0
2 oz-wt	Kelloggs Corn Flakes Cereal	0.86	9.98	1.02	0	30.05	1.98
1 each	Banana--Medium size	0.12	0.64	0.68	0	10.74	0
1/2 cup	Skim Milk-Vitamin A Added	0.17	0.11	0.05	0.46	1.20	1.23
1 piece	Whole Wheat Bread-Toasted	0.05	0.97	0.05	0.00	0	0.05
2 tsp	Jelly	0.00	0.00	0.00	0	0.11	0
1 each	White Pita Pocket Bread 6 1/2"diameter	0.20	2.78	0.02	0	0	0
1/2 cup	Tuna Salad	0.07	6.87	0.08	1.23	2.25	3.31
1/4 cup	Alfalfa Sprouts-Raw	0.01	0.04	0.00	0	0.68	0
2 piece	Fresh Tomato Wedge(1/4 of Medium Tomato)	0.03	0.39	0.05	0	11.84	0
8 oz-wt	Diet soda pop - average assorted	0	0	0	0	0	0
1 each	Medium Apple w/Peel	0.02	0.11	0.07	0	7.87	0
4 oz-wt	Chicken light meat - roasted	0.11	11.91	0.61	0.35	0	0.34
1 each	Baked Potato w/skin - medium	0.04	2.01	0.42	0	15.74	0
1 oz-wt	Cheddar Cheese-Shredded	0.11	0.02	0.02	0.23	0	0.09
4 oz-wt	Broccoli Pieces-Steamed	0.13	0.69	0.16	0	89.70	0
1/2 cup	Rich Vanilla Ice Cream	0.12	0.06	0.03	0.27	0.52	0.07
1/2 cup	Fresh Strawberries-Slices-Cup	0.05	0.19	0.05	0	47.06	0
2 tbs	Frozen Dessert Topping-Semi Solid	0	0	0	0	0	0
1 cup	Brewed Coffee	0	0.53	0	0	0	0
1 tsp	White Granulated Sugar	0.00	0	0	0	0	0
	Totals	2.11	37.54	3.37	2.55	266.19	7.07

Amount	Food Item	E-aTE (mg)	Fola (mcg)	Panto (mg)	Calc (mg)	Copp (mg)	Iron (mg)
1/2 cup	Orange Juice prepared from frozen	0.24	54.53	0.20	11.21	0.05	0.12
2 oz-wt	Kelloggs Corn Flakes Cereal	0.14	200.15	0.10	1.70	0.04	3.58
1 each	Banana--Medium size	0.32	22.54	0.31	7.08	0.12	0.37
1/2 cup	Skim Milk-Vitamin A Added	0.05	6.37	0.40	150.68	0.01	0.05
1 piece	Whole Wheat Bread-Toasted	0.23	9.75	0.10	20.25	0.08	0.93
2 tsp	Jelly	0	0.13	0.02	1.01	0.00	0.03
1 each	White Pita Pocket Bread 6 1/2"diameter	0.02	14.40	0.24	51.60	0.10	1.57
1/2 cup	Tuna Salad	0.97	7.48	0.27	17.42	0.15	1.02
1/4 cup	Alfalfa Sprouts-Raw	0.00	2.97	0.05	2.64	0.01	0.08
2 piece	Fresh Tomato Wedge(1/4 of Medium Tomato)	0.24	9.30	0.15	3.10	0.05	0.28
8 oz-wt	Diet soda pop - average assorted	0	0	0	0	0	0
1 each	Medium Apple w/Peel	0.44	3.86	0.08	9.66	0.06	0.25
4 oz-wt	Chicken light meat - roasted	0.30	3.40	1.03	14.74	0.05	1.22
1 each	Baked Potato w/skin - medium	0.06	13.42	0.68	12.20	0.37	1.66
1 oz-wt	Cheddar Cheese-Shredded	0.10	5.16	0.12	204.40	0.01	0.19
4 oz-wt	Broccoli Pieces-Steamed	0.54	68.27	0.58	54.32	0.05	1.00
1/2 cup	Rich Vanilla Ice Cream	0	3.70	0.27	86.58	0.02	0.04
1/2 cup	Fresh Strawberries-Slices-Cup	0.12	14.69	0.28	11.62	0.04	0.32
2 tbs	Frozen Dessert Topping-Semi Solid	0.02	0	0	0.59	0.00	0.01
1 cup	Brewed Coffee	0	0.24	0.00	4.74	0.02	0.12
1 tsp	White Granulated Sugar	0	0	0	0.04	0.00	0.00
	Totals	3.79	440.36	4.87	665.59	1.24	12.83

From Vivian H. Heyward, 2006, *Advanced Fitness Assessment and Exercise Prescription*, 5th ed. (Champaign, IL: Human Kinetics).

Amount	Food Item	Magn (mg)	Mang (mg)	Phos (mg)	Potas (mg)	Sel (mcg)	Sod (mg)
1/2 cup	Orange Juice prepared from frozen	12.45	0.02	19.92	236.55	0.25	1.25
2 oz-wt	Kelloggs Corn Flakes Cereal	6.80	0.05	35.72	52.16	2.89	580.04
1 each	Banana--Medium size	34.22	0.18	23.60	467.28	1.18	1.18
1/2 cup	Skim Milk-Vitamin A Added	13.97	0.00	123.73	203.35	1.23	63.09
1 piece	Whole Wheat Bread-Toasted	24.25	0.65	64.50	70.75	10.25	148.00
2 tsp	Jelly	0.76	0.02	0.63	8.11	0.25	4.56
1 each	White Pita Pocket Bread 6 1/2"diameter	15.60	0.29	58.20	72.00	18.00	321.60
1/2 cup	Tuna Salad	19.47	0.04	182.45	182.45	70.01	412.05
1/4 cup	Alfalfa Sprouts-Raw	2.23	0.02	5.78	6.52	--	0.50
2 piece	Fresh Tomato Wedge(1/4 of Medium Tomato)	6.82	0.07	14.88	137.64	0.25	5.58
8 oz-wt	Diet soda pop - average assorted	0	0	90.72	34.02	0	113.40
1 each	Medium Apple w/Peel	6.90	0.06	9.66	158.70	0.41	0
4 oz-wt	Chicken light meat - roasted	26.08	0.02	246.08	267.62	28.92	57.83
1 each	Baked Potato w/skin - medium	32.94	0.28	69.54	509.96	1.95	9.76
1 oz-wt	Cheddar Cheese-Shredded	7.88	0.00	145.15	27.90	4.03	176.05
4 oz-wt	Broccoli Pieces-Steamed	28.35	0.25	74.73	367.42	--	30.62
1/2 cup	Rich Vanilla Ice Cream	8.14	0.01	70.30	117.66	4.00	41.44
1/2 cup	Fresh Strawberries-Slices-Cup	8.30	0.24	15.77	137.78	0.75	0.83
2 tbs	Frozen Dessert Topping-Semi Solid	0.17	0.01	0.72	1.71	--	2.37
1 cup	Brewed Coffee	11.85	0.06	2.37	127.98	0.11	4.74
1 tsp	White Granulated Sugar	0	0.00	0.08	0.08	0.01	0.04
	Totals	267.18	2.25	1254.53	3187.63	144.48	1974.93

Amount	Food Item	Zinc (mg)
1/2 cup	Orange Juice prepared from frozen	0.06
2 oz-wt	Kelloggs Corn Flakes Cereal	0.16
1 each	Banana--Medium size	0.19
1/2 cup	Skim Milk-Vitamin A Added	0.49
1 piece	Whole Wheat Bread-Toasted	0.55
2 tsp	Jelly	0.01
1 each	White Pita Pocket Bread 6 1/2"diameter	0.50
1/2 cup	Tuna Salad	0.57
1/4 cup	Alfalfa Sprouts-Raw	0.08
2 piece	Fresh Tomato Wedge(1/4 of Medium Tomato)	0.06
8 oz-wt	Diet soda pop - average assorted	0
1 each	Medium Apple w/Peel	0.06
4 oz-wt	Chicken light meat - roasted	0.88
1 each	Baked Potato w/skin - medium	0.39
1 oz-wt	Cheddar Cheese-Shredded	0.88
4 oz-wt	Broccoli Pieces-Steamed	0.45
1/2 cup	Rich Vanilla Ice Cream	0.30
1/2 cup	Fresh Strawberries-Slices-Cup	0.11
2 tbs	Frozen Dessert Topping-Semi Solid	0.00
1 cup	Brewed Coffee	0.05
1 tsp	White Granulated Sugar	0.00
	Totals	5.78

The Food Processor® Nutrition Analysis program from ESHA Research, Salem, Oregon.

From Vivian H. Heyward, 2006, *Advanced Fitness Assessment and Exercise Prescription*, 5th ed. (Champaign, IL: Human Kinetics).

Physical Activity Log

Name: _____ Date: _____

Day and date	Activity	Duration (min)	X	kcal · min⁻¹	= Total (kcal)

Gross Energy Expenditure for Conditioning Exercises, Sports, and Recreational Activities

METs	Description
Conditioning Exercises	
5.0	Aerobic dancing, low impact
8.5	Aerobics, step, with 6-8 in. step
10.0	Aerobics, step, with 10-12 in. step
3.0	Bicycling, stationary, 50 W, very light effort
5.5	Bicycling, stationary, 100 W, light effort
7.0	Bicycling, stationary, 150 W, moderate effort
10.5	Bicycling, stationary, 200 W, vigorous effort
12.5	Bicycling, stationary, 250 W, very vigorous effort
8.0	Calisthenics (e.g., push-ups, pull-ups, jumping jacks, sit-ups), vigorous
3.5	Calisthenics, light or moderate effort
8.0	Circuit resistance training, including some aerobic activity and minimal rest (e.g., super circuit resistance training)
8.0	Elliptical training, machine, 125 strides $\cdot$ min^{-1} with resistance
3.5	Rowing (machine), 50 W, light effort
7.0	Rowing (machine), 100 W, moderate effort
8.5	Rowing (machine), 150 W, vigorous effort
12.0	Rowing (machine), 200 W, very vigorous effort
8.0	Running, 5 mph (12 min $\cdot$ mile^{-1})
9.0	Running, 5.2 mph (11.5 min $\cdot$ mile^{-1})
10.0	Running, 6.0 mph (10 min $\cdot$ mile^{-1})
11.0	Running, 6.7 mph (9 min $\cdot$ mile^{-1})
11.5	Running, 7.0 mph (8.5 min $\cdot$ mile^{-1})
12.5	Running, 7.5 mph (8 min $\cdot$ mile^{-1})
13.5	Running, 8 mph (7.5 min $\cdot$ mile^{-1})
14.0	Running, 8.6 mph (7 min $\cdot$ mile^{-1})
15.0	Running, 9 mph (6.5 min $\cdot$ mile^{-1})
16.0	Running, 10 mph (6 min $\cdot$ mile^{-1})
18.0	Running, 10.9 mph (5.5 min $\cdot$ mile^{-1})
9.0	Running, cross country
7.0	Jogging, general
6.0	Jogging/walking combination (jogging component less than 10 min)

From Vivian H. Heyward, 2006, *Advanced Fitness Assessment and Exercise Prescription,* 5th ed. (Champaign, IL: Human Kinetics).

4.5	Jogging on a mini-trampoline
12.5	Rollerblading, in-line skating, vigorous effort
8.0	Rope skipping, slow
10.0	Rope skipping, moderate
12.0	Rope skipping, fast
9.5	Skiing, Nordic (machine)
6.0	Slimnastics, Jazzercize
9.0	Stair-climbing (machine), step ergometer
2.5	Stretching, hatha yoga
10.0	Swimming, laps, freestyle, fast, vigorous effort
7.0	Swimming, laps, freestyle, slow, moderate or light effort
7.0	Swimming, backstroke
10.0	Swimming, breaststroke
11.0	Swimming, butterfly
11.0	Swimming, crawl, fast, vigorous effort
8.0	Swimming, crawl, slow, moderate or light effort
8.0	Swimming, sidestroke
4.0	Swimming, treading water, moderate effort
4.0	Tai chi
5.0	Treading™, walking, variable speed 2.5-4.0 mph and grade 0-10%
11.0	Treading™, running, variable speed 5.8-7.5 mph and grade 0-10%
2.5	Walking, 2.0 mph
3.0	Walking, 2.5 mph
3.3	Walking, 3.0 mph
3.8	Walking, 3.5 mph
5.0	Walking, 4.0 mph
6.3	Walking, 4.5 mph
4.0	Water aerobics, water calisthenics
8.0	Water jogging
3.0	Weightlifting (free weights/machines), light to moderate effort
6.0	Weightlifting (free weights/machines), powerlifting, bodybuilding, vigorous effort

Sports and recreational activities

3.5	Archery (non-hunting)
7.0	Badminton, competitive
4.5	Badminton, social singles or doubles
5.0	Baseball, general
8.0	Basketball, game
4.5	Basketball, shooting baskets
6.5	Basketball, wheelchair
8.5	Bicycling, BMX or mountain
4.0	Bicycling, <10 mph, leisure, pleasure

(continued)

From Vivian H. Heyward, 2006, *Advanced Fitness Assessment and Exercise Prescription*, 5th ed. (Champaign, IL: Human Kinetics).

6.0	Bicycling, 10-11.9 mph
8.0	Bicycling, 12-13.9 mph
10.0	Bicycling, 14-15.9 mph
12.0	Bicycling, 16-19 mph
16.0	Bicycling, ≥ 20 mph
5.0	Bicycling, unicycle
2.5	Billiards, pool
2.5	Bird watching
3.0	Bowling
3.0	Bowling, lawn
12.0	Boxing, in ring
6.0	Boxing, punching bag
9.0	Boxing, sparring
7.0	Broomball
12.0	Boxing, in run
6.0	Boxing, punching bag
9.0	Boxing, sparring
7.0	Broomball
3.0	Canoeing, 2.0-3.9 mph, light effort
7.0	Canoeing, 4.0-5.9 mph, moderate effort
12.0	Canoeing, ≥ 6.0 mph, vigorous effort
5.0	Children's games, hopscotch, dodgeball, T-ball, tetherball, playground
5.0	Cricket (batting and bowling)
2.5	Croquet
4.0	Curling
4.8	Dancing, ballet or modern, twist, jazz, tap, jitterbug
4.5	Dancing, Greek, Middle Eastern, belly, hula, flamenco, swing
4.5	Dancing, ballroom, fast, disco, folk, square, line dancing, Irish step dancing, polka, contra, country
3.0	Dancing, slow, waltz, foxtrot, samba, tango, mamgo, cha-cha
5.5	Dancing, traditional American Indian dancing
2.5	Darts, wall or lawn
3.0	Diving, springboard or platform
6.0	Fencing
4.0	Fishing and hunting from riverbank and walking
2.5	Fishing and hunting from boat, sitting
6.0	Fishing in stream, in waders
2.0	Fishing, ice, sitting
2.5	Fishing and hunting, bow and arrow, crossbow
2.5	Fishing and hunting, pistol shooting, trap shooting, standing
9.0	Football, competitive
2.5	Football or baseball, playing catch
8.0	Football, touch, flag
3.0	Frisbee, playing, general
8.0	Frisbee, ultimate
3.0	Gardening, lawn work, general

From Vivian H. Heyward, 2006, *Advanced Fitness Assessment and Exercise Prescription*, 5th ed. (Champaign, IL: Human Kinetics).

     APPENDIX E.4

4.5	Golfing, walking and carrying clubs
3.0	Golfing, miniature, driving range
4.3	Golfing, walking and pulling clubs
3.5	Golfing, power cart
4.0	Gymnastics, general
4.0	Hacky sack
12.0	Handball, general
8.0	Handball, team
3.5	Hang gliding
6.0	Hiking, cross country
8.0	Hockey, field
8.0	Hockey, ice
4.0	Horseback riding, general
3.0	Horseshoe pitching, quoits
12.0	Jai alai
10.0	Judo, jujitsu, kick boxing, tae kwon do
4.0	Juggling
5.0	Kayaking and whitewater rafting
7.0	Kickball
8.0	Lacrosse
4.0	Motor-cross
9.0	Orienteering
10.0	Paddleball, competitive
6.0	Paddleball, casual, general
4.0	Paddle boating
8.0	Polo
6.5	Race walking
10.0	Racquetball, competitive
7.0	Racquetball, casual, general
11.0	Rock climbing, ascending
8.0	Rock climbing, rappelling
10.0	Rugby
3.0	Sailing, boat and board sailing, wind surfing, ice surfing
7.0	Scuba diving, skin diving
3.0	Shuffleboard
5.0	Skateboarding
7.0	Skating, roller or ice
15.0	Skating, speed skating
7.0	Skiing, cross-country, 2.5 mph, light effort
8.0	Skiing, cross-country, 4.0-4.9 mph, moderate effort
9.0	Skiing, cross-country, 5.0-7.9 mph, vigorous effort

(continued)

From Vivian H. Heyward, 2006, *Advanced Fitness Assessment and Exercise Prescription*, 5th ed (Champaign, IL: Human Kinetics).

(continued)

14.0	Skiing, cross-country, >8.0 mph, racing
5.0	Skiing, downhill, light effort
6.0	Skiing, downhill, moderate effort
8.0	Skiing, downhill, vigorous effort, racing
6.0	Skiing, water
7.0	Skimobiling
3.5	Skydiving
7.0	Sledding, tobogganing, bobsledding, luge
5.0	Snorkeling
8.0	Snow shoeing
10.0	Soccer, competitive
7.0	Soccer, casual, general
5.0	Softball, fast or slow pitch
6.0	Softball, pitching
12.0	Squash
3.0	Surfing, body or board
6.0	Swimming, leisurely, not laps
8.0	Swimming, synchronized
4.0	Table tennis, Ping-Pong
7.0	Tennis, general
5.0	Tennis, doubles
8.0	Tennis, singles
4.0	Track and field, shot, discus, hammer throw
6.0	Track and field, high jump, long jump, triple jump, javelin, pole vault
10.0	Track and field, steeplechase, hurdles
3.5	Trampoline
8.0	Volleyball, competitive
8.0	Volleyball, beach
3.0	Volleyball, noncompetitive
10.0	Water polo
3.0	Water volleyball
7.0	Wallyball
6.0	Wrestling

From Vivian H. Heyward, 2006, *Advanced Fitness Assessment and Exercise Prescription,* 5th ed. (Champaign, IL: Human Kinetics). Data from Ainsworth, B.E., et al. (2000). Compendium of physical activities: An update of activity codes and MET intensities. *Medicine & Science in Sports & Exercise* 32(supplement): S498-S516.

APPENDIX E.4

Healthy Eating Pyramids

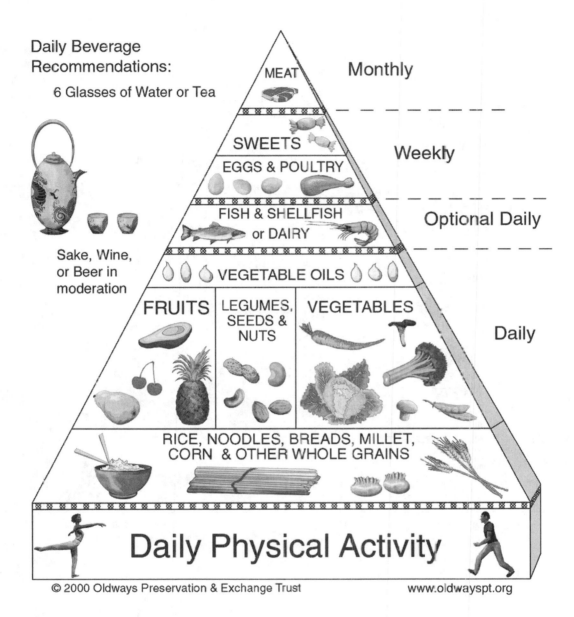

Daily Beverage Recommendations:

6 Glasses of Water or Tea

Sake, Wine, or Beer in moderation

Monthly

MEAT

SWEETS

Weekly

EGGS & POULTRY

FISH & SHELLFISH or DAIRY

Optional Daily

VEGETABLE OILS

FRUITS

LEGUMES, SEEDS & NUTS

VEGETABLES

Daily

RICE, NOODLES, BREADS, MILLET, CORN & OTHER WHOLE GRAINS

Daily Physical Activity

© 2000 Oldways Preservation & Exchange Trust   www.oldwayspt.org

Figure E.5.1 Asian diet pyramid.

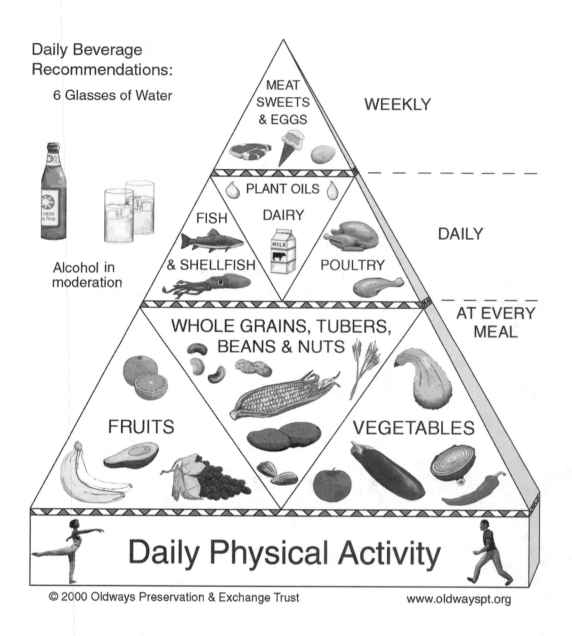

Daily Beverage Recommendations:

6 Glasses of Water

Alcohol in moderation

MEAT SWEETS & EGGS — WEEKLY

PLANT OILS

FISH & SHELLFISH

DAIRY

POULTRY — DAILY

WHOLE GRAINS, TUBERS, BEANS & NUTS — AT EVERY MEAL

FRUITS

VEGETABLES

Daily Physical Activity

© 2000 Oldways Preservation & Exchange Trust

www.oldwayspt.org

Figure E.5.2 Latin American diet pyramid.

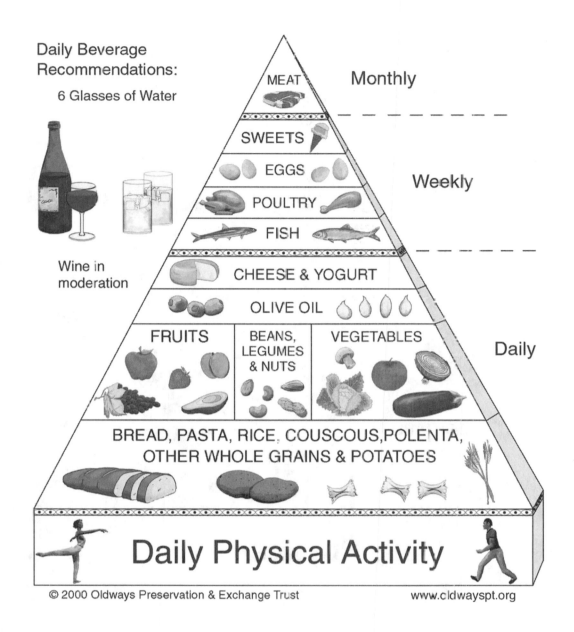

Figure E.5.3 Mediterranean diet pyramid.

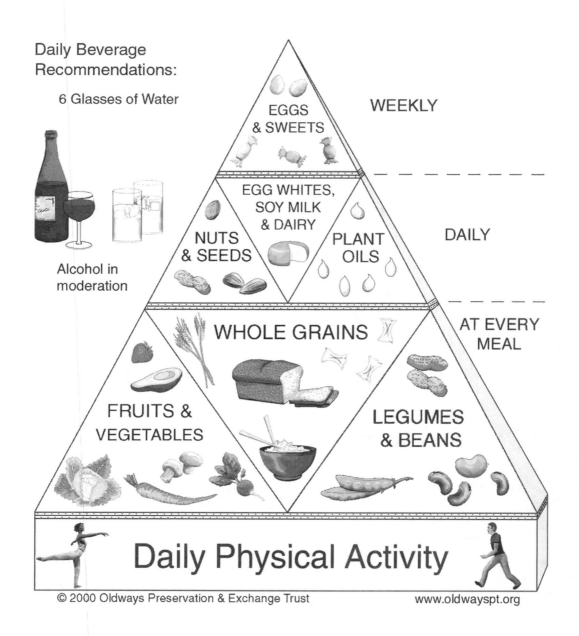

Daily Beverage Recommendations:

6 Glasses of Water

Alcohol in moderation

WEEKLY

EGGS & SWEETS

EGG WHITES, SOY MILK & DAIRY

NUTS & SEEDS

PLANT OILS

DAILY

WHOLE GRAINS

AT EVERY MEAL

FRUITS & VEGETABLES

LEGUMES & BEANS

Daily Physical Activity

© 2000 Oldways Preservation & Exchange Trust   www.oldwayspt.org

Figure E.5.4 Vegetarian diet pyramid.

Flexibility and Low Back Care Exercises

Appendix F.1 describes and illustrates selected static stretching exercises for flexibility. This information is organized by body region and muscle groups. Appendix F.2 summarizes Exercise Do's and Don'ts. For each contraindicated exercise, a safe alternative exercise is presented.

Recommended exercises for low back care programs are illustrated in appendix F.3. This appendix provides a description and identifies muscle groups involved for each exercise.

Selected Flexibility Exercises

ANTERIOR THIGH REGION

Muscle Groups: Quadriceps and Hip Flexors

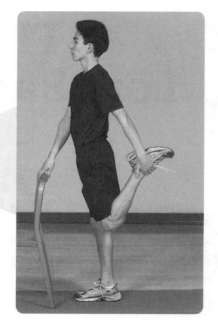

Exercise 1

Description: From a standing position, raise one foot toward hips and grasp ankle. Pull leg upward toward buttocks.

Exercise 2

Description: Lying on your side, flex the knee and grasp the ankle. Press the foot into the hand and squeeze the pelvis forward. Do not pull the foot.

Exercise 3

Description: In a prone position, flex the knee and grasp ankle or foot with both hands. Do not pull on the foot. Keep knees on the floor and do not arch the back.

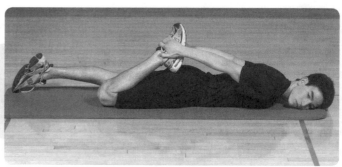

From Vivian H. Heyward, 2006, *Advanced Fitness Assessment and Exercise Prescription*, 5th ed. (Champaign, IL: Human Kinetics).

APPENDIX F.1

POSTERIOR THIGH REGION

Muscle Groups: Hamstrings and Hip Extensors

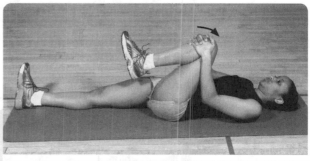

Exercise 1

Description: In a supine position, grasp knee and pull knee toward chest, then flex head to knee.

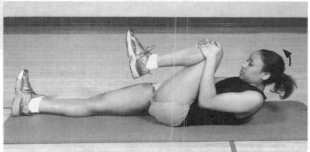

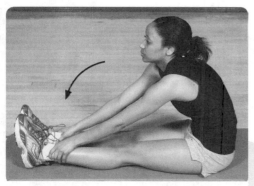

Exercise 2

Description: From a long-sitting position, grasp ankles and flex trunk to legs.

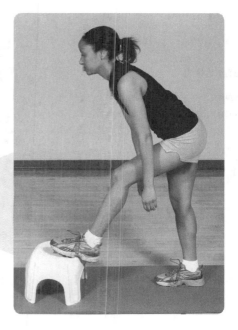

Exercise 3

Description: From a standing position, place your foot on a low step, keep the knee flexed slightly, and bend from the hips until you feel the stretch.

From Vivian H. Heyward, 2006, *Advanced Fitness Assessment and Exercise Prescription*, 5th ed. (Champaign, IL: Human Kinetics).

APPENDIX F.1

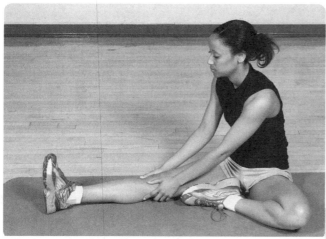

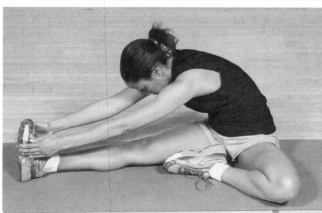

Exercise 4

Description: From a sitting position, with one knee flexed, flex the trunk keeping the spine extended until you feel tension.

Exercise 5

Description: From a lying position, with one leg extended and the other leg flexed, grasp leg with both hands and flex thigh to trunk.

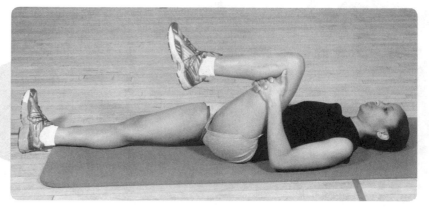

From Vivian H. Heyward, 2006, *Advanced Fitness Assessment and Exercise Prescription*, 5th ed. (Champaign, IL: Human Kinetics).

Muscle Groups: Hip Adductors

Exercise 1

Description: From a tailor-sitting position, with soles of feet together, place hands on inside of knees and push downward slowly.

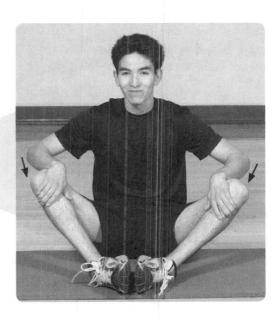

Exercise 2

Description: From a straddle-standing position, flex one knee and hip, lowering body closer to floor.

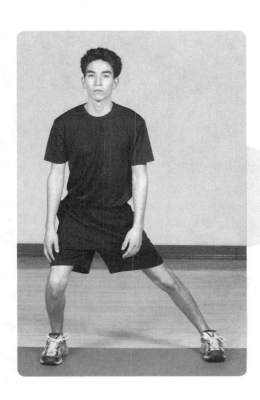

Exercise 3

Description: Standing on one leg while supporting yourself against wall or chair abduct hip, keeping leg straight. Have partner grasp ankle and passively stretch the muscle further.

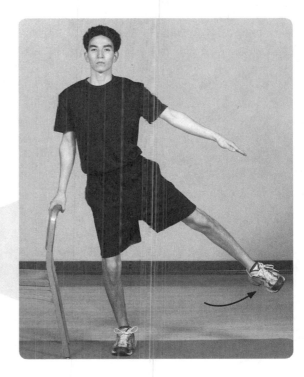

From Vivian H. Heyward, 2006, *Advanced Fitness Assessment and Exercise Prescription*, 5th ed. (Champaign, IL: Human Kinetics).

Muscle Groups: Hip Abductors and Trunk Lateral Flexors

Exercise 1

Description: From standing position, with arms overhead, clasp hands together and laterally flex trunk to side no more than 20°.

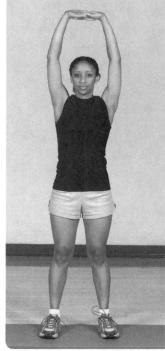
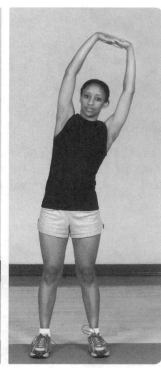

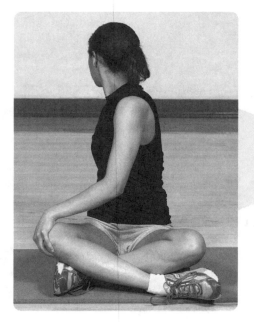

Exercise 2

Description: From a crossed-leg sitting position, rotate trunk to the right. Place hands on right side of thigh and pull. Repeat to opposite side.

From Vivian H. Heyward, 2006, *Advanced Fitness Assessment and Exercise Prescription*, 5th ed. (Champaign, IL: Human Kinetics).

Muscle Group: Plantar Flexors

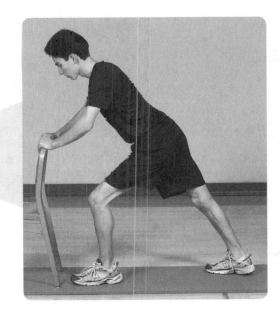

Exercise 1

Description: Assume front-leaning position against wall or chair with one foot ahead of the other. Flex hip, knee and ankle to lower your body closer to the ground, keeping feet flat on floor.

Exercise 2

Description: Standing with balls of feet on stairs, curb, or wood block, lower heels to floor.

From Vivian H. Heyward, 2006, *Advanced Fitness Assessment and Exercise Prescription*, 5th ed. (Champaign, IL: Human Kinetics).

ANTERIOR LEG REGION

Muscle Group: Dorsiflexors

Exercise 1

Description: Standing with ankle of the nonsupporting leg fully extended, stretch the dorsiflexors by slowly flexing the knee of the supporting leg.

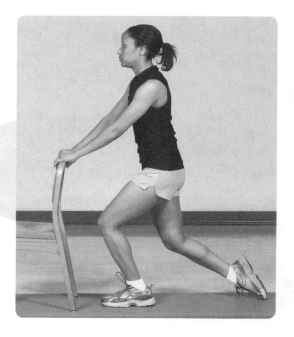

UPPER AND LOWER BACK REGIONS

Muscle Group: Trunk Extensors

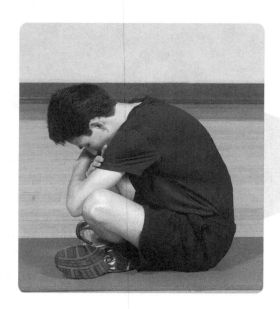

Exercise 1

Description: Sit with legs crossed and arms relaxed. Tuck chin and curl forward attempting to touch forehead to knees.

From Vivian H. Heyward, 2006, *Advanced Fitness Assessment and Exercise Prescription,* 5th ed. (Champaign, IL: Human Kinetics).

APPENDIX F.1

Exercise 2

Description: In a supine position, with knees flexed, grasp thighs below the knee caps and bring knees to chest. Flatten lower back to floor.

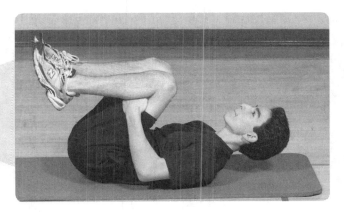

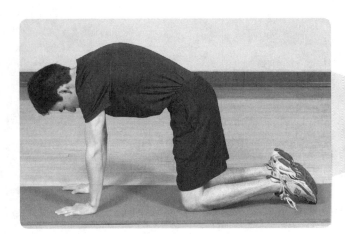

Exercise 3

Description: From a kneeling position, bring chin to chest. Contract abdomen and buttocks muscles while rounding lower back.

ANTERIOR CHEST, SHOULDER, AND ABDOMINAL REGIONS

Muscle Groups: Shoulder Flexors and Adductors, Trunk Flexors

Exercise 1

Description: In a prone position, push up until elbows are fully extended. Keep pelvis and hips on floor.

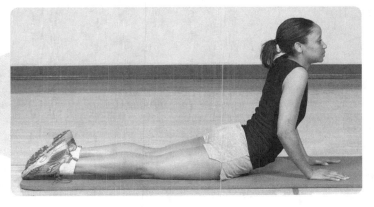

From Vivian H. Heyward. 2006, *Advanced Fitness Assessment and Exercise Prescription*, 5th ed. (Champaign, IL: Human Kinetics).

Exercise 2

Description: Grasp towel or rope with both hands. Rotate arms overhead behind trunk.

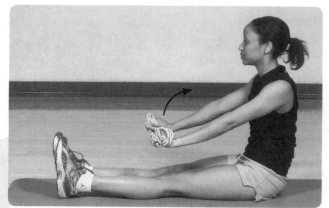

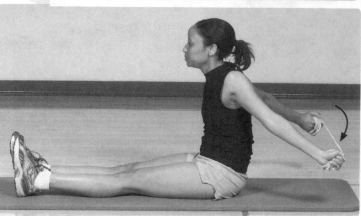

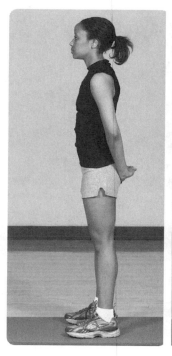

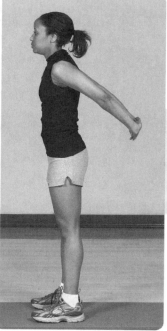

Exercise 3

Description: Clasp hands together behind trunk with elbows extended. Slowly raise arms upward.

From Vivian H. Heyward, 2006, *Advanced Fitness Assessment and Exercise Prescription*, 5th ed. (Champaign, IL: Human Kinetics).

Exercise Do's and Don'ts

DON'T: Neck Hyperextension

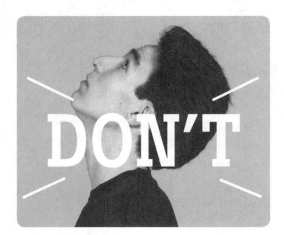

DO: Neck Lateral Flexion

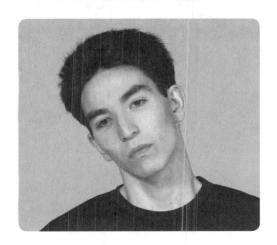

DON'T: Head Throws in a Crunch

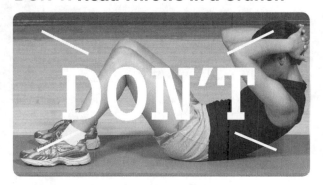

DO: Partial Sit-Up

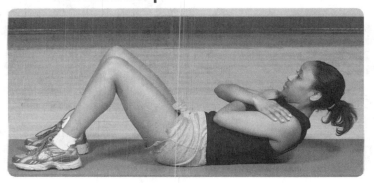

DON'T: Unsupported Hip/Trunk Flexion

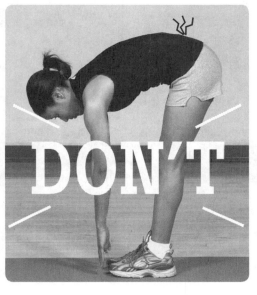

DO: Seated Hip/Trunk Flexion

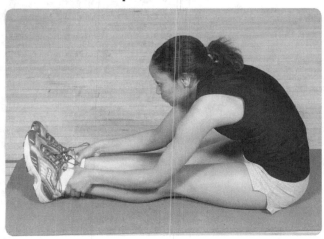

From Vivian H. Heyward, 2006, *Advanced Fitness Assessment and Exercise Prescription*, 5th ed. (Champaign, IL: Human Kinetics).

DON'T: The Plow

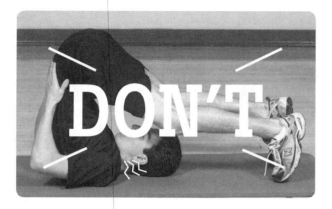

DO: Camel

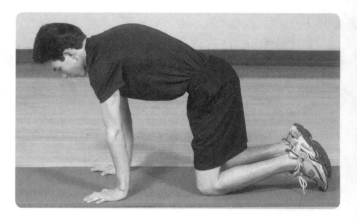

DON'T: Swan Lifts

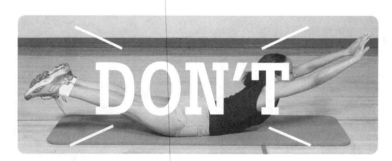

DO: Trunk Extensions

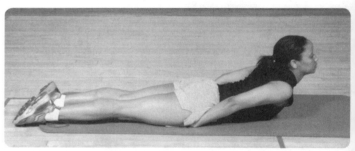

DON'T: V-Sits

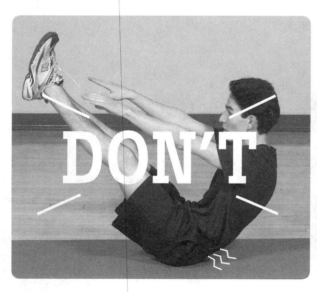

DO: Partial Sit-Up

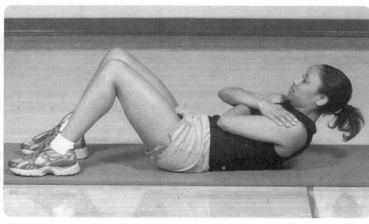

From Vivian H. Heyward, 2006, *Advanced Fitness Assessment and Exercise Prescription,* 5th ed. (Champaign, IL: Human Kinetics).

APPENDIX F.2

DON'T: Leg Lifts With Trunk Hyperextended

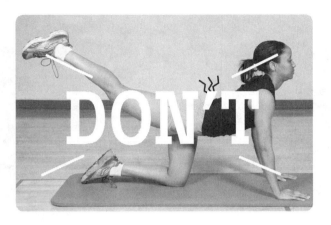

DO: Leg Lifts With Trunk and Leg in Straight Line

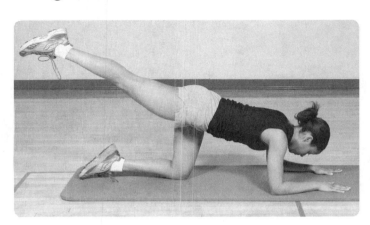

DON'T: Hamstring Stretch— Leg on Bar

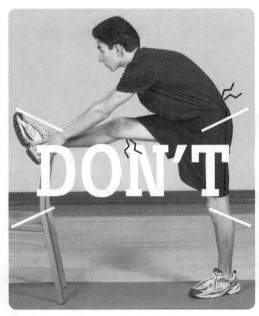

DO: Hamstring Stretch—Knee to Chest

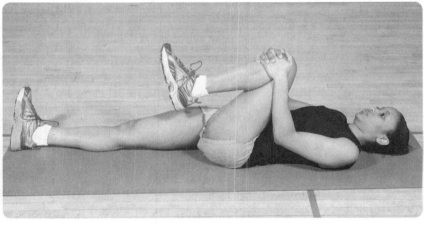

DON'T: Hurdler's Stretch

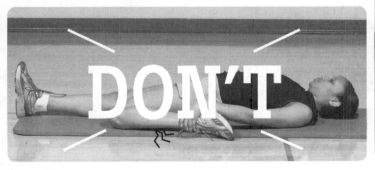

DO: Quad Stretch

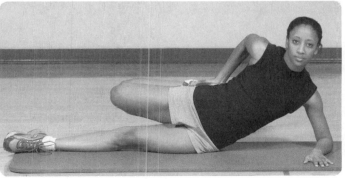

From Vivian H. Heyward, 2006, *Advanced Fitness Assessment and Exercise Prescription,* 5th ed (Champaign IL: Human Kinetics).

APPENDIX F.2

DON'T: Squats & Deep Knee Bends

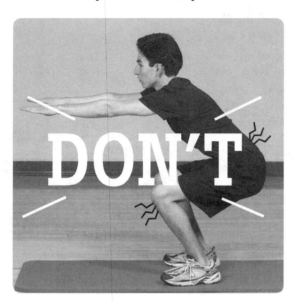

DO: Half-Squats

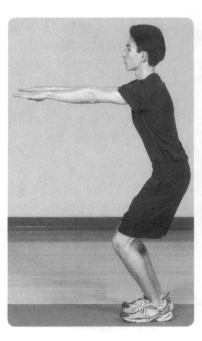

DON'T: Lunges (with knee forward of supporting foot)

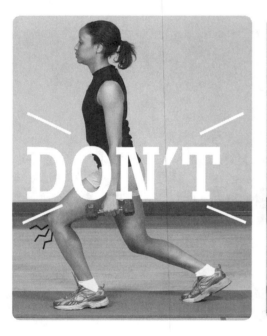

DO: Lunges (with knee in line with supporting hee

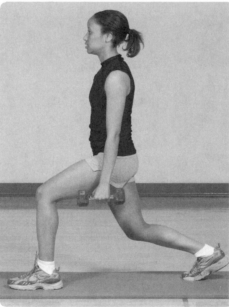

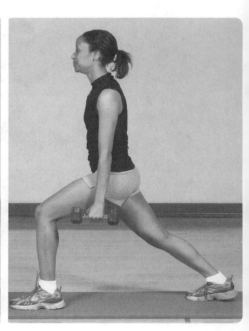

From Vivian H. Heyward, 2006, *Advanced Fitness Assessment and Exercise Prescription*, 5th ed. (Champaign, IL: Human Kinetics).

DON'T: Fast Twists & Jump Twists

DO: Jump Without Twist

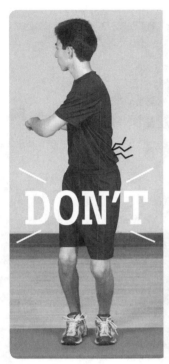 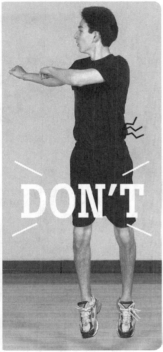 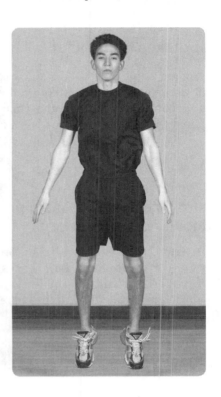

Exercises for Low Back Care

Pelvic Tilt (stretches abdominal muscles)

Lie on your back with knees bent, feet flat on the floor, and arms at your sides. Flatten the small of your back against the floor. (Your hips will tilt upward.) Hold.

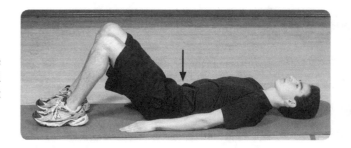

Double Knee to Chest (stretches hip, buttock, and lower back muscles)

Lie on your back with knees bent, feet flat on the floor, and arms at your sides. Raise both knees, one at a time, to your chest and hold with your hands. Lower your legs, one at a time, to the floor and rest briefly.

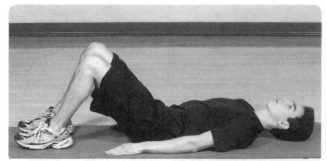

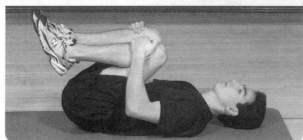

Trunk Flex (stretches back, abdominal, and leg muscles)

On your hands and knees, tuck in your chin and arch your back. Slowly sit back on your heels, letting your shoulders drop toward the floor. Hold.

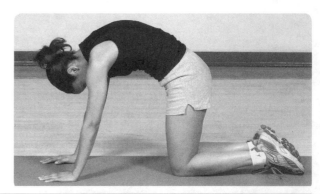

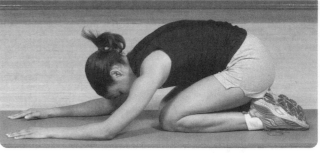

From Vivian H. Heyward, 2006, *Advanced Fitness Assessment and Exercise Prescription*, 5th ed. (Champaign, IL: Human Kinetics).

Cat and Camel (strengthens back and abdominal muscles)

On your hands and knees with your head parallel to the floor, arch your back and then let it slowly sag toward the floor. Try to keep your arms straight.

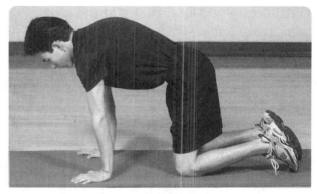

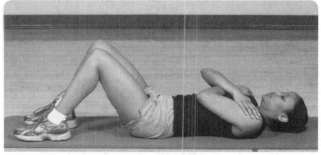

Partial Sit-Up (strengthens abdominal muscles)

Lie on your back with knees bent, feet flat on the floor, and arms crossed over your chest. Keeping your middle and lower back flat on the floor, raise your head and shoulders off the floor, and hold. Gradually increase your holding time.

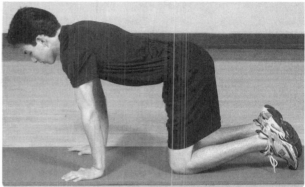

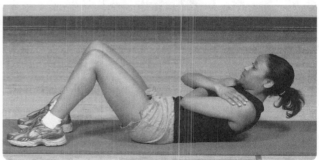

From Vivian H. Heyward, 2006, *Advanced Fitness Assessment and Exercise Prescription*, 5th ed. (Champaign, IL: Human Kinetics).

Single-Leg Extension (strengthens hip and buttock muscles, and stretches abdominal and leg muscles)

Lie on your stomach with your arms folded under your chin. Slowly lift one leg—not too high—without bending it, while keeping your pelvis flat on the floor. Slowly lower your leg and repeat with the other leg.

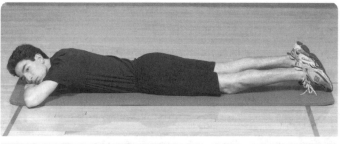
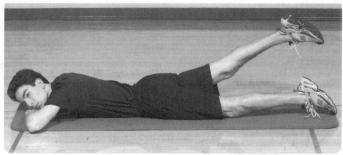

Single Leg-Extension Hold (strengthens the trunk extensors)

On your hands and knees with your head parallel to the floor, extend your thigh and leg and hold this position. Raising the contralateral arm simultaneously is more difficult and increases the extensor muscle activity and spinal compression.

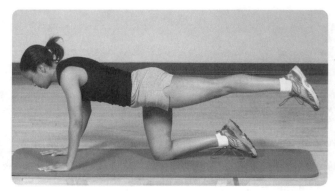

Curl-Up with Leg Extended (strengthens abdominal muscles)

Lie on your back with one knee flexed (foot flat on floor) and the other knee extended. Place your hands under the lumbar spine to preserve the neutral spine position. Slowly raise your head and shoulders off the floor.

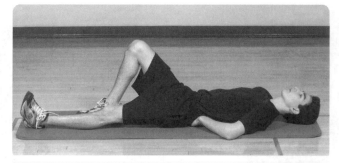
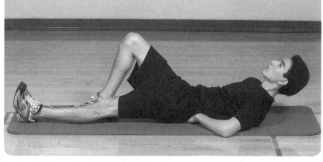

From Vivian H. Heyward, 2006, *Advanced Fitness Assessment and Exercise Prescription*, 5th ed. (Champaign, IL: Human Kinetics).

Isometric Side Support or Side Bridge (strengthens the lateral muscles of trunk and abdomen)

Assume a side support position with body supported by the knee, thigh, and forearm (flexed to 90°), and hold this position. Supporting the body with the feet, instead of the knee and thigh, increases the muscle activity and spinal load.

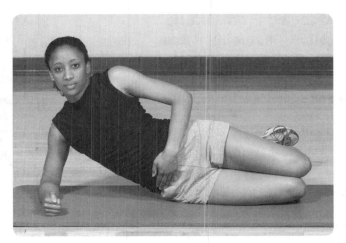

Standing Cat and Camel (strengthens back and abdominal muscles)

Stand with feet shoulder-width apart and with hands on knees. Straighten back and hold this position. Perform 10 to 20 repetitions.

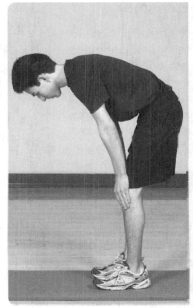
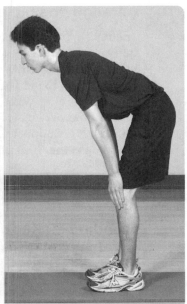

Bent-Knee Curl-Up (strengthens abdominal muscles)

Lie on your back with one knee bent and with foot flat on the floor. Place arms across chest. Lift shoulders off ground and hold this position momentarily. Perform 10 to 20 repetitions.

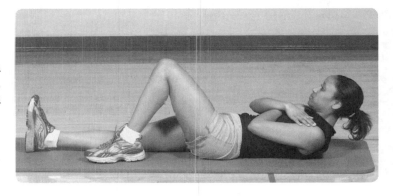

From Vivian H. Heyward, 2006, *Advanced Fitness Assessment and Exercise Prescription*, 5th ed. (Champaign, IL: Human Kinetics).

Modified Front Bridge (strengthens back and abdominal muscles)

Assume a front support position with the body supported by the forearms (elbows flexed to 90°), knees, and toes. Hold this position for 10 to 20 counts.

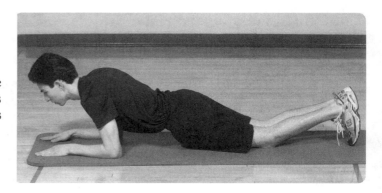

Modified Bird Dog (strengthens hip extensors)

Assume a front support position with the body supported by both hands (shoulder-width apart and elbows extended), one knee, and one foot. Extend unsupported leg so that thigh is parallel with the trunk. Hold this position momentarily. Perform 10 repetitions for each leg. Support the body with one arm to increase the difficulty of this exercise.

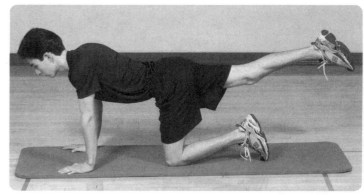

Standing McKenzie Exercise (stretches abdominal muscles and strengthens back extensors)

Assume a standing position with feet shoulder-width apart and with hands placed on hips. Extend the trunk and hold this position momentarily. Perform 10 repetitions.

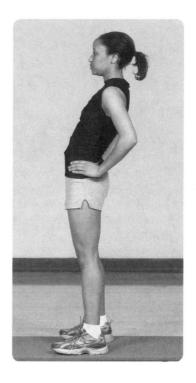

From Vivian H. Heyward, 2006, *Advanced Fitness Assessment and Exercise Prescription*, 5th ed. (Champaign, IL: Human Kinetics).

List of Abbreviations

Terms	
%BF	Relative body fat
AAHPERD	American Alliance for Health, Physical Education, Recreation and Dance
ACSM	American College of Sports Medicine
ADL	Activities of daily living
AI	Adequate intake
ATP	Adenosine triphosphate
AV	Atrioventricular
BIA	Bioelectrical impedance analysis
BM	Body mass
BMI	Body mass index
BMR	Basal metabolic rate
BP	Blood pressure
BSA	Body surface area
BV	Body volume
BW	Body weight
C	Circumference
CDC	Centers for Disease Control
CE	Constant error
CHD	Coronary heart disease
CP	Creatine phosphate
CRAC	Contract-relax with agonist contraction
CSA	Cross-sectional area
CSEP	Canadian Society for Exercise Physiology
CV	Cardiovascular
CVD	Cardiovascular disease
D	Skeletal diameter
Db	Body density
DOMS	Delayed-onset muscle soreness
DXA	Dual-energy X-ray absorptiometry
ECG	Electrocardiogram
EMG	Electromyography
F	Force
FFB	Fat-free body

Terms	
FFM	Fat-free mass
FM	Fat mass
FRC	Functional residual lung capacity
GH	Growth hormone
GI	Glycemic index
GV	Volume of air in gastrointestinal tract
GXT	Graded exercise test
HDL	High-density lipoprotein
HDL-C	High-density lipoprotein cholesterol
HMB	β-hydroxy-β-methylbutyrate
HR	Heart rate
HRmax	Maximal heart rate
HRrest	Resting heart rate
HRA	Health risk appraisal
HRR	Heart rate reserve
HT	Standing height
HT^2/R	Resistance index
HW	Hydrostatic weighing
LDL	Low-density lipoprotein
LDL-C	Low-density lipoprotein cholesterol
LP	Linear periodization
MET	Metabolic equivalent
MRI	Magnetic resonance imaging
MVC	Maximal voluntary contraction
N	Sample size
NCEP	National Cholesterol Education Program
NIDDM	Non-insulin-dependent diabetes mellitus
NIH	National Institutes of Health
NIR	Near-infrared interactance
P	Power output
p	Specific resistivity
PAL	Physical activity level
PAR-Q	Physical Activity Readiness Questionnaire

Terms

PARmed-X	Physical Activity Readiness Medical Examination Questionnaire
PEI	Physical efficiency index
$\dot{Q}$	Cardiac output
R	Resistance for bioimpedance analysis
r	Pearson product-moment correlation
RDA	Recommended dietary allowance
rep	Repetition
RER	Respiratory exchange ratio
RLP	Reverse linear periodization
RM	Repetition maximum
R_{mc}	Multiple correlation coefficient
RMR	Resting metabolic rate
ROM	Range of motion
RPE	Rating of perceived exertion
RV	Residual lung volume
SAD	Sagittal abdominal diameter
SEE	Standard error of estimate
SKF	Skinfold
SV	Stroke volume
TBW	Total body water
TC	Total cholesterol
TC/HDL-C	Ratio of total cholesterol to HDL-cholesterol
TE	Total error
TEE	Total energy expenditure
TGV	Thoracic gas volume
TLC	Total lung capacity
TLCNS	Total lung capacity, head not submerged
UWW	Underwater weight
UP	Undulating periodization
VC	Vital capacity
VLDL	Very low-density lipoprotein
$\dot{V}O_2$	Volume of oxygen consumed per minute
$\dot{V}O_2max$	Maximal oxygen uptake
$\dot{V}O_2R$	Oxygen uptake reserve
WHR	Waist-to-hip ratio
X_c	Reactance
YMCA	Young Men's Christian Association
Z	Impedance
ΣSKF	Sum of skinfolds

Units of Measure

bpm	beats per minute
C	Celsius
cc	cubic centimeter
cm	centimeter
dl	deciliter
F	Fahrenheit
ft-lb	foot-pound
g	gram
hr	hour
in.	inch
kcal	kilocalorie
kg	kilogram
kgm	kilogram-meter
km	kilometer
L	liter
lb	pound
m	meter
meq	milli-equivalent
mg	milligram
min	minute
ml	milliliter
mm	millimeter
mmHg	millimeters of mercury
mph	miles per hour
Nm	newton-meter
rpm	revolutions per minute
sec	second
W	watt
wk	week
yr	year
µg	microgram
µg RE	retinol equivalent
Ω	ohm

Glossary

absolute $\dot{V}O_2$—Measure of rate of oxygen consumption and energy cost of non-weight-bearing activities; measured in $L \cdot min^{-1}$ or $ml \cdot min^{-1}$.

accommodating-resistance exercise—Type of exercise in which fluctuations in muscle force throughout the range of motion are matched by an equal counterforce as the speed of limb movement is kept at a constant velocity; isokinetic exercise.

acquired immune deficiency syndrome (AIDS)—Disease characterized as a deficiency in the body's immune system, caused by human immunodeficiency virus (HIV).

active stretching—Stretching technique that involves moving a body part without external assistance; voluntary muscle contraction.

active-assisted stretching—Stretching technique that involves voluntarily moving a body part to the end of its active range of motion followed by an assistant moving the body part beyond its active range of motion.

activities of daily living (ADL)—Normal everyday activities such as getting out of a chair or car, climbing stairs, shopping, dressing, bathing, and so on.

acute-onset muscle soreness—Soreness or pain occurring during or immediately after exercise; caused by ischemia and accumulation of metabolic waste products in the muscle.

air displacement plethysmography (ADP)—Densitometric method to estimate body volume using air displacement and pressure–volume relationships.

android obesity—Type of obesity in which excess body fat is localized in the upper body; upper-body obesity; apple-shaped body.

aneurysm—Dilation of a blood vessel wall causing a weakness in the vessel's wall; usually caused by atherosclerosis and hypertension.

angina pectoris—Chest pain.

ankylosis—Limited range of motion at a joint.

anorexia nervosa—Eating disorder characterized by excessive weight loss.

anthropometry—Measurement of body size and proportions including skinfold thicknesses, circumferences, bony widths and lengths, stature, and body weight.

aortic stenosis—Narrowing of the aortic valve that obstructs blood flow from the left ventricle into the aorta.

Archimedes' principle—Principle stating that weight loss underwater is directly proportional to the volume of water displaced by the body's volume.

arrhythmia—Abnormal heart rhythm.

arteriosclerosis—Hardening of the arteries, or thickening and loss of elasticity in the artery walls, that obstruct blood flow; caused by deposits of fat, cholesterol, and other substances.

asthma—Respiratory disorder characterized by difficulty in breathing and wheezing due to constricted bronchi.

at risk for overweight—Children with a body mass index between the 85th and 94th percentiles for age and sex.

ataxia—Impaired ability to coordinate movement characterized by staggering gait or postural imbalance.

atherosclerosis—Buildup and deposition of fat and fibrous plaque in the inner walls of the coronary arteries.

atrial fibrillation—Cardiac dysrhythmia in which the atria quiver instead of pumping in an organized fashion.

atrial flutter—Type of atrial tachycardia in which the atria contract at rates of 230 to 380 bpm.

at risk for overweight—Children with a body mass index between the 85th and 94th percentiles for age and sex.

atrophy—A wasting or decrease in size of a body part.

attenuation—Weakening of X-ray energy as it passes through fat, lean tissue, and bone.

augmented unipolar leads—Three ECG leads (aVF, aVL, aVR) that compare voltage across each limb lead to the average voltage across the two opposite electrodes.

auscultation—Method used to measure heart rate or blood pressure by listening to heart and blood sounds.

β-hydroxy-β-methyl butyrate (HMB)—Dietary supplement known to increase lean body mass and strength of individuals engaging in resistance training.

ballistic stretching—Type of stretching exercise that uses a fast bouncing motion to produce stretch and increase range of motion.

basal metabolic rate (BMR)—Measure of minimal amount of energy needed to maintain basic and essential physiological functions.

behavior modification model—Psychological theory of change; clients become actively involved with the change process by setting short- and long-term goals.

bias—In regression analysis, a systematic over- or underestimation of actual scores caused by technical error or biological variability between validation and cross-validation samples; constant error.

biaxial joint—Joint allowing movement in two planes; condyloid and saddle joints.

bioelectrical impedance analysis (BIA)—Field method for estimating the total body water or fat-free mass using measures of impedance to current flowing through the body.

Bland and Altman method—Statistical approach used to assess the degree of agreement between methods by calculating the 95% limits of agreement and confidence intervals; used to judge accuracy of a prediction equation or method for estimating measured values of individuals in a group.

body composition—A component of physical fitness; absolute and relative amounts of muscle, bone, and fat tissues composing body mass.

body density (Db)—Overall density of fat, water, mineral, and protein components of the human body; total body mass expressed relative to total body volume.

body mass (BM)—Measure of the size of the body; body weight.

body mass index (BMI)—Crude index of obesity; body mass (kg) divided by height squared (m²).

body surface area—Amount of surface area of the body estimated from the client's height and body weight.

body volume (BV)—Measure of body size estimated by water or air displacement.

body weight (BW)—Mass or size of the body; body mass.

bone strength—Function of mineral content and density of bone tissue; related to risk of bone fracture.

Boyle's law—Isothermal gas law stating that volume and pressure are inversely related.

bradycardia—Resting heart rate < 60 bpm.

bronchitis—Acute or chronic inflammation of the bronchi of lungs.

caloric threshold—Method to estimate duration of exercise based on the caloric cost of the exercise and to estimate the total amount of exercise needed per week for health benefits.

cardiac arrest—Sudden loss of heart function usually caused by ventricular fibrillation.

cardiomyopathy—Any disease that affects the structure and function of the heart.

cardiorespiratory endurance—Ability of heart, lungs, and circulatory system to supply oxygen to working muscles efficiently.

cardiovascular disease—Disease of the heart and/or blood vessels; types of cardiovascular disease include atherosclerosis, hypertension, coronary heart disease, congestive heart failure, and stroke.

chest leads—Six ECG leads (V_1 to V_6) used to measure voltage across specific areas of the chest.

cholesterol—Waxy, fatlike substance found in all animal products (i.e., meats, dairy products, and eggs).

chylomicron—Type of lipoprotein derived from intestinal absorption of triglycerides.

circumference (C)—Measure of the girth of body segments.

cirrhosis—Chronic, degenerative disease of the liver in which the lobes are covered with fibrous tissue; associated with chronic alcohol abuse.

claudication—Cramp like pain in the calves due to poor circulation to leg muscle.

complex carbohydrates—Macronutrient found in plant-based foods, whole grains, and low-fat dairy products; for example, starch and cellulose.

compound sets—Advanced resistance training system in which two sets of exercises for the same muscle group are performed consecutively, with little or no rest between sets.

concentric contraction—Type of dynamic muscle contraction in which muscle shortens as it exerts tension.

congestive heart failure—Impaired cardiac pumping caused by myocardial infarction, ischemic heart disease, or cardiomyopathy.

constant error (CE)—Average difference between measured and predicted values for cross-validation group; bias.

constant-resistance exercise—Type of exercise in which the external resistance remains the same throughout the range of motion (e.g., lifting free weights or dumbbells).

continuous exercise test—Type of graded exercise test that is performed with no rest between workload increments.

continuous training—One continuous, aerobic exercise bout performed at low-to-moderate intensity.

contract-relax agonist contract (CRAC) technique—Type of proprioceptive neuromuscular facilitation technique in which the target muscle is isometrically contracted and then stretched; stretching is assisted by a submaximal contraction of the agonistic muscle group.

contract-relax (CR) technique—Type of proprioceptive neuromuscular facilitation technique in which the target muscle is isometrically contracted and then stretched.

contracture—Shortening of resting muscle length caused by disuse or immobilization.

core stability—Ability to maintain ideal alignment of neck, spine, scapulae, and pelvis while exercising.

core strengthening—Strengthening core muscle groups (erector spinae and abdominal movers and stabilizers) used for core stability.

coronary heart disease (CHD)—Disease of the heart caused by a lack of blood flow to heart muscle, resulting from atherosclerosis.

criterion method—Gold standard or reference method; typically a direct measure of a component used to validate other tests.

cross training—Type of training in which the client participates in a variety of exercise modes to develop one or more components of physical fitness.

cuff hypertension—Overestimation of blood pressure caused by using a bladder that is too small for the arm circumference.

cyanosis—Bluish discoloration of skin caused by lack of oxygenated hemoglobin in the blood.

delayed-onset muscle soreness (DOMS)—Soreness in the muscle occurring 24 to 48 hr after exercise.

densitometry—Measurement of total body density; hydrodensitometry and air displacement plethysmography are densitometry methods.

diabetes—Complex disorder of carbohydrate, fat, and protein metabolism resulting from a lack of insulin secretion (type 1) or defective insulin receptors (type 2).

diastolic blood pressure (DBP)—Lowest pressure in the artery during the cardiac cycle.

dietary thermogenesis—Energy needed for digesting, absorbing, transporting, and metabolizing foods.

digital activity log—A hand computer used to record the type and duration of physical activities performed during the day.

diminishing return principle—Training principle; as genetic ceiling is approached, rate of improvement slows or evens off.

discontinuous exercise test—Type of graded exercise test that is performed with 5 to 10 min of rest between increments in workload.

discontinuous training—Several intermittent, low- to high-intensity aerobic exercise bouts interspersed with rest or relief intervals.

dose-response relationship—The volume of physical activity is directly related to health benefits from that activity.

dual-energy X-ray absorptiometry (DXA)—Method used to measure total body bone mineral density, bone mineral content, fat, and lean soft-tissue mass.

dynamic contraction—Type of muscle contraction producing visible joint movement; concentric, eccentric, or isokinetic contraction.

dynamic flexibility—Measure of the rate of torque or resistance developed during stretching throughout the range of joint motion.

dyslipidemia—Abnormal blood lipid profile.

dyspnea—Shortness of breath or difficulty breathing caused by certain heart conditions, anxiety, or strenuous exercise.

eccentric contraction—Type of muscle contraction in which the muscle lengthens as it produces tension to resist gravity or decelerate a moving body segment.

edema—Accumulation of interstitial fluid in tissues such as pericardial sac and joint capsules.

elastic deformation—Deformation of the muscle-tendon unit that is proportional to the load or force applied during stretching.

electrocardiogram (ECG)—A composite record of the electrical events in the heart during the cardiac cycle.

electromyography (EMG)—Method used to measure muscle activity during rest and exercise.

embolism—Piece of tissue or thrombus that circulates in the blood until it lodges in a vessel.

emphysema—Pulmonary disease causing damage in alveoli and loss of lung elasticity.

exercise-induced hypertrophy—Increase in size of muscle as a result of resistance training.

factorial method—Method used to assess energy needs; the sum of the resting metabolic rate and the additional calories expended during work, household chores, personal daily activities, and exercise.

false negative—Describes individuals who are incorrectly identified as having no risk factors when in fact they do have risk factors.

false positive—Describes individuals who are incorrectly identified as having risk factors even though they have no risk factors.

fat-free body (FFB)—All residual, lipid-free chemicals and tissues in the body, including muscle, water, bone, connective tissue, and internal organs.

fat-free mass (FFM)—See fat-free body; weight or mass of the fat-free body.

fat mass (FM)—All extractable lipids from adipose and other tissues in the body.

flexibility—Ability to move joints fluidly through complete range of motion without injury.

flexibility training—Systematic program of stretching exercises designed to progressively increase the range of motion of joints over time.

flexometer—Device for measuring range of joint motion using a weighted 360° dial and pointer.

free-motion machines—Resistance exercise machines that have adjustable seats, lever arms, and cable pulleys for exercising muscle groups in multiple planes.

functional fitness—Ability to perform everyday activities safely and independently without fatigue; requires aerobic endurance, flexibility, balance, agility, and muscular strength.

functional training—System describing exercise progressions for specific muscle groups using a stepwise approach that increases the difficulty level (strength) and skill (balance and coordination) required for each exercise in the progression.

generalized prediction equations—Prediction equations that are applicable to a diverse, heterogeneous group of individuals.

glucose intolerance—Inability of body to metabolize glucose.

glycemic index (GI)—Rating of the body's glycemic response to a food compared to the reference value (GI = 100 for white bread or glucose).

goniometer—Protractor-like device used to measure joint angle at the extremes of the range of motion.

graded exercise test (GXT)—A multistage submaximal or maximal exercise test requiring the client to exercise at gradually increasing workloads; may be continuous or discontinuous; used to estimate $\dot{V}O_2$max.

Graves disease—Disease associated with an overactive thyroid gland that secretes greater-than-normal amounts of thyroid hormones; also known as hyperthyroidism or thyrotoxicosis.

gross $\dot{V}O_2$—Total rate of oxygen consumption, reflecting the caloric cost of both rest and exercise.

Group I aerobic activities—Aerobic exercise modalities that provide constant intensity and are not skill dependent.

Group II aerobic activities—Aerobic exercise modalities that provide constant or variable intensity, depending on skill.

Group III aerobic activities—Aerobic exercise modalities that provide variable intensity and are highly skill dependent.

gynoid obesity—Type of obesity in which excess fat is localized in the lower body; lower-body obesity; pear-shaped body.

HDL-cholesterol (HDL-C)—Cholesterol transported in the blood by high-density lipoproteins.

healthy body weight—Body mass index from 18.5 to 25 kg/m².

heart block—Interference in the normal conduction of electrical impulses that control normal contraction of the heart muscle; may occur at sinoatrial node, atrioventricular node, bundle of HIS, or at combination of these sites.

heart rate reserve (HRR)—Maximal heart rate minus the resting heart rate.

hepatitis—Inflammation of the liver characterized by jaundice and gastrointestinal discomfort.

high blood pressure—Hypertension; chronic elevation of blood pressure.

high CHD risk—One or more signs/symptoms of cardiovascular and pulmonary disease; or characterizing individuals with known cardiovascular, pulmonary, or metabolic disease.

high intensity–low repetitions—Optimal training stimulus for strength development; 85% to 100% 1-RM or 1- to 6-RM.

high-density lipoprotein (HDL)—Type of lipoprotein involved in the reverse transport of cholesterol to the liver.

hydrodensitometry—Method used to estimate body volume by measuring weight loss when the body is fully submerged; underwater weighing.

hydrostatic weighing (HW)—See hydrodensitometry.

hypercholesterolemia—Excess of total cholesterol and/or LDL-cholesterol in blood.

hyperlipidemia—Excess lipids in blood.

hypermobility—Excessive range of motion at a joint.

hyperplasia—Increase in number of cells.

hypertension—High blood pressure; chronic elevation of blood pressure.

hyperthyroidism—Overactive thyroid gland that secretes greater-than-normal amounts of thyroid hormones; also known as thyrotoxicosis or Graves disease.

hypertrophy—Increase in size of cells.

hypoglycemia—Low blood glucose level.

hypokalemia—Inadequate amount of potassium in the blood characterized by an abnormal ECG, weakness, and flaccid paralysis.

hypomagnesemia—Inadequate amount of magnesium in the blood resulting in nausea, vomiting, muscle weakness, and tremors.

hypothyroidism—Underactive thyroid gland that secretes lower-than-normal amounts of thyroid hormones; also known as myxedema.

hypoxia—Inadequate oxygen at the cellular level.

impedance (Z)—Measure of total amount of opposition to electrical current flowing through the body; function of resistance and reactance.

improvement stage—Stage of exercise program in which client improves most rapidly; frequency, intensity, duration are systematically increased; usually lasting 16 to 20 weeks.

inclinometer—Gravity-dependent goniometer used to measure the angle between the long axis of the moving segment and the line of gravity.

initial conditioning stage—Stage of exercise program used as primer to familiarize client with exercise training; usually lasting four weeks.

initial values principle—Training principle; the lower the initial value of a component, the greater the relative gain and the faster the rate of improvement in that component; the higher the initial value, the slower the improvement rate.

insulin dependent diabetes mellitus—Type 1 diabetes caused by lack of insulin production by the pancreas.

interindividual variability principle—Training principle; individual responses to training stimulus are variable and depend on age, initial fitness level, and health status.

interval training—A repeated series of exercise work bouts interspersed with rest or relief periods.

ischemia—Decreased supply of oxygenated blood to body part or organ.

ischemic heart disease—Pathologic condition of the myocardium caused by lack of oxygen to the heart muscle.

isokinetic contraction—Maximal contraction of a muscle group at a constant velocity throughout entire range of motion.

isometric contraction—Type of muscle contraction in which there is no visible joint movement; static contraction.

isotonic contraction—Type of muscle contraction producing visible joint movement; dynamic contraction.

joint laxity—Looseness or instability of a joint, increasing risk of musculoskeletal injury.

Karvonen method—Method to prescribe exercise intensity as a percentage of the heart rate reserve added to the resting heart rate; percent heart rate reserve method.

kilocalorie (kcal)—Amount of heat needed to raise the temperature of 1 kg of water 1 °C; measure of energy need and expenditure.

LDL-cholesterol (LDL-C)—Cholesterol transported in the blood by low-density lipoproteins.

limb leads—Three ECG leads (I, II, III) measuring the voltage differential between left and right arms (I) and between the left leg and right (II) and left (III) arms.

limits of agreement—Statistical method used to assess the degree of agreement between methods; also known as the Bland and Altman method.

line of best fit—Regression line depicting relationship between reference measure and predictor variables in an equation.

line of identity—Straight line with a slope equal to 1 and an intercept equal to 0; used in a scatterplot to illustrate the differences in the measured and predicted scores of a cross-validation sample.

linear periodization (LP)—Strength training method that progressively increases training intensity as training volume decreases between microcycles.

lipoprotein—Molecule used to transport and exchange lipids among the liver, intestine, and peripheral tissues.

low back pain—Pain produced by muscular weakness or imbalance resulting from lack of physical activity.

low CHD risk—Characterizing younger individuals (men < 45 years and women < 55 years) who are asymptomatic and have no more than one risk factor.

low-density lipoprotein (LDL)—Primary transporter of cholesterol in the blood; product of very low-density lipoprotein metabolism.

lower-body obesity—Type of obesity in which excess body fat is localized in the lower body; gynoid obesity; pear-shaped body.

low intensity–high repetitions—Optimal training stimulus for development of muscular endurance; ≤60% 1-RM or 15- to 20-RM.

lumbar stabilization—Maintaining a static position of the lumbar spine by isometrically co-contracting the abdominal wall and low back muscles during exercise.

macrocycle—Phase of periodized resistance training program usually lasting 9 to 12 mo.

maintenance stage—Stage of exercise program designed to maintain level of fitness achieved by end of improvement stage; should be continued on a regular, long-term basis.

maximal exercise test—Graded exercise test in which exercise intensity increases gradually until the $\dot{V}O_2$ plateaus or fails to rise with a further increase in workload.

maximum oxygen consumption—Maximum rate of oxygen utilization by muscles during exercise; $\dot{V}O_2$max.

maximum oxygen uptake ($\dot{V}O_2$max)—Maximum rate of oxygen utilization of muscles during aerobic exercise.

McArdle's syndrome—Inherited metabolic disease characterized by inability to metabolize muscle glycogen, resulting in excessive amounts of glycogen stored in skeletal muscles.

mesocycle—Phase of a periodized resistance training program usually lasting 3 to 4 mo.

metabolic syndrome—Describes a combination of cardiovascular disease risk factors associated with hypertension, dyslipidemia, insulin resistance, and abdominal obesity.

microcycle—Phase of a periodized resistance training program usually lasting 1 to 4 wk.

miscuffing—Source of blood pressure measurement error caused by using a blood pressure cuff that is not appropriately scaled for the client's arm circumference.

moderate CHD risk—Characterizing older individuals (men ≥45 years and women ≥55 years), or individuals of any age having two or more risk factors.

multicomponent model—Body composition model that takes into account interindividual variations in water, protein, and mineral content of the fat-free body.

multimodal exercise program—Type of exercise program that uses a variety of aerobic exercise modalities.

multiple correlation coefficient (R_{mc})—Correlation between reference measure and predictor variables in a prediction equation.

murmur—Low-pitched fluttering or humming sound.

muscle balance—Ratio of strength between opposing muscle groups, contralateral muscle groups, and upper- and lower-body muscle groups.

muscular endurance—Ability of muscle to maintain submaximal force levels for extended periods.

muscular strength—Maximal force or tension level produced by a muscle or muscle group.

musculoskeletal fitness—Ability of skeletal and muscular systems to perform work.

myocardial infarction—Heart attack.

myocardial ischemia—Lack of blood flow to the coronary arteries.

myocarditis—Inflammation of the heart muscle caused by viral, bacterial, or fungal infection.

myxedema—Disease associated with an underactive thyroid gland that secretes lower-than-normal amounts of thyroid hormones; also known as hypothyroidism.

near-infrared interactance (NIR)—Field method that estimates %BF based on optical density of tissues at the measurement site; presently, validity of this method is questionable.

negative energy balance—Excess of energy expenditure in relation to energy intake.

net $\dot{V}O_2$—Rate of oxygen consumption in excess of the resting $\dot{V}O_2$; used to describe the caloric cost of exercise.

nonaxial joint—Type of joint allowing only gliding, sliding, or twisting rather than movement about an axis of rotation; gliding joint.

non-insulin dependent diabetes mellitus (NIDDM)—Type 2 diabetes caused by decreased insulin receptor sensitivity.

normotensive—Normal blood pressure, defined as values less than 120/80 mmHg.

obesity—Excessive amount of body fat relative to body mass; BMI of 30 kg/m^2 or more.

objectivity—Intertester reliability; ability of test to yield similar scores for given individual when same test is administered by different technicians.

objectivity coefficient—Correlation between pairs of test scores measured on same individuals by two different technicians.

occlusion—Blockage of blood flow to body part or organ.

omnikinetic exercise—Type of accommodating-resistance exercise that adjusts for fluctuations in both muscle force and speed of joint rotation throughout range of motion.

one-repetition maximum (1-RM)—Maximal weight that can be lifted for one complete repetition of a movement.

optical density—Measure of the amount of near-infrared light reflected by the body's tissues at specific wavelengths.

oscillometry—Method for measuring blood pressure that uses an automated electronic manometer to measure oscillations in pressure when the cuff is deflated.

osteoarthritis—Degenerative disease of the joints characterized by excessive amounts of bone and cartilage in the joint.

osteopenia—Low bone mineral mass; precursor to osteoporosis.

osteoporosis—Disorder characterized by low bone mineral and bone density; occurring most frequently in postmenopausal women and sedentary individuals.

overcuffing—Using a blood pressure cuff with a bladder too large for the arm circumference, leading to an underestimation of blood pressure.

overload principle—Training principle; physiological systems must be taxed beyond normal to stimulate improvement.

overweight—Adults with BMI between 25 to 29.9 kg/m$_2$; children with BMI greater than or equal to 95th percentile for age and sex.

pallor—Unnatural paleness or absence of skin color.

palpation—Method used to measure heart rate by feeling the pulse at specific anatomical sites.

palpitations—Racing or pounding of the heart.

passive stretching—Stretching technique that involves a body part being moved by an assistant as the client relaxes the target muscle group.

pelvic stabilization—Maintaining a static position of the pelvis while performing exercises for the low back extensor muscles.

percent body fat (%BF)—Fat mass expressed relative to body mass; relative body fat.

percent heart rate maximum (%HRmax)—Method used to prescribe exercise intensity as a percentage of the measured or age-predicted maximum heart rate.

percent heart rate reserve (%HRR)—Method used to prescribe exercise intensity as a percentage of the heart rate reserve (HRR = HRmax – HRrest) added to the resting heart rate; Karvonen method.

percent $\dot{V}O_2$reserve ($\%\dot{V}O_2R$)—Method used to prescribe exercise intensity as a percentage of $\dot{V}O_2$reserve ($\dot{V}O_2R$ = $\dot{V}O_2$max – $\dot{V}O_2$rest) added to the resting $\dot{V}O_2$.

pericarditis—Inflammation of the pericardium caused by trauma, infection, uremia, or heart attack.

periodization—Advanced form of training that systematically varies the volume and intensity of the training exercises.

physical activity level (PAL)—The ratio of total energy expenditure to basal metabolic rate; PAL = TEE/BMR.

physical fitness—Ability to perform occupational, recreational, and daily activities without undue fatigue.

population-specific equations—Prediction equations intended only for use with individuals from a specific homogeneous group.

positive energy balance—Excess of energy intake in relation to energy expenditure.

prehypertension—Systolic blood pressure of 120 to 139 mmHg or diastolic pressure of 80 to 89 mmHg.

PR interval—Part of ECG tracing that indicates delay in the impulse at the atrioventricular node.

progression principle—Training principle; training volume must be progressively increased to overload and stimulate further improvements.

proprioceptive neuromuscular facilitation (PNF)—Mode of stretching designed to increase range of joint motion through spinal reflex mechanisms such as reciprocal inhibition.

prosthesis—An artificial replacement of a missing body part, such as an artificial limb or joint.

pulmonary ventilation—Movement of air into and out of the lungs.

pulse pressure—Difference between the systolic and diastolic blood pressures.

P wave—Part of ECG tracing that reflects depolarization of the atria.

pyramiding—Advanced resistance training system in which a relatively light weight is lifted in the first set and progressively heavier weights are lifted in subsequent sets; light-to-heavy system.

QRS complex—Part of ECG tracing reflecting ventricular depolarization and contraction.

ramp protocols—Graded exercise tests that are individualized and provide for continuous, frequent (every 10-20 sec) increments in work rate so that $\dot{V}O_2$ increases linearly.

range of motion (ROM)—Degree of movement at a joint; measure of static flexibility.

rating of perceived exertion (RPE)—A scale used to measure a client's subjective rating of exercise intensity.

reactance (X_c)—Measure of opposition to electrical current flowing through body due to the capacitance of cell membranes; a vector of impedance.

reciprocal inhibition—Reflex that inhibits the contraction of antagonistic muscles when the prime mover is voluntarily contracted.

reference method—Gold standard or criterion method; typically a direct measure of a component used to validate other tests.

regression line—Line of best fit depicting relationship between reference measure and predictor variables.

relative body fat (%BF)—Fat mass expressed as a percentage of total body mass; percent body fat.

relative strength—Muscular strength expressed relative to the body mass or lean body mass; 1-RM/BM.

relative $\dot{V}O_2$max—Rate of oxygen consumption expressed relative to the body mass or lean body mass; measured in $ml \cdot kg^{-1} \cdot min^{-1}$.

reliability—Ability of test to yield consistent and stable scores across trials and over time.

reliability coefficient—Correlation depicting relationship between trial 1 and trial 2 scores or day 1 and day 2 scores of a test.

repetition maximum (RM)—Measure of intensity for resistance exercise expressed as maximum weight that can be lifted for a given number of repetitions.

repetitions—Number of times a specific exercise movement is performed in a set.

residual score—Difference between the actual and predicted scores (Y – Y').

residual volume (RV)—Volume of air remaining in lungs following a maximal expiration.

resistance (R)—Measure of pure opposition to electrical current flowing through body; a vector of impedance.

resistance index (ht^2/R)—Predictor variable in some BIA regression equations that is calculated by dividing standing height squared by resistance.

respiratory exchange ratio (RER)—Ratio of expired CO_2 to inspired O_2.

resting energy expenditure (REE)—Energy required to maintain essential physiological processes at rest; resting metabolic rate.

resting metabolic rate (RMR)—Energy required to maintain essential physiological processes in a relaxed, awake, and reclined state; resting energy expenditure.

reverse linear periodization (RLP)—Strength training method that progressively decreases training intensity as training volume increases between microcycles.

reversibility principle—Training principle; physiological gains from training are lost when individual stops training (detraining).

rheumatic heart disease—Condition in which the heart valves are damaged by rheumatic fever, contracted from a streptococcal infection (strep throat).

rheumatoid arthritis—Chronic, destructive disease of the joints characterized by inflammation and thickening of the synovial membranes and swelling of the joints.

sagittal abdominal diameter (SAD)—Measure of the anteroposterior thickness of the abdomen at the umbilical level.

self-efficacy—Individuals' perception of their ability to perform a task and their confidence in making a specific behavioral change.

sensitivity—Probability of a test correctly identifying individuals with risk factors for a specific disease.

set—Defines the number of times a specific number of repetitions of a given exercise is repeated; single or multiple sets.

simple carbohydrates—Simple sugars (e.g., glucose and fructose) found in fruits, berries, table sugar, honey, and some vegetables.

skeletal diameter (D)—Measure of the width of bones.

skinfold (SKF)—Measure of the thickness of two layers of skin and the underlying subcutaneous fat.

social cognitive model—Psychological theory of behavior change; based on concepts of self-efficacy and outcome expectation.

specificity—Measure of a test's ability to correctly identify individuals with no risk factors for a specific disease.

specificity principle—Training principle; physiological and metabolic responses and adaptations to exercise training are specific to type of exercise and muscle groups involved.

sphygmomanometer—Device used to measure blood pressure manually, consisting of a blood pressure cuff and a manometer.

spinning—Group-led exercise that involves stationary cycling at various cadences and resistances.

split routine—Advanced resistance training system in which different muscle groups are targeted on consecutive days to avoid overtraining.

stages of motivational readiness for change model—Psychological theory of behavior change; ability to make long-term behavioral change is based on client's emotional and intellectual readiness; stages of readiness are precontemplation, contemplation, preparation, action, and maintenance.

standard error of estimate (SEE)—Measure of error for prediction equation; quantifies the average deviation of individual data points around the line of best fit.

static contraction—Type of muscle contraction in which there is no visible joint movement; isometric contraction.

static flexibility—Measure of the total range of motion at a joint.

static stretching—Mode of exercise used to increase range of motion by placing the joint at the end of its range of motion and slowly applying torque to the muscle to stretch it further.

stress relaxation—Decreased tension within musculotendinous unit when it is held at a fixed length during static stretching.

stretch tolerance—Measure of the amount of resistive force to stretch within target muscles that can be tolerated before experiencing pain.

stroke—Rupture or blockage of blood flow to the brain caused by a blood clot or some other particle.

ST segment—Part of ECG tracing reflecting ventricular repolarization; used to detect coronary occlusion and myocardial infarct.

submaximal exercise test—Graded exercise test in which exercise is terminated at some predetermined submaximal heart rate or workload; used to estimate $\dot{V}O_2$max.

super circuit resistance training—Type of circuit resistance training that intersperses a short, aerobic exercise bout between each resistance training exercise station.

supersetting—Advanced resistance training system in which exercises for agonistic and antagonistic muscle groups are done consecutively without rest.

syncope—Brief lapse in consciousness caused by lack of oxygen to the brain.

systolic blood pressure (SBP)—Highest pressure in the arteries during systole of the heart.

tachycardia—Resting heart rate >100 bpm.

talk test—Method to monitor exercise intensity; measure of the client's ability to converse comfortably while exercising; based on the relationship between exercise intensity and pulmonary ventilation.

tare weight—Weight of chair or platform and its supporting equipment used in hydrostatic weighing.

thoracic gas volume (TGV)—Volume of air in the lungs and thorax.

thrombophlebitis—Inflammation of a vein often accompanied by formation of a blood clot.

thrombus—Lump of cellular elements of the blood attached to inner walls of an artery or vein, sometimes blocking blood flow through the vessel.

thyrotoxicosis—Overactive thyroid gland that secretes greater-than-normal amounts of thyroid hormones; also known as Graves disease or hyperthyroidism.

tonic vibration reflex—Reflex that activates muscle spindles and alpha motor neurons of muscles stimulated by vibration loading.

total cholesterol (TC)—Absolute amount of cholesterol in the blood.

total energy expenditure (TEE)—Sum of energy expenditures for resting metabolic rate, dietary thermogenesis, and physical activity.

total energy expenditure (TEE) method—Method for determining energy expenditure measured by doubly-labeled water or predicted from equations.

total error (TE)—Average deviation of individual scores of the cross-validation sample from the line of identity.

training volume—Total amount of training as determined by the number of sets and exercises for a muscle group, intensity, and frequency of training.

treading—Type of group-led interval training that involves walking, jogging, and running at various speeds and grades on a treadmill with relief intervals interspersed.

triaxial joint—Type of joint allowing movement in three planes; ball-and-socket joint.

tri-sets—Advanced resistance training system in which three different exercises for the same muscle group are performed consecutively with little or no rest between the exercises.

T wave—Part of ECG tracing corresponding to ventricular repolarization.

two-component model—Body composition model that divides the body into fat and fat-free body components.

type 1 diabetes—Insulin-dependent diabetes caused by lack of insulin production by the pancreas.

type 2 diabetes—Non-insulin-dependent diabetes caused by decreased insulin receptor sensitivity.

undercuffing—Using a blood pressure cuff with a bladder too small for the arm circumference, leading to an overestimation of blood pressure.

underwater weight (UWW)—Method used to estimate body volume by measuring weight loss when the body is fully submerged; hydrostatic weighing.

underweight—BMI < 18.5 kg/m^2.

undulating periodization (UP)—Strength training method that varies training intensity and volume weekly or even daily.

uniaxial joint—Type of joint allowing movement in one plane; hinge or pivot joint.

upper-body obesity—Type of obesity in which excess fat is localized to the upper body; android obesity; apple-shaped body.

uremia—Excessive amounts of urea and other nitrogen waste products in the blood associated with kidney failure.

validity—Ability of a test to accurately measure, with minimal error, a specific component.

validity coefficient—Correlation between reference measure and predicted scores.

valvular heart disease—Congenital disorder of a heart valve characterized by obstructed blood flow, valvular degeneration, and regurgitation of blood.

variable-resistance exercise—Type of exercise in which resistance changes during the range of motion due to levers, pulleys, and cams.

ventilatory threshold—Point at which there is an exponential increase in pulmonary ventilation relative to exercise intensity and rate of oxygen consumption.

ventricular ectopy—Premature (out of sequence) contraction of the ventricles.

ventricular fibrillation—Cardiac dysrhythmia marked by rapid, uncoordinated, and unsynchronized contractions of the ventricles, so that no blood is pumped by the heart.

vertigo—Dizziness or inability to maintain normal balance in a standing or seated position.

very low-density lipoprotein (VLDL)—Lipoprotein made in the liver for transporting triglycerides.

vibration training—Training method that uses whole-body mechanical vibration to increase strength, balance, and bone integrity.

viscoelastic properties—Tension within the muscle-tendon unit caused by the elastic and viscous deformation of the unit when force is applied during stretching.

viscous deformation—Deformation of the muscle-tendon unit that is proportional to the speed at which tension is applied during stretching.

$\dot{V}O_2$max—Maximum rate of oxygen utilization of muscles during exercise.

$\dot{V}O_2$peak—Measure of highest rate of oxygen consumption during an exercise test regardless of whether or not a $\dot{V}O_2$ plateau is reached.

$\dot{V}O_2$reserve—The $\dot{V}O_2$max minus the $\dot{V}O_2$rest.

waist-to-hip ratio (WHR)—Waist circumference divided by hip circumference; used as a measure of upper-body or abdominal obesity.

white coat hypertension—Condition describing individuals who have normal blood pressure but become hypertensive when blood pressure is measured by a health professional.

References

Abraham, W.M. 1977. Factors in delayed muscle soreness. *Medicine and Science in Sports* 9: 11–20.

Adams, J., Mottola, M., Bagnall, K.M., and McFadden, K.D. 1982. Total body fat content in a group of professional football players. *Canadian Journal of Applied Sport Sciences* 7: 36-44.

Adamovich, D.R. 1984. *The heart.* East Moriches, NY: Sports Medicine Books.

Ahlback, S.O., and Lindahl, O. 1964. Sagittal mobility of the hip-joint. *Acta Orthopaedica Scandinavica* 34: 310–313.

Ainsworth, B.E., Haskell, W.L., Whitt, M.C., Irwin, M.L., Swartz, A.M., Strath, S.J., O'Brien, W.L., Bassett, D.R. Jr., Schmitz, K.H., Emplaincourt, P.O., Jacobs, D.R., and Leon, A.S. 2000. Compendium of physical activities: An update of activity codes and MET intensities. *Medicine & Science in Sports & Exercise* 32(Suppl.): S498–S516.

Albert, W.J., Bonneau, J., Stevenson, J.M., and Gledhill, N. 2001. Back fitness and back health assessment considerations for the Canadian Physical Activity, Fitness and Lifestyle Appraisal. *Canadian Journal of Applied Physiology* 26: 291–317.

Alter, M.J. 1996. *Science of flexibility and stretching.* Champaign, IL: Human Kinetics.

Alway, S.E., Grumbt, W.H., Gonyea, W.J., and Stray-Gundersen, J. 1989. Contrasts in muscle and myofibers of elite male and female bodybuilders. *Journal of Applied Physiology* 67: 24–31.

American Alliance for Health, Physical Education, Recreation and Dance. 1988. *The AAHPERD physical best program.* Reston, VA: Author.

American College of Sports Medicine. 1996. Position stand on exercise and fluid replacement. *Medicine & Science in Sports & Exercise* 28(1): i-vii.

American College of Sports Medicine (ACSM). 2000. *ACSM's guidelines for exercise testing and prescription,* 6th ed. Philadelphia: Lippincott Williams & Wilkins.

American College of Sports Medicine (ACSM). 2001. American College of Sports Medicine Position Stand. Appropriate intervention strategies for weight loss and prevention of weight regain for adults. *Medicine & Science in Sports & Exercise* 33: 2145-2156.

American College of Sports Medicine (ACSM). 2004. NCCA accreditation. *ACSM's Certified News* 14(3): 1.

American College of Sports Medicine (ACSM). 2006. *ACSM's guidelines for exercise testing and prescription,* 7th ed. Philadelphia: Lippincott Williams & Wilkins.

American College of Sports Medicine and American Diabetes Association. 1997. Joint position statement on diabetes mellitus and exercise. *Medicine & Science in Sports & Exercise* 27(12): i-vi.

American Council on Exercise. 1997. Absolute certainty: Do abdominal trainers work any better than the average crunch? *ACE Fitness Matters* 3(2): 1-2.

American Dietetic Association. 2000. Position of the American Dietetic Association, Dietitians of Canada, and the American College of Sports Medicine: Nutrition and athletic performance. *Journal of American Dietetic Association* 100: 1543-1556.

American Dietetic Association. 2003. *Let the evidence speak: Indirect calorimetry and weight management guides.* Chicago: Author.

American Fitness Professionals and Associates. 2004. AFPA news flash: What is the National Board of Fitness Examiners (NBFE) and how does it work? www. afpafitness.com.

American Heart Association. 1999. *2000 heart and stroke statistical update.* Dallas: Author.

American Heart Association. 2001. *International cardiovascular disease statistics.* Dallas: Author.

American Heart Association. 2004. *Heart disease and stroke statistics—2004 update.* Dallas: Author.

American Medical Association. 1988. *Guides to the evaluation of permanent impairment,* 3rd ed. Chicago, IL: Author.

American Psychiatric Association. 1994. *Diagnostic and statistical manual of mental disorders: IV,* 4th ed. Washington, D.C.: Author.

American Society of Exercise Physiologists. 2004. Standards of professional practice. www.css.edu/ASEP/StandardsofProfessionalPractice.

Anderson, B., and Burke, E.R. 1991. Scientific, medical, and practical aspects of stretching. *Clinics in Sports Medicine* 10: 63-86.

Anderson, G.S. 1992. The 1600-m and multistage 20-m shuttle run as predictive tests of aerobic capacity in children. *Pediatric Exercise Science* 4: 312–318.

Anderson, R. 1980. *Stretching.* Fullerton, CA: Shelter.

Antonio, J., and Gonyea, W.J. 1993. Skeletal muscle fiber hyperplasia. *Medicine & Science in Sports & Exercise* 25: 1333–1345.

Ardern, C.I., Katzmarzyk, P.T., and Ross, R. 2003. Discrimination of health risk by combined body mass index and waist circumference. *Obesity Research* 11: 135-142.

Armsey, T.D., and Grime, T.E. 2002. Protein and amino acid supplementation in athletes. *Current Sports Medicine Reports* 4: 253-256.

Armstrong, R.B. 1984. Mechanisms of exercise-induced delayed onset muscular soreness: A brief review. *Medicine & Science in Sports & Exercise* 16: 529-538.

Ashwell, M., McCall, S.A., Cole, T.J., and Dixon, A.K. 1985. Fat distribution and its metabolic complications: Interpretations. In *Human body composition and fat distribution,* ed. N.G. Norgan, 227-242. Wageningen, Netherlands: Euronut.

Åstrand, I. 1960. Aerobic capacity in men and women with special reference to age. *Acta Physiologica Scandinavica* 49(Suppl. 169): 1-92.

Åstrand, P.O. 1956. Human physical fitness with special reference to age and sex. *Physiological Reviews* 36: 307-335.

Åstrand, P.O. 1965. *Work tests with the bicycle ergometer.* Varberg, Sweden: AB Cykelfabriken Monark.

Åstrand, P.O., and Rodahl, K. 1977. *Textbook of work physiology.* New York: McGraw-Hill.

Åstrand, P.O., and Ryhming, I. 1954. A nomogram for calculation of aerobic capacity (physical fitness) from pulse rate during submaximal work. *Journal of Applied Physiology* 7: 218-221.

Atterhog, J.H., Jonsson, B., and Samuelsson, R. 1979. Exercise testing: A prospective study of complication rates. *American Heart Journal* 98: 572-580.

Axler, C.T., and McGill, S.M. 1997. Low back loads over a variety of abdominal exercises: Searching for the safest abdominal challenge. *Medicine & Science in Sports & Exercise* 29: 804-810.

Baechle, T.R. 1994. *Essentials of strength training and conditioning.* Champaign, IL: Human Kinetics.

Baechle, T.R., Earle, R.W., and Wathen, D. 2000. Resistance training. In *Essentials of strength training and conditioning,* eds. T.R. Baechle and R.W. Earle. Champaign, IL: Human Kinetics.

Bahr, R., Ingnes, I., Vaage, O., Sjersted, O.M., and Newsholme, E.A. 1987. Effect of duration of exercise on excess post-exercise O_2 consumption. *Journal of Applied Physiology* 62: 485-490.

Baker, D., Wilson, G., and Carlyon, R. 1994. Periodization: The effect on strength of manipulating volume and intensity. *Journal of Strength and Conditioning Research* 8: 235-242.

Balke, B. 1963. A simple field test for the assessment of physical fitness. *Civil Aeromedical Research Institute Report,* 63-18. Oklahoma City: Federal Aviation Agency.

Balke, B., and Ware, R. 1959. An experimental study of physical fitness of Air Force personnel. *US Armed Forces Medical Journal* 10: 675-688.

Ball, T.E., and Rose, K.S. 1991. A field test for predicting maximum bench press lift of college women. *Journal of Applied Sport Science Research* 5: 169-170.

Ballor, D.L., and Keesey, R.E. 1991. A meta-analysis of the factors affecting exercise-induced changes in body mass, fat mass, and fat-free mass in males and females. *International Journal of Obesity* 15: 717-726.

Bandura, A. 1982. Self-efficacy mechanism in human agency. *American Psychologist* 37: 122-147.

Bandy, W.D., and Irion, J.M. 1994. The effect of time on static stretch on the flexibility of the hamstring muscles. *Physical Therapy* 74: 845-851.

Baumgartner, R.N., Heymsfield, S.B., and Roche, A.F. 1995. Human body composition and the epidemiology of chronic disease. *Obesity Research* 3: 73-95.

Baumgartner, R.N., Heymsfield, S.B., Lichtman, S., Wang, J., and Pierson, R.N. 1991. Body composition in elderly people: Effect of criterion estimates on predictive equations. *American Journal of Clinical Nutrition* 53: 1-9.

Baumgartner, T.A. 1978. Modified pull-up test. *Research Quarterly* 49: 80-84.

Baumgartner, T.A., and Jackson, A.S. 1975. *Measurement for evaluation in physical education.* Boston: Houghton Mifflin.

Baumgartner, T.A., East, W.B., Frye, P.A., Hensley, L.D., Knox, D.F., and Norton, C.J. 1984. Equipment improvements and additional norms for the modified pull-up test. *Research Quarterly for Exercise and Sport* 55: 64-68.

Baun, W.B., and Baun, M.R. 1981. A nomogram for the estimate of percent body fat from generalized equations. *Research Quarterly for Exercise and Sport* 52: 380-384.

Beaulieu, J.E. 1980. *Stretching for all sports.* Pasadena, CA: Athletic Press.

Beevers, G., Lip, G.Y.H., and O'Brien, E. 2001a. ABC of hypertension. Blood pressure measurement. Part I—Sphygmomanometry: Factors common to all techniques. *British Medical Journal* 322: 981-985.

Beevers, G., Lip, G.Y.H., and O'Brien, E. 2001b. ABC of hypertension. Blood pressure measurement. Part II—Conventional sphygmomanometry: Technique of auscultatory blood pressure measurement. *British Medical Journal* 322: 1043-1047.

Behnke, A.R. 1961. Quantitative assessment of body build. *Journal of Applied Physiology* 16: 960-968.

Behnke, A.R., and Wilmore, J.H. 1974. *Evaluation and regulation of body build and composition.* Englewood Cliffs, NJ: Prentice Hall.

Benardot, D., Clarkson, P., Coleman, E., and Manore, M. 2001. Can vitamin supplements improve sport performance? *Gatorade Sports Science Exchange Roundtable* 12(3): 1-4.

Bergsma-Kadijk, J.A., Baumeister, B., and Deurenberg, P. 1996. Measurement of body fat in young and elderly women: Comparison between a four-compartment model and widely used reference methods. *British Journal of Nutrition* 75: 649-657.

Berlin, J.A., and Colditz, G.A. 1990. A meta-analysis of physical activity in the prevention of coronary heart disease. *American Journal of Epidemiology* 132: 612-628.

Berry, M.J., Cline, C.C., Berry, C.B., and Davis, M. 1992. A comparison between two forms of aerobic dance and treadmill running. *Medicine & Science in Sports & Exercise* 24: 946-951.

Bielinski, R., Schultz, Y., and Jequier, E. 1985. Energy metabolism during the postexercise recovery in man. *American Journal of Clinical Nutrition* 42: 69–82.

Birk, T.J., and Birk, C.A. 1987. Use of ratings of perceived exertion for exercise prescription. *Sports Medicine* 4: 1–8.

Bjorntorp, P. 1988. Abdominal obesity and the development of non-insulin diabetes mellitus. *Diabetes and Metabolism Reviews* 4: 615–622.

Blair, D., Habricht, J.P., Sims, E.A., Sylwester, D., and Abraham, S. 1984. Evidence of an increased risk for hypertension with centrally located body fat, and the effect of race and sex on this risk. *American Journal of Epidemiology* 119: 526–540.

Blair, S.N., LaMonte, M.J., and Nichaman, M.Z. 2004. The evolution of physical activity recommendations: How much is enough? *American Journal of Clinical Nutrition* 79 (Suppl.): 913S–920S.

Bland, J.M., and Altman, D.G. 1986. Statistical methods for assessing agreement between two methods of clinical measurement. *The Lancet* 12: 307–310.

Blessing, D.L., Wilson, D.G., Puckett, J.R., and Ford, H.T. 1987. The physiological effects of 8 weeks of aerobic dance with and without hand-held weights. *American Journal of Sports Medicine* 15: 508–510.

Blum, V., Carriere, E.G.J., Kolsters, W., Mosterd, W.L., Schiereck, P., and Wesseling, K.H. 1997. Aortic and peripheral blood pressure during isometric and dynamic exercise. *International Journal of Sports Medicine* 18: 30–34.

Bohe, J., Low, A., Wolfe, R.R., and Rennie, M.J. 2003. Human muscle protein synthesis is modulated by extracellular, not intramuscular amino acid availability: A dose-response study. *Journal of Physiology* 552: 315–324.

Bompa, T.O., DiPasquale, M.D., and Cornacchia, L.J. 2003. *Serious strength training.* 2nd ed. Champaign, IL: Human Kinetics.

Bonge, D., and Donnelly, J.E. 1989. Trials to criteria for hydrostatic weighing at residual volume. *Research Quarterly for Exercise and Sport* 60: 176–179.

Borg, G. 1998. *Borg's perceived exertion and pain scales.* Champaign, IL: Human Kinetics.

Borg, G.V., and Linderholm, H. 1967. Perceived exertion and pulse rate during graded exercise in various age groups. *Acta Medica Scandinavica* 472(Suppl.): 194–206.

Borms, J., Van Roy, P., Santens, J.P., and Haentjens, A. 1987. Optimal duration of static stretching exercises for improvement of coxo-femoral flexibility. *Journal of Sports Science* 5: 39–47.

Bosco, C.M., Colli, R., Introini, E., Cardinale, M., Tsarpela, O., Madella, A., Tihanyi, J., and Viru, A. 1999. Adaptive responses of human skeletal muscle to vibration exposure. *Clinical Physiology* 19: 183–187.

Bouchard, C. 2001. Physical activity and health: Introduction to the dose-response symposium. *Medicine & Science in Sports & Exercise* 33 (Suppl.): S347–S350.

Bouchard, C., Perusse, L., Leblanc, C., Tremblay, A., and Theriault, G. 1988. Inheritance of the amount and distribution of human body fat. *International Journal of Obesity* 12: 205–215.

Bouchard, C., Shephard, R.J., and Stephens, T., eds. 1994. *Physical activity, fitness, and health. International proceedings and conference statement.* Champaign, IL: Human Kinetics.

Bouchard, C., Tremblay, A., Despres, J.P., Nadeau, A., Lupien, P.J., Theriault, G., Dussault, J., Moorjani, S., Pinault, S., and Fournier, G. 1990. The response of long-term overfeeding in identical twins. *New England Journal of Medicine* 322: 1477–1482.

Bracko, M.R. 2002. Can stretching prior to exercise and sports improve performance and prevent injury. *ACSM's Health & Fitness Journal* 6(5): 17-22.

Bracko, M.R. 2004. Can we prevent back injuries? *ACSM's Health & Fitness Journal* 8(4): 5–11.

Brahler, C.J., and Blank, S.E. 1995. VersaClimbing elicits higher $\dot{V}O_2$max than does treadmill running or rowing ergometry. *Medicine & Science in Sports & Exercise* 27: 249–254.

Braith, R.W., Graves, J.E, Leggett, S.H., and Pollock, M.L. 1993. Effect of training on the relationship between maximal and submaximal strength. *Medicine & Science in Sports & Exercise* 25: 132–138.

Branch, J.D. 2003. Effect of creatine supplementation on body composition and performance: A meta-analysis. *International Journal of Sport Nutrition and Exercise Metabolism* 13: 198–226.

Bravata, D.M., Sanders, L., Huang, J., Krumholz, H.M., Olkin, I., Gardner, C.D., Bravata, D.M. 2003. Efficacy and safety of low-carbohydrate diets: A systematic review. *Journal of the American Medical Association* 289: 1837-1850.

Bray, G.A. 1978. Definitions, measurements and classifications of the syndromes of obesity. *International Journal of Obesity* 2: 99–113.

Bray, G.A., and Gray, D.S. 1988a. Anthropometric measurements in the obese. In *Anthropometric standardization reference manual,* ed. T.G. Lohman, A.F. Roche, and R. Martorell, 131–136. Champaign, IL: Human Kinetics.

Bray, G.A., and Gray, D.S. 1988b. Obesity. Part I—Pathogenesis. *Western Journal of Medicine* 149: 429–441.

Brehm, B.A. 1988. Elevation of metabolic rate following exercise—implications for weight loss. *Sports Medicine* 6: 72–78.

British Heart Foundation. 2004. Statistics database. www.heartstats.org/temp/bloodspressures2004.pdf.

Brooks, G.A., Butte, N.F., Rand, W.M., Flatt, J.P., and Caballero, B. 2004. Chronicle of the Institute of Medicine physical activity recommendation: How a physical activity recommendation came to be among dietary recommendations. *American Journal of Clinical Nutrition* 79 (Suppl.): 921S–930S.

Brose, A., Parise, G., and Tarnopolsky, M.A. 2003. Creatine supplementation enhances isometric strength and body composition improvements following strength exercise training in older adults. *Journals of Gerontology Series A: Biological Sciences and Medical Sciences* 58: 11-19.

Brown, D.A., and Miller, W.C. 1998. Normative data for strength and flexibility of women throughout life. *European Journal of Applied Physiology* 78: 77-82.

Brozek, J., Grande, F., Anderson, J.T., and Keys, A. 1963. Densiometric analysis of body composition: Revision of some quantitative assumptions. *Annals of the New York Academy of Sciences* 110: 113-140.

Bruce, R.A., Kusumi, F., and Hosmer, D. 1973. Maximal oxygen intake and nomographic assessment of functional aerobic impairment in cardiovascular disease. *American Heart Journal* 85: 546-562.

Bryner, R.W., Ullrich, I.H., Sauers, J., Donley, D., Hornsby, G., Kolar, M., and Yeater, R. 1999. Effects of resistance vs. aerobic training combined with an 800 calorie liquid diet on lean body mass and resting metabolic rate. *Journal of the American College of Nutrition* 18(2): 115-121.

Brynteson, P., and Sinning, W.E. 1973. The effects of training frequencies on the retention of cardiovascular fitness. *Medicine and Science in Sports* 5: 29-33.

Brzycki, M. 1993. Strength testing—predicting a one-rep max from reps-to-fatigue. *Journal of Physical Education, Recreation and Dance* 64 (1): 88-90.

Brzycki, M. 2000. Assessing strength. *Fitness Management* 16(7): 34-37.

Buchholz, A.C., and Schoeller, D.A. 2004. Is a calorie a calorie? *American Journal of Clinical Nutrition* 79 (Suppl.): 899S-906S.

Bundred, P., Kitchiner, D., and Buchan, I. 2001. Prevalence of overweight and obese children between 1989 and 1998: Population based series of cross sectional studies. *British Medical Journal* 322: 326-328.

Bunt, J.C., Lohman, T.G., and Boileau, R.A. 1989. Impact of total body water fluctuations on estimation of body fat from body density. *Medicine & Science in Sports & Exercise* 21: 96-100.

Buresh, R., and Berg, K. 2002. Scaling oxygen uptake to body size and several practical applications. *Journal of Strength and Conditioning Research* 16: 461-465.

Burke, D.G., Culligan, C.J., and Holt, L.E. 2000. The theoretical basis of proprioceptive neuromuscular facilitation. *Journal of Strength and Conditioning Research* 14: 496-500.

Burke, L.M., Kiens, B., and Ivy, J.L. 2004. Carbohydrates and fat for training and recovery. *Journal of Sports Science* 22: 15-30.

Byrnes, W.C., Clarkson, P.M., and Katch, F.I. 1985. Muscle soreness following resistive exercise with and without eccentric contraction. *Research Quarterly for Exercise and Sport* 56: 283-285.

Cable, A., Nieman, D.C., Austin, M., Hogen, E., and Utter, A.C. 2001. Validity of leg-to-leg bioelectrical impedance measurement in males. *Journal of Sports Medicine and Physical Fitness* 41: 411-414.

Callaway, C.W., Chumlea, W.C., Bouchard, C., Himes, J.H., Lohman, T.G., Martin, A.D., Mitchell, C.D., Mueller, W.H., Roche, A.F., and Seefeldt, V.D. 1988. Circumferences. In *Anthropometric standardization reference manual*, ed. T.G. Lohman, A.F. Roche, and R. Martorell, 39-54. Champaign, IL: Human Kinetics.

Campaigne, B.N. 1998. Exercise and diabetes mellitus. In *ACSM's resource manual for guidelines for exercise testing and prescription*, ed. J.L. Roitman (3rd ed.), 267-274. Philadelphia: Lippincott Williams & Wilkins.

Campbell, W.W., and Geik, R.A. 2004. Nutritional considerations for the older athlete. *Nutrition* 20: 603-608.

Canadian Society for Exercise Physiology. 2003. *The Canadian physical activity, fitness and lifestyle approach: CSEP-Health & Fitness Program's Health-Related Appraisal and Counselling Strategy*. 3rd ed. Ottawa, ON: Author.

Canning, P.M., Courage, M.L., and Frizzell, L.M. 2004. Prevalence of overweight and obesity in a provincial population of Canadian preschool children. *Canadian Medical Association Journal* 171: 240-242.

Carns, M.L., Schade, M.L., Liba, M.R., Hellebrandt, F.A., and Harris, C.W. 1960. Segmental volume reduction by localized and generalized exercise. *Human Biology* 32: 370-376.

Carpenter, D.M., and Nelson, B.W. 1999. Low back strengthening for the prevention and treatment of low back pain. *Medicine & Science in Sports & Exercise* 31: 18-24.

Casa, D.L., Armstrong, L.E., Hillman, S.K., Montain, S.J., Reiff, R.V., Rich, B.S.E., Roberts, W.O., and Stone, J.A. 2002. National Athletic Trainers' Association position statement: Fluid replacement for athletes. *Journal of Athletic Training* 35(2): 21-224.

Cassady, S.L., Nielsen, D.H., Janz, K.F., Wu, Y., Cook, J.S., and Hansen, J.R. 1993. Validity of near infrared body composition analysis in children and adolescents. *Medicine & Science in Sports & Exercise* 25: 1185-1191.

Cataldo, D., and Heyward, V. 2000. Pinch an inch: A comparison of several high-quality and plastic skinfold calipers. *ACSM's Health & Fitness Journal* 4(3): 12-16.

Caton, J.R., Mole, P.A., Adams, W.C., and Heustis, D.S. 1988. Body composition analysis by bioelectrical impedance: Effect of skin temperature. *Medicine & Science in Sports & Exercise* 20: 489-491.

Centers for Disease Control. 2001. Physical activity trends—United States, 1990-1998. *Morbidity and Mortality Weekly Report* 50: 166-169.

Centers for Disease Control. 2003a. Diabetes prevalence among American Indians and Alaskan Natives and the overall population—United States, 1994-2002. *Morbidity and Mortality Weekly* 52(30): 702-704.

Centers for Disease Control. 2003b. Prevalence of physical activity, including lifestyle activities among adults—United States, 2000-2001. *Morbidity and Mortality Weekly* 52(32): 764-769.

Chalmers, G. 2004. Re-examination of the possible role of Golgi tendon organ and muscle spindle reflexes in proprioceptive neuromuscular facilitation muscle stretching. *Sports Biomechanics* 3: 159-183.

Chapman, E.A., deVries, H.A., and Swezey, R. 1972. Joint stiffness: Effects of exercise on young and old men. *Journal of Gerontology* 27: 218–221.

Charette, S.L., McEvoy, L., Pyka, G., Snow-Harter, C., Guido, D., Wiswell, R.A., and Marcus, R. 1991. Muscle hypertrophy response to resistance training in older women. *Journal of Applied Physiology* 70: 1912–1916.

Chewning, B., Yu, T., and Johnson, J. 2000. T'ai chi (part 2): Effects on health. *ACSM's Health & Fitness Journal* 4(3): 17–19, 28, 30.

Chobanian, A.V., Bakris, G.L., Black, H.R., Cushman, W.C., Green, L.A., Izzo, J.L., Jones, D.W., Materson, B.J., Oparil, S., Wright, J.T. Jr., Roccella, E.J., and the National High Blood Pressure Education Coordinating Committee. 2003. The seventh report of the Joint National Committee on prevention, detection, evaluation, and treatment of high blood pressure. *Hypertension* 42: 1206–1252. Also available in *Journal of the American Medical Association* 289 (2003): 2560–2572.

Chung, I., and Lip, G.Y.H. 2003. White coat hypertension: Not so benign after all? *Journal of Human Hypertension* 17: 807–809.

Cipriani, D., Abel, B., and Pirrwitz, D. 2003. A comparison of two stretching protocols on hip range of motion: Implications for total daily stretch duration. *Journal of Strength and Conditioning Research* 17: 274–278.

Clark, N. 1997. *Sports nutrition guidebook.* Champaign, IL: Human Kinetics.

Clarke, D.H. 1975. *Exercise physiology.* Englewood Cliffs, NJ: Prentice Hall.

Clarke, H.H. 1966. *Muscular strength and endurance in man.* Englewood Cliffs, NJ: Prentice Hall.

Clarke, H.H., and Monroe, R.A. 1970. *Test manual: Oregon cable-tension strength test batteries for boys and girls from fourth grade through college.* Eugene, OR: University of Oregon.

Clarkson, P.M. 1990. Tired blood: Iron deficiency in athletes and effects of iron supplementation. *Sports Science Exchange* 3(28). Gatorade Sports Science Institute, Quaker Oats Co.

Clarkson, P.M., and Haymes, E.M. 1994. Trace mineral requirements for athletes. *International Journal of Sport Nutrition* 4: 104–119.

Clarkson, P.M., Byrnes, W.C., McCormick, K.M., Turcotte, L.P., and White, J.S. 1986. Muscle soreness and serum creatine kinase activity following isometric, eccentric and concentric exercise. *International Journal of Sports Medicine* 7: 152–155.

Clarys, J.P., Martin, A.D., Drinkwater, D.T., and Marfell-Jones, M.J. 1987. The skinfold: Myth and reality. *Journal of Sports Sciences* 5: 3–33.

Clemons, J.M., Duncan, C.A., Blanchard, O.E., Gatch, W.H., Hollander, D.B., and Doucet, J.L. 2004. Relationships between the flexed-arm hang and select measures of muscular fitness. *Journal of Strength and Conditioning Research* 18: 630-636.

Colberg, S.R. 2001. *The diabetic athlete.* Champaign, IL: Human Kinetics.

Cole, T.J., Bellizzi, M.C., Flegal, K.M., and Dietz, W.H. 2000. Establishing a standard definition for child overweight and obesity worldwide: International survey. *British Medical Journal* 320: 1240-1245.

Collins, M., Millard-Stafford, M., Sparling, P., Snow, T., Rosskopf, L., Webb, S., and Omer, J. 1999. Evaluation of the Bod Pod for assessing body fat in collegiate football players. *Medicine & Science in Sports & Exercise* 31: 1350–1356.

Conley, D., Cureton, K., Dengel, D., and Weyand, P. 1991. Validation of the 12-min swim as a field test of peak aerobic power in young men. *Medicine & Science in Sports & Exercise* 23: 766–773.

Conley, D., Cureton, K., Hinson, B., Higbie, E., and Weyand, P. 1992. Validation of the 12-minute swim as a field test of peak aerobic power in young women. *Research Quarterly for Exercise and Sport* 63: 153–161.

Conover, M.B. 1992. *Understanding electrocardiography.* St. Louis: Mosby Year Book.

Cooper Institute for Aerobics Research. 1992. *The Prudential FITNESSGRAM test administration manual.* Dallas: Author.

Cooper Institute for Aerobics Research. 1994. *Fitnessgram user's manual.* Dallas: Author.

Cooper Institute for Aerobics Research. 2005. *The fitness specialist certification manual.* Dallas: Author.

Cooper, K.H. 1968. A means of assessing maximal oxygen intake. *Journal of the American Medical Association* 203: 201–204.

Cooper, K.H. 1977. *The aerobics way.* New York: Evans.

Corbin, C.B., Dowell, L.J., Lindsey, R., and Tolson, H. 1978. *Concepts in physical education.* Dubuque, IA: Brown.

Costill, D.L., and Fox, E.L. 1969. Energetics of marathon running. *Medicine and Science in Sports* 1: 81–86.

Costill, D.L., Coyle, E.F., Fink, W.F., Lesmes, G.R., and Witzmann, F.A. 1979. Adaptations in skeletal muscle following strength training. *Journal of Applied Physiology* 46: 96–99.

Costill, D.L., Thomason, H., and Roberts, E. 1973. Fractional utilization of the aerobic capacity during distance running. *Medicine and Science in Sports* 5: 248–252.

Cote, C., Simoneau, J.A., Lagasse, P., Bouley, M., Thibault, M.C., Marcotte, M., and Bouchard, C. 1988. Isokinetic strength training protocols: Do they induce skeletal muscle fiber hypertrophy? *Archives of Physical Medicine and Rehabilitation* 69: 281–285.

Cote, D.K., and Adams, W.C. 1993. Effect of bone density on body composition estimates in young adult black and white women. *Medicine & Science in Sports & Exercise* 25: 290–296.

Cotten, D.J. 1972. A comparison of selected trunk flexibility tests. *American Corrective Therapy Journal* 26: 24.

Coyle, E.F. 1995. Fat metabolism during exercise. *Sports Science Exchange* 8(6). Gatorade Sports Science Institute, Quaker Oats Co.

Coyle, E.F., Feiring, D.C., Rotkis, T.C., Cote, R.W. III, Roby, F.B., Lee, W., and Wilmore, J.H. 1981. Specificity of power improvements through slow and fast isokinetic training. *Journal of Applied Physiology* 51: 1437–1442.

Crommett, A., Kravitz, L., Wongsathikun, J., and Kemerly, T. 1999. Comparison of metabolic and subjective response of three modalities in college-age subjects. *Medicine & Science in Sports & Exercise* 31(Suppl.): S158 [abstract].

Cullinen, K., and Caldwell, M. 1998. Weight training increases fat-free mass and strength in untrained young women. *Journal of the American Dietetic Association* 98(4): 414–418.

Cureton, K.J., Collins, M.A., Hill, D.W., and McElhannon, F.M. Jr. 1988. Muscle hypertrophy in men and women. *Medicine & Science in Sports & Exercise* 20: 338–344.

Cureton, K.J., Sloniger, M., O'Bannon, J., Black, D., and McCormack, W. 1995. A generalized equation for prediction of VO_2peak from 1-mile run/walk performance. *Medicine & Science in Sports & Exercise* 27: 445–451.

Cureton, K.J., Sparling, P.B., Evans, B.W., Johnson, S.M., Kong, U.D., and Purvis, J.W. 1978. Effect of experimental alterations in excess weight on aerobic capacity and distance running performance. *Medicine and Science in Sports* 10: 194–199.

Cureton, T.K., and Sterling, L.F. 1964. Interpretation of the cardiovascular component resulting from the factor analysis of 104 test variables measured in 100 normal young men. *Journal of Sports Medicine and Physical Fitness* 4: 1–24.

Day, J.R., Rossiter, H.B., Coats, E.M., Skasick, A., and Whipp, B.J. 2003. The maximally attainable VO_2 during exercise in humans: The peak vs. maximum issue. *Journal of Applied Physiology* 95: 1901-1907.

del Rio-Navarro, B.E., Velazquez-Monroy, O., Sanchez-Castillo, C.P., Lara-Esqueda, A., Berber, A., Fanghanel, G., Violante, R., Tapia-Conyer, R., and James, W.P.T. 2004. The high prevalence of overweight and obesity in Mexican children. *Obesity Research* 12: 215-223.

Delecluse, C., Roelants, M., and Verschueren, S. 2003. Strength increase after whole-body vibration compared with resistance training. *Medicine & Science in Sports & Exercise* 35: 1033-1041.

Demerath, E.W., Guo, S.S., Chumlea, W.C., Towne, B., Roche, A.F., and Siervogel, R.M. 2002. Comparison of percent body fat estimates using air displacement plethysmography and hydrodensitometry in adults and children. *International Journal of Obesity and Related Metabolic Disorders* 26: 389-397.

Demont, R.G., Lephart, S.M., Giraldo, J.L., Giannantonio, F.P., Yuktanandana, P., and Fu, F.H. 1999. Comparison of two abdominal training devices with an abdominal crunch using strength and EMG measurements. *Journal of Sports Medicine and Physical Fitness* 39: 253-258.

Dempster, P., and Aitkens, S. 1995. A new air displacement method for the determination of human body composition. *Medicine & Science in Sports & Exercise* 27: 1692–1697.

Demura, S., Yamaji, S., Goshi, F., Kobayashi, H., Sato, S., and Nagasawa, Y. 2002. The validity and reliability of relative body fat estimates and the construction of new

prediction equations for young Japanese adult males. *Journal of Sports Sciences* 20: 153-164.

Deschenes, M.R., and Kraemer, W.J. 2002. Performance and physiologic adaptations to resistance training. *American Journal of Physical Medicine and Rehabilitation* 8 (Suppl.): S3-S16.

Despres, J.P., and Lamarche, B. 1994. Low-intensity endurance training, plasma lipoproteins, and the risk of coronary heart disease. *Journal of Internal Medicine* 236: 7–22.

Despres, J.P., Bouchard, C., Tremblay, A., Savard, R., and Marcotte, M. 1985. Effects of aerobic training on fat distribution in male subjects. *Medicine & Science in Sports & Exercise* 17: 113–118.

Deurenberg, P. 2001. Universal cut-off BMI points for obesity are not appropriate. *British Journal of Nutrition* 85: 135-136.

Deurenberg, P., and Deurenberg-Yap, M. 2001. Differences in body-composition assumptions across ethnic groups: Practical consequences. *Current Opinion in Clinical Nutrition and Metabolic Care* 4: 377-383.

Deurenberg, P., and Deurenberg-Yap, M. 2002. Validation of skinfold thickness and hand-held impedance measurements for estimation of body fat percentage among Singaporean Chinese, Malay and Indian subjects. *Asia Pacific Journal of Clinical Nutrition* 11: 1-7.

Deurenberg, P., van der Kooy, K., and Leenan, R. 1989. Differences in body impedance when measured with different instruments. *European Journal of Clinical Nutrition* 43: 885-886.

Deurenberg, P., van der Kooy, K., Evers, P., and Hulshof, T. 1990. Assessment of body composition by bioelectrical impedance in a population aged >60 y. *American Journal of Clinical Nutrition* 51: 3-6.

Deurenberg, P., Weststrate, J.A., Paymans, I., and van der Kooy, K. 1988. Factors affecting bioelectrical impedance measurements in humans. *European Journal of Clinical Nutrition* 42: 1017–1022.

Deurenberg, P., Yap, M., and van Staveren, W.A. 1998. Body mass index and percent body fat: A meta analysis among different ethnic groups. *International Journal of Obesity* 22: 1164-1171.

Deurenberg. P., Weststrate, J.A., and Seidell, J.C. 1991. Body mass index as a measure of body fatness: Age- and sex-specific prediction formulas. *British Journal of Nutrition* 65: 105–114.

Deurenberg-Yap, M., Schmidt, G., van Staveren, W.A., Hautvast, J.G.A.J., and Deurenberg, P. 2001. Body fat measurement among Singaporean Chinese, Malays and Indians: A comparative study using a four-compartment model and different two-compartment models. *British Journal of Nutrition* 85: 491-498.

deVries, H.A. 1961. Prevention of muscular distress after exercise. *Research Quarterly* 32: 177–185.

deVries, H.A. 1962. Evaluation of static stretching procedures for improvement of flexibility. *Research Quarterly* 33: 222–229.

deVries, H.A., and Klafs, C.E. 1965. Prediction of maximal oxygen intake from submaximal tests. *Journal of Sports Medicine and Physical Fitness* 5: 207–214.

deWeijer, V.C., Gorniak, G.C., and Shamus, E. 2003. The effect of static stretch and warm-up exercise on hamstring length over the course of 24 hours. *Journal of Orthopaedic and Sports Physical Therapy* 33: 727-733.

Dewit, O., Fuller, N.J., Fewtrell, M.S., Elia, M., and Wells, J.C.K. 2000. Whole body air displacement plethysmography compared with hydrodensitometry for body composition analysis. *Archives of Disease in Childhood* 82: 159-164.

Dickinson, R.V. 1968. The specificity of flexibility. *Research Quarterly* 39: 792–793.

Disch, J., Frankiewicz, R., and Jackson, A. 1975. Construct validation of distance run tests. *Research Quarterly* 46: 169–176.

Dishman, R.K. 1994. Prescribing exercise intensity for healthy adults using perceived exertion. *Medicine & Science in Sports & Exercise* 26: 1087–1094.

Dolezal, B.A., and Potteiger, J.A. 1998. Concurrent resistance and endurance training influence basal metabolic rate in nondieting individuals. *Journal of Applied Physiology* 85: 695–700.

Donahue, C.P., Lin, D.H., Kirschenbaum, D.S., and Keesey, R.E. 1984. Metabolic consequence of dieting and exercise in the treatment of obesity. *Journal of Counseling and Clinical Psychology* 52: 827–836.

Donnelly, J.R., Brown, T.E., Israel, R.G., Smith-Sintek, S., O'Brien, K.F., and Caslavka, B. 1988. Hydrostatic weighing without head submersion: Description of a method. *Medicine & Science in Sports & Exercise* 20: 66–69.

Dons, B., Bollerup, K., Bonde-Petersen, F., and Hancke, S. 1979. The effect of weight-lifting exercise related to muscle fiber composition and muscle cross-sectional area in humans. *European Journal of Applied Physiology* 40: 95–106.

Dubin, D. 1980. *Rapid interpretation of EKGs*. Tampa: Cover.

Ducimetier, P., Richard, J., and Cambien, F. 1989. The pattern of subcutaneous fat distribution in middle-aged men and the risk of coronary heart disease: The Paris prospective study. *International Journal of Obesity* 10: 229–240.

Dudley, G.A., and Fleck, S.J. 1987. Strength and endurance training: Are they mutually exclusive? *Sports Medicine* 4: 79–85.

Dunbar, C.C., Robertson, R.J., Baun, R., Blandin, M.F., Metz, K., Burdett, R., and Goss, F.L. 1992. The validity of regulating exercise intensity by ratings of perceived exertion. *Medicine & Science in Sports & Exercise* 24: 94–99.

Dunn, A.L., Marcus, B.H., Kampert, J.B., Garcia, M.E., Kohl, H.W. III, and Blair, S.N. 1999. Project Active—A 24-month randomized trial to compare lifestyle and structured physical activity interventions. *Journal of the American Medical Association* 281: 327-334.

Durstine J.L., Grandjean, F.W., Cox, C.A., and Thompson, P.D. 2002. Lipids, lipoproteins, and exercise. *Journal of Cardiopulmonary Rehabilitation* 22: 385-398.

Ebbeling, C., Ward, A., Puleo, E., Widrick, J., and Rippe, J. 1991. Development of a single-stage submaximal treadmill walking test. *Medicine & Science in Sports & Exercise* 23: 966–973.

Eckert, S., and Horstkotte D. 2002. Comparison of Portapres non-invasive blood pressure measurement in the finger with intra-aortic pressure measurement during incremental bicycle exercise. *Blood Pressure Monitoring* 7: 179-183.

Edgerton, V.R. 1970. Morphology and histochemistry of the soleus muscle from normal and exercised rats. *American Journal of Anatomy* 127: 81–88.

Edgerton, V.R. 1973. Exercise and the growth and development of muscle tissue. In *Physical activity, human growth and development*, ed. G.L. Rarick, 1-31. New York: Academic Press.

Edwards, D.A., Hammond, W.H., Healy, M.J., Tanner, J.M., and Whitehouse, R.H. 1955. Design and accuracy of calipers for measuring subcutaneous tissue thickness. *British Journal of Nutrition* 9: 133–143.

Elia, M., Parkinson, S.A., and Diaz, E. 1990. Evaluation of near infra-red interactance as a method for predicting body composition. *European Journal of Clinical Nutrition* 44: 113–121.

Ellis, K.J., Bell, S.J., Chertow, G.M., Chumlea, W.C., Knox, T.A., Kotler, D.P., Lukaski, H.C., and Schoeller, D.A. 1999. Bioelectrical impedance methods in clinical research: A follow-up to the NIH technology assessment conference. *Nutrition* 15: 874-880.

Elsen, R., Siu, M.L., Pineda, O., and Solomons, N.W. 1987. Sources of variability in bioelectrical impedance determinations in adults. In *In vivo body composition studies*, ed. K.J. Ellis, S. Yasamura, and W.D. Morgan, 184–188. London: Institute of Physical Sciences in Medicine.

Enwemeka, C.S. 1986. Radiographic verification of knee goniometry. *Scandinavian Journal of Rehabilitation Medicine* 18: 47–49.

Esmark, B., Andersen, J.L., Olsen, S., Richter, E.A., Mizuno, M., and Kjaer, M. 2001. Timing of postexercise protein intake is important for muscle hypertrophy with resistance training in elderly humans. *Journal of Physiology*, 535:301-311.

Etnyre, B.R., and Abraham, L.D. 1986. H-reflex changes during static stretching and two variations of proprioceptive neuromuscular facilitation techniques. *Electroencephalography and Clinical Neurophysiology* 63: 174-179.

Ettinger, B., Genault H.K., and Cann, C.E. 1987. Postmenopausal bone loss is prevented by treatment with low-dosage estrogen with calcium. *Annals of Internal Medicine* 106: 40-45.

Evans, W., and Rosenberg, I. 1992. *Biomarkers*. New York: Simon & Schuster.

Fagard, R.H. 1999. Physical activity in the prevention and treatment of hypertension in the obese. *Medicine & Science in Sports & Exercise* 31(Suppl.): S624–S630.

Fahey, T.D., Rolph, R., Moungmee, P., Nagel, J., and Mortara, S. 1976. Serum testosterone, body composition, and strength of young adults. *Medicine and Science in Sports* 8: 31–34.

Faigenbaum, A.D. 2003. Youth resistance training. *President's Council on Physical Fitness and Sports Research Digest,* September: 1-8.

Faigenbaum, A.D., Milliken, L.A., and Westcott, W.L. 2003. Maximal strength testing in healthy children. *Journal of Strength and Conditioning Research* 17: 162-166.

Faigenbaum, A.D., Westcott, W.L., Loud, R.L., and Long, C. 1999. The effects of different resistance training protocols on muscular strength and endurance development in children. *Pediatrics* 104(1): e5.

Feigenbaum, M.S., and Pollock, M.L. 1999. Prescription of resistance training for health and disease. *Medicine & Science in Sports & Exercise* 31: 38–45.

Feland, J.B., Myrer, J.W., Schulthies, S.S., Fellingham, G.W., and Measom, G.W. 2001. The effect of duration of stretching of the hamstring muscle group for increasing range of motion in people aged 65 years or older. *Physical Therapy* 81: 1110-1117.

Fenstermaker, K., Plowman, S., and Looney, M. 1992. Validation of the Rockport walking test in females 65 years and older. *Research Quarterly for Exercise and Sport* 63: 322–327.

Ferber, R., Osternig, L., and Gravelle, D. 2002. Effect of PNF stretch techniques on knee flexor muscle EMG activity in older adults. *Journal of Electromyography and Kinesiology* 12: 391-397.

Ferland, M., Despres, J.P., Tremblay, A., Pinault, S., Nadeau, A., Moorjani, S., Lupien, P.J., Theriault, G., and Bouchard, C. 1989. Assessment of adipose distribution by computed axial tomography in obese women: Association with body density and anthropometric measurements. *British Journal of Nutrition* 61: 139-148.

Fess, E.E. 1992. Grip Strength. In *Clinical assessment recommendations,* American Society of Hand Therapists, 41–45, Chicago, IL: American Society of Hand Therapists.

Fiatarone, M.A., Marks, E.C., Ryan, N.D., Meredith, C.N., Lipsitz, L.A., and Evans, W.J. 1991. High-intensity strength training in nonagenarians. Effects on skeletal muscle. *Journal of the American Medical Association* 263: 3029–3034.

Fields, D.A., and Goran, M.I. 2000. Body composition techniques and the four-compartment model in children. *Journal of Applied Physiology* 89: 6113-620.

Fields, D.A., Goran, M.I., and McCrory, M.A. 2002. Body-composition assessment via air-displacement plethysmography in adults and children: A review. *American Journal of Clinical Nutrition* 75: 453-467.

Fields, D.A., Hunter, G.R., and Goran, M.I. 2000. Validation of the Bod Pod with hydrostatic weighing: Influence of body clothing. *International Journal of Obesity* 24: 200-205.

Fields, D.A., Wilson, G.D., Gladden, L.B., Hunter, G.R., Pascoe, D.D., and Goran, M.I. 2001. Comparison of the Bod Pod with the four-compartment model in adult females. *Medicine & Science in Sports & Exercise* 33: 1605-1610.

Fitness Canada. 1986. *Canadian standardized test of fitness (CSTF) operations manual,* 3rd ed., Ottawa, ON: Fitness and Amateur Sport Canada.

Fleck, S.J. 1999. Periodized strength training: A critical review. *Journal of Strength and Conditioning Research* 13(1): 82–89.

Fleck, S.J., and Falkel, J.E. 1986. Value of resistance training for the reduction of sports injuries. *Sports Medicine* 3: 61–68.

Fleck, S.J., and Kraemer, W.J. 1997. *Designing resistance training programs.* Champaign, IL: Human Kinetics.

Flegal, K.M., Carroll, M.D., Kuczmarski, R.J., and Johnson, C.L. 1998. Overweight and obesity in the United States: Prevalence and trends, 1960-1994. *International Journal of Obesity* 22: 39–47.

Flegal, K.M., Carroll, M.D., Ogden, C.L., and Johnson, C.L. 2002. Prevalence and trends in obesity among U.S. adults, 1999-2000. *Journal of the American Medical Association* 288(14): 1723-1727.

FMpulse. 2004. Standards sought for personal trainers. *Fitness Management* 20(6): 16.

Fogelholm, G.M., Sievanan, H.T., Kukkonen-Harjula, K. Oja, P. and Vuori, I. 1993. Effects of a meal and its electrolytes on bioelectrical impedance. In *Human body composition: In vivo methods, models and assessment,* ed. K.J. Ellis and J.D. Eastman, 331-332. New York: Plenum Press.

Fohlin, L. 1977. Body composition, cardiovascular and renal function in adolescent patients with anorexia nervosa. *Acta Paediatrica Scandinavica* 268(Suppl.): 7–20.

Forbes, G.B. 1976. Adult decline in the lean body mass. *Human Biology* 48: 151–173.

Fornetti, W.C., Pivarnik, J.M., Foley, J.M., and Fiechtner, J.J. 1999. Reliability and validity of body composition measures in female athletes. *Journal of Applied Physiology* 87: 1114-1122.

Foster, C., Jackson, A.S., Pollock, M.L., Taylor, M.M., Hare, J., Sennett, S.M., Rod, J.L., Sarwar, M., and Schmidt, D.H. 1984. Generalized equations for predicting functional capacity from treadmill performance. *American Heart Journal* 107: 1229–1234.

Foster, C., Pollock, M.L., Rod, J.L., Dymond, D.S., Wible, G., and Schmidt, D.H. 1983. Evaluation of functional capacity during exercise radionuclide angiography. *Cardiology* 70: 85–93.

Foster, G.D., Wyatt, H.R., Hill, J.O., McGuckin, B.G., Brill, C., Selma Mohammed, B., Szapary, P.O., Rader, D.J., Edman, J.S., and Klien, S. 2003. A randomized trial of a low-carbohydrate diet for obesity. *New England Journal of Medicine* 348: 2082-2090.

Foster-Powell, K., and Miller, J. 1995. International tables of glycemic index. *American Journal of Clinical Nutrition* 62: 871S–893S.

Fowles, J.R., Sale, D.G., and MacDougall, J.D. 2000. Reduced strength after passive stretch of the human plantar flexors. *Journal of Applied Physiology* 89: 1179-1188.

Fox, E.L. 1973. A simple, accurate technique for predicting maximal aerobic power. *Journal of Applied Physiology* 35: 914–916.

Fox, E.L., and Mathews, D.K. 1974. *Interval training: Conditioning for sports and general fitness.* Philadelphia: Saunders.

Francis, P.R., Kolkhorst, F.W., Pennuci, M., Pozos, R.S., and Buono, M.J. 2001. An electromyographic approach to the evaluation of abdominal exercises. *ACSM's Health & Fitness Journal* 5(4): 8-14.

Friden, J. 2002. Delayed onset muscle soreness. *Scandinavian Journal of Medicine and Science in Sports* 12: 327-328.

Friden, J., Sjostrom, M., and Ekblom, B. 1983. Myofibrillar damage following intense eccentric exercise in man. *International Journal of Sports Medicine* 4: 170–176.

Friedl, K.E., DeLuca, J.P., Marchitelli, L.J., and Vogel, J.A. 1992. Reliability of body-fat estimations from a four-compartment model by using density, body water, and bone mineral measurements. *American Journal of Clinical Nutrition* 55: 764-770.

Frisancho, A.R. 1984. New standard of weight and body composition by frame size and height for assessment of nutritional status of adults and the elderly. *American Journal of Clinical Nutrition* 40: 808–819.

Frontera, W.R., Meredith, C.N., O'Reilly, K.P., Knuttgen, H.G., and Evans, W.J. 1988. Strength conditioning in older men: Skeletal muscle hypertrophy and improved function. *Journal of Applied Physiology* 64: 1038–1044.

Fuller, N.J., Sawyer, M.B., and Elia, M. 1994. Comparative evaluation of body composition methods and predictions, and calculation of density and hydration fraction of fat-free mass, in obese women. *International Journal of Obesity* 18: 503-512.

Gajdosik, R.L., Vander Linden, D.W., and Williams, A.K. 1999. Influence of age on length and passive elastic stiffness characteristics of the calf muscle-tendon unit of women. *Physical Therapy* 79: 827–838.

Gallagher, D., Visser, M., Sepulveda, D., Pierson, R.N., Harris, T., and Heymsfield, S.B. 1996. How useful is body mass index for comparison of body fatness across age, sex, and ethnic groups? *American Journal of Epidemiology* 143: 228-239.

Gallagher, M.R., Walker, K.Z., and O'Dea, K. 1998. The influence of a breakfast meal on the assessment of body composition using bioelectrical impedance. *European Journal of Clinical Nutrition* 52: 94-97.

Gardner, G.W. 1963. Specificity of strength changes of the exercised and non-exercised limb following isometric training. *Research Quarterly* 34: 98–101.

Genton, L., Hans, D., Kyle, U.G., and Pichard, C. 2002. Dual-energy X-ray absorptiometry and body composition: Differences between devices and comparison with reference methods. *Nutrition* 18: 66-70.

Genton, L., Karsegard, V.L., Kyle, U.G., Hans, D.B., Michel, J.P., and Pichard, C. 2001. Comparison of four bioelectrical impedance analysis formulas in healthy elderly subjects. *Gerontology* 47: 315-323.

George, J., Vehrs, P., Allsen, P., Fellingham, G., and Fisher, G. 1993. VO$_2$max estimation from a submaximal 1-mile track jog for fit college-age individuals. *Medicine & Science in Sports & Exercise* 25: 401-406.

Gettman, L.R., and Pollock, M.L. 1981. Circuit weight training: A critical review of its physiological benefits. *The Physician and Sportsmedicine* 9: 44-60.

Gettman, L.R., Ayres, J.J., Pollock, M.L., and Jackson, A. 1978. The effect of circuit weight training on strength, cardiorespiratory function, and body composition of adult men. *Medicine and Science in Sports* 10: 171-176.

Gibbons, R.J., Balady, G.J., Bricker, J.T., Chaitman, B.R., Fletcher, G.F., Froelicher, V.F., Mark, D.B., McCallister, B.D., Mooss, A.N., O'Reilly, M.G., and Winters, W.L. Jr. 2002. *ACC/AHA* 2002 guideline update for exercise testing: A report of the American College of Cardiology/American Heart Association Task Force on Practice Guidelines (Committee on Exercise Testing). www.acc.org/clinical/guidelines/exercise/dirIndex.htm.

Gibson, A., Heyward, V., and Mermier, C. 2000. Predictive accuracy of Omron Body Logic Analyzer in estimating relative body fat of adults. *International Journal of Sport Nutrition and Exercise Metabolism* 10: 216–227.

Girouard, C.K., and Hurley, B.F. 1995. Does strength training inhibit gains in range of motion from flexibility training in older adults? *Medicine & Science in Sports & Exercise* 27: 1444–1449.

Gledhill, N., and Jamnik, R. 1995. Determining power outputs for cycle ergometers with different sized flywheels. *Medicine & Science in Sports & Exercise* 27: 134–135.

Gleichauf, C.N., and Rose, D.A. 1989. The menstrual cycle's effect on the reliability of bioimpedance measurements for assessing body composition. *American Journal of Clinical Nutrition* 50: 903–907.

Goldberg, A., Etlinger, J., Goldspink, D., and Jablecki, C. 1975. Mechanism of work-induced hypertrophy of skeletal muscle. *Medicine and Science in Sports* 7: 185–198.

Goldberger, A.L., and Goldberger, E. 1981. *Clinical electrocardiography: A simplified approach.* St. Louis: Mosby.

Golding, L. 2000. *The Y's way to physical fitness.* Champaign, IL: Human Kinetics.

Goldman, M.J. 1982. *Principles of clinical electrocardiography.* Cambridge, MD: Lange Medical.

Gonyea, W.J., Ericson, G.C., and Bonde-Petersen, F. 1977. Skeletal muscle fiber splitting induced by weight-lifting exercise in cats. *Acta Physiologica Scandinavica* 99: 105–109.

Goran, M.I., Allison, D.B., and Poehlman, E.T. 1995. Issues relating to normalization of body fat content in men and women. *International Journal of Obesity* 19: 638-643.

Goran, M.I., Toth, M.J., and Poehlman, E.T. 1998. Assessment of research-based body composition techniques in healthy elderly men and women using the 4-component model as a criterion method. *International Journal of Obesity* 22: 135-142.

Graves, J.D., Webb, M., Pollock, M.L., Matkozich, J., Leggett, S.H., Carpenter, D.M., Foster, D.N., and Cirulli, J. 1994. Pelvic stabilization during resistance training: Its effect on the development of lumbar extension strength. *Archives of Physical Medicine and Rehabilitation* 75: 211-215.

Graves, J.E., Pollock, M.L., Colvin, A.B., Van Loan, M., and Lohman, T.G. 1989. Comparison of different bioelectrical impedance analyzers in the prediction of body composition. *American Journal of Human Biology* 1: 603–611.

Gray, D.S., Bray, G.A., Gemayel, N., and Kaplan, K. 1989. Effect of obesity on bioelectrical impedance. *American Journal of Clinical Nutrition* 50: 255–260.

Greene, W.B., and Heckman, J.D. 1994. *The clinical measurement of joint motion.* Rosemont, IL: American Academy of Orthopaedic Surgeons.

Grembowski, D., Patrick, D., Diehr, P., Durham, M., Beresford, S., Kay, E., and Hecht, J. 1993. Self-efficacy and health behavior among older adults. *Journal of Health and Social Behavior* 34(6): 89–104.

Grenier, S.G., Russell, C., and McGill, S.M. 2003. Relationships between lumbar flexibility, sit-and-reach test, and a previous history of low back discomfort in industrial workers. *Canadian Journal of Applied Physiology* 28: 165-177.

Grier, T.D., Lloyd, L.K., Walker, J.L., and Murray, T.D. 2002. Metabolic cost of aerobic dance bench stepping at varying cadences and bench heights. *Journal of Strength and Conditioning Research* 16: 242-249.

Griffin, S., Roberts, R., and Heyward, V. 1997. Assessment of exercise blood pressure: A review. *Medicine & Science in Sports & Exercise* 29: 149–159.

Gruber, J.J., Pollock, M.L., Graves, J.E., Colvin, A.B., and Braith, R.W. 1990. Comparison of Harpenden and Lange calipers in predicting body composition. *Research Quarterly for Exercise and Sport* 61: 184-190.

Grundy, S., Blackburn, G., Higgins, M., Lauer, R., Perri, M., and Ryan, D. 1999. Roundtable consensus statement: Physical activity in the prevention and treatment of obesity and its comorbidities: Evidence report of independent panel to assess the role of physical activity in the treatment of obesity and its comorbidities. *Medicine & Science in Sports & Exercise* 31(Suppl.): S502-S508.

Gudivaka, R., Schoeller, D., and Kushner, R.F. 1996. Effect of skin temperature on multifrequency bioelectrical impedance analysis. *Journal of Applied Physiology* 81: 838-845.

Gustavsen, P.H., Hoegholm, A., Bang, L.E., and Kristensen, K.S. 2003. White coat hypertension is a cardiovascular risk factor. A 10-year follow-up study. *Journal of Human Hypertension* 17: 811-817.

Guy, J.A., and Micheli, L.J. 2001. Strength training for children and adolescents. *Journal of the American Academy of Orthopaedic Surgeons* 9: 29-36.

Habash, D. 2002. Tactile and interpersonal techniques for fatfold anthropometry. School of Medicine. Ohio State University. Unpublished paper.

Hagberg, J.M. 1990. Exercise, fitness, and hypertension. In *Exercise, fitness, and health: A consensus of current knowledge,* ed. C. Bouchard, R.J. Shephard, T. Stephens, J.R. Sutton, and B.D. McPherson, 455–466. Champaign, IL: Human Kinetics.

Hagerman, F. 1993. *Concept II rowing ergometer nomogram for prediction of maximal oxygen consumption* [abstract]. Morrisville, VT: Concept II.

Hanson, P. 1988. Clinical exercise testing. In *Resource manual for guidelines for exercise testing and prescription,* ed. S.N. Blair, P. Painter, R. Pate, L.K. Smith, and C.B. Taylor, 248–255. Philadelphia: Lea & Febiger.

Harris, J.A., and Benedict, F.G. 1919. *A biometric study of basal metabolism in man* (publication no. 279). Washington, D.C.: Carnegie Institute.

Harris, M.L. 1969. A factor analytic study of flexibility. *Research Quarterly* 40: 62–70.

Harrison, G.G., Buskirk, E.R., Carter, L.J.E., Johnston, F.E., Lohman, T.G., Pollock, M.L., Roche, A.F., and Wilmore, J.H. 1988. Skinfold thicknesses and measurement technique. In *Anthropometric standardization reference manual,* ed. T.G. Lohman, A.F. Roche, and R. Martorell, 55–70. Champaign, IL: Human Kinetics.

Hartley, L.H. 1975. Growth hormone and catecholamine response to exercise in relation to physical training. *Medicine and Science in Sports* 7: 34–36.

Hartley, L.H., Mason, J.W., Hogan, R.P., Jones, L.G., Kotchen, T.A., Mougey, E.H., Wherry, R., Pennington, L., and Ricketts, P. 1972. Multiple hormonal responses to graded exercise in relation to physical conditioning. *Journal of Applied Physiology* 33: 602–606.

Hartley-O'Brien, S.J. 1980. Six mobilization exercises for active range of hip flexion. *Research Quarterly for Exercise and Sport* 51: 625–635.

Harvard School of Public Health. 2004. Food Pyramids. www.hsph.harvard.edu/nutritionsource/pyramids.html.

Hass, C.J., Garzarella, L., De Hoyas, D., and Pollock, M. 2000. Single versus multiple sets in long-term recreational weightlifters. *Medicine & Science in Sports & Exercise* 32: 235–242.

Hather, B.M., Tesch, P.A., Buchanan, P., and Dudley, G.A. 1991. Influence of eccentric actions on skeletal muscle adaptations to resistance training. *Acta Physiologica Scandinavica* 143: 177–185.

Hayes, P.A., Sowood, P.J., Belyavin, A., Cohen, J.B., and Smith, F.W. 1988. Sub-cutaneous fat thickness measured by magnetic resonance imaging, ultrasound, and calipers. *Medicine & Science in Sports & Exercise* 20: 303–309.

Health Canada. 2003. Canada's physical activity guide to healthy active living. Version 9. www.hc-sc.ca/english/lifestyles/index.html.

Hedley, A.A., Ogden, C.L., Johnson, C.L., Carroll, M.D., Curtin, L.R., and Flegal, K.M. 2004. Prevalence of overweight and obesity among U.S. children, adolescents, and adults, 1999-2002. *Journal of the American Medical Association* 291(23): 2847-2850.

Heil, D.P. 1997. Body mass scaling of peak oxygen uptake in 20- to 79-year-old adults. *Medicine & Science in Sports & Exercise* 29: 1602-1608.

Heitmann, B.L., Kondrup, J., Engelhart, M., Kristensen, J.H., Podenphant, J., Hoie, L.H., and Andersen, V. 1994.

Changes in fat free mass in overweight patients with rheumatoid arthritis on a weight reducing regimen. A comparison of eight different body composition methods. *International Journal of Obesity* 18: 812-819.

Henwood, T.R., and Taaffe, D.R. 2003. Beneficial effects of high-velocity resistance training in older adults. *Medicine & Science in Sports & Exercise* 35 (Suppl.): S292 [abstract].

Herbert, D.L. 1995. First state licenses exercise physiologists. *Fitness Management,* October, 26–27.

Herbert, D.L. 2004. New law to regulate personal trainers proposed in Oregon. *The Exercise Standards and Malpractice Reporter* 18(2): 17, 20-24.

Herbert, R.D., and Gabriel, M. 2002. Effects of stretching on muscle soreness and risk of injury: A meta-analysis. *British Medical Journal* 325: 468-471.

Hermansen, L., and Saltin, B. 1969. Oxygen uptake during maximal treadmill and bicycle exercise. *Journal of Applied Physiology* 26: 31–37.

Hettinger, T., and Muller, E.A. 1953. Muskelleistung und muskeltraining. *European Journal of Applied Physiology* 15: 111–126.

Heymsfield, S.B., Wang, J., Lichtman, S., Kamen, Y., Kehayias, J., and Pierson, R.N. 1989. Body composition in elderly subjects: A critical appraisal of clinical methodology. *American Journal of Clinical Nutrition* 50: 1167–1175.

Heyward, V.H., Cook, K.L., Hicks, V.L., Jenkins, K.A., Quatrochi, J.A., and Wilson, W. 1992. Predictive accuracy of three field methods for estimating relative body fatness of nonobese and obese women. *International Journal of Sport Nutrition* 2: 75–86.

Heyward, V.H., and Wagner, D.R. 2004. *Applied body composition assessment,* 2nd ed. Champaign, IL: Human Kinetics.

Hickson, R.C., and Rosenkoetter, M.A. 1981. Reduced training frequencies and maintenance of increased aerobic power. *Medicine & Science in Sports & Exercise* 13: 13–16.

Higgins, P.B., Fields, D.A., Hunter, G.R., and Gower, B.A. 2001. Effect of scalp and facial hair on air displacement plethysmography estimates of percentage of body fat. *Obesity Research* 9: 326-330.

Hill, J.O., and Melanson, E.L. 1999. Overview of the determinants of overweight and obesity: Current evidence and research issues. *Medicine & Science in Sports & Exercise* 31(Suppl.): S515–S521.

Himes, J.H., and Frisancho, R.A. 1988. Estimating frame size. In *Anthropometric standardization reference manual,* ed. T.G. Lohman, A.F. Roche, and R. Martorell, 121-124. Champaign, IL: Human Kinetics.

Hirsh, J. 1971. Adipose cellularity in relation to human obesity. *Advances in Internal Medicine* 17: 289–300.

Hoeger, W.W.K. 1989. *Lifetime physical fitness and wellness.* Englewood Cliffs, NJ: Morton.

Hoeger, W.W.K., and Hopkins, D.R. 1992. A comparison of the sit-and-reach and the modified sit-and-reach in the measurement of flexibility in women. *Research Quarterly for Exercise and Sport* 63: 191–195.

Hoeger, W.W.K., Hopkins, D.R., Button, S., and Palmer, T.A. 1990. Comparing the sit and reach with the modified sit and reach in measuring flexibility in adolescents. *Pediatric Exercise Science* 2: 156–162.

Holt, L.E., Travis, T.M., and Okita, T. 1970. Comparative study of three stretching techniques. *Perceptual and Motor Skills* 31: 611–616.

Houtkooper, L.B., Going, S.G., Lohman, T.G., Roche, A.F., and VanLoan, M. 1992. Bioelectrical impedance estimation of fat-free body mass in children and youth: A cross-validation study. *Journal of Applied Physiology* 72: 366-373.

Houtkooper, L.B., Going, S.B., Westfall, C.H., Lohman, T.G. 1989. Prediction of fat-free body corrected for bone mass from impedance and anthropometry in adult females. *Medicine & Science in Sports & Exercise* 21: 539 [abstract].

Howley, E.T., Colacino, D.L., and Swensen, T.C. 1992. Factors affecting the oxygen cost of stepping on an electronic stepping ergometer. *Medicine & Science in Sports & Exercise* 24: 1055–1058.

Hubley-Kozey, C.L. 1991. Testing flexibility. In *Physiological testing of the high-performance athlete,* ed. J.D. MacDougall, H.A. Wenger, and H.J. Green, 309–359. Champaign, IL: Human Kinetics.

Hui, S.C., and Yuen, P.Y. 2000. Validity of the modified back-saver sit-and-reach test: A comparison with other protocols. *Medicine & Science in Sports & Exercise* 32: 1655–1659.

Hui, S.C., Yuen, P.Y., Morrow, J.R., and Jackson, A.W. 1999. Comparison of the criterion-related validity of sit-and-reach tests with and without limb length adjustment in Asian adults. *Research Quarterly for Exercise and Sport* 70: 401–406.

Hultborn, H., Illert, M., and Santini, M. 1974. Disynaptic inhibition of the interneurons mediating the reciprocal Ia inhibition of motor neurones. *Acta Physiologica Scandinavica* 91: 14A-16A.

Human Kinetics. 1995. *Practical body composition kit.* Champaign, IL: Author.

Human Kinetics. 1999. *Assessing body composition.* Champaign, IL: Author.

Hunter, G.R., Wetzstein, C.J., McLafferty, C.L., Zuckerman, P.A., Landers, K.A., and Bamman, M.M. 2001. High-resistance versus variable-resistance training in older adults. *Medicine & Science in Sports & Exercise* 33: 1759-1764.

Idema, R.N., van den Meiracker, A.H., and Imholz, B.P.M. 1989. Comparison of Finapres non-invasive beat-to-beat finger blood pressure with intrabrachial artery pressure during and after bicycle ergometry. *Journal of Hypertension* 7 (Suppl. 6): S58-S59.

Ikai, M., and Fukunaga, T. 1968. Calculation of muscle strength per unit cross-sectional area of human muscle by means of ultrasonic measurement. *European Journal of Applied Physiology* 26: 26–32.

Institute of Medicine. 2002. *Dietary reference intakes for energy, carbohydrates, fiber, fat, fatty acids, cholesterol, protein, and amino acids.* Washington, D.C.: National Academies Press.

International Dance and Exercise Association. 2004. Personal fitness trainer certification. *IDEA Health & Fitness Source,* March: 15.

International Obesity Task Force. 2005. EU platform on diet, physical activity and health: Obesity in Europe. www.iotf.org.

Invergo, J.J., Ball, T.E., and Looney, M. 1991. Relationship of pushups and absolute muscular endurance to bench press strength. *Journal of Applied Sport Science Research* 5: 121–125.

Jackson, A. 1984. Research design and analysis of data procedures for predicting body density. *Medicine & Science in Sports & Exercise* 16: 616–620.

Jackson, A.S., and Pollock, M.L. 1976. Factor analysis and multivariate scaling of anthropometric variables for the assessment of body composition. *Medicine & Science in Sports & Exercise* 8: 196–203.

Jackson, A.S., and Pollock, M.L. 1978. Generalized equations for predicting body density of men. *British Journal of Nutrition* 40: 497–504.

Jackson, A.S., and Pollock, M.L. 1985. Practical assessment of body composition. *The Physician and Sportsmedicine* 13: 76–90.

Jackson, A.S., Pollock, M.L., and Ward, A. 1980. Generalized equations for predicting body density of women. *Medicine & Science in Sports & Exercise* 12: 175–182.

Jackson, A.S., Pollock, M.L., Graves, J.E., and Mahar, M.T. 1988. Reliability and validity of bioelectrical impedance in determining body composition. *Journal of Applied Physiology* 64: 529–534.

Jackson, A.W., and Langford, N.J. 1989. The criterion-related validity of the sit-and-reach test: Replication and extension of previous findings. *Research Quarterly for Exercise and Sport* 60: 384–387.

Jackson, A.W., Morrow, J.R., Brill, P.A., Kohl, H.W., Gordon, N.F., and Blair, S.N. 1998. Relations of sit-up and sit-and-reach tests to low back pain in adults. *Journal of Orthopaedic and Sports Physical Therapy* 27: 22–26.

Janssen, I., Heymsfield, S.B., Allison, D.B., Kotler, D.P., and Ross, R. 2002. Body mass index and waist circumference independently contribute to the prediction of nonabdominal, abdominal subcutaneous, and visceral fat. *American Journal of Clinical Nutrition* 75: 683–688.

Janssen, I., Katzmarzyk, P.T., and Ross, R. 2004. Waist circumference and not body mass index explain obesity-related health risk. *American Journal of Clinical Nutrition* 79: 379–384.

Jenkins, W.L., Thackaberry, M., and Killian, C. 1984. Speed-specific isokinetic training. *Journal of Orthopaedic and Sports Physical Therapy* 6: 181–183.

Johns, R.J., and Wright, V. 1962. Relative importance of various tissues in joint stiffness. *Journal of Applied Physiology* 17: 824–828.

Johnson, B.L., and Nelson, J.K., eds. 1986. *Practical measurements for evaluation in physical education.* Minneapolis: Burgess.

Jones, B.H., and Knapik, J.J. 1999. Physical training and exercise-related injuries. *Sports Medicine* 27: 111–125.

Jones, C.J., Rikli, R.E., Max, J., and Noffal, G. 1998. The reliability and validity of a chair sit-and-reach test as a measure of hamstring flexibility in older adults. *Research Quarterly for Exercise and Sport* 69: 338–343.

Jones, D.W., Frohlich, E.D., Grim, C.M., Grim, C.E., and Taubert, K.A. 2001. Mercury sphygmomanometers should not be abandoned: An advisory statement from the Council for High Blood Pressure Research, American Heart Association. *Hypertension* 37: 185-186.

Juker, D., McGill, S., Kropf, P., and Steffen, T. 1998. Quantitative intramuscular myoelectric activity of lumbar portions of psoas and the abdominal wall during a wide variety of tasks. *Medicine & Science in Sports & Exercise* 30: 301-310.

Kaminsky, L.A., and Whaley, M.H. 1998. Evaluation of a new standardized ramp protocol: The BSU/Bruce ramp protocol. *Journal of Cardiopulmonary Rehabilitation* 18: 438-444.

Katch, F.I., Clarkson, P.M., Kroll, W., McBride, T., and Wilcox, A. 1984. Effects of sit-up exercise training on adipose cell size and adiposity. *Research Quarterly for Exercise and Sport* 55: 242–247.

Katch, F.I., McArdle, W.D., Czula, R., and Pechar, G.S. 1973. Maximal oxygen intake, endurance running performance, and body composition in college women. *Research Quarterly* 44: 301–312.

Kattus, A.A., Hanafee, W.N., Longmire, W.P., MacAlpin, R.N., and Rivin, A.U. 1968. Diagnosis, medical and surgical management of coronary insufficiency. *Annals of Internal Medicine* 69: 115–136.

Keim, N.L., Blanton, C.A., and Kretsch, M.J. 2004. America's obesity epidemic: Measuring physical activity to promote an active lifestyle. *Journal of the American Dietetic Association* 104: 1398-1409.

Kelley, D.E., and Goodpaster, B.H. 1999. Effects of physical activity on insulin action and glucose tolerance in obesity. *Medicine & Science in Sports & Exercise* 31(Suppl.): S619–S623.

Kesaniemi, Y.K., Danforth, E., Jensen, M.D., Kopelman, P.G., Lefebvre, P., and Reeder, B.A. 2001. Dose-response issues concerning physical activity and health: An evidenced-based symposium. *Medicine & Science in Sports & Exercise* 33 (Suppl.): S351–S358.

Keys, A., and Brozek, J. 1953. Body fat in adult man. *Physiological Reviews* 33: 245–325.

Khaled, M.A., McCutcheon, M.J., Reddy, S., Pearman, P.L., Hunter, G.R., and Weinsier, R.L. 1988. Electrical impedance in assessing human body composition: The BIA method. *American Journal of Clinical Nutrition* 47: 789–792.

Kim, P.S., Mayhew, J.L., and Peterson, D.F. 2002. A modified bench press test as a predictor of 1 repetition maximum bench press strength. *Journal of Strength and Conditioning Research* 16: 440-445.

Kimball, S.R., and Jefferson, L.S. 2002. Control of protein synthesis by amino acid availability. *Current Opinions in Clinical Nutrition and Metabolic Care* 5: 63-67.

Kirby, R.L., Simms, F.C., Symington, V.J., and Garner, J.B. 1981. Flexibility and musculoskeletal symptomatology in female gymnasts and age-matched controls. *American Journal of Sports Medicine* 9: 160–164.

Kline, G.M., Porcari, J.P., Hintermeister, R., Freedson, P.S., Ward, A., McCarron, R.F., Ross, J. and Rippe, J.M. 1987. Estimation of VO$_2$max from a one-mile track walk, gender, age, and body weight. *Medicine & Science in Sports & Exercise* 19: 253–259.

Knowler, W.C., Barrett-Conner, E., Fowler, S.E., Hamman, R.F., Lachin, J.M., Walker, E.A., and Nathan, D.M. 2002. Reduction in incidence of type 2 diabetes with lifestyle intervention or metaformin. Diabetes Prevention Program Research Group. *New England Journal of Medicine* 346: 393-403.

Knudson, D. 2001. The validity of recent curl-up tests in young adults. *Journal of Strength and Conditioning Research* 15: 81-85.

Knudson, D., and Johnston, D. 1995. Validity and reliability of a bench trunk-curl test of abdominal endurance. *Journal of Strength and Conditioning Research* 9: 165-169.

Knudson, D., and Johnston, D. 1998. Analysis of three test durations of the bench trunk-curl. *Journal of Strength and Conditioning Research* 12: 150-151.

Knudson, D.V. 1999. Issues in abdominal fitness: Testing and technique. *Journal of Physical Education, Recreation & Dance* 70(3): 49-55.

Knudson, D.V., Magnusson, P., and McHugh, M. 2000. Current issues in flexibility fitness. *President's Council on Physical Fitness and Sports Research Digest* 3(10): 1–8.

Knuttgen, H.G., and Kraemer, W.J. 1987. Terminology and measurement in exercise performance. *Journal of Applied Sport Science Research* 1: 1–10.

Knutzen, K.M., Brilla, L.R., and Caine, D. 1999. Validity of 1RM prediction equations for older adults. *Journal of Strength and Conditioning Research* 13: 242-246.

Kohrt, W.M. 1998. Preliminary evidence that DEXA provides an accurate assessment of body composition. *Journal of Applied Physiology* 84: 372-377.

Kohrt, W.M., Bloomfield, S.A., Little, K.D., Nelson, M.E., and Yingling, V.R. 2004. American College of Sports Medicine position stand: Physical activity and bone health. *Medicine & Science in Sports & Exercise* 36: 1985-1996.

Kohrt, W.M., Spina, R.J., Holloszy, J.O., and Ehsani, A.A. 1998. Prescribing exercise intensity for older women. *Journal of the American Geriatric Society* 46: 129-133.

Kokkinos, P.F., and Fernhall, B. 1999. Physical activity and high density lipoprotein cholesterol levels: What is the relationship? *Sports Medicine* 28: 307-314.

Kokkinos, P.F., Hurley, B.F., Smutok, M.A., Farmer, C., Reece, C., Shulman, R., Charabogos, C., Patterson, J., Will, S., Devane-Bell, J., and Goldberg, A.P. 1991. Strength training does not improve lipoprotein-lipid profiles in men at risk for CHD. *Medicine & Science in Sports & Exercise* 23: 1134–1139.

Komi, P.V., Viitasalo, J.T., Rauramaa, R., and Vihko, V. 1978. Effect of isometric strength training on mechanical, electrical, and metabolic aspects of muscle function. *European Journal of Applied Physiology* 40: 45–55.

Koulmann, N., Jimenez, C., Regal, D., Bolliet, P., Launay, J., Savourey, G., and Melin, B. 2000. Use of bioelectrical impedance analysis to estimate body fluid compartments after acute variations of the body hydration level. *Medicine & Science in Sports & Exercise* 32: 857-864.

Kraemer, W.J. 2003. Strength training basics. *The Physician and Sportsmedicine* 31(8) 39-45.

Kraemer, W.J., Adams, K., Cafarelli, E., Dudley, G.A., Dooly, C., Feigenbaum, M.S., Fleck, S.J., Franklin, B., Fry, A.C., Hoffman, J.R., Newton, R.U., Potteiger, J., Stone, M.H., Ratamess, N.A., and Triplett-McBride, T. 2002. ACSM Position Stand: Progression models in resistance training for healthy adults. *Medicine & Science in Sports & Exercise* 34: 364-380.

Kraemer, W.J., Deschenes, M.R., and Fleck, S.J. 1988. Physiological adaptations to resistance exercise: Implications for athletic conditioning. *Sports Medicine* 6: 246–256.

Kraemer, W.J., and Fleck, S.J. 1993. *Strength training for young athletes.* Champaign IL: Human Kinetics.

Kraemer, W.J., Fleck, S.J., and Evans, W.J. 1996. Strength and power training: Physiological mechanisms of adaptation. In *Exercise and Sport Sciences Reviews,* ed. J.O. Holloszy, 24: 363-397. Baltimore: Williams & Wilkins.

Kraemer, W.J., Gordon, S.J., Fleck, S.J., Marchitelli, L.J., Mello, R., Dziados, J.E., Friedl, K., Harman, E., Maresh, C., and Fry, A.C. 1991. Endogenous anabolic hormonal and growth factor responses to heavy resistance exercise in males and females. *International Journal of Sports Medicine* 12: 228-235.

Kraemer, W.J., Häkkinen, K., Newton, R.U., Nindl, B.C., Volek, J.S., McCormick, M., Gotshalk, L.A., Gordon, S.E., Fleck, S.J., Campbell, W.W., Putukian, M., and Evans, W.J. 1999. Effects of heavy-resistance training on hormonal response patterns in younger vs. older men. *Journal of Applied Physiology* 87: 982–992.

Kraemer, W.J., Nindl, B.C., Ratamess, N.A., Gotshalk, L.A., Volek, J.S., Fleck, S.J., Newton, R.U., and Hakkinen, K. 2004. Changes in muscle hypertrophy in women with periodized resistance training. *Medicine & Science in Sports & Exercise* 36: 697-708.

Kraemer, W.J., Noble, B.J., Clark, M.J., and Culver, B.W. 1987. Physiologic responses to heavy-resistance exercise with very short rest periods. *International Journal of Sports Medicine* 8: 247–252.

Kraemer, W.J., Patton, J., Gordon, S.E., Harman, E.A., Deschenes, M.R., Reynolds, K., Newton, R.U., Triplett, N.T., and Dziados, J.E. 1995. Compatibility of high intensity strength and endurance training on hormonal and skeletal muscle adaptations. *Journal of Applied Physiology* 78: 976–989.

Kraemer, W.J., and Ratamess, N.A. 2004. Fundamentals of resistance training: Progression and exercise prescription. *Medicine & Science in Sports & Exercise* 36: 674-688.

Kraemer, W.J., Volek, J.S., Clark, K.L., Gordon, S.E., Puhl, S.M., Koziris, L.P., McBride, J.M., Triplett-McBride, N.T., Putukian, M., Newton, R.U., Häkkinen, K., Bush, J.A., and Sabastianelli, W.J. 1999. Influence of exercise training on physiological and performance changes with weight loss in men. *Medicine & Science in Sports & Exercise* 31: 1320-1329.

Kravitz, L., and Heyward, V.H. 1995. Flexibility training. *Fitness Management* 11(2): 32-38.

Kravitz, L., Cizar, C., Christensen, C., and Setterlund, S. 1993. The physiological effects of step training with and without handweights. *Journal of Sports Medicine and Physical Fitness* 33: 348-358.

Kravitz, L., Heyward, V., Stolarczyk, L., and Wilmerding, V. 1997. Effects of step training with and without hand-weights on physiological profiles of women. *Journal of Strength and Conditioning Research* 11: 194-199.

Kravitz, L., Roberms, R., and Heyward, V. 1996. Are all aerobic exercise modes equal? *Idea Today* 14: 51-58.

Kravitz, L., Roberms, R.A., Heyward, V.H., Wagner, D.R., and Powers, K. 1997. Exercise mode and gender comparisons of energy expenditure at self-selected intensities. *Medicine & Science in Sports & Exercise* 29: 1028-1035.

Kravitz, L., Wax, B., Mayo, J.J., Daniels, R., and Charette, K. 1998. Metabolic response of elliptical exercise training. *Medicine & Science in Sports & Exercise* 30(Suppl.): S169 [abstract].

Kreider, R.B., Melton, C., Rasmussen, C.J., Greenwood, M., Lancaster, S., Cantler, E.C., Milnor, P., and Almada, A.L. 2003. Long-term creatine supplementation does not significantly affect clinical markers of health in athletes. *Molecular and Cellular Biochemistry* 244: 95-104.

Kreighbaum, E., and Barthels, K.M. 1981. *Biomechanics: A qualitative approach for studying human movement.* Minneapolis: Burgess.

Kretsch, M.J., Blanton, C.A., Baer, D., Staples, R., Horn, W.F., and Keim, N. 2004. Measuring energy expenditure with simple, low-cost tools. *Journal of the American Dietetic Association* 104: A-13.

Kriska, A.M., Blair, S.N., and Pereira, M.A. 1994. The potential role of physical activity in the prevention of non-insulin dependent diabetes mellitus: The epidemiological evidence. In *Exercise and Sport Sciences Reviews,* ed. J.O. Holloszy, 22: 121-143.

Krotkiewski, M., Gudmundsson, M., Backstrom, P., and Mandroukas, K. 1982. Zinc and muscle strength and endurance. *Acta Physiologica Scandinavica* 116: 309-311.

Kubo, K., Kaneshisa, H., Takeshita, D., Kawakami, Y., Fukashiro, S., and Fukunaga, T. 2000. In vivo dynamics of human medial gastrocnemius muscle-tendon complex curing stretch-shortening cycle exercise. *Acta Physiologica Scandinavica* 170: 127-135.

Kubo, K., Kawakami, Y., and Fukunaga, T. 1999. Influence of elastic properties of tendon structures on jump performance in humans. *Journal of Applied Physiology* 87: 2090-2096.

Kuntzelman, B.A. 1979. *The complete guide to aerobic dancing.* Skokie, IL: Publications International.

Kuramoto, A.K., and Payne, V.G. 1995. Predicting muscular strength in women: A preliminary study. *Research Quarterly for Exercise and Sport* 66: 168-172.

Kushner, R.F. 1992. Bioelectrical impedance analysis: A review of principles and applications. *Journal of the American College of Nutrition* 11: 199-209.

Kushner, R.F., Gudivaka, R., and Schoeller, D.A. 1996. Clinical characteristics influencing bioelectrical impedance analysis measurements. *American Journal of Clinical Nutrition* 64: 423S-427S.

Kushner, R.F., and Schoeller, D.A. 1986. Estimation of total body water in bioelectrical impedance analysis. *American Journal of Clinical Nutrition* 44: 417-424.

Kyle, U.G., Genton, L., Karsegard, L., Slosman, D.O., and Pichard, C. 2001. Single prediction equation for bioelectrical impedance analysis in adults aged 20-94 years. *Nutrition* 17: 248-253.

Lan, C., Lai, J., Chen, S., and Wong, M. 1998. 12-month tai chi training in the elderly: Its effects on health fitness. *Medicine & Science in Sports & Exercise* 30: 345-351.

Larsen, G.E., George, J.D., Alexander, J.L., Fellingham, G.W., Aldana, S.G., and Parcell, A.C. 2002. Prediction of maximum oxygen consumption from walking, jogging, or running. *Research Quarterly for Exercise and Sport* 73: 66-72.

Latin, R., and Elias, B. 1993. Predictions of maximum oxygen uptake from treadmill walking and running. *Journal of Sports Medicine and Physical Fitness* 33: 34-39.

Layne, J.E., and Nelson, M.E. 1999. The effects of progressive resistance training on bone density: A review. *Medicine & Science in Sports & Exercise* 31:25-30.

Leger, L.A., Lambert, J., and Martin, P. 1982. Validity of plastic skinfold caliper measurements. *Human Biology* 54: 667-675.

Leger, L.A., Mercier, D., Gadoury, C., and Lambert, J. 1988. The multistage 20-metre shuttle run test for aerobic fitness. *Journal of Sports Sciences* 6: 93-101.

Leighton, J.R. 1955. An instrument and technique for measurement of range of joint motion. *Archives of Physical Medicine and Rehabilitation* 36: 571-578.

Lemieux, S., Prud'homme, D., Bouchard, C., Tremblay, A., and Despres, J-P. 1996. A single threshold value of waist girth identifies normal-weight and overweight subjects with excess visceral adipose tissue. *American Journal of Clinical Nutrition* 64: 685-693.

Lemon, P.W. 2000. Beyond the Zone: Protein needs of active individuals. *Journal of the American College of Nutrition* 19: 513S-521S.

Lermen, J., Bruce, R.A., Sivarajan, E., Pettet, G., and Trimble, S. 1976. Low-level dynamic exercises for earlier cardiac rehabilitation: Aerobic and hemodynamic responses. *Archives of Physical Medicine and Rehabilitation* 57: 355-360.

Lesmes, G.R., Costill, D.L., Coyle, E.F., and Fink, W.J. 1978. Muscle strength and power changes during maximal isokinetic training. *Medicine and Science in Sports* 10: 266-269.

Levine, B., Zuckerman, J., and Cole, C. 1998. Medical complications of exercise. In *ACSM's resource manual for guidelines for exercise testing and prescription,* ed. J.L. Roitman, 488-498. Philadelphia: Lippincott Williams & Wilkins.

Liang, M.T.C., Su, H., and Lee, N. 2000. Skin temperature and skin blood flow affect bioelectrical impedance study of female fat-free mass. *Medicine & Science in Sports & Exercise* 32: 221-227.

Liang, M.Y., and Norris, S. 1993. Effects of skin blood flow and temperature on bioelectrical impedance after exercise. *Medicine & Science in Sports & Exercise* 25: 1231-1239.

Litchell, H., and Boberg, J. 1978. The lipoprotein lipase activity of adipose tissue from different sites in obese women and relationship to cell size. *International Journal of Obesity* 2: 47-52.

Lockner, D., Heyward, V., Baumgartner, R., and Jenkins, K. 2000. Comparison of air-displacement plethysmography, hydrodensitometry, and dual X-ray absorptiometry for assessing body composition of children 10 to 18 years of age. *Annals of the New York Academy of Sciences* 904: 72-78.

Lohman, T.G. 1981. Skinfolds and body density and their relation to body fatness: A review. *Human Biology* 53: 181-115.

Lohman, T.G. 1987. *Measuring body fat using skinfolds* [videotape]. Champaign, IL: Human Kinetics.

Lohman, T.G. 1989. Bioelectrical impedance. In *Applying new technology to nutrition: Report of the ninth roundtable on medical issues*, 22-25. Columbus, OH: Ross Laboratories.

Lohman, T.G. 1992. *Advances in body composition assessment. Current issues in exercise science series.* Monograph no. 3. Champaign, IL: Human Kinetics.

Lohman, T.G. 1996. Dual energy X-ray absorptiometry. In *Human body composition,* ed. A.F. Roche, S.B. Heymsfield, and T.G. Lohman, 63-78. Champaign, IL: Human Kinetics.

Lohman, T.G., Boileau, R.A., and Slaughter, M.H. 1984. Body composition in children and youth. In *Advances in pediatric sport sciences,* ed. R.A. Boileau, 29-57. Champaign, IL: Human Kinetics.

Lohman, T.G., Going, S.B., and Metcalfe, L. 2004. Seeing ourselves through the obesity epidemic. *President's Council on Physical Fitness and Sports Research Digest Series* 5(3): 1-8.

Lohman, T.G., Going, S., Pamenter, R., Hall, M., Boyden, T., Houtkooper, L., Ritenbaugh, C., Bare, L., Hill, A., and Aickin, M. 1995. Effects of resistance training on regional and total bone mineral density in premenopausal women: A randomized prospective study. *Journal of Bone Mineral Research* 10: 1015-1024.

Lohman, T.G., Harris, M., Teixeira, P.J., and Weiss, L. 2000. Assessing body composition and changes in body composition: Another look at dual-energy X-ray absorptiometry. *Annals of the New York Academy of Sciences* 904: 45-54.

Lohman, T.G., Houtkooper, L., and Going, S. 1997. Body fat measurement goes high-tech: Not all are created equal. *ACSM's Health & Fitness Journal* 7: 30-35.

Lohman, T.G., Pollock, M.L., Slaughter, M.H., Brandon, L.J., and Boileau, R.A. 1984. Methodological factors and the prediction of body fat in female athletes. *Medicine & Science in Sports & Exercise* 16: 92-96.

Lohman, T.G., Roche, A.F., and Martorell, R., eds. 1988. *Anthropometric standardization reference manual.* Champaign, IL: Human Kinetics.

Lokey, E.A., and Tran, Z.V. 1989. Effects of exercise training on serum lipids and lipoprotein concentrations in women: A meta-analysis. *International Journal of Sports Medicine* 10: 424-429.

Londeree, B., and Moeschberger, M. 1984. Influence of age and other factors on maximal heart rate. *Journal of Cardiac Rehabilitation* 4: 44-49.

Loy, S., Likes, E., Andrews, P., Vincent, W., Holland, G.J., Kawai, H., Cen, S., Swenberger, J., VanLoan, M., Tanaka, K., Heyward, V., Stolarczyk, L., Lohman, T.G., and Going, S.B. 1998. Easy grip on body composition measurements. *ACSM's Health & Fitness Journal* 2(5): 16-19.

Lozano, A., Rosell, J., and Pallas-Areny, R. 1995. Errors in prolonged electrical impedance measurements due to electrode repositioning and postural changes. *Physiological Measurement* 16: 121-130.

Ludwig, D.S., and Eckel, R.H. 2002. The glycemic index at 20 y. *American Journal of Clinical Nutrition* 76 (Suppl.): 264S-265S.

Lukaski, H.C. 1986. Use of the tetrapolar bioelectrical impedance method to assess human body composition. In *Human body composition and fat patterning,* ed. N.G. Norgan, 143-158. Wageningen, Netherlands: Euronut.

Lukaski, H.C. 1993. Soft tissue composition and bone mineral status: Evaluation by dual-energy X-ray absorptiometry. *Journal of Nutrition* 123: 438-443.

Lukaski, H.C., and Bolonchuk, W.W. 1988. Estimation of body fluid volumes using tetrapolar impedance measurements. *Aviation, Space, and Environmental Medicine* 59: 1163-1169.

Lukaski, H.C., Johnson, P.E., Bolonchuk, W.W., and Lykken, G.I. 1985. Assessment of fat-free mass using bioelectric impedance measurements of the human body. *American Journal of Clinical Nutrition* 41: 810-817.

Luthi, J.M., Howald, H., Claasen, H., Rosler, K., Vock, P., and Hoppeler, H. 1986. Structural changes in skeletal muscle tissue with heavy resistance exercise. *International Journal of Sports Medicine* 7: 123-127.

MacDougall, J.D., Sale, D.G., Moroz, J.R., Elder, G.C., Sutton, J.R., and Howalk, H. 1979. Mitochondrial volume density in human skeletal muscle following heavy resistance training. *Medicine and Science in Sports* 11: 164-166.

Magarey, A.M., Daniels, L.A., and Boulton, T.J. 2001. Prevalence of overweight and obesity in Australian children and adolescents: Reassessment of 1985 and 1995 data against new standard international definitions. *Medical Journal of Australia* 174: 561-564.

Magel, J.R., Foglia, G.F., McArdle, W.D., Gutin, B., Pechard, G.S., and Katch F.I. 1974. Specificity of swim training on maximum oxygen uptake. *Journal of Applied Physiology* 38: 151-155.

Magnusson, S.P. 1998. Passive properties of human skeletal muscle during stretch maneuvers. A review. *Scandinavian Journal of Medicine and Science in Sports* 8(2): 65-77.

Magnusson, S.P., Simonsen, E.B., Aagaard, P., Bueson, J., Johannson, F., and Kjaer, M. 1997. Determinants of musculoskeletal flexibility: Visoelastic properties, cross-sectional area, EMG and stretch tolerance. *Scandinavian Journal of Medicine and Science in Sports* 7: 195–202.

Mahar, M.T., Jackson, A.S., Ross, R.M., Pivarnik, J.M., and Pollock, M.L. 1985. Predictive accuracy of single and double stage submax treadmill work for estimating aerobic capacity. *Medicine & Science in Sports & Exercise* 17: 206–207.

Maksud, M.G., and Coutts, K.D. 1971. Comparison of a continuous and discontinuous graded treadmill test for maximal oxygen uptake. *Medicine and Science in Sports* 3: 63–65.

Malek, M.H., Nalbone, D.P., Berger, D.E., and Coburn, J.W. 2002. Importance of health science education for personal fitness trainers. *Journal of Strength and Conditioning Research* 16: 19-24.

Manore, M.M. 2004. Nutrition and physical activity: Fueling the active individual. *President's Council on Physical Fitness and Sports Research Digest* 5(1): 1-8.

Manson, J.E., Nathan, D.M., Krolewski, A.S., Stampfer, M.J., Willett, W.C., and Hennekens, C.H. 1992. A prospective study of exercise and incidence of diabetes among US male physicians. *Journal of the American Medical Association* 268: 63–67.

Manson, J.E., Rimm, E.B., Stampfer, M.J., Rosner, B., Hennekens, C.H., Speizer, F.E., Colditz, G.A., Willett, W.C., and Krolewski, A.S. 1991. Physical activity incidence of non-insulin dependent diabetes mellitus in women. *Lancet* 338: 774–778.

Marcus, B.H., Bock, B.C., Pinto, B.M., Forsyth, L.H., Roberts, M.B., and Traficante, R.M. 1998. Efficacy of an individualized, motivationally tailored physical activity intervention. *Annals of Behavioral Medicine* 20: 174-180.

Marcus, B.H., and Forsyth, L.H. 2003. *Motivating people to be physically active.* Champaign, IL: Human Kinetics.

Marcus, B.H., and Lewis, B.A. 2003. Physical activity and the stages of motivational readiness for change model. *President's Council on Physical Fitness and Sports Research Digest* 4(1): 1-8.

Markandu, N.D., Whitcher, F., Arnold, A., and Carney, C. 2000. The mercury sphygmomanometer should be abandoned before it is proscribed. *Journal of Human Hypertension* 14: 31-36.

Marks, B.L., Ward, A., Morris, D.H., Castellani, J., and Rippe, J.M. 1995. Fat-free mass is maintained in women following a moderate diet and exercise program. *Medicine & Science in Sports & Exercise* 27: 1243–1251.

Marley, W., and Linnerud, A. 1976. A three-year study of the Åstrand-Ryhming step test. *Research Quarterly* 47: 211–217.

Martin, A.D., Drinkwater, D.T., and Clarys, J.P. 1992. Effects of skin thickness and skinfold compressibility on skinfold thickness measurements. *American Journal of Human Biology* 4: 453–460.

Martin, A.D., Ross, W.D., Drinkwater, D.T., and Clarys, J.P. 1985. Prediction of body fat by skinfold caliper: Assumptions and cadaver evidence. *International Journal of Obesity* 9 (Suppl. 1): 31–39.

Martin, S.B., Jackson, A.W., Morrow, J.R., and Liemohn, W. 1998. The rationale for the sit and reach test revisited. *Measurement in Physical Education and Exercise Science* 2: 85–92.

Marx, J.O., Ratamess, N.A., Nindl, B.C., Gotshalk, L.A., Volek, J.S., Dohi, K., Bush, J.A., Gomez, A.L., Mazzetti, S.A., Fleck, S.J., Hakkinen, K., Newton, R.U., and Kraemer, W.J. 2001. Low-volume circuit versus high-volume periodized resistance training in women. *Medicine & Science in Sports & Exercise* 33: 635-643.

Mayer, J. 1968. *Overweight: Causes, costs and control.* Englewood Cliffs, NJ: Prentice Hall.

Mayer, T.G., Tencer, A.F., and Kristoferson, S. 1984. Use of noninvasive technique for quantification of spinal range-of-motion in normal subjects and chronic low back dysfunction patients. *Spine* 9: 588–595.

Mayhew, J.L., Ball, T.E., Arnold, M.D., and Bowen, J.C. 1992. Relative muscular endurance performance as a predictor of bench press strength in college men and women. *Journal of Applied Sport Science Research* 6: 200–206.

Mazess, R.B., Barden, H.S., and Ohlrich, E.S. 1990. Skeletal and body-composition effects of anorexia nervosa. *American Journal of Clinical Nutrition* 52: 438–441.

McArdle, W.D., Katch, F.I., and Katch, V.L. 1996. *Exercise physiology: Energy, nutrition and human performance,* 4th ed. Baltimore: Williams & Wilkins.

McArdle, W.D., Katch, F.I., and Pechar, G.S. 1973. Comparison of continuous and discontinuous treadmill and bicycle tests for VO$_2$max. *Medicine and Science in Sports* 5: 156–160.

McArdle, W.D., Katch, F.I., Pechar, G.S., Jacobson, L., and Ruck, S. 1972. Reliability and interrelationships between maximal oxygen intake, physical working capacity and step-test scores in college women. *Medicine and Science in Sports* 4: 182–186.

McConnell, T., and Clark, B. 1987. Prediction of maximal oxygen consumption during handrail-supported treadmill exercise. *Journal of Cardiopulmonary Rehabilitation* 7: 324–331.

McCrory, M.A., Gomez, T.D., Bernauer, E.M., and Mole, P.A. 1995. Evaluation of a new displacement plethysmograph for measuring human body composition. *Medicine & Science in Sports & Exercise* 27: 1686–1691.

McCrory, M.A., Mole, P.A., Gomez, T.D., Dewey, K.G., and Bernauer, E.M. 1998. Body composition by air displacement plethysmography using predicted and measured thoracic gas volumes. *Journal of Applied Physiology* 84: 1475-1479.

McCue, B.F. 1953. Flexibility of college women. *Research Quarterly* 24: 316–324.

McGill, S. 2002. *Low back disorders: Evidence-based prevention and rehabilitation.* Champaign, IL: Human Kinetics.

McGill, S.M. 1998. Low back exercises: Prescription for the healthy back and when recovering from injury. In *ACSM's resource manual for guidelines for exercise testing and prescription,* 3rd ed., Senior ed. J. Roitman.116-126. Philadelphia: Lippincott, Williams & Wilkins.

McGill, S.M. 2001. Low back stability: From formal description to issues for performance and rehabilitation. *Exercise and Sport Sciences Reviews* 29(1): 26–31.

McGill, S.M., Childs, A., and Liebenson, D.C. 1999. Endurance times for low back stabilization exercises: Clinical targets for testing and training from a normal database. *Archives of Physical Medicine and Rehabilitation* 80: 941-944.

McHugh, M.P. Kremenic, I.J., Fox, M.B., and Gleim, G.W. 1998. The role of mechanical and neural restraints to joint range of motion during passive stretch. *Medicine & Science in Sports & Exercise* 30: 928–932.

McHugh, M.P., Magnusson, S.P., Gleim, G.W., and Nicholas, J.A. 1992. Viscoelastic stress relaxation in human skeletal muscle. *Medicine & Science in Sports & Exercise* 24: 1375–1382.

McInnis, K., and Balady, G. 1994. Comparison of submaximal exercise responses using the Bruce vs modified Bruce protocols. *Medicine & Science in Sports & Exercise* 26: 103–107.

Mcrae, I.F., and Wright, V. 1969. Measurement of back movement. *Annals of Rheumatic Diseases* 28: 584–589.

McTiernan, A., Kooperberg, C., White, E., Wilcox, S., Coates, R., Adams-Campbell, L.L., Woods, N. and Okene, J. 2003. Recreational physical activity and the risk of breast cancer in postmenopausal women: The Women's Health Initiative Cohort Study. *Journal of the American Medical Association* 290(10): 1331-1336.

Messier, S.P., Royer, T.D., Craven, T.E., O'Toole, M.L., Burns, R., and Ettinger W.H. Jr. 2000. Long-term exercise and its effect on balance in older, osteoarthritic adults: Results from the Fitness, Arthritis, and Seniors Trial (FAST). *Journal of the American Geriatrics Society* 48: 131-138.

Metropolitan Life Insurance Company. 1995. *Your guide to physical activity for health.* New York: Author.

Micozzi, M.S., Albanes, D., Jones, Y., and Chumlea, W.C. 1986. Correlations of body mass indices with weight, stature, and body composition in men and women in NHANES I and II. *American Journal of Clinical Nutrition* 44: 725–731.

Mifflin, M.D., St. Jeor, S.T., Hill, L.A., Scott, B.J., Daugherty, S.A., and Koh, Y.O. 1990. A new predictive equation for resting energy expenditure in healthy individuals. *American Journal of Clinical Nutrition* 51: 241-247.

Mikesky, A.E., Giddings, C.J., Matthews, W., and Gonyea, W.J. 1991. Changes in fiber size and composition in response to heavy-resistance exercise. *Medicine & Science in Sports & Exercise* 23: 1042–1049.

Milburn, S., and Butts, N.K. 1983. A comparison of the training responses to aerobic dance and jogging in college females. *Medicine & Science in Sports & Exercise* 15: 510–513.

Millard-Stafford, M.L., Collins, M.A., Evans, E.M. Snow, T.K., Cureton, K.J., and Rosskopf, L.B. 2001. Use of air displacement plethysmography for estimating body fat in a four-component model. *Medicine & Science in Sports & Exercise* 33: 1311-1317.

Miller, J.B. 2001. GI research. http://www.glycemicindex. com.

Minkler, S., and Patterson, P. 1994. The validity of the modified sit-and-reach test in college-age students. *Research Quarterly for Exercise and Sport* 65: 189-192.

Moffatt, R.J., Stamford, B.A., and Neill, R.D. 1977. Placement of tri-weekly training sessions: Importance regarding enhancement of aerobic capacity. *Research Quarterly* 48: 583-591.

Moffroid, M.T., and Whipple, R.H. 1970. Specificity of speed of exercise. *Physical Therapy* 50: 1699-1704.

Mole, P.A., Oscai, L.B., and Holloszy, J.O. 1971. Adaptation of muscle to exercise: Increase in levels of palmityl CoA synthetase, carnitine palmityl-transferase, and palmityl CoA dehydrogenase and the capacity to oxidize fatty acids. *Journal of Clinical Investigation* 50: 2323-2329.

Montoye, H.J., and Faulkner, J.A. 1964. Determination of the optimum setting of an adjustable grip dynamometer. *Research Quarterly* 35: 29-36.

Mooney, V., Kron, M., Rummerfield, P., and Holmes, B. 1995. The effect of workplace based strengthening on low back injury rates: A case study in the strip mining industry. *Journal of Occupational Rehabilitation* 5: 157-167.

Moore, M.A., and Hutton, R.S. 1980. Electromyographic investigation of muscle stretching techniques. *Medicine & Science in Sports & Exercise* 12: 322-329.

Morehouse, L.E. 1972. *Laboratory manual for physiology of exercise.* St. Louis: Mosby.

Moritani, T., and deVries, H.A. 1979. Neural factors versus hypertrophy in the time course of muscle strength gain. *American Journal of Physical Medicine* 58: 115-130.

Morris, N., Gass, G., Thompson, M., Bennett, G., Basic, D., and Morton H. 2002. Rate and amplitude of adaptation to intermittent and continuous exercise in older men. *Medicine & Science in Sports & Exercise* 34: 471-477.

Morrow, J.R., Jackson, A.S., Bradley, P.W., and Hartung, G.H. 1986. Accuracy of measured and predicted residual lung volume on body density measurement. *Medicine & Science in Sport & Exercise* 18: 647-652.

Muller, M.J., Bosy-Westphal, A., Klaus, S., Kreymann, G., Luhrmann, P.M., Neuhauser-Berthold, M., Noack, R., Pirke, K.M., Platte, P., Selberg, O., and Steiniger, J. 2004. World Health Organization equations have shortcomings for predicting resting energy expenditure in persons from a modern, affluent population: Generation of a new reference standard from a retrospective analysis of a German database of resting energy expenditure. *American Journal of Clinical Nutrition* 80: 1379-1390.

Munroe, R.A. and Romance, T.J. 1975. Use of the Leighton flexometer in the development of a short flexibility test battery. *American Corrective Therapy Journal* 29: 22.

Nagle, F.S., Balke, B., and Naughton, J.P. 1965. Gradational step tests for assessing work capacity. *Journal of Applied Physiology* 20: 745-748.

National Academy of Sciences. 2000. *Dietary reference intakes.* Washington, D.C.: National Academy Press.

National Cholesterol Education Program. 2001. Executive summary of the third report of the National Cholesterol Education Program (NCEP) Expert Panel on detection, evaluation, and treatment of high blood cholesterol in adults (Adult Treatment Panel III). *Journal of the American Medical Association* 285(19): 2486–2497.

National Institutes of Health and National Heart, Lung, and Blood Institute. 1998. Clinical guidelines on the identification, evaluation, and treatment of overweight and obesity in adults: The evidence report. *Obesity Research* 6 (Suppl. 2): S51–S209.

National Institutes of Health Consensus Development Panel. 1985. Health implications of obesity: National Institutes of Health Consensus development statement. *Annals of Internal Medicine* 103: 1073–1079.

National Osteoporosis Foundation. 2004. America's bone health: The state of osteoporosis and low bone mass. www.nof.org/advocacy/prevalence/.

Naughton, J., Balke, B., and Nagle, F. 1964. Refinement in methods of evaluation and physical conditioning before and after myocardial infarction. *American Journal of Cardiology* 14: 837.

Ng, J.K., Kippers, V., Richardson, C.A., and Parnianpour, M. 2001. Range of motion and lordosis of the lumbar spine: Reliability of measurement and normative values. *Spine* 26: 53-60.

Nichols, D.L., Sanborn, C.F., and Love, A.M. 2001. Resistance training and bone mineral density in adolescent females. *Journal of Pediatrics* 139: 494-499.

Nichols, J.F., Sherman, C.L., and Abbott, E. 2000. Treading is new and hot: 30 minutes meets the ACSM recommendations for cardiorespiratory fitness and caloric expenditure. *ACSM's Health & Fitness Journal* 4(2): 12–17.

Nissen, S.L., and Sharp, R.L. 2003. Effect of dietary supplements on lean mass and gains with resistance training: A meta-analysis. *Journal of Applied Physiology* 94: 651-659.

Noland, M., and Kearney, J.T. 1978. Anthropometric and densitometric responses of women to specific and general exercise. *Research Quarterly* 49: 322–328.

Norkin, C.C., and White, D.J. 1995. *Measurement of joint motion: A guide to goniometry.* Philadelphia: Davis.

Norris, C. 2000. *Back stability.* Champaign, IL: Human Kinetics.

Norton, K., Marfell-Jones, M., Whittingham, N., Kerr, D., Carter, L., Saddington, K., and Gore, C. 2000. Anthropometric assessment protocols. In *Physiological tests for elite athletes,* ed. C. Gore, 66–85. Champaign, IL: Human Kinetics.

Nunez, C., Kovera, A., Pietrobelli, A., Heshka, S., Horlick, M., Kehayias, J., Wang, Z., and Heymsfield, S. 1999. Body composition in children and adults by air displacement plethysmography. *European Journal of Clinical Nutrition* 53: 382–387.

O'Brien, E. 2003. Demise of the mercury sphygmomanometer and the dawning of a new era in blood pressure measurement. *Blood Pressure Monitoring* 8: 19-21.

O'Brien, E., Pickering, T., Asmar, R., Myers, M., Parati, G., Staessen, J., Mengden, T., Imai, Y., Waeber, B., and Palantini, P. 2002. Working group on blood pressure monitoring of the European Society of Hypertension International Protocol for validation of blood pressure measuring devices in adults. *Blood Pressure Monitoring* 7: 3-17.

O'Brien, E., Waeber, B., Parati, G., Staessen, J., and Myers, M.G. 2001. Blood pressure measuring devices: Recommendations of the European Society of Hypertension. *British Medical Journal* 322: 531- 536.

Ogden, C.L., Flegal, K.M., Carroll, M.D., and Johnson, C.L. 2002. Prevalence and trends in overweight among U.S. children and adolescents, 1999-2000. *Journal of the American Medical Association* 288(14): 1728-1732.

Ohrvall, M., Berglund, L., and Vessby, B. 2000. Sagittal abdominal diameter compared with other anthropometric measurements in relation to cardiovascular risk. *International Journal of Obesity* 24: 497-501.

Olson, M.S., Williford, H.N., Blessing, D.L., and Greathouse, R. 1991. The cardiovascular and metabolic effects of bench stepping exercise in females. *Medicine & Science in Sports & Exercise* 23: 1311–1318.

Oppliger, R.A., Nielsen, D.H., and Vance, C.G. 1991. Wrestlers' minimal weight: Anthropometry, bioimpedance, and hydrostatic weighing compared. *Medicine & Science in Sports & Exercise* 23: 247–253.

Ornish, D. 2004. Was Dr Atkins right? *Journal of the American Medical Association* 104: 537-542.

Ortiz, O., Russell, M., Daley, T.L., Baumgartner, R.N., Waki, M., Lichtman, S., Wang, S., Pierson, R.N., and Heymsfield, S.B. 1992. Differences in skeletal muscle and bone mineral mass between black and white females and their relevance to estimates of body composition. *American Journal of Clinical Nutrition* 55: 8–13.

Ostchega, Y., Prineas, R.J., Dillon, C., McDowell, M., and Carroll, M. 2004. Estimating equations and tables for adult mid-arm circumference based on measured height and weight: Data from the third National Health and Nutrition Examination Survey (NHANES III) and NHANES 1999-2000. *Blood Pressure Monitoring* 9: 123-131.

Paffenbarger, R.S., Jung, D.L., Leung, R.W., and Hyde, R.T. 1991. Physical activity and hypertension: An epidemiological view. *Annals of Medicine* 23: 319–327.

Paffenbarger, R.S., and Olsen, E. 1996. *LifeFit: An effective exercise program for optimal health and a longer life.* Champaign, IL: Human Kinetics.

Painter, J., Rah, J.H., and Lee, Y.K. 2002. Comparison of international food guide pictorial representations. *Journal of the American Dietetic Association* 102: 483-489.

Panotopoulos, G., Ruiz, J.C., Guy-Grand, B., and Basdevant, A. 2001. Dual x-ray absorptiometry, bioelectrical impedance, and near-infrared interactance in obese women. *Medicine & Science in Sports & Exercise* 33: 665-670.

Parker, S.B., Hurley, B.F., Hanlon, D.P., and Vaccaro, P. 1989. Failure of target heart rate to accurately monitor intensity during aerobic dance. *Medicine & Science in Sports & Exercise* 21: 230–234.

Partnership for Essential Nutrition. 2004. *The impact of the low-carb craze on attitudes about eating and weight loss: A national opinion survey conducted for the Partnership for Essential Nutrition.* http://www.essentialnutrition. org/survey.php.

Pate, R.R., Pratt, M., Blair, S.N., Haskell, W.L., Macera, C.A., Bouchard, C., Buchner, D., Ettinger, W., Heath, G.W., and King, A.C. 1995. Physical activity and public health: A recommendation from the Centers for Disease Control and Prevention and the American College of Sports Medicine. *Journal of the American Medical Association* 273: 402-407.

Patterson, P., Wiksten, D.L., Ray, L., Flanders, C., and Sanphy, D. 1996. The validity and reliability of the back-saver sit-and-reach test in middle school girls and boys. *Research Quarterly for Exercise and Sport* 67: 448-451.

Paulsen, G., Myklested, D., and Reestad, T. 2003. The influence of volume of exercise on early adaptations to strength training. *Journal of Strength and Conditioning Research* 17: 115-120.

Pavlou, K.N., Steffee, W.P., Lerman, R.H., and Burrows, B.A. 1985. Effects of dieting and exercise on lean body mass, oxygen uptake, and strength. *Medicine & Science in Sports & Exercise* 17: 466-471.

Payne, N., Gledhill, N., Kazmarzyk, P.T., Jamnik, V., and Keir, P.J. 2000. Canadian musculoskeletal fitness norms. *Canadian Journal of Applied Physiology* 25: 430-442.

Perrin, D.H. 1993. *Isokinetic exercise and assessment.* Champaign, IL: Human Kinetics.

Persinger, R., Foster, C., Gibson, M., Fater, D.C.W., and Porcari, J.P. 2004. Consistency of the talk test for exercise prescription. *Medicine & Science in Sports & Exercise* 36: 1632-1636.

Pescatello, L.S., Franklin, B.A., Fagard, R., Farquhar, W.B., Kelley, G.A, and Ray, C.A. 2004. American College of Sports Medicine position stand. Exercise and hypertension. *Medicine & Science in Sports & Exercise* 36: 533-553.

Peters, D., Fox, K., Armstrong, N., Sharpe, P., and Bell, M. 1992. Assessment of children's abdominal fat distribution by magnetic resonance imaging and anthropometry. *International Journal of Obesity* 16(Suppl. 2): S35 [abstract].

Petersen, T., Verstraete, D., Schultz, W., and Stray-Gundersen, J. 1993. Metabolic demands of step aerobics. *Medicine & Science in Sports & Exercise* 25: S79 [abstract].

Peterson, M.D., Rhea, M.R., and Alvar, B.A. 2004. Maximizing strength development in athletes: A meta-analysis to determine the dose-response relationship. *Journal of Strength and Conditioning Research* 18: 377-382.

Pietrobelli, A., Formica, C., Wang, Z., and Heymsfield, S.B. 1996. Dual-energy X-ray absorptiometry body composition model: Review of physical concepts. *American Journal of Physiology* 271: E941-E951.

Pi-Sunyer, F.X. 1999. Comorbidities of overweight and obesity: Current evidence and research issues. *Medicine & Science in Sports & Exercise* 31: S602-S608.

Pi-Sunyer, F.X. 2002. Glycemic index and disease. *American Journal of Clinical Nutrition* 76 (Suppl.): 290S-298S.

Plowman, S.A. 1992. Physical activity, physical fitness, and low-back pain. *Exercise and Sport Sciences Reviews* 20: 221-242.

Pollock, M.L. 1973. The quantification of endurance training programs. In *Exercise and Sport Sciences Reviews,* ed. J.H. Wilmore, 1: 155-188. New York: Academic Press.

Pollock, M.L., Bohannon, R.L., Cooper, K.H., Ayres, J.J., Ward, A., White, S.R., and Linnerud, A.C. 1976. A comparative analysis of four protocols for maximal treadmill stress testing. *American Heart Journal* 92: 39-46.

Pollock, M.L., Broida, J., and Kendrick, Z. 1972. Validity of the palpation technique of heart rate determination and its estimation of training heart rate. *Research Quarterly* 43: 77-81.

Pollock, M.L., Cureton, T.K., and Greninger, L. 1969. Effects of frequency of training on working capacity, cardiovascular function, and body composition of adult men. *Medicine and Science in Sports* 1: 70-74.

Pollock, M.L., Dimmick, J., Miller, H.S., Kendrick, Z., and Linnerud, A.C. 1975. Effects of mode of training on cardiovascular function and body composition of middle-aged men. *Medicine and Science in Sports* 7: 139-145.

Pollock, M.L., Foster, C., Schmidt, D., Hellman, C., Linnerud, A.C., and Ward, A. 1982. Comparative analysis of physiologic responses to three different maximal graded exercise test protocols in healthy women. *American Heart Journal* 103: 363-373.

Pollock, M.L., Gaesser, G.A., Butcher, J.D., Despres, J.P., Dishman, R.K., Franklin, B.A., and Garber, C.E. 1998. The recommended quantity and quality of exercise for developing and maintaining cardiorespiratory and muscular fitness, and flexibility in healthy adults. *Medicine & Science in Sports & Exercise* 30: 975-991.

Pollock, M.L., Garzarella, L., and Graves, J. 1992. Effects of isolated lumbar extension resistance training on BMD of the elderly. *Medicine & Science in Sports & Exercise* 24: S66 [abstract].

Pollock, M.L., Gettman, L., Milesis, C., Bah, M., Durstine, L., and Johnson, R. 1977. Effects of frequency and duration of training on attrition and incidence of injury. *Medicine and Science in Sports* 9: 31-36.

Pollock, M.L., and Jackson, A.S. 1984. Research progress in validation of clinical methods of assessing body composition. *Medicine & Science in Sports & Exercise* 16: 606-613.

Pollock, M.L., Miller, H.S., Janeway, R., Linnerud, A.C., Robertson, B., and Valentino, R. 1971. Effects of walking on body composition and cardiovascular function of middle-aged men. *Journal of Applied Physiology* 30: 126-130.

Pollock, M.L., Miller, H.S., Linnerud, A.C., and Cooper, K.H. 1975. Frequency of training as a determinant for improvement in cardiovascular function and body composition of middle-aged men. *Archives of Physical Medicine and Rehabilitation* 56: 141-145.

Pollock, M.L., Wilmore, J.H., and Fox, S.M. III. 1978. *Health and fitness through physical activity.* New York: Wiley.

Poortmans, J.R., and Francaux, M. 2000. Adverse effects of creatine supplementation: Fact or fiction? *Sports Medicine* 30: 155-170.

Pope R.P., Herbert, R.D., Kirwan, J.D., and Graham, B.J. 2000. A randomized trial of preexercise stretching for prevention of lower limb injury. *Medicine & Science in Sports & Exercise* 32: 271–277.

Porcari, J., Foster, C., and Schneider, P. 2000. Exercise response to elliptical trainers. *Fitness Management* 16(9): 50–53.

Porszasz, J., Casaburi, R., Somfay, A., Woodhouse, L.J., and Whipp, B.J. 2003. A treadmill ramp protocol using simultaneous changes in speed and grade. *Medicine & Science in Sports & Exercise* 35: 1596-1603.

Porter, G.H. 1988. Case study evaluation for exercise prescription. In *Resource manual for guidelines for exercise testing and prescription*, ed. S.N. Blair, P. Painter, R.R. Pate, L.K. Smith, and C.B. Taylor, 248–255. Philadelphia: Lea & Febiger.

Powell, K.E., Thompson, P.D., Casperson, C.J., and Kendrick, J.S. 1987. Physical activity and the incidence of coronary heart disease. *Annual Review of Public Health* 8: 253–287.

President's Council on Physical Fitness and Sports. 1997. *The presidential physical fitness award program.* Washington, D.C.: author.

Prevalence of leisure-time physical activity among overweight adults—United States, 1998. 2000. *Morbidity and Mortality Weekly Report* 49(15), April 21.

Prior, B.M., Cureton, K.J., Modlesky, C.M., Evans, E.M., Sloniger, M.A., Saunders, M., and Lewis, R.D. 1997. In vivo validation of whole body composition estimates from dual-energy X-ray absorptiometry. *Journal of Applied Physiology* 83: 623-630.

Prochaska, J.O., and DiClemente, C.C. 1982. Trans-theoretical therapy: Toward a more integrative model of change. *Psychotherapy: Theory, Research, and Practice* 19: 276–288.

Proske, U., and Morgan, D.L. 2001. Muscle damage from eccentric exercise: Mechanism, mechanical signs, adaptation, and clinical applications. *Journal of Physiology* 537: 333-345.

Pruitt, L.A., Jackson, R.D., Bartels, R.L., and Lehnhard, H.J. 1992. Weight-training effects on bone mineral density in early postmenopausal women. *Journal of Bone Mineral Research* 7: 179–185.

Pruitt, L.A., Taaffe, D.R., and Marcus, R. 1995. Effects of a one-year high-intensity versus low-intensity resistance training program on bone mineral density in older women. *Journal of Bone Mineral Research* 10: 1788–1795.

Quatrochi, J.A., Hicks, V.L., Heyward, V.H., Colville, B.C., Cook, K.L., Jenkins, K.A., and Wilson, W. 1992. Relationship of optical density and skinfold measurements: Effects of age and level of body fatness. *Research Quarterly for Exercise and Sport* 63: 402-409.

Rajaram, S., Weaver, C.M., Lyle, R.M., Sedlock, D.A., Martin, B., Templin, T.J., Beard, J.L., and Percival, S.S. 1995. Effects of long-term moderate exercise on iron status in young women. *Medicine & Science in Sports & Exercise* 27: 1105–1110.

Ratamess, N.A., Kraemer, W.J., Volek, J.S., Rubin, M.R., Gomez, A.L., French, D.N., Sharman, M.J., McGuigan, M.M., Scheett, T., Hakkinen, K., Newton, R.U., and Dioguardi, F. 2003. The effects of amino acid supplementation on muscular performance during resistance training overreaching. *Journal of Strength and Conditioning Research* 17: 250-258.

Rawson, E.S., and Clarkson, P.M. 2003. Scientifically debatable: Is creatine worth its weight? *Gatorade Sport Science Exchange 91* 16(4): 1-13.

Rawson, E.S., Gunn, B., and Clarkson, P.M. 2001. The effects of creatine supplementation on exercise-induced muscle damage. *Journal of Strength and Conditioning Research* 15: 178-184.

Reaven, P.D., Barrett-Connor, E., and Edelstein, S. 1991. Relation between leisure-time physical activity and blood pressure in older women. *Circulation* 83: 559–565.

Rebuffe-Scrive, M. 1985. Adipose tissue metabolism and fat distribution. In *Human body composition and fat distribution,* ed. N.G. Norgan, 212–217. Wageningen, Netherlands: Euronut.

Recalde, P.T., Foster, C., Skemp-Arlt, K.M., Fater, D.C.W., Neese, C.A., Dodge, C., and Porcari, J.P. 2002. The talk test as a simple marker of ventilatory threshold. *South African Journal of Sports Medicine* 8: 5-8.

Reese, N.B., and Bandy, W.D. 2003. Use of an inclinometer to measure flexibility of the iliotibial band using the Ober test and the modified Ober test: Differences in magnitude and reliability of measurements. *Journal of Orthopaedic and Sports Physical Therapy* 33: 326-330.

Reeves, R.A. 1995. Does this patient have hypertension? How to measure blood pressure. *Journal of the American Medical Association* 273: 1211–1218.

Rhea, M.R., Alvar, B.A., Burkett, L.N., and Ball, S.D. 2003. A meta-analysis to determine the dose response for strength development. *Medicine & Science in Sports & Exercise* 35: 456-464.

Rhea, M.R., Ball, S.D., Phillips, W.T., and Burkett, L.N. 2002. A comparison of linear and daily undulating periodized programs with equated volume and intensity for strength. *Journal of Strength and Conditioning Research* 16: 250-255.

Rhea, M.R., Phillips, W.T., Burkett, L.N., Stone, W.J., Ball, S.D., Alvar, B.A., and Thomas, A.B. 2003. A comparison of linear and daily undulating periodized programs with equated volume and intensity for local muscular endurance. *Journal of Strength and Conditioning Research* 17: 82-87.

Riebe, D., and Niggs, C. 1998. Setting the stage for healthy living. *ACSM's Health & Fitness Journal* 2(3): 11–15.

Rikli, R., Petray, C., and Baumgartner, T. 1992. The reliability of distance run tests for children in grades K-4. *Research Quarterly for Exercise and Sport* 63: 270–276.

Rikli, R.E., and Jones, C.J. 1999. Development and validation of a functional fitness test for community-residing older adults. *Journal of Aging and Physical Activity* 7: 127-159.

Rikli, R.E, and Jones, C.J. 2001. *Senior fitness test manual.* Champaign, IL: Human Kinetics.

Roberts, J.M., and Wilson, K. 1999. Effect of stretching duration on active and passive range of motion in the lower extremity. *British Journal of Sports Medicine* 33: 259-263.

Roby, R.B. 1962. Effect of exercise on regional subcutaneous fat accumulations. *Research Quarterly* 33: 273–278.

Rochmis, P., and Blackburn, H. 1971. Exercise tests. A survey of procedures, safety and litigation experience in approximately 170,000 tests. *Journal of the American Medical Association* 217: 1061–1066.

Rockport Walking Institute. 1986. *Rockport fitness walking test.* Marlboro, MA: Author.

Rodd, D., Ho, L., and Enzler, D. 1999. Validity of Tanita TBF-515 bioelectrical impedance scale for estimating body fat in young adults. *Medicine & Science in Sports & Exercise* 31(Suppl.): S201 [abstract].

Roelants, M., Delecluse, C., Goris, M., and Verschueren, S. 2004. Effects of 24 weeks of whole body vibration training on body composition and muscle strength in untrained females. *International Journal of Sports Medicine* 25: 1-5.

Ross, J., and Pate, R. 1987. The national children and youth fitness study II: A summary of findings. *Journal of Physical Education, Recreation and Dance* 58: 51–56.

Ross, R., and Janssen, I. 2001. Physical activity, total and regional obesity: Dose-response considerations. *Medicine & Science in Sports & Exercise* 33 (Suppl.): S521-S527.

Ross, W.D., and Marfell-Jones, M.J. 1991. Kinanthropometry. In *Physiological testing of the high-performance athlete,* ed. J.D. MacDougall, H.A. Wenger, and H.J. Green, 75–115, Champaign, IL: Human Kinetics.

Rowlands, A.V., Marginson, V.F., and Lee, J. 2003. Chronic flexibility gains: Effect of isometric contraction duration during proprioceptive neuromuscular facilitation stretching techniques. *Research Quarterly for Exercise and Sport* 74: 47-51.

Roy, J.L.P., Smith, J.F., Bishop, P.A., Hallinan, C., Wang, M., and Hunter, G.R. 2004. Prediction of maximal $\dot{V}O_2$ from a submaximal StairMaster test in young women. *Journal of Strength and Conditioning Research* 18: 92-96.

Roza, A.M., and Shizgal, H.M. 1984. The Harris Benedict equation reevaluated: Resting energy requirements and the body cell mass. *American Journal of Clinical Nutrition.* 40: 168–182.

Rubin, C., Recker, R., Cullen, D., Ryaby, J., and McLeod, K. 1998. Prevention of bone loss in a post-menopausal population by low-level biomechanical intervention. *Bone* 23: S174 [abstract].

Runge, M., Rehfeld, G., and Resnicek, E. 2000. Balance training and exercise in geriatric patients. *Journal of Musculoskeletal and Neuronal Interactions* 1: 61-65.

Rush, E.C., Plank, L.D., Laulu, M.S., and Robinson, S.M. 1997. Prediction of percentage body fat from anthropometric measurements: Comparison of New Zealand European and Polynesian young women. *American Journal of Clinical Nutrition* 66: 2-7.

Russell, P.J. 1983. Aerobic dance programs: Maintaining quality and effectiveness. *Physical Educator* 40: 114–120.

Sale, D. 1988. Neural adaptation to resistance training. *Medicine & Science in Sports & Exercise* 20: S135–S145.

Sale, D., MacDougall, J.D., Jacobs, I., and Garner, S. 1987. Interaction between concurrent strength and endurance training. *Journal of Applied Physiology* 68: 260–270.

Salem, J.G., Wang, M.Y., and Sigward, S. 2002. Measuring lower extremity strength in older adults: The stability of isokinetic versus 1RM measures. *Journal of Aging and Physical Activity* 10: 489-503.

Sallis, J.F., and Owen, N. 1999. *Physical activity and behavioral medicine.* Thousand Oaks, CA: Sage.

Samaha, F.F., Iqbal, N., Seshadri, P., Chicano, K.L., Daily, D.A., McGrory, J., Williams, T., Williams, M., Gracely, E.J., and Stern, L. 2003. A low-carbohydrate as compared with a low-fat diet in severe obesity. *New England Journal of Medicine* 348: 2074-2081.

Sanborn, C.F. 1990. Exercise, calcium, and bone density. *Sports Science Exchange* 2(24). Gatorade Sports Science Institute, Quaker Oats Co.

Saris, W.H.M., Blair, S.N., van Baak, M.A., Eaton, S.B., Davies, P.S.W., Di Pietro, L., Fogelholm, M., Rissanen, A., Schoeller, D., Swinburn, B., Tremblay, A., Westerterp, K.R., and Wyatt, H. 2003. How much physical activity is enough to prevent unhealthy weight gain? Outcome of the IASO 1st Stock Conference and consensus statement. *Obesity Reviews* 4: 101-114.

Schade, M., Hellebrandt, F.A., Waterland, J.C., and Carns, M.L. 1962. Spot reducing in overweight college women: Its influence on fat distribution as determined by photography. *Research Quarterly* 33: 461–471.

Schaefer, E.J. 2002. Lipoproteins, nutrition, and heart disease. *American Journal of Clinical Nutrition* 75: 191-212.

Schlicht, J., Godin, J., and Camaione, D.C. 1999. How to help your client stick with an exercise program: Build self-efficacy to promote exercise adherence. *ACSM's Health & Fitness Journal* 3(6): 27–31.

Schmidt, P.K., and Carter, J.E.L. 1990. Static and dynamic differences among five types of skinfold calipers. *Human Biology* 62: 369-388.

Schot, P.K., Knutzen, K.M., Poole, S.M., and Mrotek, L.A. 2003. Sit-to-stand performance of older adults following strength training. *Research Quarterly for Exercise and Sport* 74: 1-8.

Schutte, A.E., Huisman, H.W., van Rooyen, J.M., Malan, N.T., and Schutte, R. 2004. Validation of the Finometer device for measurement of blood pressure in black women. *Journal of Human Hypertension* 18: 79-84.

Schwane, J.A., Johnson, S.R., Vandenakker, C.B., and Armstrong R.B. 1983. Delayed-onset muscular soreness and plasma CPK and LDH activities after downhill running. *Medicine & Science in Sports & Exercise* 15: 51–56.

Segal, K.R., Van Loan, M., Fitzgerald, P.I., Hodgdon, J.A., and Van Italie, T.B. 1988. Lean body mass estimation by bioelectrical impedance analysis: A four-site cross-validation study. *American Journal of Clinical Nutrition* 47: 7–14.

Seip, R., and Weltman, A. 1991. Validity of skinfold and girth based regression equations for the prediction of body composition in obese adults. *American Journal of Human Biology* 3: 91–95.

Sell, K.E., Verity, T.M., Worrell, T.W., Pease, B.J., and Wigglesworth, J. 1994. Two measurement techniques for assessing subtalar joint position: A reliability study. *Journal of Orthopaedic and Sports Physical Therapy* 19: 162–167.

Serdula, M.K., Williamson, D.F., Anda, R.F., Levy, A., Heaton, A., and Byers, T. 1994. Weight control practices in adults: Results of a multistate telephone survey. *American Journal of Public Health* 84: 1821–1824.

Seshadri, P. 2004. A calorie by any name is still a calorie. *Archives of Internal Medicine* 164: 1702-1703.

Sharkey, B.J. 1979. *Physiology of fitness.* Champaign, IL: Human Kinetics.

Sharkey, B.J. 1990. *Physiology of fitness,* 3rd ed. Champaign, IL: Human Kinetics.

Shaw, C.E., McCully, K.K., and Posner, J.D. 1995. Injuries during the one repetition maximum assessment in the elderly. *Journal of Cardiopulmonary Rehabilitation* 15: 283-287.

Shephard, R.J. 1972. *Alive man: The physiology of physical activity.* Springfield, IL: Charles C Thomas.

Shephard, R.J. 1977. Do risks of exercise justify costly caution? *The Physician and Sportsmedicine* 5: 58–65.

Shoenhair, C.L., and Wells, C.L. 1995. Women, physical activity, and coronary heart disease: A review. *Medicine, Exercise, Nutrition and Health* 4: 200–206.

Shrier, I. 1999. Stretching before exercise does not reduce the risk of local muscle injury: A critical review of the clinical and basic science literature. *Clinical Journal of Sport Medicine* 9: 221-227.

Shrier, I. 2000. Stretching before exercise: An evidence based approach. *British Journal of Sports Medicine* 34: 324-325.

Shrier, I., and Gossal, K. 2000. Myths and truths of stretching: Individualized recommendations for healthy muscles. *The Physician and Sportsmedicine* 28: 57-63.

Sinning, W. 1975. *Experiments and demonstrations in exercise physiology.* Philadelphia: Saunders.

Siri, W.E. 1961. Body composition from fluid space and density. In *Techniques for measuring body composition,* ed. J. Brozek and A. Henschel, 223–224. Washington, D.C.: National Academy of Sciences.

Sjodin, A.M., Forslund, A.H., Westerterp, K.R., Andersson, A.B., Forslund, J.M., and Hambraeus, L.M. 1996. The influence of physical activity on BMR. *Medicine & Science in Sports & Exercise* 28: 85–91.

Sjostrom, M., Lexell, J., Eriksson, A., and Taylor, C.C. 1992. Evidence of fiber hyperplasia in human skeletal muscles from healthy young men? *European Journal of Applied Physiology* 62: 301–304.

Skinner, J. 1993. *Exercise testing and exercise prescription for special cases.* Philadelphia: Lea & Febiger.

Slaughter, M.H., Lohman, T.G., Boileau, R.A., Horswill, C.A., Stillman, R.J., Van Loan, M.D., and Bemben, D.A. 1988. Skinfold equations for estimation of body fatness in children and youth. *Human Biology* 60: 709–723.

Smith, D.B., Johnson, G.O., Stout, J.R., Housh, T.J., Housh, D.J., and Evetovich, T.K. 1997. Validity of near-infrared interactance for estimating relative body fat in female high school gymnasts. *International Journal of Sports Medicine* 18: 531-537.

Smith, L.L. 1991. Acute inflammation: The underlying mechanism in delayed onset muscle soreness? *Medicine & Science in Sports & Exercise* 23: 542–551.

Smith, U., Hammerstein, J., Bjorntorp, P., and Kral, J.G. 1979. Regional differences and effect of weight reduction on human fat cell metabolism. *European Journal of Clinical Investigation* 9: 327–332.

Smutok, M.A., Skrinar, G.S., and Pandolf, K.B. 1980. Exercise intensity: Subjective regulation by perceived exertion. *Archives of Physical Medicine and Rehabilitation* 61: 569–574.

Smye, S.W., Sutcliffe, J., and Pitt, E. 1993. A comparison of four commercial systems used to measure whole-body electrical impedance. *Physiological Measurement* 14: 473-478.

Snijder, M.B., Kuyf, B.E., and Deurenberg, P. 1999. Effect of body build on the validity of predicted body fat from body mass index and bioelectrical impedance. *Annals of Nutrition and Metabolism* 43: 277- 285.

Society of Actuaries and Association of Life Insurance Medical Directors of America. 1980. *1979 build study.* New York: Metropolitan Life Insurance.

Staron, R.S., Karapondo, D.L., Kraemer, W.J., Fry, A.C., Gordon, S.E., Falkel, J.E., Hagerman, F.C., and Hikida, R.S. 1994. Skeletal muscle adaptations during the early phase of heavy-resistance training in men and women. *Journal of Applied Physiology* 76: 1247-1255.

Stolarczyk, L.M., Heyward, V.H., Hicks, V.L., and Baumgartner, R.N. 1994. Predictive accuracy of bioelectrical impedance in estimating body composition of Native American women. *American Journal of Clinical Nutrition* 59: 964-970.

Stout, J.R., Eckerson, J.M., Housh, T.J., and Johnson, G.O. 1994. Validity of methods for estimating percent body fat in black males. *Journal of Strength and Conditioning Research* 8: 243-246.

Stout, J.R., Eckerson, J.M., Housh, T.J., Johnson, G.O., and Betts, N.M. 1994. Validity of percent body fat estimations in males. *Medicine & Science in Sports & Exercise* 26: 632-636.

Stout, J.R., Housh, T.J., Eckerson, J.M., Johnson, G.O., and Betts, N.M. 1996. Validity of methods for estimating percent body fat in young women. *Journal of Strength and Conditioning Research* 10: 25-29.

Stuhr, R.M. 1998. Strategies for beating the barriers to exercise in women. *ACSM's Health & Fitness Journal* 2(5): 20–29, 51.

Sung, R.Y.T., Lau, P., Yu, C.W., Lam, P.K.W., and Nelson, E.A.S. 2001. Measurement of body fat using leg to leg bioimpedance. *Archives of Disease in Childhood* 85: 263-267.

Svendsen, O.L., Hassager, C., Bergmann, I., and Christiansen, C. 1992. Measurement of abdominal and intra-abdominal fat in postmenopausal women by dual energy X-ray absorptiometry and anthropometry: Comparison with computerized tomography. *International Journal of Obesity* 17: 45- 51.

Swain, D.P. 1999. $\dot{V}O_2$ reserve: A new method for exercise prescription. *ACSM's Health & Fitness Journal* 3(5): 10–14.

Swain, D.P., and Franklin, B.A. 2002. $\dot{V}O_2$ reserve and the minimal intensity for improving cardiorespiratory fitness. *Medicine & Science in Sports & Exercise* 34: 152-157.

Swain, D.P., and Leutholtz, B.C. 1997. Heart rate reserve is equivalent to % $\dot{V}O_2$ reserve, not to $\dot{V}O_2$max. *Medicine & Science in Sports & Exercise* 29: 410–414.

Swain, D.P., Leutholtz, B.C., King, M.E., Haas, L.A., and Branch, J.D. 1998. Relationship between % heart rate reserve and % $\dot{V}O_2$reserve in treadmill exercise. *Medicine & Science in Sports & Exercise* 30: 318–321.

Swain, D.P., Parrott, J.A., Bennett, A.R., Branch, J.D., and Dowling, E.A. 2004. Validation of a new method for estimating $\dot{V}O_2$max based on $\dot{V}O_2$ reserve. *Medicine & Science in Sports & Exercise* 36: 1421-1426.

Swank, A.M., Funk, D.C., Durham, M.P., and Roberts, S. 2003. Adding weights to stretching exercise increases passive range of motion for healthy elderly. *Journal of Strength and Conditioning Research* 17: 374-378.

Taaffe, D.R., Duret, C., Wheeler, S., and Marcus, R. 1999. Once-weekly resistance exercise improves muscle strength and neuromuscular performance in older adults. *Journal of the American Geriatrics Society* 47: 1208-1214.

Takeshima, N., Rogers, M.E., Watanabe, E., Brechue, W.F., Okada, A., Yamada, T., Islam, M.M., and Hayano, J. 2002. Water-based exercise improves health-related aspects of fitness in older women. *Medicine & Science in Sports & Exercise* 34: 544-551.

Talag, T.S. 1973. Residual muscular soreness as influenced by concentric, eccentric, and static contractions. *Research Quarterly* 44: 458–469.

Tanaka, H., Monahan, K.D., and Seals, D.R. 2001. Age-predicted maximal heart rate revisited. *Journal of the American College of Cardiology* 37: 153-156.

Taylor, D.C., Dalton, J.D., Seaber, A.V., and Garrett, W.E. 1990. Viscoelastic properties of muscle-tendon units. The biomechanical effects of stretching. *American Journal of Sports Medicine* 18: 300-309.

Taylor, N.A.S., and Wilkinson, J.G. 1986. Exercise-induced skeletal muscle growth: Hypertrophy or hyperplasia? *Sports Medicine* 3: 190–200.

Taylor, W.D., George, J.D., Allsen, P.E., Vehrs, P.R. Hager, R.L., and Roberts, M.P. 2002. Estimation of $\dot{V}O_2$max from a 1.5-mile endurance test. *Medicine & Science in Sports & Exercise* 35 (Suppl.): S257 [abstract].

Telford, R., Catchpole, E., Deakin, V., Hahn, A., and Plank, A. 1992. The effect of 7 to 8 months of vitamin/mineral supplementation on athletic performance. *International Journal of Sport Nutrition* 2: 135–153.

Terry, J.W., Tolson, H., Johnson, D.J., and Jessup, G.T. 1977. A work load selection procedure for the Åstrand-Ryhming test. *Journal of Sports Medicine and Physical Fitness* 17: 361–366.

Tesch, P.A. 1988. Skeletal muscle adaptations consequent to long-term heavy resistance exercise. *Medicine & Science in Sports & Exercise* 20: S132–S134.

Tesch, P.A. 1992. Short- and long-term histochemical and biochemical adaptations in muscle. In *Strength and power in sports. The encyclopaedia of sports medicine,* ed. P. Komi, 239–248. Oxford: Blackwell.

Thacker, S.B., Gilchrist, J., Stroup, D.F., and Kimsey, C.D. 2004. The impact of stretching on sports injury risk: A systematic review of the literature. *Medicine & Science in Sports & Exercise* 36: 371-378.

Thomas, T.R., and Etheridge, G.L. 1980. Hydrostatic weighing at residual volume and functional residual capacity. *Journal of Applied Physiology* 49: 157–159.

Thomas, T.R., Ziogas, G., Smith, T., Zhang, Q., and Londeree, B.R. 1995. Physiological and perceived exertion responses to six modes of submaximal exercise. *Research Quarterly for Exercise and Sport* 66: 239–246.

Thompson, J., Manore, M. and Thomas, J. 1996. Effects of diet and diet-plus-exercise programs on resting metabolic rate: A meta-analysis. *International Journal of Sport Nutrition* 6: 41–61.

Thompson, P.D. 1993 The safety of exercise testing and participation. In *ACSM's resource manual for guidelines for exercise testing and prescription,* ed. S.N. Blair, P. Painter, R. Pate, L.K. Smith, and C.B. Taylor, 361–370. Philadelphia: Lea & Febiger.

Thorstensson, A., Hulten, B., vonDobeln, W., and Karlsson, J. 1976. Effect of strength training on enzyme activities and fibre characteristics in human skeletal muscle. *Acta Physiologica Scandinavica* 96: 392–398.

Timson, B.F., and Coffman, J.L. 1984. Body composition by hydrostatic weighing at total lung capacity and residual volume. *Medicine & Science in Sports & Exercise* 16: 411–414.

Tipton, C.M., Matthes, R.D., Maynard, J.A., and Carey, R.A. 1975. The influence of physical activity on ligaments and tendons. *Medicine and Science in Sports* 7: 165–175.

Tipton, K.D., Rasmussen, B.B., Miller, S.L., Wolfe, S.E., Owens-Stovall, S.K., Petrini, B.E., and Wolfe, R.R. 2001. Timing of amino acid-carbohydrate ingestion alters anabolic responose of muscle to resistance exercise. *American Journal of Physiology, Endocrinology and Metabolism* 281: E197-206.

Tipton, K.D., and Wolfe, R.R. 2004. Protein and amino acids for athletes. *Journal of Sports Science* 22: 65-79.

Torvinen, S., Karinus, P., Sievanen, H., Jarvinen, T.A.H., Pasanen, M., Kontulainen, S., Jarvinen, T.L.N., Jarvinen, M., Oja, P., and Vuori, I. 2002. Effect of four-month vertical whole body vibration on performance and balance. *Medicine & Science in Sports & Exercise* 34: 1523-1528.

Tothill, P., and Hannan, W.J. 2000. Comparisons between Hologic QDR 1000W, QDR 4500A, and Lunar Expert dual-energy X-ray absorptiometry scanners used for measuring total body bone and soft tissue. *Annals of the New York Academy of Sciences* 904: 63-71.

Town, G.P., Sol, N., and Sinning, W. 1980. The effect of rope skipping rate on energy expenditure of males and females. *Medicine & Science in Sports & Exercise* 12: 295–298.

Tran, Z.V., and Weltman, A. 1988. Predicting body composition of men from girth measurements. *Human Biology* 60: 167–175.

Tran, Z.V., and Weltman, A. 1989. Generalized equation for predicting body density of women from girth measurements. *Medicine & Science in Sports & Exercise* 21: 101–104.

Tremblay, M.S., Katzmarzyk, P.T., and Willms, J.D. 2002. Temporal trends in overweight and obesity in Canada, 1981-96. *International Journal of Obesity and Related Metabolic Disorders* 26: 538-543.

Tremblay, M.S., and Willms, J.D. 2000. Secular trends in the body mass index of Canadian children. *Canadian Medical Association Journal* 163: 1429-1433. Published erratum in *Canadian Medical Association Journal* (2001) 164: 970.

Trost, S.G., Owen, N., Bauman, A.E., Sallis, J.F., and Brown, W. 2002. Correlates of adults' participation in physical activity: Review and update. *Medicine & Science in Sports & Exercise* 34: 1996-2001.

Turcato, E., Bosello, O., Francesco, V.D., Harris, T.B., Zoico, E., Bissoli, L., Fracassi, E., and Zamboni, M. 2000. Waist circumference and abdominal sagittal diameter as surrogates of body fat distribution in the elderly: Their relation with cardiovascular risk factors. *International Journal of Obesity* 24: 1005-1010.

Tyrrell, V.J., Richards, G., Hofman, P., Gillies, G.F., Robinson, E., and Cutfield, W.S. 2001. Foot-to-foot bioelectrical impedance analysis: A valuable tool for the measurement of body composition in children. *International Journal of Obesity* 25: 273-278.

U.S. Department of Health and Human Services. 1996. *Physical activity and health: A report of the Surgeon General—At a glance.* Atlanta: U.S. Department of Health and Human Services, Centers for Disease Control and Prevention, National Center for Chronic Disease Prevention and Health Promotion.

U.S. Department of Health and Human Services. 2000a. *Healthy people 2010—conference edition: Physical activity and fitness (22).* Atlanta: Author.

U.S. Department of Health and Human Services. 2000b. *Healthy people 2010: Understanding and improving health—overweight and obesity.* Washington, D.C.: U.S. Government Printing Office.

U.S. Department of Health and Human Services. 2004. *2005 Dietary Guidelines Advisory Committee report: Translating the science into dietary guidance.* Washington, D.C.: U.S. Government Printing Office.

U.S. Department of Health and Human Services. 2005a. *Dietary Guidelines for Americans 2005.* Executive Summary. www.health.gov/dietaryguidelines/dga2005/document/html/executivesummary.

U.S. Department of Health and Human Services. 2005b. MyPyramid. www.MyPyramid.com.

Utter, A.C., Nieman, D.C., Ward, A.N., and Butterworth, D.E. 1999. Use of the leg-to-leg bioelectrical impedance method in assessing body-composition change in obese women. *American Journal of Clinical Nutrition* 69: 603-607.

Utter, A.C., Scott, J.R., Oppliger, R.A., Visich, P.S., Goss, F.L., Marks, B.L., Nieman, D.C., and Smith, B.W. 2001. A comparison of leg-to-leg bioelectrical impedance and skinfolds in assessing body fat in collegiate wrestlers. *Journal of Strength and Conditioning Research* 15: 157-160.

Vaisman, N., Corey, M., Rossi, M.F., Goldberg, E., and Pencharz, P. 1988. Changes in body composition during refeeding of patients with anorexia nervosa. *Journal of Pediatrics* 113: 925–929.

Vaisman, N., Rossi, M.F., Goldberg, E., Dibden, L.J., Wykes, L.J., and Pencharz, P.B. 1988. Energy expenditures and body composition in patients with anorexia nervosa. *Journal of Pediatrics* 113: 919–924.

Van Adrichem, J.A.M., and van der Korst, J.K. 1973. Assessment of flexibility of the lumbar spine: A pilot study in children and adolescents. *Scandinavian Journal of Rheumatology* 2: 87–91.

van der Kooy, K., Leenen, R., Seidell, J.C., Deurenberg, P., Droop, A., and Bakker, C.J.G. 1993. Waist-hip ratio is a poor predictor of changes in visceral fat. *American Journal of Clinical Nutrition* 57: 327-333.

Vanhelder, W.P., Radomski, M.W., and Goode, R.C. 1984. Growth hormone responses during intermittent weight lifting exercise in men. *European Journal of Applied Physiology* 53: 31–34.

Van Loan, M.D., and Mayclin, P.L. 1987. Bioelectrical impedance analysis: Is it a reliable estimator of lean body mass and total body water? *Human Biology* 59: 299–309.

Van Loan, M.D., and Mayclin, P.L. 1992. Body composition assessment: Dual-energy X-ray absorptiometry (DEXA) compared to reference methods. *European Journal of Clinical Nutrition* 46: 125–130.

Van Mechelen, W., Holbil, H., and Kemper, H.C. 1986. Validation of two running tests as estimates of maximal aerobic power in children. *European Journal of Applied Physiology and Occupational Physiology* 55: 503–506.

Vehrs, P.R., Drummond, M., Fellingham, D.K., and Brigham, G.W. 2002. Accuracy of five heart rate monitors during exercise. *Medicine & Science in Sports & Exercise* 34 (Suppl.): S272 [abstract].

Velasquez, K.S., and Wilmore, J.H. 1992. Changes in cardiorespiratory fitness and body composition after a 12-week bench step training program. *Medicine & Science in Sports & Exercise* 24: S78 [abstract].

Vera-Garcia, F.J., Grenier, S.G., and McGill, S.M. 2000. Abdominal muscle responses during curl-ups on both stable and labile surfaces. *Physical Therapy* 80: 564-569.

Vescovi, J.D., Zimmerman, S.L., Miller, W.C., Hildebrandt, L., Hammer, R.L., and Fernhall, B. 2001. Evaluation of the Bod Pod for estimating percentage body fat in a heterogeneous group of adult humans. *European Journal of Applied Physiology* 85: 326-332.

Vincent, K.R., Braith, R.W., Feldman, R.A., Magyari, P.M., Cutler, R.B., Persin, S.A., Lennon, S.L., Gabr, A.H., and Lowenthal, D.T. 2002. Resistance exercise and physical performance in adults aged 60 to 83. *Journal of the American Geriatrics Society* 50: 1100-1107.

Voelker, S.A., Foster, C., Skemp-Arlt, K.M., Brice, G., and Backes, R. 2002. Relationship between the talk test and ventilatory threshold in cardiac patients. *Clinical Exercise Physiology* 4: 120-123.

Volek, J. 1999. Update: What we know about creatine. *ACSM's Health & Fitness Journal* 3(3): 27–33.

Wagner, D.R., and Heyward, V.H. 2001. Validity of two-component models of estimating body fat of Black men. *Journal of Applied Physiology* 90: 649-656.

Wagner, D.R., and Heyward, V.H. 2004. *Applied body composition assessment*. Champaign, IL: Human Kinetics.

Wagner, D., Heyward, V., and Gibson, A. 2000. Validation of air displacement plethysmography for assessing body composition. *Medicine & Science in Sports & Exercise* 32: 1339-1344.

Wallick, M.E., Porcari, J.P., Wallick, S.B., Berg, K.M., Brice, G.A., and Arimond, G.R. 1995. Physiological responses to in-line skating compared to treadmill running. *Medicine & Science in Sports & Exercise* 27: 242-248.

Wallin, D., Ekblom, B., Grahn, R., and Nordenborg, T. 1985. Improvement of muscle flexibility. A comparison between two techniques. *American Journal of Sports Medicine* 13: 263-268.

Wang, J., Thornton, J.C., Russell, M., Burastero, S., Heymsfield, S., and Pierson, R.N. 1994. Asians have lower body mass index (BMI) but higher percent body fat than do Whites: Comparison of anthropometric measurements. *American Journal of Clinical Nutrition* 60: 23-28.

Ward, R., and Anderson, G.S. 1998. Resilience of anthropometric data assembly strategies to imposed error. *Journal of Sports Sciences* 16: 755-759.

Ward, R., Rempel, R., and Anderson, G.S. 1999. Modeling dynamic skinfold compression. *American Journal of Human Biology* 11: 521–537.

Wathen, D. 1994a. Load assignment. In *Essentials of strength testing*, ed. T.R. Baechle, 435-446. Champaign, IL: Human Kinetics.

Wathen, D. 1994b. Periodization: Concepts and applications. In *Essentials of strength training and conditioning*, ed. T.R. Baechle, 459–472. Champaign, IL: Human Kinetics.

Watsford, M.L., Murphy, A.J., Spinks, W.L., and Walshe, A.D. 2003. Creatine supplementation and its effect on musculotendinous stiffness and performance. *Journal of Strength and Conditioning Research* 17: 26- 33.

Wattles, M.G. 2002. The dissection of exercise certifications. *Professionalization of Exercise Physiology*online 5(3): 1-13.

Weiss, L.W., Cureton, K.J., and Thompson, F.N. 1983. Comparison of serum testosterone and androstenedione responses to weight lifting in men and women. *European Journal of Applied Physiology* 50: 413–419.

Weits, T., Van der Beek, E.J., Wedel, M., and Ter Haar Romeny, B.M. 1988. Computed tomography measurement of abdominal fat deposition in relation to anthropometry. *International Journal of Obesity* 12: 217-225.

Weldon, S.M., and Hill, R.H 2003. The efficacy of stretching for prevention of exercise-related injury: A systematic review of the literature *Manual Therapy* 8: 141-150.

Wells, C.L. 1996. Physical activity and women's health. In *Physical Activity and Fitness Research Digest*, ed. C. Corbin and B. Pangrazi, series 2, no. 5, 1–6. Washington, D.C.: President's Council on Physical Fitness and Sports.

Weltman, A., Levine, S., Seip, R.L., and Tran, Z.V. 1988. Accurate assessment of body composition in obese females. *American Journal of Clinical Nutrition* 48: 1179–1183.

Weltman, A., Seip, R.I., and Tran, Z.V. 1987. Practical assessment of body composition in adult obese males. *Human Biology* 59: 523–535.

Wessel, H.U., Strasburger, J.F., and Mitchell, B.M. 2001. New standards for Bruce treadmill protocol in children and adolescents. *Pediatric Exercise Science* 13: 392-401.

Whaley, M., Kaminsky, L., Dwyer, G., Getchell, L., and Norton, J. 1992. Predictors of over- and underachievement of age-predicted maximal heart rate. *Medicine & Science in Sports & Exercise* 24: 1173–1179.

Willett, W.C. 2001. *Eat, drink and be healthy: The Harvard Medical School guide to healthy eating*. New York: Simon & Schuster Adult Publishing.

Williams, D.P., Going, S.B., Massett, M.P., Lohman, T.G., Bare, L.A., and Hewitt, M.J. 1993. Aqueous and mineral fractions of the fat-free body and their relation to body fat estimates in men and women aged 49-82 years. In *Human body composition: In vivo methods, models and assessment*, ed. K.J. Ellis and J.D. Eastman, 109–113. New York: Plenum Press.

Williams, M.H. 1992. *Nutrition for fitness and sport*. Dubuque, IA: Brown & Benchmark.

Williams, M.H. 1993. Nutritional supplements for strength trained athletes. *Sports Science Exchange* 6(6). Gatorade Sports Science Institute, Quaker Oats Co.

Williams, P.T. 2001. Physical fitness and activity as separate heart disease risk factors: A meta-analysis. *Medicine & Science in Sports & Exercise* 33: 754-761.

Williams R., Binkley, J., Bloch, R., Goldsmith, C.H., and Minuk, T. 1993. Reliability of the modified-modified Schober and double inclinometer methods for measuring lumbar flexion and extension. *Physical Therapy* 73: 26–37.

Williford, H.N , Blessing, D.L., Barksdale, J.M., and Smith, F.H. 1988. The effects of aerobic dance training on serum lipids, lipoproteins, and cardiopulmonary function. *Journal of Sports Medicine and Physical Fitness* 28: 151–157.

Wilmore, J.H. 1974. Alterations in strength, body composition, and anthropometric measurements consequent to a 10-week weight training program. *Medicine and Science in Sports* 6: 133–138.

Wilmore, J.H., and Behnke, A.R. 1969. An anthropometric estimation of body density and lean body weight in young men. *Journal of Applied Physiology* 27: 25–31.

Wilmore, J.H., and Behnke, A.R. 1970. An anthropometric estimation of body density and lean body weight in young women. *American Journal of Clinical Nutrition* 23: 267–274.

Wilmore, J.H., Davis, J.A., O'Brien, R.S., Vodak, P.A., Walder, G.R., and Amsterdam, E.A. 1980. Physiological alterations consequent to 20-week conditioning programs of bicycling, tennis and jogging. *Medicine & Science in Sports & Exercise* 12: 1–9.

Wilmore, J.H., Frisancho, R.A., Gordon, C.C., Himes, J.H., Martin, A.D., Martorell, R., and Seefeldt, R.D. 1988. Body breadth equipment and measurement techniques. In *Anthropometric standardization reference manual,* ed. T.G. Lohman, A.F. Roche, and R. Martorell, 27–38. Champaign, IL: Human Kinetics.

Wilmore, J.H., Parr, R.B., Girandola, R.N., Ward, P., Vodak, P.A., Barstow, T.J., Pipes, T.V., Romero, G.T., and Leslie, P. 1978. Physiological alterations consequent to circuit weight training. *Medicine and Science in Sports* 10: 79–84.

Wilmore, J.H., Royce, J., Girandola, R.N., Katch, F.I., and Katch, V.L. 1970. Body composition changes with a 10-week program of jogging. *Medicine and Science in Sports* 2: 113–119.

Wilmoth, S.K. 1986. *Leading aerobic dance-exercise.* Champaign, IL: Human Kinetics.

Wilson, P.K., Winga, E.R., Edgett, J.W., and Gushiken, T.J. 1978. *Policies and procedures of a cardiac rehabilitation program—immediate to long term care.* Philadelphia: Lea & Febiger.

Withers, R.T., LaForgia, J., Pillans, R.K., Shipp, N.J., Chatterton, B.E., Schultz, C.G., and Leaney, F. 1998. Comparisons of two-, three-, and four-compartment models of body composition analysis in men and women. *Journal of Applied Physiology* 85: 238-245.

Witten, C. 1973. Construction of a submaximal cardiovascular step test for college females. *Research Quarterly* 44: 46–50.

Wolfe, B.L., LeMura, L.M., and Cole, P.J. 2004. Quantitative analysis of single- vs. multiple-set programs for resistance training. *Journal of Strength and Conditioning Research* 18: 35-47.

Wolf-Maier, K., Cooper, R.S., Banegas, J.R., Giampaoli, S., Hense, H.W., Joffres, M., Kastarinen, M., Poulter, N., Primatesta, P., Rodriquez-Artalego, F., Stegmayr, B., Thamm, N., Tuomilephto, J., Vanuzzo, D., and Vescio, F. 2003. Hypertension prevalence and blood pressure levels in 6 European countries, Canada, and the United States. *Journal of the American Medical Association* 289: 2363-2369.

Women's Exercise Research Center. 1998. Based on figures published by Brown, D.A., and Miller, W.C. 1998. Normative data for strength and flexibility of women throughout life. *European Journal of Applied Physiology* 78: 77–82.

Woodby-Brown, S., Berg, K., and Latin, R.W. 1993. Oxygen cost of aerobic bench stepping at three heights. *Journal of Strength and Conditioning Research* 7: 163–167.

World Health Organization (WHO). 1998. Obesity: Preventing and managing a global epidemic. *Report of a WHO Consultation on Obesity.* Geneva: Author.

World Health Organization. 2001. Global database on obesity and body mass index (BMI) in adults. http://www.who.int/nut/db_bmi.

World Health Organization. 2002a. Diabetes: The cost of diabetes. www.who.int/mediacentre/factsheets/fs236/en/print.html.

World Health Organization. 2002b. Reducing risks, promoting healthy life. *World Health Report 2002.* www.who.int/whr/2002/chapter4/en/index4.html.

World Health Organization. 2002c. Smoking statistics. www.wpro.who.int/public/press_release/press_view.asp?id=219.

World Health Organization. 2004a. Cardiovascular disease: Prevention and control. www.who.int/dietphysicalactivity/publications/facts/cvd/en/.

World Health Organization. 2004b. Obesity and overweight. www.who.int/dietphysicalactivity/publications/facts/obesity.

Wright, J.D., Kennedy-Stephenson, J., Wang, C.Y., McDowell, M.A., and Johnson, C.L. 2004. Trends in intake of energy and macronutrients—United States, 1971-2000. *Morbidity and Mortality Weekly Report* 53(4): 80-82.

Yamanoto, K. 2002. Omron Institute of Life Science [personal communication].

Yee, A.J., Fuerst, T., Salamone, L., Visser, M., Dockrell, M., Van Loan, M., and Kern, M. 2001. Calibration and validation of an air-displacement plethysmography method for estimating percentage body fat in an elderly population: A comparison among compartmental models. *American Journal of Clinical Nutrition* 74: 637-642.

Yessis, M. 2003. Using free weights for stability training. *Fitness Management* 19(11): 26-28.

YMCA of the USA. 2000. *YMCA fitness testing and assessment manual.* 4th ed. Champaign, IL: Human Kinetics.

Yoke, M., and Kennedy, C. 2004. *Functional exercise progressions.* Monterey, CA: Healthy Learning.

Zamboni, M., Turcato, E., Armellini, F., Kahn, H.S., Zivelonghi, A., Santana, H., Bergamo-Andreis, I.A., and Bosello, O. 1998. Sagittal abdominal diameter as a practical predictor of visceral fat. *International Journal of Obesity and Related Metabolic Disorders* 22: 655-660.

Zatsiorsky, V.M. 1995. *Science and practice of strength training.* Champaign, IL: Human Kinetics.

Zeni, A.I., Hoffman, M.D., and Clifford, P.S. 1996. Energy expenditure with indoor exercise machines. *Journal of the American Medical Association* 275: 1424–1427.

Zhu, S., Heshka, S., Wang, Z., Shen, W., Allison, D.B., Ross, R., and Heymsfield, S.B. 2004. Combination of BMI and waist circumference for identifying cardiovascular risk factors in whites. *Obesity Research* 12: 633-645.

Zhu, S., Heymsfield, S.B., Toyoshima, H., Wang, Z., Petrobelli, A., and Heshka, S. 2005. Race-ethnicity-specific waist circumference cutoffs for identifying cardiovascular disease risk factors. *American Journal of Clinical Nutrition* 81: 409-415.

Zwiren, L., Freedson, P., Ward, A., Wilke, S., and Rippe, J. 1991. Estimation of $\dot{V}O_2$max: A comparative analysis of five exercise tests. *Research Quarterly for Exercise and Sport* 62: 73–78.

Index

About the Author

Vivian H. Heyward, PhD, is a Regents professor emerita, having taught physical fitness assessment and exercise prescription courses for 26 years at the University of New Mexico. In addition to the previous editions of this book, she has authored two editions of *Applied Body Composition Assessment* (Human Kinetics 1996, 2004) as well as numerous articles in research and professional journals dealing with various aspects of physical fitness assessment and exercise prescription. Dr. Heyward has received professional awards, including Distinguished Alumni Awards from the University of Illinois and the State University of New York at Cortland, and the SWACSM Recognition Award for distinguished professional service and achievement.

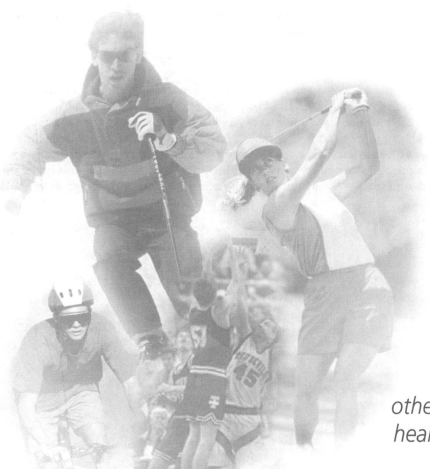

THE TIMES

A CENTURY IN

PHOTOGRAPHS

THE TIMES

A CENTURY IN

PHOTOGRAPHS

A PORTRAIT OF BRITAIN, 1900 - 1999

TIMES BOOKS
London

First published in 1999 by
Times Books
HarperCollins*Publishers*
77-85 Fulham Palace Road
London W6 8JB

British Library Cataloguing in Publication
Data:
A catalogue record for this book is available
from the British Library

Printed and bound in Great Britain by the
Bath Press Ltd

ISBN 0 7230 1082 X

Researched and written by
Joanna Hunter

Edited by
Richard Holledge
Associate Editor, *The Times*

Picture research
Tamsin Morse

Katie Baker
Mick Roffey

Picture editor
Andrew Moger

Historical consultant
Dr Michael Brock
University of Oxford

Design
Mabel Chan
Liz Brown
Kathy Gammon

Introduction

Photography, more than any other form of journalism, made 20th-century newspapers different from those that had gone before. When Queen Victoria ruled the waves, *The Times* could boast little more illustration than a "zincographic" black-and-white weather map in its grey columns of type. A hundred years later we can look back in our library at millions of powerful printed photographs. We can bring back instantly into our minds the days when Teddy Boys smoked outside the Trocadero, when stiff-capped nurses saluted the Coronation and horses vied with cars to be the best taxis in town. No words can do as much.

In planning this book we considered famous pictures of our time, Churchill acknowledging the cheers of victory on the balcony of Buckingham Palace in 1945 and the Prince and Princess of Wales on that same balcony on their wedding day in 1981. We included instead a weary Churchill picnicking on the 1945 election trail and a tentative Princess with the swans of the English National Ballet. None of these 100 images of the century, reprinted in *The Times* in 1999 to mark the century's end, is a recognised classic; but all are part of the story of ourselves; and all remind us in some small way of the years that we are leaving behind.

Peter Stothard
Editor
The Times

A poem without words

Philip Howard

L ook, stranger, at this island now. And then look back at it over the century of these pictures of each year since 1900. Photography is the most demotic of the arts. Almost anybody (except me) can take pictures. Everybody has access to cheap images of historic events. These photographs record the changing face of British society through the eyes of ordinary people and the lenses of their artisan artists, the photographers.

Great events such as world wars and national strikes are recorded here. But they are seen from the stalls, not the royal box. The children at a London street party celebrating George V's silver jubilee of 1935; Land Girls labouring in the mud of an English field; small boys playing in the ruins of a burnt-out car in Northern Ireland: these are pictures that take us under the skin of the country and the century. Many will remember with a gasp such images from our collective past. The evacuee children in baggy shorts, with rough-and-ready sacking backpacks, walking away from the camera and home to an uncertain future; the young girls sent into storms of various excitement by The Beatles. I find the boys sailing model yachts on the Round Pond in 1905 poignant. My earliest memories are of Kensington Gardens. And they still sail boats there on Sundays. Only the clothes of the sailors and the controls for steering the boats – by radio and microchip – have changed.

There have been huge changes in British society, culture and landscape down the century. One of the biggest has been in the art of photography itself. At the beginning of the century our recording angels, the snappers, were a handful of middle-aged men in suits deferentially holding small box-cameras, as though apologising for their presence. Today the scrum of photographers with their stepladders, Big Bertha lenses and recording booms for the television pictures dominate any public event. We scribblers who write the captions to go with their pictures call them "the monkeys". There may be irritation or jealousy in this professional insult. But the snappers' slogan, "a picture is worth a thousand words", is true.

These pictures tell the story of this century more vividly and economically than a dozen written histories. Great Aunt Fanny's photo album is usually more interesting than Great Aunt Fanny's diaries. And the potency of pictures ruled long before Fox Talbot started mucking about with chemicals at Lacock Abbey in order to print black-and-white pictures on paper. Van Dyck's portraits of the doomed court of Charles I show vivid causes of our Civil War inexpressible in words. The Romans had a proverb for the power of pictures: "Mutum est pictura poema" – a picture is a poem without words. At the beginning of their national epic, *The Aeneid*, the story of the birth of a nation, their greatest poet, Virgil, expressed the value of pictures. Aeneas and his refugees from Troy have been driven off course to Carthage in North Africa. He sets out with his friend Achates to explore this barbarian land. And in the great temple under construction, he discovers pictures of the Trojan War, from which they are the shipwrecked survivors. So he says: "Sunt lacrimae rerum et mentem mortalia tangunt" – Even here there are tears and men are moved by mortality.

Long before photography, *The Times* recognised the power of pictures. From its beginning the paper carried woodcuts of the latest fashions, ground plans of houses where there had been sensational murders, visionary schemes for garden cities, the plans of Nelson's catafalque and tomb. For Queen Victoria's diamond jubilee in 1897, we were the first newspaper to publish a colour plate of her. But it was Lord Northcliffe, "the Chief", who introduced photographs systematically in *The Times*, in the teeth of shellbacked opposition from staff and readers. He was lucky enough to find U.V. Bogaerde, a man skilled in the new technology of photography, an artist and somebody ready to try something new. Bogaerde's part in the press photography of this century was as dramatic as some of the parts that his son, Dirk Bogarde, played on screen. Bogaerde was installed in an iron birdcage in the basement of Printing House Square to experiment with mechanical screens and photogravure cameras. His work was so secret that only he and his assistant had keys to the photocage.

On March 1, 1922, the Chief decided to go ahead with his picture revolution at *The Times*. As usual, he did so in a theatrical way that would have excited the admiration of that artistic Emperor, Nero. He rang Bogaerde at eight in the morning and instructed him to prepare a full page of topical news pictures for publication in the next day's *Times*. The page proof, complete with captions, was to be submitted for approval to Lord Northcliffe at his house in Carlton House Gardens by midday. The proof was still wet, and Bogaerde was five minutes late. But the Chief approved, and ordered a full page of pictures in *The Times* every day from then on. Bogaerde obeyed orders (it was prudent to do so with the Chief) with the help of only one photographer and a printer.

That was how *The Times* started publishing those photographs of the changing English scene that caught the eye of artists as well as of the general reader. Roger Fry remarked that the pictures in *The Times* showed "the unerring sense of interval [i.e. spacing] that marked the work of great landscape artists". War, pestilence, famine and politics might rage on the news pages. On the picture page you could always be sure of finding a beautiful image of, say, swans on the Avon, steam trains puffing clouds or East Enders harvesting hops in Kent. Bogaerde's title of Art Editor was serious, not journalistic hyberbole.

The pictures in this book were commissioned, photographed and printed by these pioneers of popular photography. Today the art has expanded enormously. For any news event anywhere in the world we can summon immediately on screen a thousand images. Editors can select the picture that suits their story or prejudice. Modern techniques and superfluity offer readers far better pictures and choice of pictures faster than ever before. It is not just the English vice – nostalgia – that makes old pictures fascinate us more than tomorrow's. They are not just vivid records of our national and personal histories. They are part of them.

On choosing a picture

RICHARD HOLLEDGE

It was a word used rather too often as we trawled through the years: "great". That's a great photograph we'd say, as we swooped on a picture of respectable matrons supping tea from saucers or a French farmer pouring a glass of wine for a soldier from the Hampshire regiment near the D-Day beaches or a pair of Cambridge undergraduates in 1920 on pogo sticks. As the selectors of this collection of photographs, we reached for that inevitable shorthand of people making instinctive judgments: great. We could have chosen quirky, nostalgic, provoking, improbable, a complete Roget's Thesaurus of adjectives, but great helped us through the nigh-impossible task of picking 100 pictures to celebrate the century.

What, then, does make a photograph great? When you turn to the experts you get answers as varied as the number of adjectives we could have used. They are in agreement on one thing: it is, they say in unison, totally subjective. Take Colin Harding, the curator of photographic technology at the Bradford Museum of Film and Photography: "You can take a picture which is technically brilliant but which leaves you cold and unmoved, whereas something which is short on technique can sometimes touch a nerve which transcends its failings. Some of the great pictures give you a sense of what went before the shutter clicked and a feeling for what came after. What is also important is a sense of immediacy and reality."

Achieving a precise emotional effect is often essential to this process. "People have been playing with the image since 1839," says Harding. "Sometimes by overtly superimposing one image on another to achieve a particular effect but even without something as deliberate as that we have to remember that taking a picture is not merely a mechanical act. There is always a decision about what to include and what to leave out and in that sense it is not the camera that takes the picture but the photographer."

Hamish Crooks, the archive director at the picture agency Magnum says: "Photography was once about offering an objective truth, but now people know about manipulation and what we are often looking at is an individual interpretation of events. Photo essays are now not objective but subjective, for the photographer and the consumer. We still interpret photography by our own culture, there is no right or wrong. Photography is more widely used than ever before. With all the new technology it is easier to be a competent photographer now but to be very good takes as much hard work as it ever did. There are a lot of competent photographers but not many really good ones."

Mark Hayworth-Booth, the curator of photographs at the Victoria and Albert Museum, agrees: "There is no common denominator which defines what makes a good picture. If you gave someone a collection of English verse and asked which poems were the best you would have as many replies as there were individuals. Taking a good picture is very like writing; we can all do it some of the time, but we cannot do it well consistently."

Terence Pepper, the curator of photography at the National Portrait Gallery, is carefully vague on the definition of a good picture. "It has to do with the subject being interesting," he says, "and, of course, it is a matter of composition. The subject matter is critical and so too is the act of collaboration between the subject and the photographer. You need some sort of chemistry between them: it is as if the taking of the picture is a defining moment for them both."

For David Bailey, whose work covered the decades from the sixties, photography has replaced art. "The first half of the century belonged to Picasso. From 1973 it belonged to photography. Now that a private sale of Man Ray's work has gone for more than a million it is definitely art. When Picasso died we found a new way of seeing and photography was at the leading edge of that."

The immediacy, the tension, a sense of nostalgia and a need for knowledge plays a role in what makes a photograph compelling and that as much as, maybe more than, technique was persuasive in making this selection. In the process it became clear that it was easier to choose pictures with which we were not directly implicated. The further away in time and the less we knew, the clearer the vision. Much easier, for example, than choosing 100 of one's own family snaps.

Nowadays the ubiquity of the "happy snap" and the ease of using a camera has made the photograph not just the proof of the experience but the experience itself. Tourists use the camera or camcorder as a third eye. Instead of looking, they film. Within seconds of seeing a pride of lions on a safari holiday or the Duomo in Florence, you can play back the scene to reassure yourself that you were indeed there.

Sometimes you need not even be present. On a cruise off Alaska a couple who were too late to witness whales off the port side rushed to the on-board shop where a video of the scene was for sale. They simply videoed the video. To the folks back home in Kyoto it would have looked like the real thing. What we have in this book is absolutely the real thing. Not a video in sight.

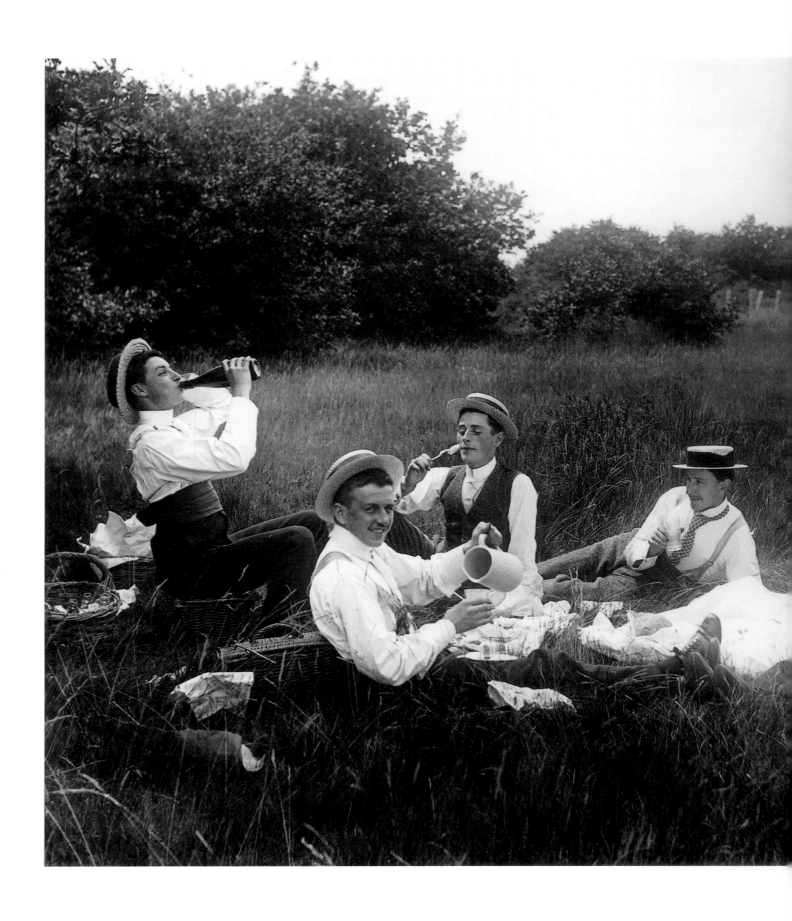

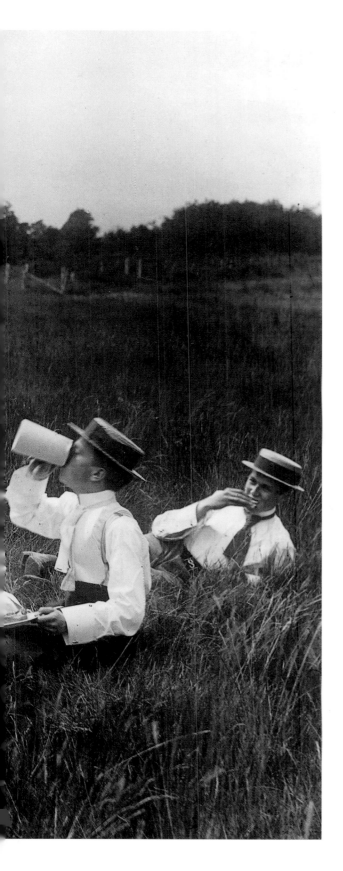

Boaters and ale as the century beckons

A group of shirtsleeved men enjoy a picnic in a field, drinking their ale from mugs or straight from the bottle as the Victorian era nears its end and a new century beckons. This picture was taken by Francis James Mortimer (1874–1944) who went on to become an influential photographer in Britain and editor of Amateur Photographer and Photograms of the Year. The photograph would have been taken with a technical camera using movements to correct for distortion and a magnesium powder flash.

Despite the informality of the occasion, the men in the photograph are all dressed in boaters, stiff collars and ties. This was typical of the decorum and propriety of the Victorian era. The group's confident manner reflects their status as members of the most powerful nation on earth. By 1900 the British Empire, the largest the world had known, was at its height, its rule encompassing India, Canada, Australasia, the British West Indies and vast areas of Africa, among them South Africa, Rhodesia, the Anglo-Egyptian Sudan, Nigeria and Sierra Leone. It was an era in which Europeans generally – and Britons above all – looked out upon the wider world confident that what they offered was civilization and technical progress. They saw the world in their own image.

Picnics were a French invention that evolved around the mid-18th century and harked back to an idealised pre-industrial bucolic lifestyle. In Britain, the world's first industrialised nation, which by 1900 had 80 per cent of its population living in towns, eating al fresco became the height of fashion, whatever the vagaries of the weather.

Also this year...

The Labour Representation Committee, forerunner of the Labour Party, is formed under Ramsay MacDonald

The first weekly long-distance bus service – a two-day journey between London and Leeds – begins

The "Tuppenny Tube" from Shepherd's Bush to Bank opens

Thousands die in an influenza epidemic

In Paris, British tennis player Charlotte Cooper becomes the first woman to win an Olympic title

Coca-Cola is introduced to the UK and proves instantly popular

Great celebrations in London when the sieges of Ladysmith and Mafeking are lifted by British forces in South Africa

Lady Elizabeth Bowes Lyon – the Queen Mother – is born.

Deaths: John Ruskin, Gottlieb Daimler, Fredrich Nietzsche

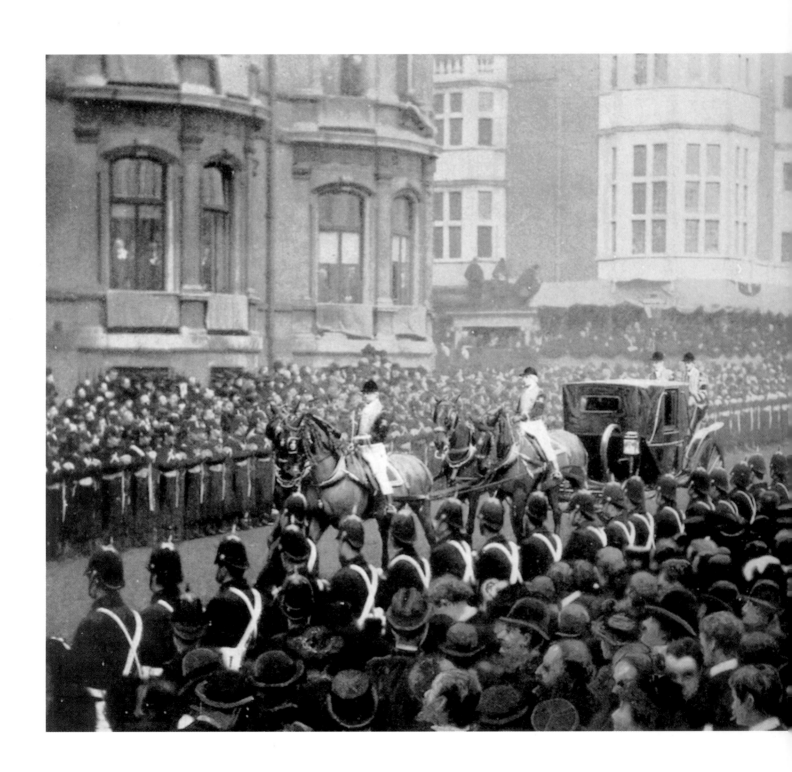

The death of Victoria and the end of an era

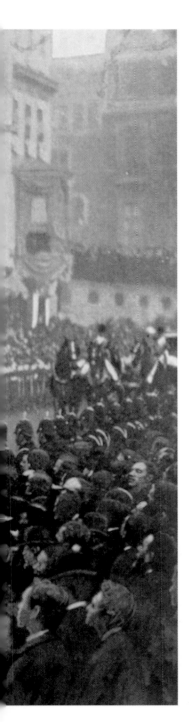

The nation mourns as Victoria, sovereign for nearly 64 years and Queen-Empress of the British Empire, is carried three and a half miles through the streets of London. The Queen, aged 82, died at Osborne, the royal residence on the Isle of Wight. King Edward VII decreed that her coffin be carried through London to allow the nation to pay its respects.

On Saturday, February 2, the body was taken by train from Portsmouth to Victoria Station. The procession travelled via The Mall, Piccadilly and Hyde Park to Paddington before being taken to Windsor by train. The roads were lined with what was believed to be the largest crowds seen in London; at Marble Arch and Albemarle Street the crowd was "dangerous in its mere mass". Nearly 40 princes attended the funeral, including the German Emperor, the Grand Duke Michael of Russia, and the kings of Greece, Portugal and the Belgians.

Memorial services were held at cathedrals and churches around the world. *The Times* reported from St Paul's Cathedral: "It was one of those occasions on which the Church of England shows itself even more than usual to be the true interpreter of the deepest feelings of English people. From the opening sentence ... all was perfectly attuned to the national mood of grief at the loss of a revered and beloved Sovereign; of gratitude for the benefits and blessings of that Sovereign's long and noble reign." After a service at St George's Chapel, Windsor, the Queen was buried two days later in the Royal Mausoleum at Frogmore, next to her late husband, Prince Albert.

Also this year...

Guglielmo Marconi transmits one of the earliest wireless messages, from Cornwall to Newfoundland

London's telephone system is completed

Electric trams introduced in London

The first diesel motor goes on show and the first British submarine is launched, at Barrow

British astronomers photograph a total eclipse of the Sun from Mauritius

The census reveals that the population of England and Wales has grown to 32,525,716, with the biggest increases in northern industrial towns and London suburbs

Deaths: Giuseppe Verdi, Henri Toulouse-Lautrec, former US presidents Benjamin Harrison and William McKinley

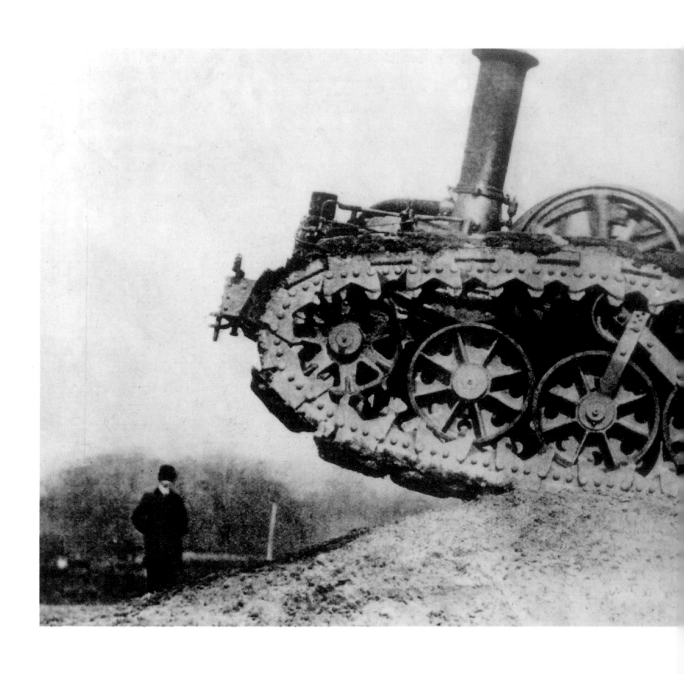

Clattering to a British revolution on the land

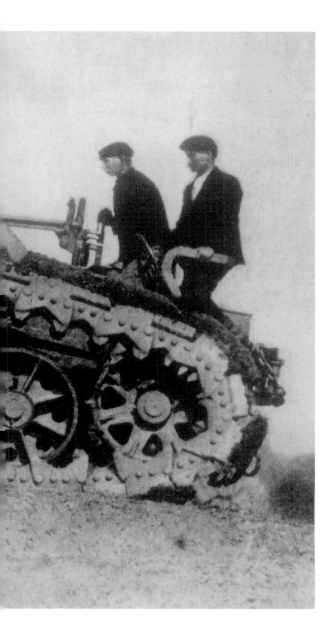

This caterpillar-track farm machine was built by the Lincolnshire-based company Rustin and Hornsby and was first used in the east of England. Machines such as this were the precursors of the modern tractor as well as of the tank. The caterpillar-track was in fact invented by Richard Edgeworth in 1770, with the American Holt Company later developing a tractor based on his design. Despite trials during the Crimean War it was not until the Killen-Strait Armoured Tractor was produced in 1915 that the caterpillar-track's full military potential was recognised and, using a design by Colonel Ernest Swinton, given the code name "tank".

In 1902, British agriculture had suffered two decades of severe depression. This had been brought about by dramatic improvements in shipping: as ships became larger, faster and cheaper to operate, so vast cargoes of wheats and other agricultural produce were imported into Britain. The advent of refrigerated ships increased the pressure on British farmers (the first refrigerated cargo reached London, from Australia, in 1880). But by the end of the 19th century, British agriculture began to see an equally dramatic transformation. Steam-driven machines had been first used on farms as early as the mid-19th century and although the earliest machines were cumbersome as well as less reliable and flexible than horses, the advantages of the new machinery soon became apparent. Unlike horses or oxen, tractors needed relatively little upkeep and required fewer men to operate them.

Machines may have eased the workers' burden but, as they gradually replaced the horse and cart, they also relieved them of their jobs. Smaller farms continued to rely on manual labour and there was seasonal work on the larger, richer estates, but many workers were forced to move to the towns and find jobs in trade and industry. Rural communities and traditions which had remained largely unchanged for centuries all but died out.

Also this year...

London's population reaches more than six and a half million

The army permits soldiers to wear spectacles

A state of emergency is declared in Ireland

The London School of Economics and Political Science is opened

The Imperial Vaccination League is founded

Edward VII crowned; 450,000 free dinners are given to the poor of London to mark the occasion

The 10th-century campanile in St Mark's Square in Venice collapses

Beatrix Potter's The Tale of Peter Rabbit *is published*

Deaths: Samuel Butler, Cecil Rhodes, Emile Zola, US jeweller Charles Tiffany

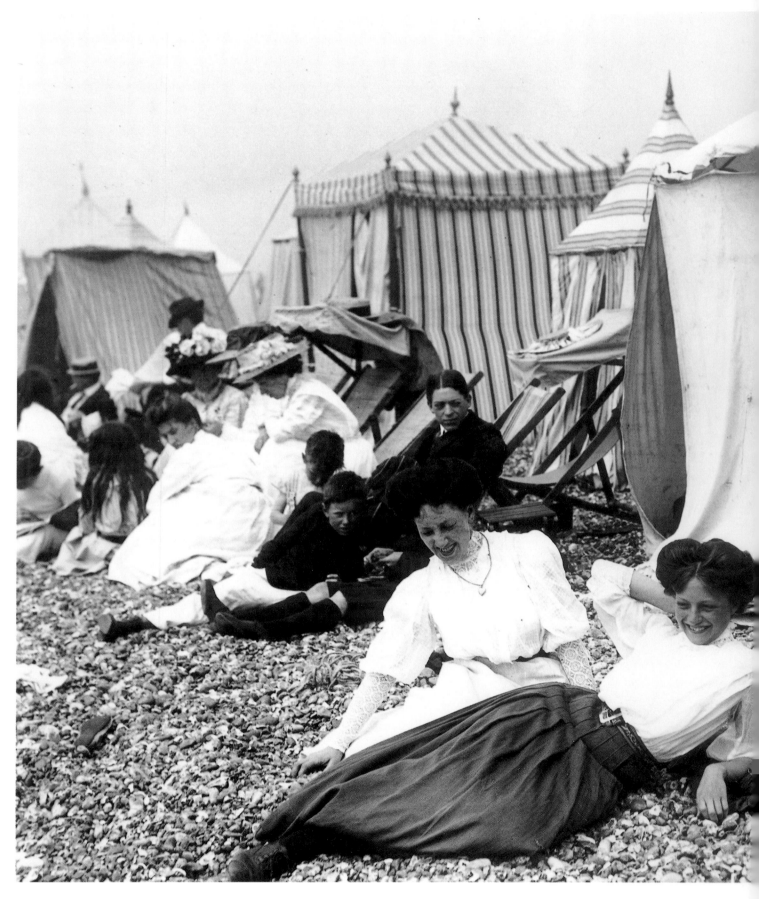

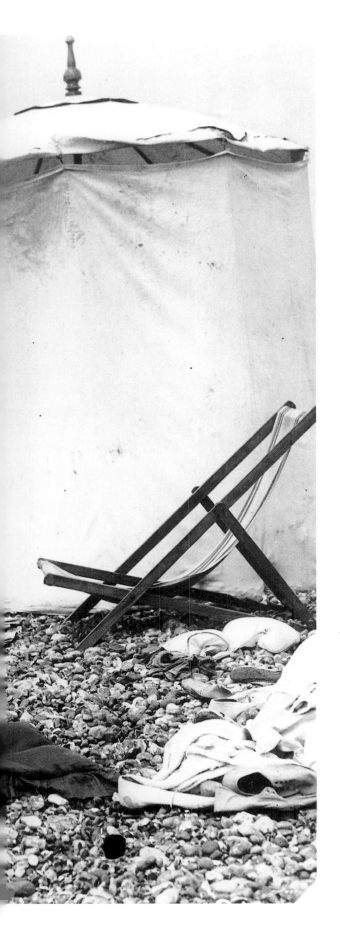

All dressed up for a day on the beach

The building of the railways and the introduction of bank holidays in 1871 allowed the middle and working classes greater mobility and leisure than ever before. Given the chance, Edwardian Britons liked nothing better than to be beside the sea. While foreign travel continued to be the preserve of the very rich, a couple of days at a domestic watering spot was a treat available to most British people. The beach was one of the few places where social classes mixed, but where you went spoke volumes about your social status: Brighton was traditionally the enclave of the aristocracy; Blackpool was regarded as downmarket. These women at Hove were on a better class of beach.

Bathers first flocked to the seaside for the sake of their health. In the 1750s Brighton-based Dr Russell declared that sea water could cure a broad range of ailments and the afflicted – and hypochondriacs – arrived in droves. While sea air was still regarded as beneficial for convalescents, most Edwardians took to the beach for more frivolous purposes. Piers, promenades, band stands and theatres were built to entertain them. Decorum demanded a certain modesty of dress but bathing was permitted – albeit strictly segregated. The beach hut offered an opportunity to protect one's modesty as well as to store a bucket and spade. Staying fully dressed also prevented holidaymakers from getting a tan – which was associated with outdoor manual work – and parasols were popular for keeping off the sun. However, as in the 19th century, nude bathing by men continued to be perfectly acceptable though not, of course, if there were women present.

Untreated and direct sewage disposal meant that bathers had to be of a determined disposition. British beaches have been much criticised in recent years but the sanitation at the turn of the century would have been far worse than it is now.

Also this year...

The Woman's Social and Political Union, headed by Emmeline Parkhurst, is formed

Letchworth becomes Britain's first "garden city"

Edward VII is made Emperor of India

A royal commission is set up to look into controlling traffic congestion

The Wright brothers make their first flight

The Ford Motor Company sells its first car

Deaths: Robert Cecil, Camille Pissarro, Paul Gaugin, James McNeill Whistler, inventor of the machine-gun Richard Gatling

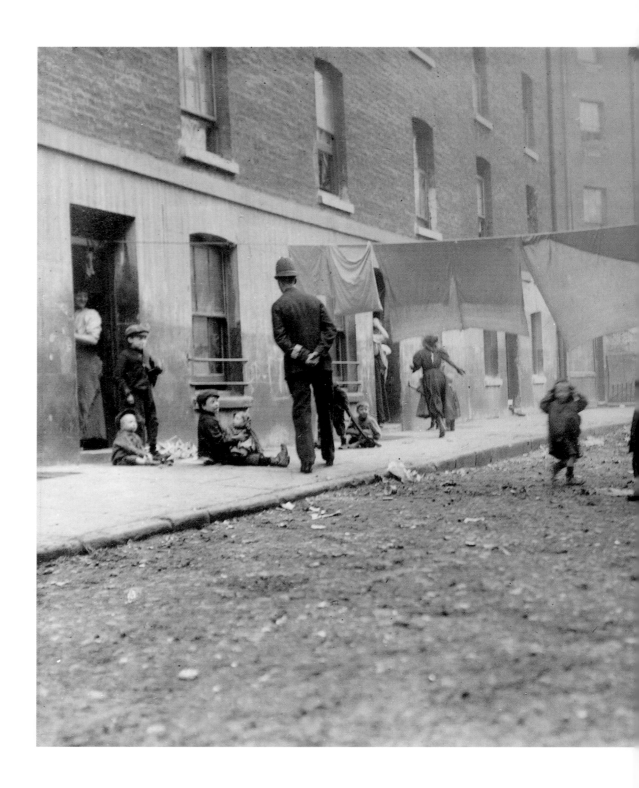

Squalor and suffering in the heart of London

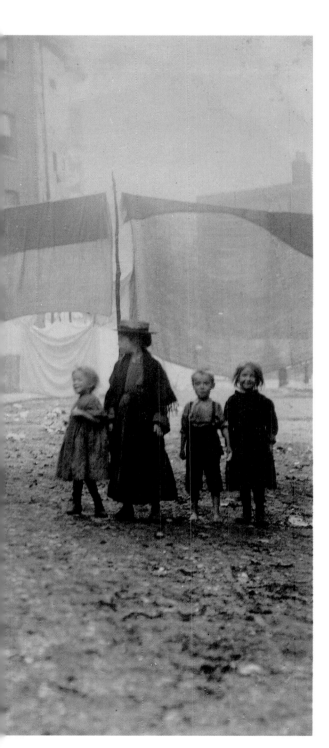

This side street off the Gray's Inn Road in central London was among the most squalid and deprived in London. It had reached such a pitch of poverty that it was disowned by two parishes, Holborn and Clerkenwell, with the result that it enjoyed no charity relief. The washing hanging up to dry may have been clean, but mud, stagnant water and general waste lay in the road. The lone policeman pictured here was braver than most – policemen generally went down the road in pairs during the day and in threes after dark.

According to figures released at the end of November this year, more than 122,000 people in London and up to 800,000 in England and Wales were receiving Poor Relief. While a fortunate few made their millions out of trade and empire, a larger section of society lived in abject poverty. Conditions in inner cities were generally considered to be the worst, with those in east and northeast of England identified as particularly deprived. Overcrowding and poor sanitation meant that disease spread quickly. Life expectancy was much shorter than today's and infant mortality correspondingly high. With little formal state support available, many people had to look to charity – often supplied by the local parish – to support them.

The last resort was the workhouse. In October 1904 an estimated 250,000 people were receiving "indoor relief". Workhouses operated on the principle that while they would cater for able-bodied poor people of working age, they in turn were to find life in the workhouse less attractive than almost any work for wages. Conditions in them were such that the following year the government established a Royal Commission to investigate the whole question of Poor Relief.

Also this year...

A freak tidal wave hits the south coast and washes away six houses in Halisands, Devon

Richmond Royal Park is opened to the public

The first attempt at talking pictures at Fulham Theatre, London

Britain and France sign the entente cordiale

London's first electric Underground train is put into service

A weather forecast from the Atlantic is transmitted by radio for the first time

A postcard craze sweeps the nation

James Barrie's Peter Pan opens

The Trans-Siberian railway is completed

Deaths: Sir Henry Morton Stanley, Anton Chekov, Theodor Herzl, Paul Kruger

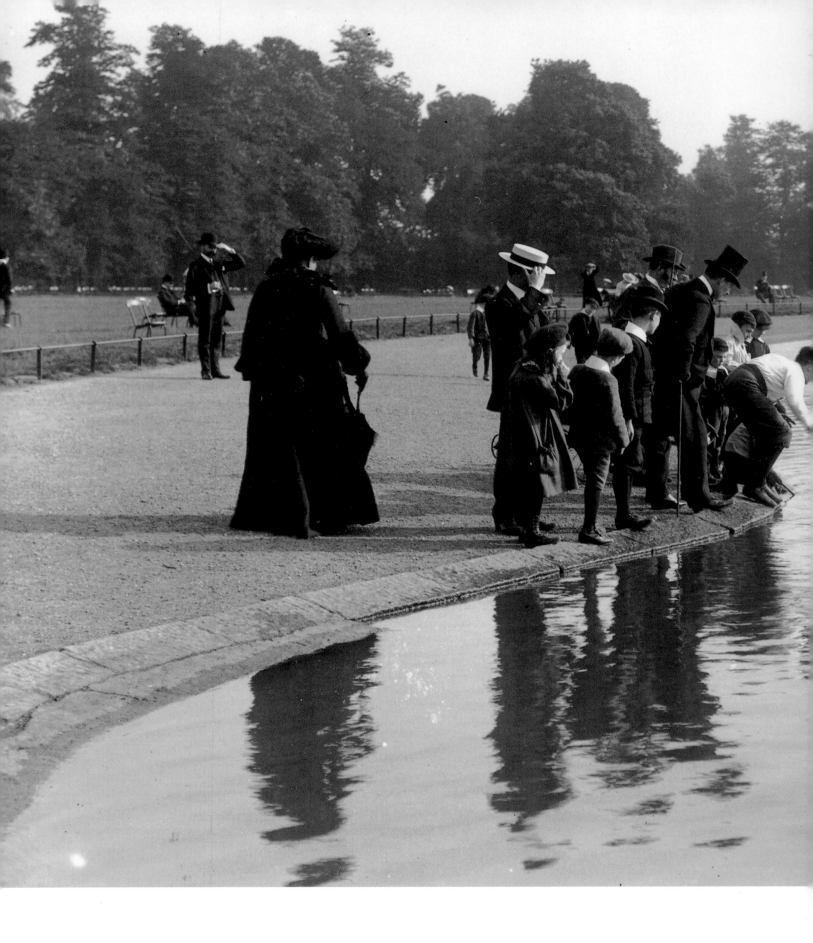

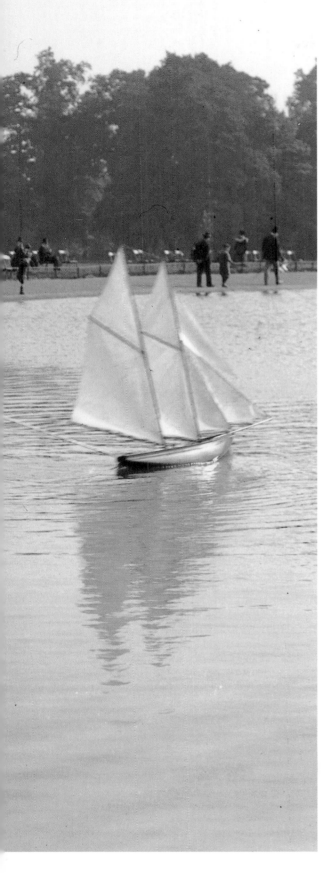

When Britannia ruled the waves

1905 saw the commissioning of HMS *Dreadnought*, the most advanced and destructive battleship of what still the world's largest and most powerful navy. But while the Royal Navy patrolled the seas, maintaining the Empire and enforcing the Pax Britannica, many Edwardians pursued water pursuits of a rather more modest nature. The group pictured here were sailing their boat on the Round Pond in Kensington Gardens.

Public parks were extremely popular in Edwardian Britain, providing natural retreats in the country's burgeoning cities, with many boasting outdoor theatres, bandstands, ice-skating rinks and boating ponds, even in some cases zoos. By Edwardian times, parks were maintained by local councils. From 1846, park-keepers had had the status of special constable, many exercising a strict hold over their domains. In some parks, visitors were not only banned from shooting but were not permitted to dance, skip, leapfrog, wash dogs in the pond, beat carpets or, of course, walk on the grass.

This picture, like the first in this book, was taken by F. J. Mortimer. The eye is naturally drawn to the boat, something that demonstrates Mortimer's familiarity with the traditional rules of painting – here that of the golden sector, which leads the eye two-thirds across and two-thirds down the picture. The photograph also appears as if were taken from the water, and is an example of how photographers in this period began to seek to compose their shots artistically as well as to document events.

Also this year...

A typhus outbreak is recorded in the east of London

Mining disasters kill 56 in south Wales

Albert Einstein publishes his General Theory of Relativity

The Automobile Association is founded

Government research suggests that the tedium of country life has apparently led to an increase in rural lunacy figures

The suffragettes Christabel Pankhurst and Annie Kenney are sent to prison

Up to 1,000 Jews are massacred in Odessa, in the Russian Empire

The Norwegian Roald Amundsen reaches the magnetic North Pole

Deaths: Dr Thomas Barnardo, founder of 112 institutes for homeless children, Jules Verne, Sir Henry Irving

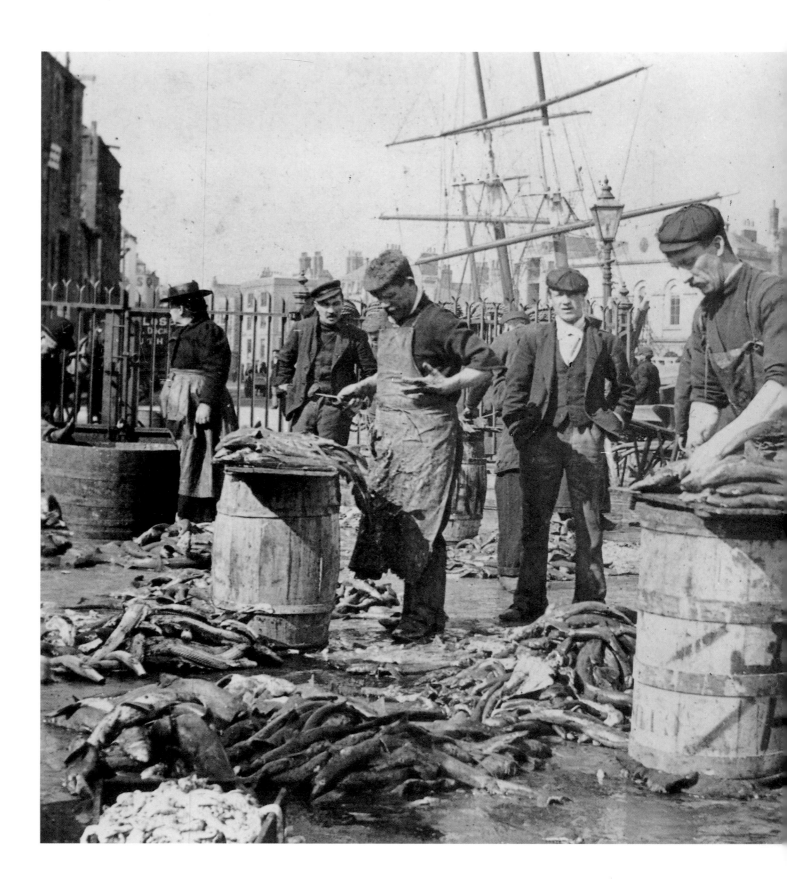

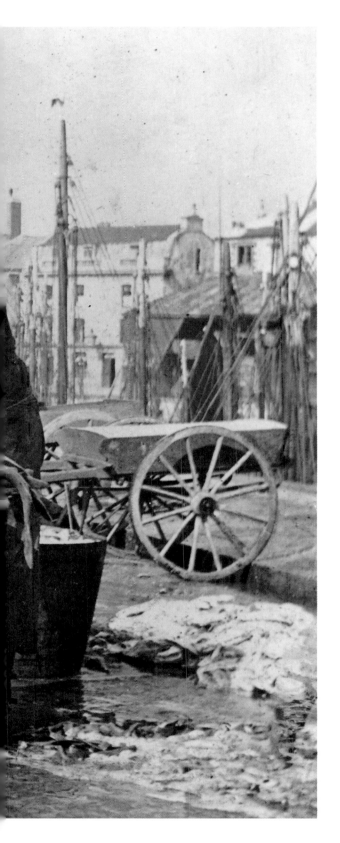

Struggling to make a living from the sea

Fishermen in Plymouth skin their catch of dogfish – often more appetisingly sold as rock salmon. Other popular catches of the time included sole, halibut, plaice, haddock and cod. Herrings and oysters were particularly popular, not least because, at a farthing each, they were very cheap.

Industrialisation by the late 19th century – and hence pollution – meant that the nation's stock of freshwater fish had been substantially reduced. As a result, the demand for sea-water fish increased enormously. Ironically it was one of the great developments of the industrial age that allowed the shortfall to be covered – the railways improved distribution dramatically. The introduction of steam trawlers in the late 19th century also allowed fishermen access to wider fishing grounds.

The fishing industry was the responsibility of the Board of Trade. Workers' welfare and discipline, shipwrecks and casualties, even the signing on of crews came under its remit. The Board of Agriculture and Fisheries, which took over some of these responsibilities in 1903, was in charge of scientific investigation, principally the maintenance of fish stocks.

While advances in technology and growing trade meant that for some sections of the population standards of living were improving, life still offered little more than bare survival for many. According to David Lloyd George – the great social reformer and future Prime Minister, who in 1906 was President of the Board of Trade – an estimated ten million workers were living in chronic destitution, despite living in the richest country in the world.

Also this year...

The Liberals win a landslide general election victory

China signs a treaty ceding control of all roads to Tibet to the British

Mount Vesuvius erupts, and hundreds of people die

The Russian parliament, the Duma, dissolved by the tsar

In America, William S. Kellogg forms the Battle Creek Toasted Corn Flake Company to make cereal as part of a new therapy for mental patients

Algeciras Conference averts European war over Morocco

San Francisco earthquake kills 1,000 and devastates the city

Olympic Games held in Athens (not subsequently recognised as official Olympiad)

SOS message becomes international distress call

Deaths: Henrik Ibsen, French historian Albert Sorel, Paul Cézanne, Pierre Curie

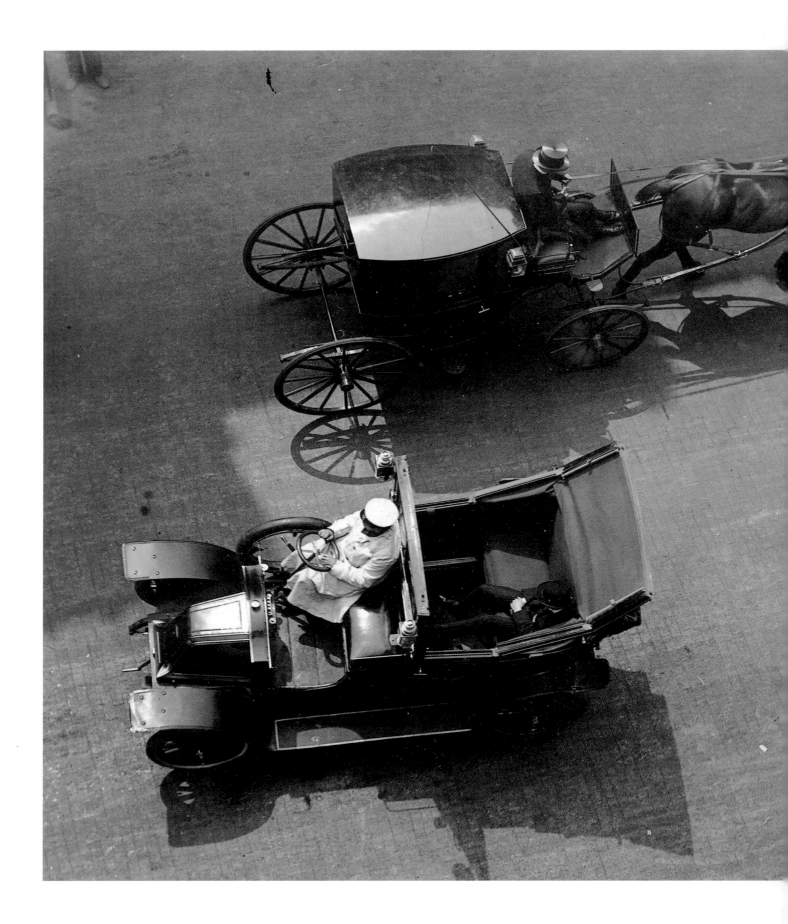

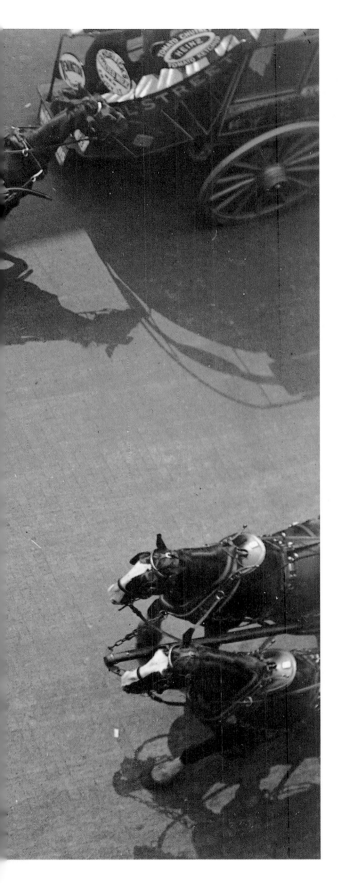

Wheels turn in the hunt for cheap transport

A motorised taxi passes a "growler", a four-wheeled, four-seater horse-driven cab at a time when the battle between horse and motor was at its height. Until the late 19th century, private transport was the domain of the rich – those who had their own carriages or could afford a hackney cab. But if only the rich could afford to travel in such style, public transport, introduced from 1831, had already revolutionised the lives of the middle and working classes. At a penny a mile, trams were seen as the people's transport, and were half the price of buses. Cheaper fares also enabled workers to commute and move to cheaper and better accommodation in the suburbs.

In 1900 there were 50,000 horses being used for transport in London. Horse-drawn taxis had been introduced to Britain from France. The name cab is derived from *cabriolet*, a leading model in the late 19th century. The main advantage of the growler, such as the one pictured here, was space: four seats and plenty of room for luggage. It was for this reason that growlers traditionally carried passengers between London's mainline rail stations.

London had seen its first motorised cab in 1903; by 1907 there were 723. The motor car did not immediately endear itself to the population. Cars were regarded as noisy and dangerous, despite the 1903 Motor Car Act which laid down a top speed of only 20 mph. But the triumph of the combustion engine had about it an inevitability. By 1914 there were 132,000 privately owned cars in Britain.

But whether travelling by horse or car, city transport was hardly less congested than today. In addition, there was little lane discipline, vast amounts of horse manure made the streets unpleasant and sometimes dangerous and it was only after 1934 that drivers were required to taking driving or eyesight tests.

Also this year...

The Boy Scouts are created and taken on their first group camp by Baden Powell

The Criminal Courts of Justice open at the Old Bailey in London

New Zealand gains autonomy within the British Empire

Rudyard Kipling becomes the first British writer to be awarded the Nobel Prize for Literature

James Thompson, from Clare, Ulster, gets out of bed after 29 years

Frenchman Paul Cornu builds and flies the world's first helicopter

Deaths: Edvard Grieg, J.K. Huysmans, Times *war correspondent Sir William Howard Russell*

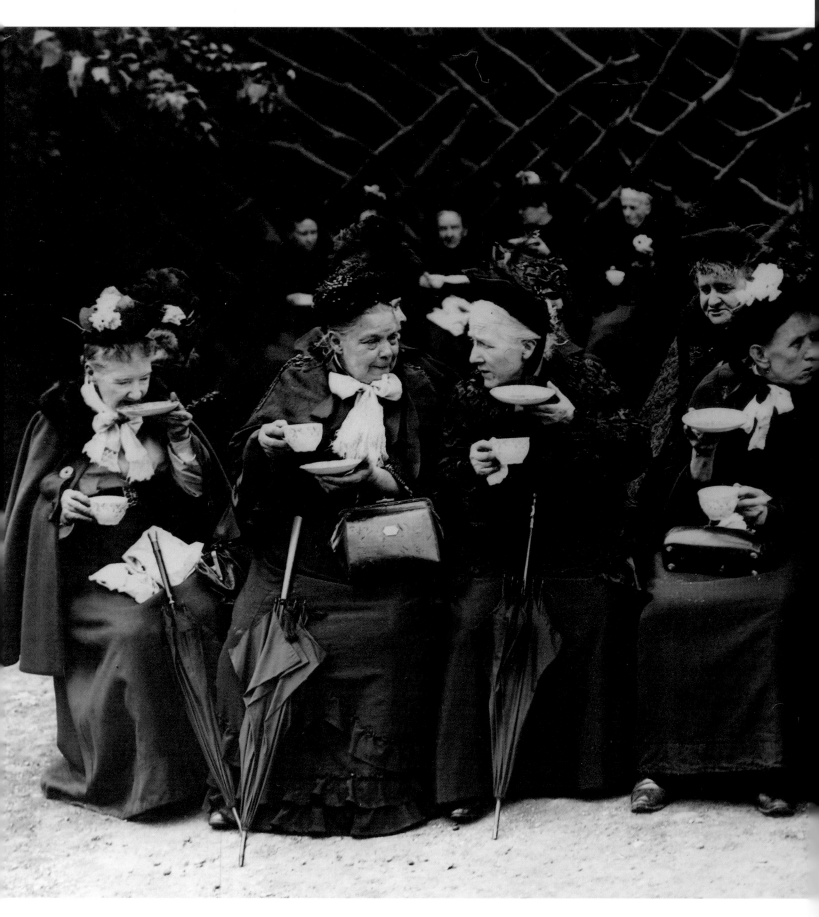

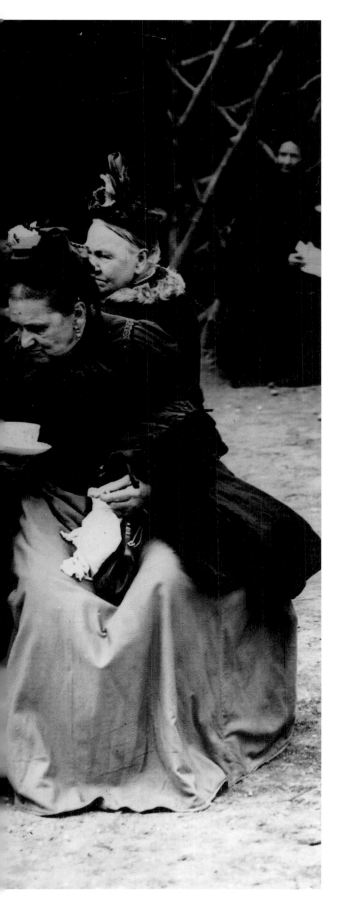

When everything stopped for tea

These women enjoying a cup of tea, and supping enthusiastically from saucers, were doing so in a good cause. They were attending a fundraising day, in June, at Loughton, near Epping Forest in Essex, organised by the Fresh Air Fund and the Ragged School Union. These charities gave children from east London the chance of a day in the country, taking up to 1,000 children away from the city's smoke and grime every day in summer. The women, apparently in their best clothes, may have been at Epping at the same time as the Prince and Princess of Wales, who visited on June 12. The future George V was one of the Fresh Air Fund's most generous benefactors.

The fashion for taking afternoon tea was reputedly started by Anna, 7th Duchess of Bedford, in the early 19th century, who, it was said, was too hungry to wait for dinner. For those at work all day, tea-time offered a chance for family togetherness. Tea itself had become known in Europe towards the end of the 16th century. In 17th-century England it rapidly became fashionable in court circles while from the early 18th century it began to enjoy wide popularity in the country at large. By the end of the 19th century Britain was importing 220 million lbs of tea a year and the average Briton drank about 6 lbs a year. In the Edwardian era tea was firmly established as the drink of the masses. The tea-bag was introduced in 1908.

Extravagant claims had originally made for the medicinal properties of tea – for example, that it was effective against diseases such as cholera. Even at the time that this photograph was taken, it was still claimed that tea could rid you of bad dreams, strengthen your bones, or act as a decongestant – even as an aphrodisiac.

Also this year...

The Children's Act forbids adults to allow children to smoke

Pit explosions kill ten miners in Somerset and 73 in Lancashire

The old-age pension is introduced for over-70s

The Olympics are held at White City in London

A new harbour opened at Dover

Asquith, the Prime Minister, introduces emergency measures to combat high unemployment

Professor Ernest Rutherford is awarded the Nobel Prize for Chemistry for his work on radioactivity and the atom

Deaths: Sir Henry Campbell-Bannerman, Stephen Grover Cleveland, Nikolai Rimsky-Korsakov

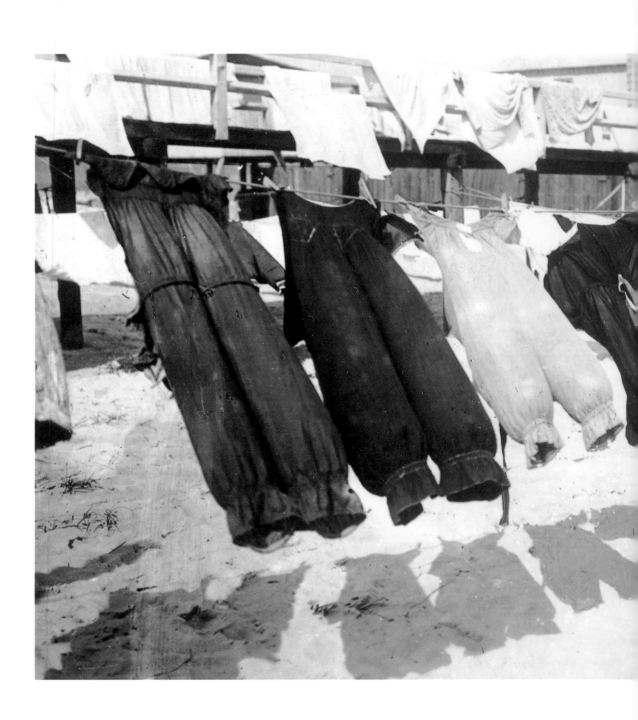

We do like to bloom beside the seaside

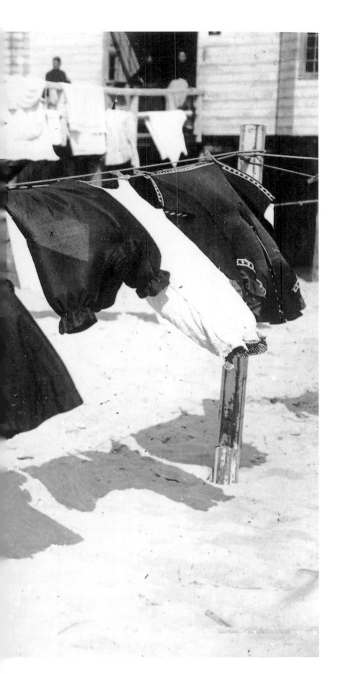

These bloomers hanging out to dry on a beach are in fact ladies' swimming costumes. On the beaches of Edwardian Britain, women were expected to keep well-covered from mid-calf upwards, whether sporting an all-in-one bathing costume or below-the-knee dress and bloomers. Men's swimming costumes were equally demure, although men were only required to cover up from the knees. Striped costumes were very popular.

"Bloomers" were named after Amelia Jenks Bloomer, a mid-19th century American campaigner for women's rights whose concerns included dress reform. Where Victorian fashion depended heavily on the corset, often worn so tight that it could cause physical deformities such as crooked spines and distorted kidneys, Amelia Bloomer advocated "rational dress": a short jacket, a skirt to below the knee and baggy, full-length trousers that gathered in at the ankle – bloomers. But in Britain, both Bloomer and the attire she advocated met with scorn and ridicule; nor did the English Rational Dress Society, which campaigned for sensible clothing, fare much better in the 1880s.

Edwardian women favoured long, full skirts with nipped-in waists. By 1910 the very narrow "hobble" skirt – so-called because of the way it made the wearer walk – was the height of fashion. Female sporting endeavours were far from encouraged – Pierre de Coubertin, founder of the modern Olympics, declared: "Women have but one task, that of the role of crowning the victor with garlands." However, women gradually infiltrated what had been male preserves, with cycling and tennis emerging as the most popular sports. But despite the obvious advantages of wearing bloomers or such-like on the playing fields, most British sportswomen kept to their corsets and wide, long skirts up to the First World War.

Also this year...

A court rules that a wife may not divorce her husband, even if he deserts her

The Victoria and Albert Museum is opened by Edward VII

Louis Blériot makes the first crossing of the Channel in an airplane

26 miners die in a South Wales pit explosion

Imprisoned suffragettes claim they have been force-fed

Selfridge's opens for business

The claim by US explorer Frederick Cook to have reached the North Pole is shown to be fake

Deaths: Apache Indian chief Geronimo, George Meredith, Algernon Charles Swinburne, John Millington Synge

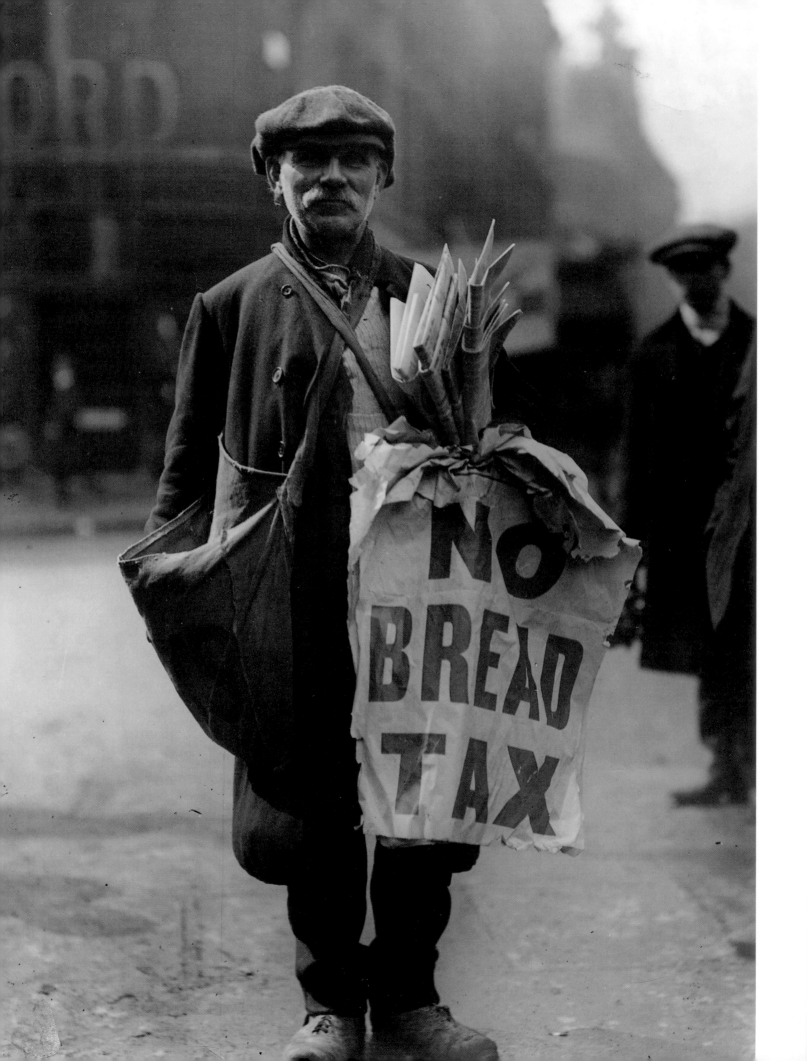

Taking to the streets to sell food and ideas

A newspaper seller plies his wares on the streets. Many salesmen and women couldn't afford shop rents, and the streets were lined with people selling, among much else, flowers, food, drinks and toys. Newspapers were the prime source of news until the general introduction of radio and, later, television. They were also cheap: in 1910 a copy of *The Times* cost 3d.

The headline on the newspaper seller's bag was a slogan of the ruling Liberal Party. 1910 was among the most tempestuous political years of the century, with two general elections, in January and December. The key issues of the day – free trade and the position of the House of Lords – deeply divided the two principal parties: the Liberals, led by H.H. Asquith; and the Conservatives, led by Bonar Law.

The arguments over free trade stemmed from a Conservative campaign for tariffs on imported goods, with wheat from the United States, on which Britain largely depended for cheap bread, a particular target. The Liberals, by contrast, argued forcefully in favour of free trade, largely for fear that British import tariffs would lead to retaliation in kind by countries importing goods from Britain, hence the Liberal slogan, No Bread Tax.

The question of the House of Lords was equally contentious. In 1909, the Lords had refused to pass Lloyd George's Budget, which introduced a nascent welfare state, and in so doing had acted illegally in the view of the Liberals who accordingly sought to abolish their right of veto. It was a move fiercely opposed by the Conservatives, not merely as an attack on the hereditary principle but because they feared it would allow the Liberals to push through Home Rule for Ireland, a measure the Lords could be relied upon to reject. In the event, neither party won an overall majority in either election. The Liberals nonetheless managed to retain their tenuous grip on office, buttressed by the support of the infant Labour Party and the Irish Nationalists.

Also this year...

Dr Crippen is sentenced to death for poisoning his wife

The first 80 labour exchanges are opened

The Girl Guides are founded

Talking pictures pioneered by Thomas Edison

Mount Etna erupts

Over 100,000 dockers sacked; 10,000 Welsh miners strike in sympathy; troops are sent in to maintain order

Halley's comet is visible

Deaths: Florence Nightingale Edward VII, Mark Twain, Count Leo Tolstoy

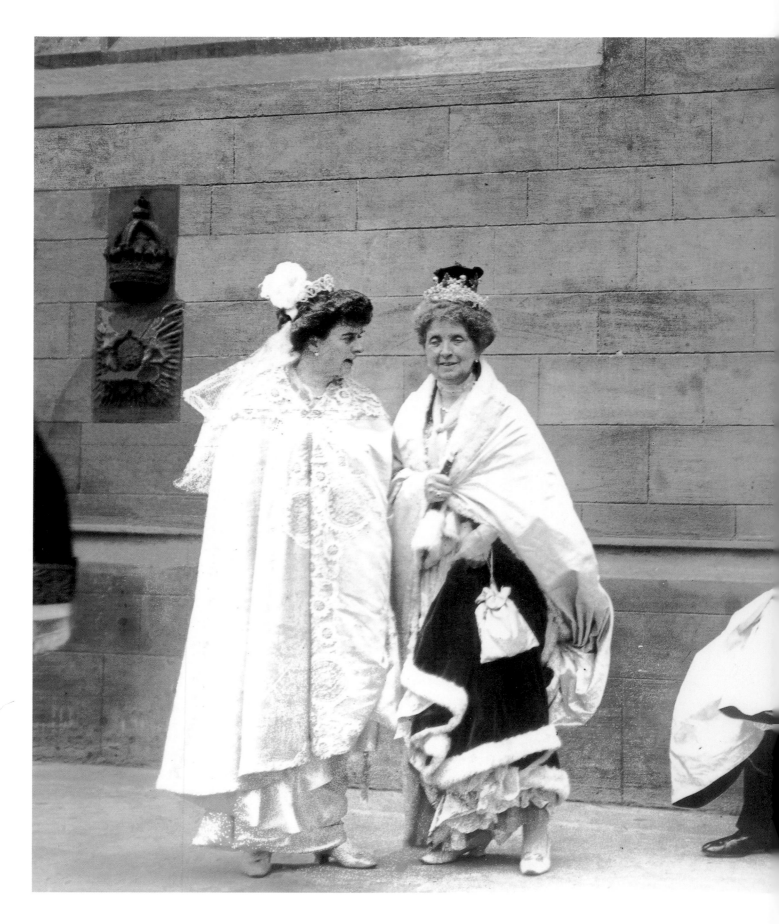

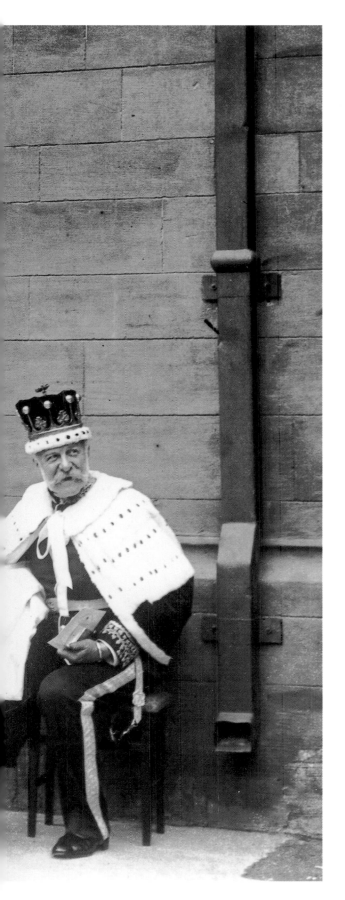

Peers and people celebrate the new King

George V's coronation ceremony, on Thursday, June 22, took seven hours. Perhaps it is hardly suprising that this peer looked somewhat fatigued, though the ladies seem to be bearing up with greater fortitude.

The new monarch's title was "King of the United Kingdom of Great Britain and Ireland and of the British Dominions beyond the seas, Defender of the Faith, Emperor of India". The coronation was attended by princes and representatives of the Empire but the next day, when the King and Queen took to the streets in an open carriage to present themselves to the people of London, was dubbed "the people's day".

The Times reported: "Such ceremonies have an undeniable power to knit the sympathies of the masses of the nation to the occupants of the Throne and it cannot be doubted that many thousands of Londoners and visitors to London who viewed yesterday's Procession will feel a warmer personal attachment to their Majesties for the future."

It looked like rain, and there was an occasional shower, but the King and Queen seemed to be accompanied by an almost unwavering sun-burst as they travelled their seven-mile route. The King accepted five addresses of loyalty from the people and a welcome to the City from the Lord Mayor of London at Temple Bar. There was some embarrassment when it was felt that not all the foreign dignitaries responded to the Mayor's greeting with the respect that it was due. Afterwards the King and Queen, accompanied by Field-Marshal Lord Roberts and a number of Indian Maharajahs and officers were given an enthusiastic welcome by the crowd. The King also gave a Coronation fête at Crystal Palace for 100,000 of the capital's children before travelling to Edinburgh.

Also this year...

Three anarchists die in the siege of Sidney Street in London's East End after a gun battle with over 1,000 troops

The Shops Act, entitling shopworkers to a mandatory half-day, is passed

Nine people are killed in Llanelli, south Wales, during riots

The hottest day for 70 years – 97 Fahrenheit – is recorded in London while across the country 2,500 children die in the heatwave

The House of Lords gives up right of veto

More than 200 suffragettes jailed

Roald Amundsen reaches the South Pole

The Mona Lisa is stolen from the Louvre

Deaths: Gustav Mahler, American temperance campaigner Carry Nation, Sir William Gilbert, American journalist Joseph Pulitzer

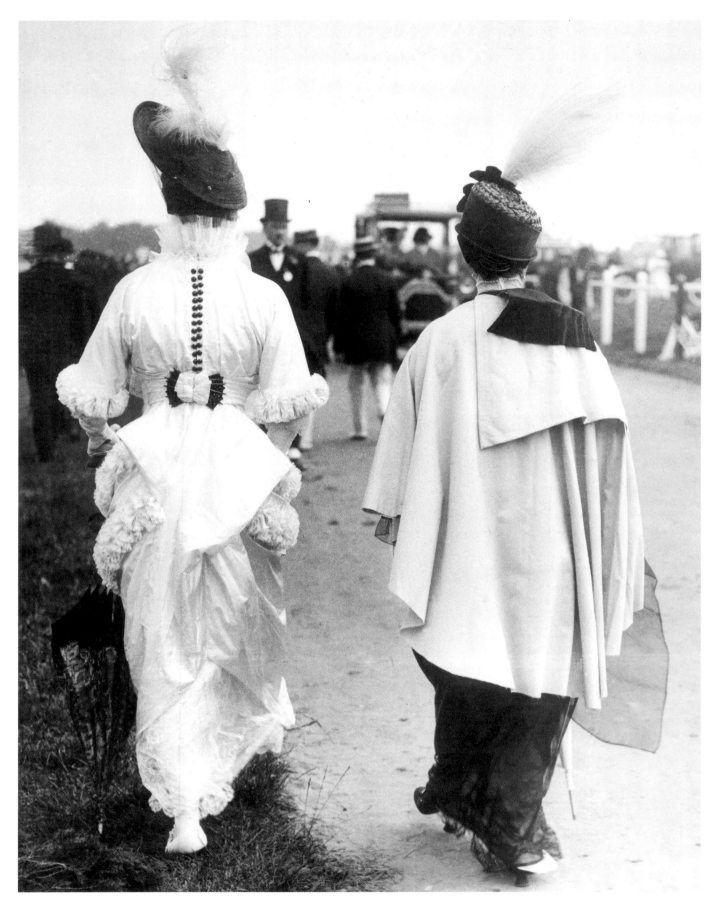

Ascot parades in hats and ironed laces

Queen Anne built the first racecourse at Ascot, in 1711. A century later, George IV ordered the Royal Enclosure to be built, but it was Edward VII, a passionate racegoer, who really made Ascot a fashionable event. (After his death in 1910, Ascot racegoers wore black in mourning for the King.) Entrance to the Royal Enclosure, itself an extension of the Court, was strictly by invitation only. As late as the early 1960s, divorcees were refused entrance. Today, only those with a known prison record or undischarged bankrupts are barred – or those who are inappropriately dressed.

The competition for suitably flamboyant hats was as fierce at Ascot in 1912 as it is today. Racegoers were expected to wear "formal daywear", which probably included hats for both sexes and full-length dresses for women, as in the photograph. However, not all guests had sartorial standards as high as those of Lieutenant-Colonel Sir Gordon Carter – appointed Clerk of the Course in 1911 – who had his shoelaces ironed every day.

The introduction of a hot water apparatus meant that 1912 was the first year when there were no complaints about the lack of hot water for making tea. It was something of a mixed blessing, however: the machine caused a small fire in May. But not everybody went to the races for toffs and tea. Racing was popular with all classes, not least for the chance to gamble. Under the 1853 Betting Houses Act, and until the Tote was legalised in 1928, gambling on horses was legal only at racecourses.

Also this year...

Captain Scott's party reach the South Pole to discover they have been beaten by Roald Amundsen; all die on the trek home

Ulster Unionists sign a covenant against Irish Home Rule

A record low temperature of -35 Fahrenheit recorded in the United Kingdom

More than 120 suffragettes are arrested after rioting in London

The Titanic sinks on her maiden voyage

A transport strike brings Britain to a halt

The voting age is set at 21 for men

Foot-and-mouth outbreaks across the country

The first fatal accident on London's Underground kills 22

The first British film censor is appointed

Deaths: Wilbur Wright, William Booth, founder of the Salvation Army, French composer Jules Massenet

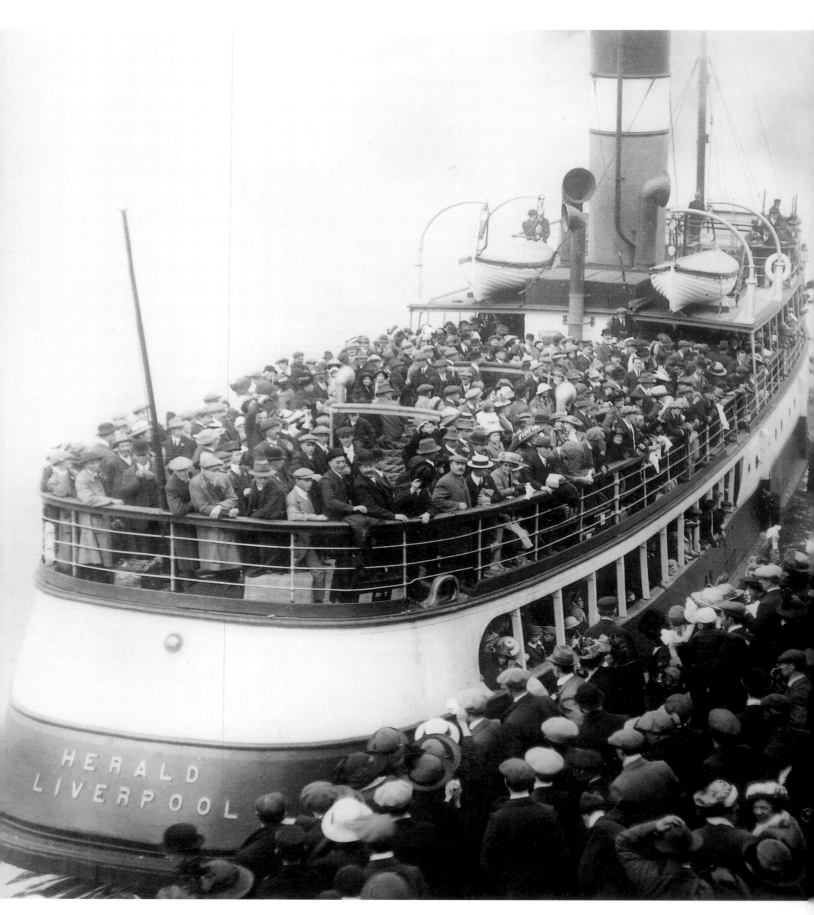

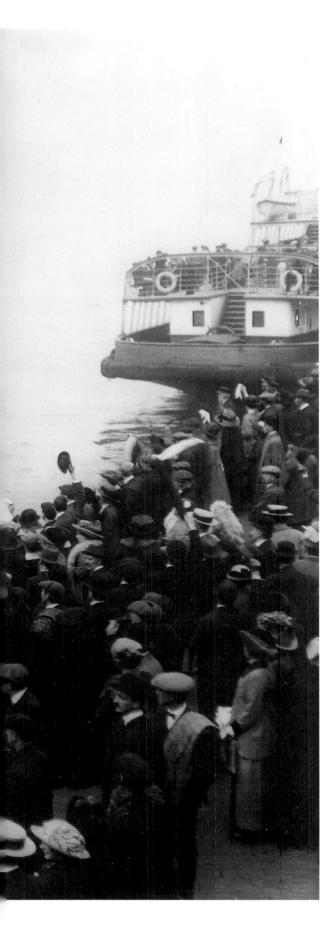

Setting sail for a better life a world away

The tender *Herald*, packed with hopeful emigrants to Australia, leaves a Liverpool landing stage for the passenger ship *Zealandic* anchored off-shore. The *Zealandic* was owned by the White Star Line, the same company which owned the doomed *Titanic*. Launched in 1911, the ship voyaged between Liverpool and Wellington, New Zealand, before being chartered by the Western Australian government as an immigrant carrier.

Until 1830, the majority of Australia's immigrants were convicts. However, by 1913 most emigrants travelled to Australia as part of a state-supported scheme. The Australian Immigration Restriction Act of 1901 allowed the Australian government to limit immigration almost entirely to Europeans; the 1911 Australian census showed that of the country's 4.4 million population, only 1.8 per cent were of non-British European extraction. Aborigines were not included in the census. British emigrants were encouraged by the offer of agricultural land, though on arrival many discovered that the land allotted to them was small and unyielding. The scheme caused trouble at home and in Australia: the British government thought the Australian immigration information was suspect, while Australian trade unions opposed the scheme, fearing it would lead to higher unemployment.

Many British immigrants returned home. Of the 237,000 people who emigrated to Victoria between 1901 and 1914, 182,000 made the long journey back to Britain. Immigration was halted during the First World War.

Also this year...

The National Insurance Act introduces maternity and sick benefits

The House of Lords twice rejects the Home Rule Bill

Emmeline and Sylvia Pankhurst are sent to prison; suffragette Emily Davidson dies after throwing herself under the King's horse at the Derby; the "Cat and Mouse" Act is passed, allowing the release and re-imprisonment of suffragettes on hunger strike; the first female JP, Emily Dawson, is appointed

Henry Ford opens the first moving assembly line in Michigan

D.H.Lawrence's Sons and Lovers *is published*

Mahatma Gandhi is jailed in South Africa for his part in the anti-British movement

In Los Angeles, Georgina Broadwick becomes the first woman to make a parachute jump

Deaths: German engineer Rudolf Diesel, J. Pierpoint Morgan, legendary American anti-slavery campaigner Harriet Tubman

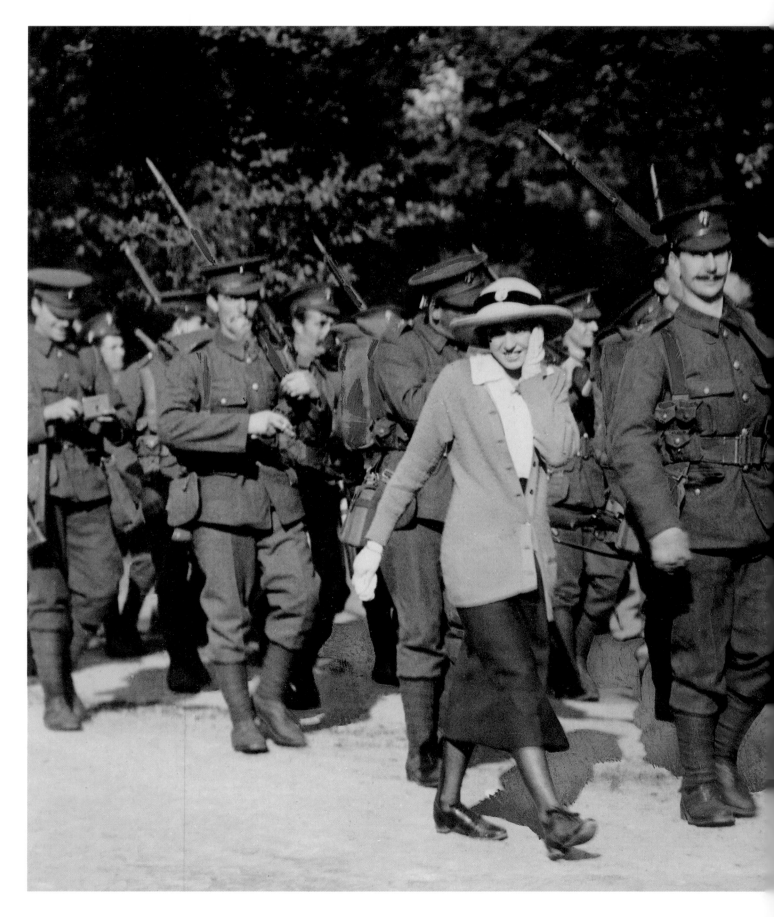

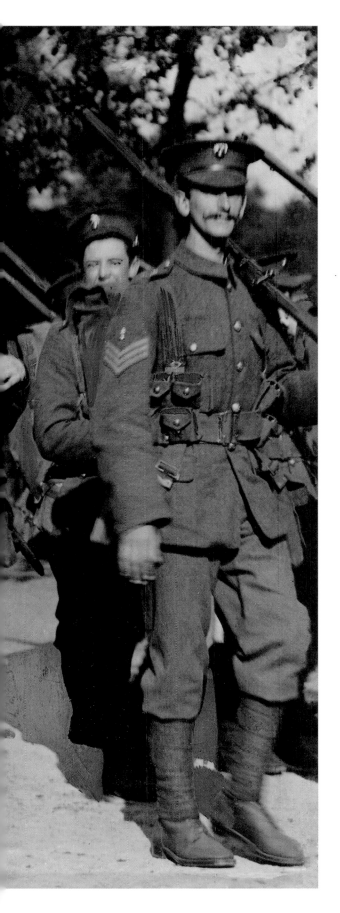

Seeing the volunteer army off to the front

A young woman marches alongside soldiers of the 1st Battalion Grenadier Guards as they leave Wellington Barracks in London for Waterloo Station on their way to the front. The outbreak of the First World War was welcomed by many. In London, euphoric crowds collected outside Downing Street and Buckingham Palace to cheer and sing the national anthem. There was a rush of volunteers, many of whom lied about their age. Field-Marshal Sir John French, who commanded the British Expeditionary Force, was quoted as saying the war would be over by Christmas.

War had been triggered on June 28 when Archduke Franz Ferdinand, heir to the Austro-Hungarian throne, was assassinated by Gavrilo Princip, a Bosnian-Serbian student in Sarajevo. Austria, allied with Germany in the Triple Alliance and anxious to increase its control of the Balkans, issued an ultimatum to Serbia, demanding a part in the investigation into the shooting and the suppression of anti-Austrian movements within Serbia. The inevitable Serb refusal was followed by an Austrian declaration of war against Serbia.

Russia, Serbia's ally, ordered a general mobilisation. Germany in turn responded and on August 1 declared war on Russia. But Berlin saw the sudden crisis as a golden opportunity to destroy not just Russia but Russia's allies in the Triple Entente – France and Britain. On August 3, the Germans declared war on France and the following day invaded Belgium. Britain promptly declared war on Germany, Austria declared war on Russia. The First World War had begun.

The British declaration of war came on August 5 at 12.15am when the Foreign Office released the following statement: "Owing to the summary rejection by the German Government of the request made by His Majesty's Government for assurances that the neutrality of Belgium will be respected, His Majesty's Ambassador at Berlin has received his passports and His Majesty's Government have declared to the German Government that a state of war exists between Great Britain and Germany as from 11pm on August 4."

Also this year...

100,000 Yorkshire miners strike for minimum wage

The zip, brain-child of US engineer Gideon Sundback, is launched

King George accused by the Liberals of siding with Ulster Unionists

Deaths: Joseph Chamberlain, Sir John Tenniel, illustrator of Alice in Wonderland, US industrialist George Westinghouse

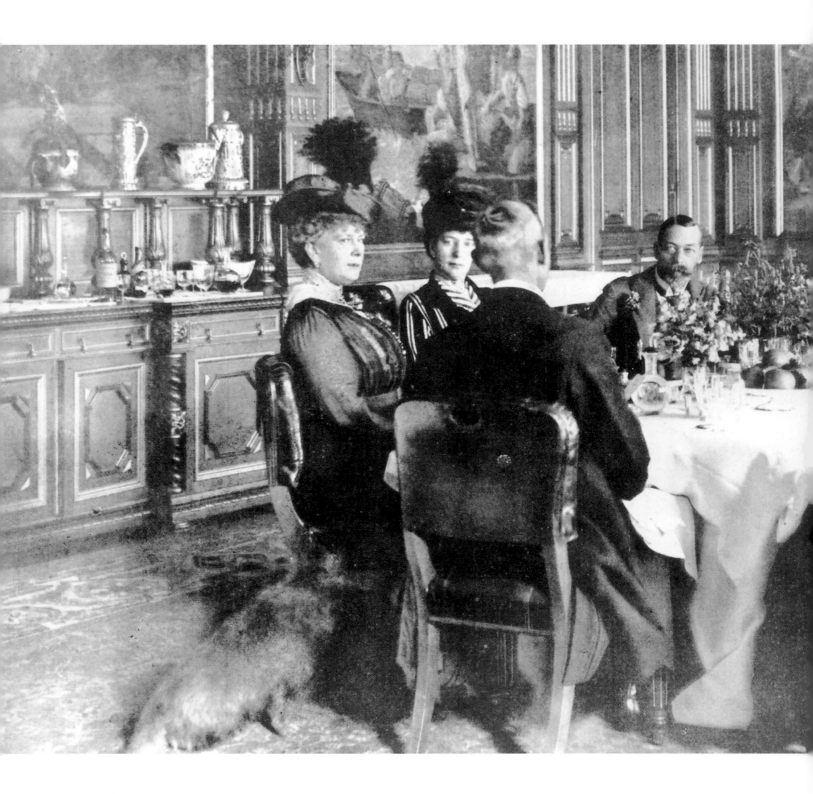

Royal family gives up alcohol for "war effort"

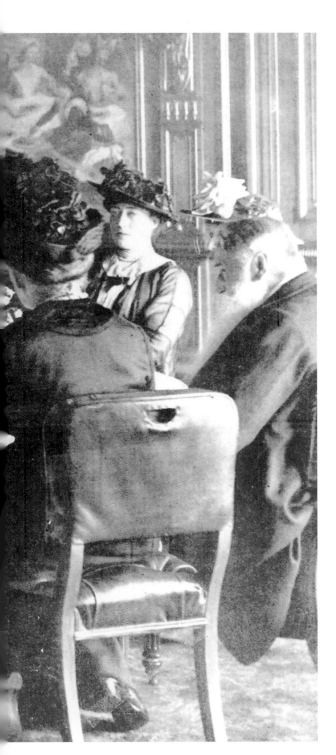

As a contribution to the war effort, in 1915 George V announced that he and the Royal Household were to abstain from alcohol for the duration. This picture, taken at Sandringham, was intended to demonstrate to the public the Royal Family's wartime abstemiousness.

The King took his responsibility seriously. Ponsonby's *Recollections of Three Reigns* tells of a courtier being berated when he called for an egg at breakfast: "If he had ordered a dozen turkeys he could not have made a bigger stir. The King accused him of being a slave to his inside, of unpatriotic behaviour, and even went so far as to hint that we should lose the war on account of his gluttony."

The King's abstention from alcohol was intended to set an example, particularly to workers in the shipyards and armaments, whose heavy drinking was said to be holding up weapons production. Lord Kitchener complained about the delay in getting arms to the front and Lloyd George, then the Chancellor, identified Britain's enemies as "Germany, Austria and drink". In October buying a round of drinks was made illegal, on pain of a £100 fine or six months' imprisonment.

Of longer lasting impact was the call for women to work. The government's Register of Women for War Service encouraged women to take up traditionally male jobs, freeing men to fight. Many women – including girls as young as 14 – worked seven days a week in factories, trades and on the farms for an average wage of 32 shillings a week. The women proved good workers: it was estimated that in some factories turnover was raised two and a half times. However, some yearned for greater involvement in the war effort: 40,000 women demonstrated in London for what they saw as their "right to serve".

Also this year...

Gas is first used as a war weapon by the Germans

1,000 British suffragettes travel to France to help with war work

The Derby is held at Newmarket after the Army requisitions Epsom

Winston Churchill resigns from the government

226 people are killed in a train crash at Gretna Green.

The Lusitania *is torpedoed by a U-Boat off the coast of Ireland with the loss of 1,198 lives*

Deaths: cricket colossus W.G. Grace, Rupert Brooke, in Gallipoli, Edith Cavell, shot by the Germans as a spy, socialist pioneer Kier Hardie

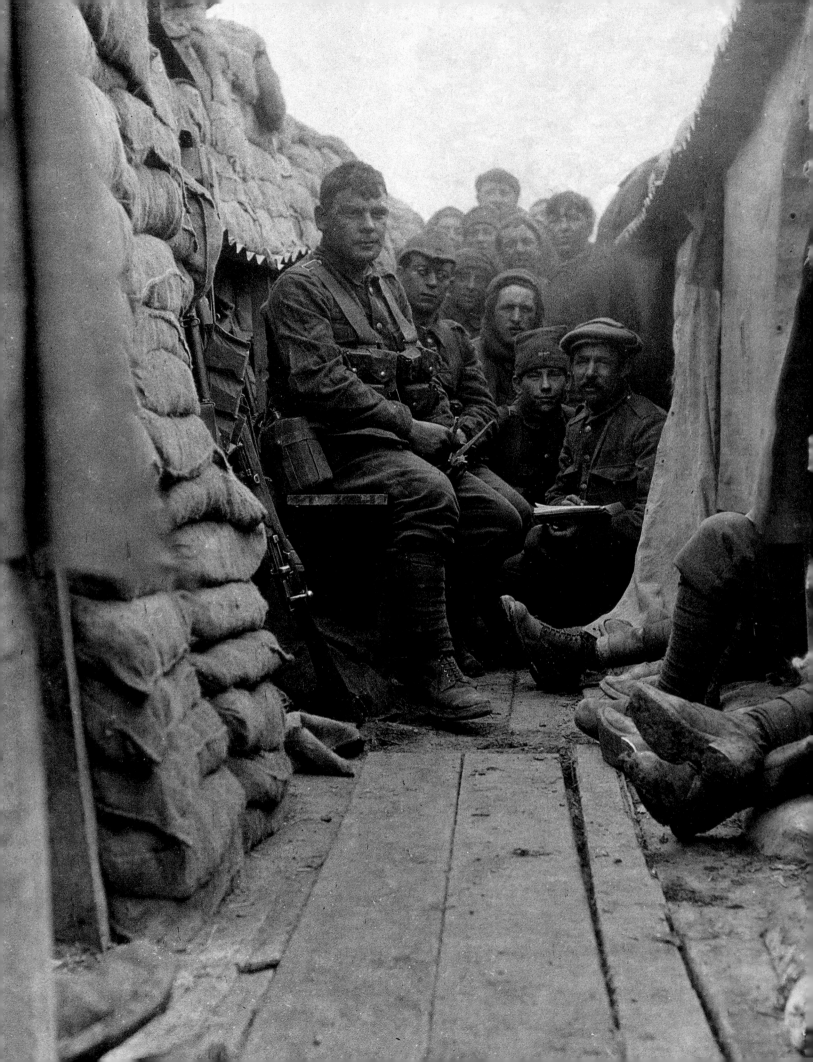

A far cry from the "romance" of war

On most fighting fronts, soldiers' lives were dominated by the trench. Conditions were at their worst on the Western Front. Prey to disease, living in damp, poorly ventilated bunkers, constantly shelled and occasionally gassed, the soldier's life was brutal and cheerless, a far cry from the glory that many envisaged when they rushed to join up. There would have been no martial romance for the troops in France pictured here. It was not just the volunteers who suffered. Conscription for single men was introduced in January this year. In April, it was extended to married men between 18 and 41.

As early as November 1914, both sides had dug in along a 400-mile front from the English Channel to Switzerland. Behind a tangle of barbed wire, machine guns and artillery, each side confronted the other for four years of grim attritional warfare. The incessant shelling caused some soldiers to go into such a severe state of shock that they could not walk; some deliberately wounded themselves in a desperate attempt to escape the horror of the front. There were limited medical facilities and the Allies were unprepared for German gas attacks, which burnt, choked and blinded. A lack of gasmasks led soldiers to improvise: they went into battle with wet cloths to their faces.

The upper and middle classes of Britain suffered disproportionately high casualties. Poor health and essential war work in the mines and factories had excluded many of the working classes from military service. France lost more than 300,000 men at the Battle of Verdun in 1916. On the opening day of the Battle of Somme, which helped relieve the desperate fighting around Verdun, the British suffered 60,000 casualties, mowed down as they advanced through the mud and barbed wire. In all, Britain mobilised almost nine million men in the war for a cost of 900,000 lives.

Also this year...

794 civilians and 521 police are killed or wounded in the Easter Rising in Dublin; the seven rebel leaders are later executed

Daylight-saving time is introduced

The last Allied troops are withdrawn from Gallipoli

Ulster Unionists vote for the partition of Ireland

Mexican revolutionary Pancho Villa launches raid against the US

John D. Rockefeller becomes the world's first billionaire

3.2 million British women are now employed in war work

Lloyd George becomes Prime Minister.

The Battle of Jutland: Germany and Britain's navies clash indecisively in the North Sea

Deaths: War Secretary Lord Kitchener is drowned, Rasputin is murdered, American writer Henry James

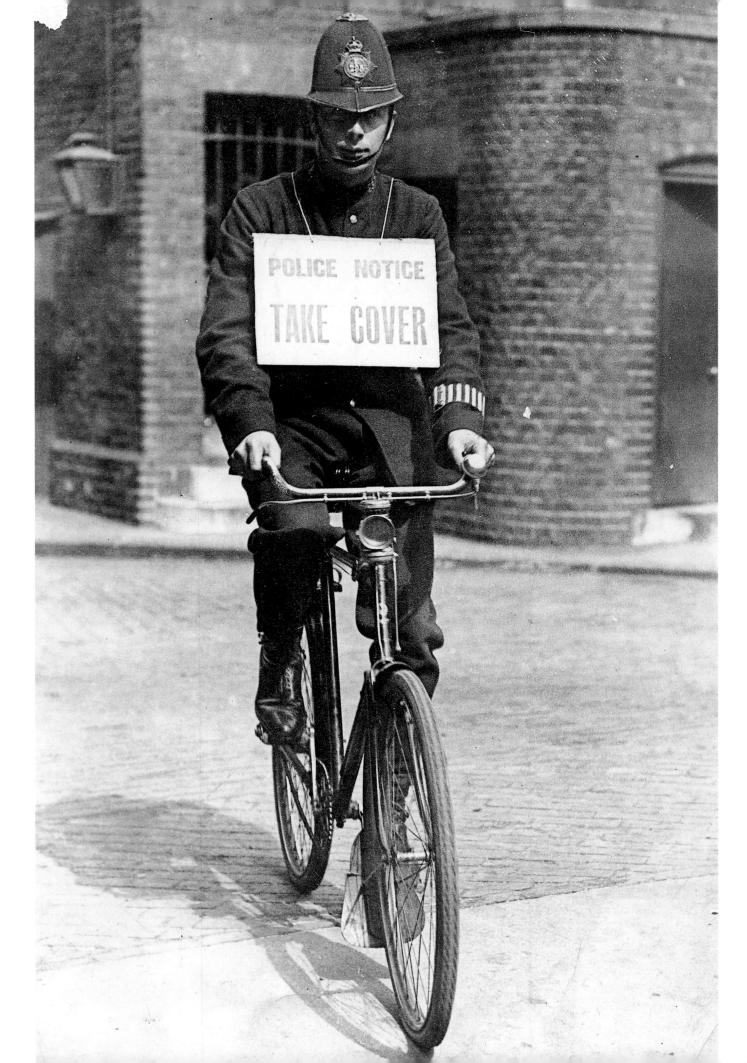

Pedal power warns London of bombs

A policeman pedals his way around London, warning civilians to take cover against an air raid. This simple method was the usual means by which air raid warnings were given.

The first German attacks against mainland Britain were seaborne. In December 1914, a small German naval force bombarded Scarborough and Whitby. The following month, the first air raid was launched, when two airships bombed the east coast, killing four and injuring 19. In May 1915, the first air raid against London, personally authorised by the Kaiser, was launched. Thirty high-explosive and 90 incendiary bombs were dropped, killing seven people and wounding 14 others.

At this stage of the war, much more was expected of airships, in which Germany enjoyed a decisive lead, than airplanes. But airships were to prove difficult to navigate and vulnerable to air attack. Overall, they inflicted little damage – in 51 raids they killed 557 people. They also sustained high losses. On a single day in October 1917, the German navy lost five airships and the following January they lost a further five, again in a single day. As the effectiveness of British air defences was demonstrated, so German airship crews became progressively more demoralised.

From the summer of 1917, the Germans supplemented raids with airships with raids by Gotha heavy bombers. Though only 27 such attacks were launched, they prompted Britain to create a separate airforce – and, in turn, from 1918 to begin the systematic bombing of Germany itself.

Also this year...

Non-military National Service for women launched

America joins the war

Women are permitted to become taxi drivers

Tsar Nicholas II abdicates and is sent to Siberia

Germany helps to repatriate Lenin, a second rebellion puts him and the Bolsheviks in power and Lenin opens negotiations with the Germans to end the war

George V asks Britons to cut back on bread

Plans for Irish Home Rule exclude Ulster

41 die in a Lancashire munitions factory explosion

The Royal Family replaces its Germanic surnames with Windsor and Mountbatten

Deaths: William Cody (Buffalo Bill), Edgar Degas, Auguste Rodin, Dutch-born adventuress Mata Hari, rag-time composer Scott Joplin, actor-manager Sir Herbert Beerbohm Tree

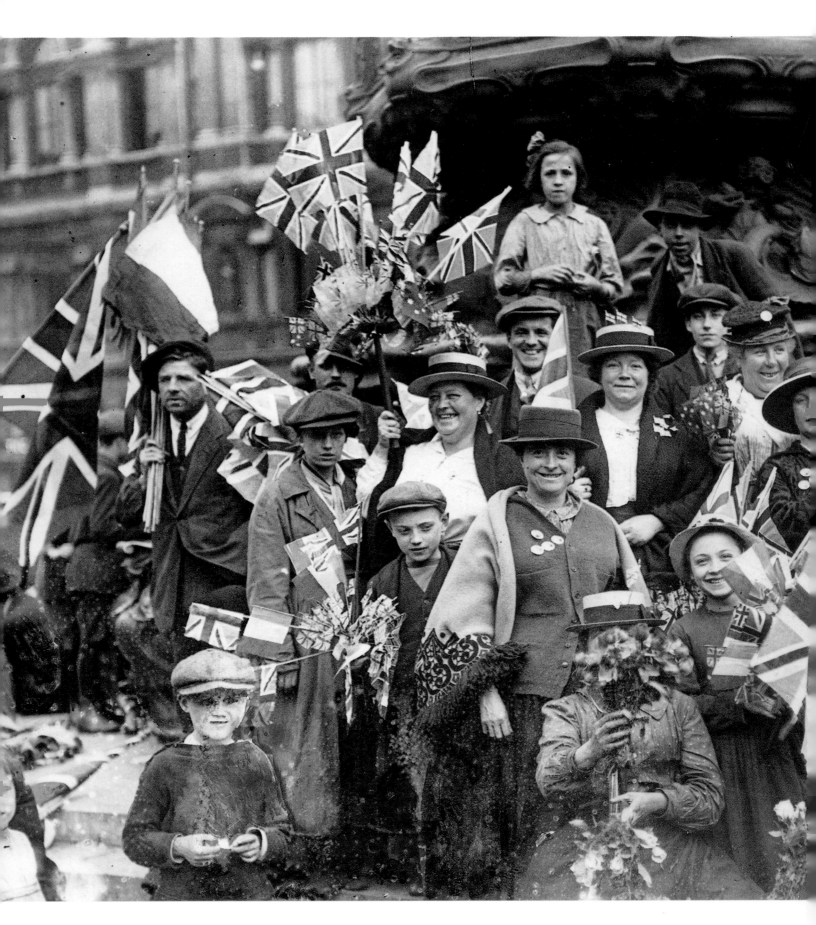

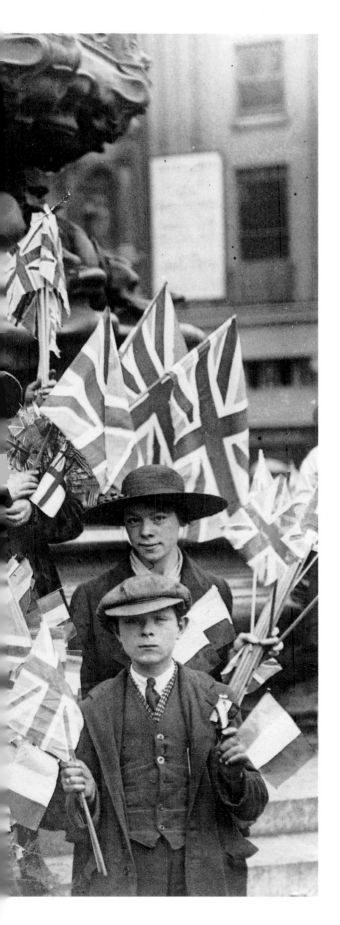

End of the war "to end all wars"

"At 11 o'clock this morning came to an end the cruellest and most terrible war that has ever scourged mankind. I hope we may say that thus, this fateful morning, came to an end all wars." With these words the Prime Minister, David Lloyd George, announced the Armistice to the House of Commons on November 11, 1918.

With over ten million dead, the Great War was effectively at an end when the Kaiser abdicated and fled with his family to Holland. *The Times* reported: "It was an inarticulate people which genuinely and with comparative soberness made the streets merry. Yet after all, this may have been the most dramatic way in which vent could be given to sudden joy after years of depression and restraint. Human nature is tongue-tied at its greatest moments; and London with a great moment to celebrate abandoned the hope of suitable words and made festival by the ringing of handbells, the hooting of motors, the screaming of whistles, the rattling of tin-trays, and the banging of anything that could be banged."

Crowds collected outside 10 Downing Street to greet the Prime Minister; others went to Buckingham Palace where a band led the crowd in *Keep The Home Fires Burning, Auld Lang Syne, Tipperary* and *Land of Hope and Glory*. The King and Queen appeared on a balcony to greet the cheering crowds. The Queen was waving a flag. November 15 was declared V-Day. Street lights were unmasked and licensing laws ignored as the pubs were packed and drunk dry. In the City, fireworks were let off. People danced in the streets and packed into and on top of cars with flags representing the Allies and the colonies.

Also this year...

US President Wilson presents his 14-point peace plan

London and Home Counties' residents are rationed to 20 ounces of meat each a week

The school leaving age is extended to 14

The Royal Flying Corps and Royal Naval Service merge to form Royal Air Force

Tsar Nicholas II and his family are murdered

Dr Marie Stopes calls for birth control

The government sets up a commission into equal pay for women after disruptive action from tram, bus, rail and Underground workers

Britain's first oil well opened at Hardstoft, Derbyshire

100 female police patrols are appointed in London

Women over 30 who are householders or the wives of householders are given the vote

Deaths: Claude Debussy, war poet Wilfred Owen, Manfred von Richthofen – the Red Baron

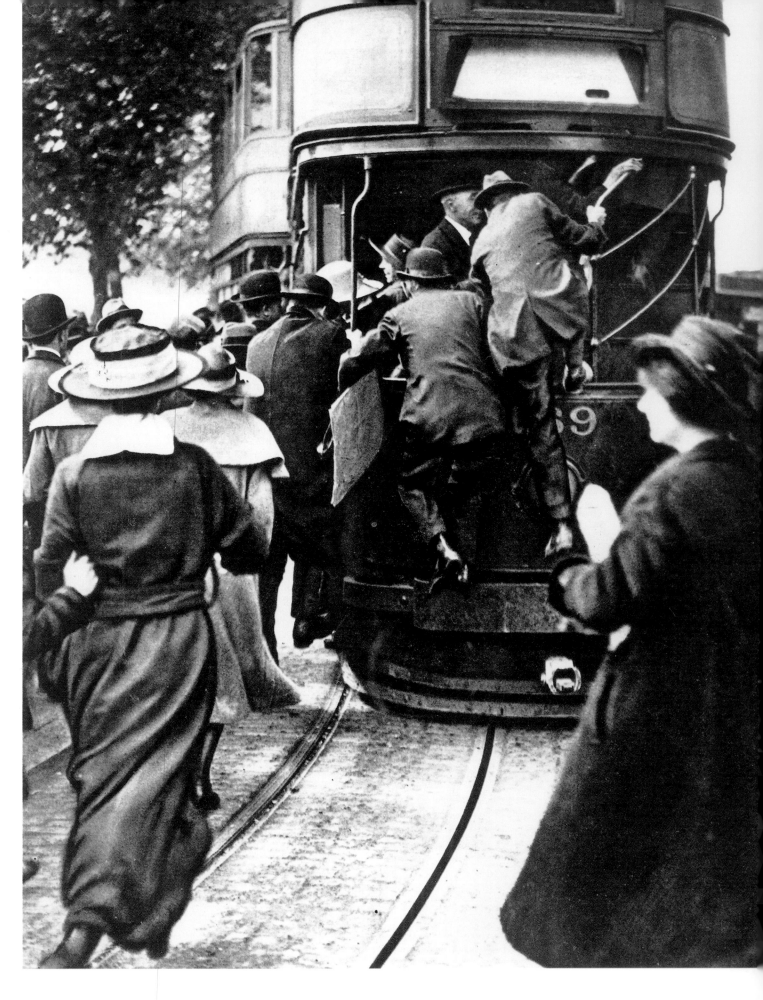

Peace brings dispute on the home front

The Armistice may have signalled the end of the war in Europe but it did not bring domestic harmony, as these commuters, scuffling to board a tram in London during the great rail strike of 1919, make clear. It was estimated that almost 35 million working days were lost to strikes this year, compared with 5.8 million the previous year.

The unrest was widespread. In Glasgow a demonstration attended by 20,000 people erupted into violence: mounted police had to be called in and 40 people were injured. When Liverpool police went on strike in August 1919, troops had to be sent in to control looters: 370 arrests were made and one man was killed. There were similar strikes by the police in London.

But it was the rail workers' strike, which began at midnight on September 27, that really paralysed the nation. Fearful that the violent unrest sweeping much of Europe would be repeated in Britain, the government viewed the strike as a declaration of war from the unions and threatened to bring in the military. Food rations were introduced for milk, butter, cheese, sugar, beef and mutton. An aerial mail service was started to help to shift the backlog. But when the strike was ended, on October 3, it was very much on the rail workers' terms.

Most of the strikes were called to demand better rates of pay and shorter working hours. Nonetheless, the revolution in Russia two years earlier had emboldened socialists and many suspected Bolshevik influence behind the disputes. So great was the government's fear that in March 1919 a Bill was prepared that would have enabled the government to refuse unions access to strike funds and to arrest their leaders. It was never passed.

Also this year...

25 Sinn Fein MPs refuse to attend Westminster and form the first Irish parliament which is later declared illegal

Professor Ernest Rutherford splits the atom

Mussolini founds the Fasci di Combattimento

A rabies scare leads to 850,000 dogs being muzzled

Alcock and Brown make the first non-stop Atlantic flight; the first daily international flights – between Paris and London – are introduced

Nancy Astor becomes first female MP to take her seat in the House of Commons

The Sex Disqualification Act allows women to enter the professions

First female student admitted to Lincoln's Inn

Deaths: former US President Theodore Roosevelt, multimillionaire and philanthrophist Andrew Carnegie, Pierre August Renoir

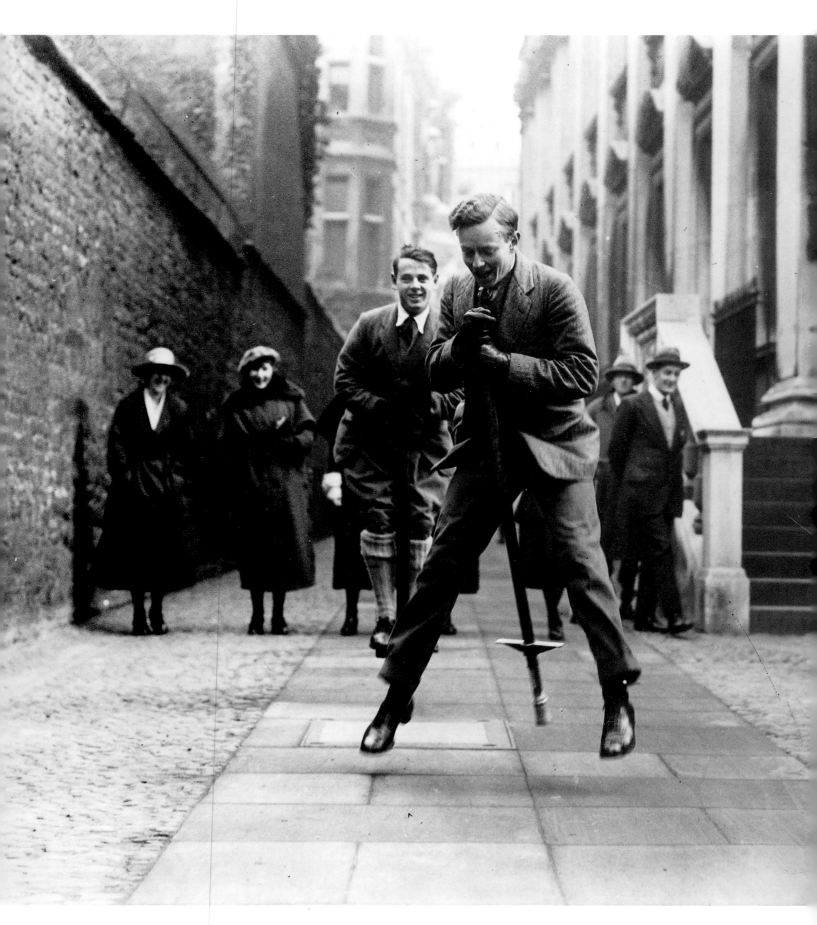

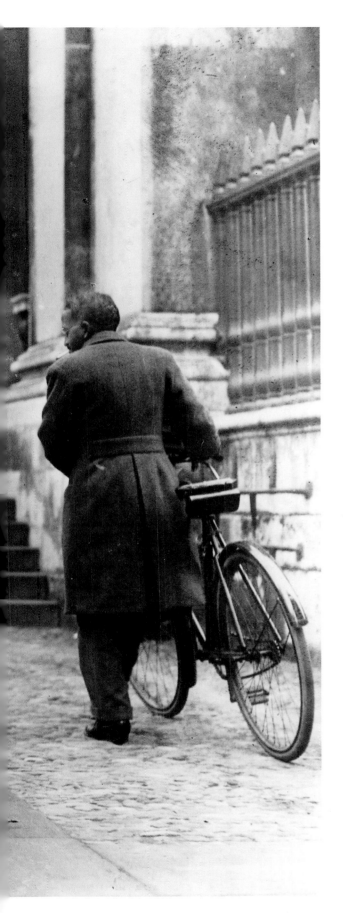

High jinks as students return to the universities

The First World War had practically emptied both Oxford and Cambridge of undergraduates. However, by 1920 many students had returned to their books, and, as demonstrated by the expertise displayed on their pogo sticks by the Cambridge undergraduates pictured here, student high jinks. Contemporary accounts record that the ex-servicemen were difficult to discipline. J.B Priestley, an undergraduate at Trinity Hall in 1919, recalled: "College rooms were loud with argument until dawn ... porters reprimanded their late commanding officers."

The diminished number of students during the war had inevitably led to a lack of income, and in 1919 Cambridge University had to turn to state support. In return, a Royal Commission was set up to investigate the structure of both Oxford and Cambridge. The Commission's findings led to lectures and practical teaching becoming more centrally organised at both universities, although colleges retained control of individual tutorials. The government also backed undergraduates by awarding grants to ex-service students and state scholarships. The result was a huge increase in students: in 1914 Cambridge had 3,263 undergraduates; by 1920 there were 5,733.

Girton and Newnham colleges – which accommodated female students – were established in the 19th century, but despite the freedoms won for women in other areas during the war women were still largely excluded from university life at Cambridge. A married woman had to act as chaperone whenever a female wished to visit a male undergraduate in his room, or entertain him in hers. Oxford was considerably more progressive and gave women full membership of the university in May 1920, when they became eligible for all degrees other than Divinity. Professorships and lectureships at Cambridge were made open to women from 1926, but it was not until 1947 that Cambridge women finally achieved equal status with their male counterparts. By way of contrast, University College, Reading, had elected its first woman professor as early as 1908.

Also this year...

Adolf Hitler publishes plan for a Third German Reich

Black and Tans sent into Ireland

Imperial War Museum opens

Foreigners are banned from most council jobs

Night bus service started in London

Scotland votes against prohibition.

Deaths: propagandist for the Russian Revolution John Reed, sociologist Max Weber, Amedeo Modigliani, Robert Peary

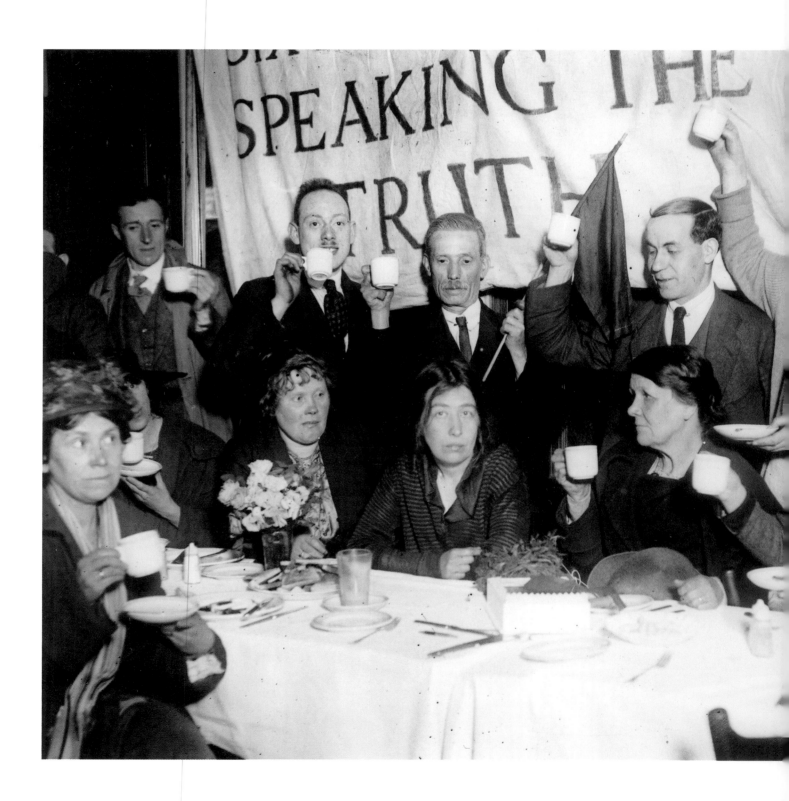

Pankhurst freedom celebrated with tea

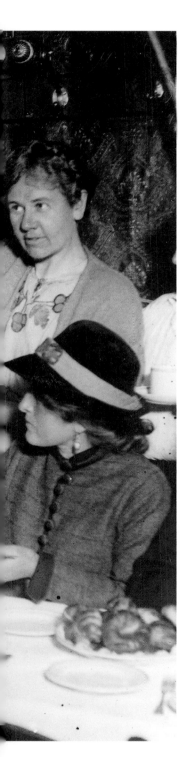

Suffragette Sylvia Pankhurst and her supporters enjoy a celebratory cup of tea following her release after six months in prison. Sylvia is the woman seated in the middle, staring directly at the camera. She was a radical figure in the movement to gain votes for women and was sent to prison a total of 15 times. In 1920 she visited Russia, where she met Lenin, and on her return was associated with Britain's most prominent Communists. The sentence was for the publication of subversive matter in *The Women's Dreadnought*, a weekly paper she produced for working-class women.

Sylvia's political career centred around the suffragette movement. Her mother, Emmeline Pankhurst, and her sister, Christabel, were founding members of the Women's Social and Political Union, established in 1903. Sylvia Pankhurst became honorary secretary. Using the slogan "Votes for Women and Chastity for Men", the suffragettes set fire to churches, blew up stations, threw bricks through windows, cut telegraph wires and tied themselves to railings. As the radical branch of feminism, the Pankhursts and their supporters were frequently the butt of music hall jokes and were sometimes physically attacked. While in prison many went on hunger strike and were subjected to force-feeding, a practice previously restricted to lunatic asylums.

Sylvia parted company from her mother and sister when war broke out in 1914. Her relatives believed their demonstrations should stop in the interests of the war effort but Sylvia promoted pacifist and socialist ideas, forming a breakaway group, the Women's Peace Army, which demanded a negotiated peace. By the time Sylvia Pankhurst emerged from yet another stretch in prison in 1921, the women's movement had made some progress: women over 30 and conforming to certain property qualifications were given the vote in 1918, and in 1921 Dr Marie Stopes opened the first birth-control clinic, in north London. In 1927 Sylvia Pankhurst went on to outrage the British public further when she became an unmarried mother.

Also this year...

British troops enter Dublin and martial law is declared before the Irish Treaty establishes the Irish Free State

Northern Ireland Parliament opens

Unemployment exceeds two million

A coal strike forces the government to declare state of emergency

Police patrols use motorbikes for the first time

DH Lawrence publishes Women in Love

Deaths: Enrico Caruso, Engelbert Humperdinck, Camille Saint-Saëns

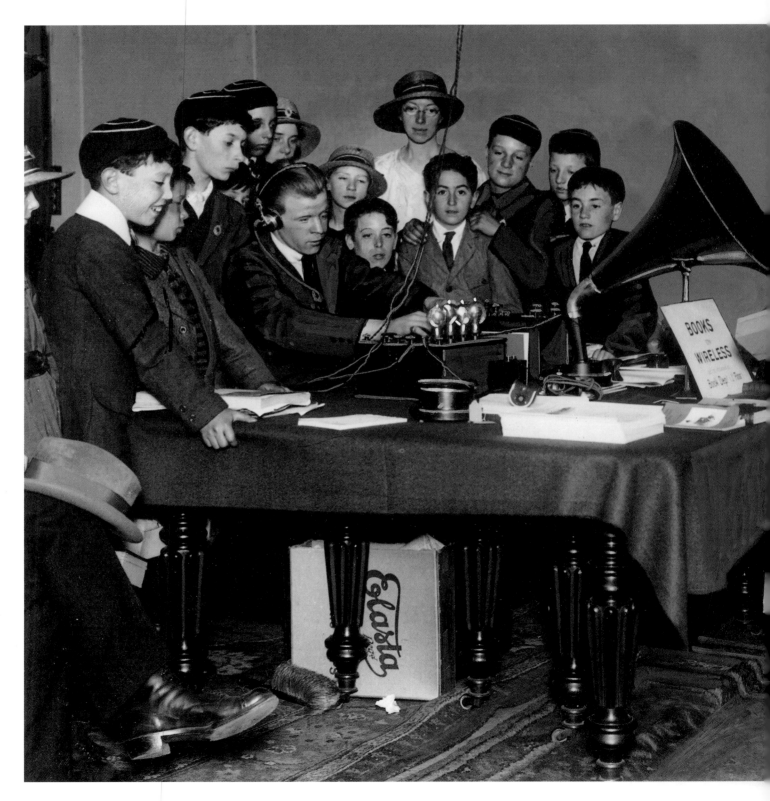

The birth of "Auntie" and a modern marvel

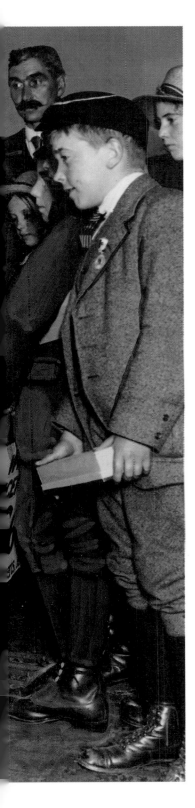

A crowd gathers around the wireless to catch a broadcast at Harrods in London. The British-based Italian Guglielmo Marconi, the leading pioneer in the field, had successfully transmitted wireless signals across the Atlantic in 1901, thereby demonstrating the practicability of radio broadcasts. Until the 1920s, however, broadcasting remained largely in the hands of the government and amateur broadcasters.

It was the newspaper magnate, Lord Northcliffe, who first saw the commercial potential of the airwaves. On June 15, 1920, a *Daily Mail* special featuring Dame Nellie Melba, who sang in English, Italian and French, was broadcast from the Marconi company's transmitter in Chelmsford. Such frivolity was frowned upon by the Postmaster General, who banned this and similar broadcasts which were "interfering with important communications". It was only when 63 wireless societies got together a petition that this ban was lifted, on January 13, 1922.

The group pictured here may have been listening to one of Marconi's weekly Tuesday night broadcasts, which started on February 14. The first programme lasted 15 minutes and was a mixture of talk and music. The licence demanded that every seven minutes of broadcasting was followed by a three-minute silence so that the operators could listen in and check that government transmissions had not been interfered with.

The British Broadcasting Company, as it was first called, was formed by six electrical companies. The first broadcast – a news bulletin – went on the air on November 14 at 6pm from 2LO, its station in London. Two days later it was followed by the first entertainment programme which lasted an hour. This opened with Leonard Hawke, a baritone, performing *Duke Goes West* and *Tick, Tock*, and concluded with Dorothy Chalmers performing *Hymn to the Sun* and Schubert's *Rosamund* on the violin. Programmes were sometimes interrupted by amateurs broadcasting on the same wave length.

Also this year...

The government offers amnesty for all Irish prisoners

The Irish parliament approves the Irish Free State; Michael Collins assassinated

Flu kills 804 in January

Thousands of cattle, sheep and pigs are slaughtered after outbreaks of foot and mouth disease

Dr Ivy Williams becomes the first woman to be called to the Bar

Conservatives under Bonar Law win general election; Ramsay MacDonald is elected Labour leader

James Joyce's Ulysses is published in Paris after being banned in America and Britain

Deaths: telephone pioneer Alexander Graham Bell, Marcel Proust, explorer Ernest Shackleton

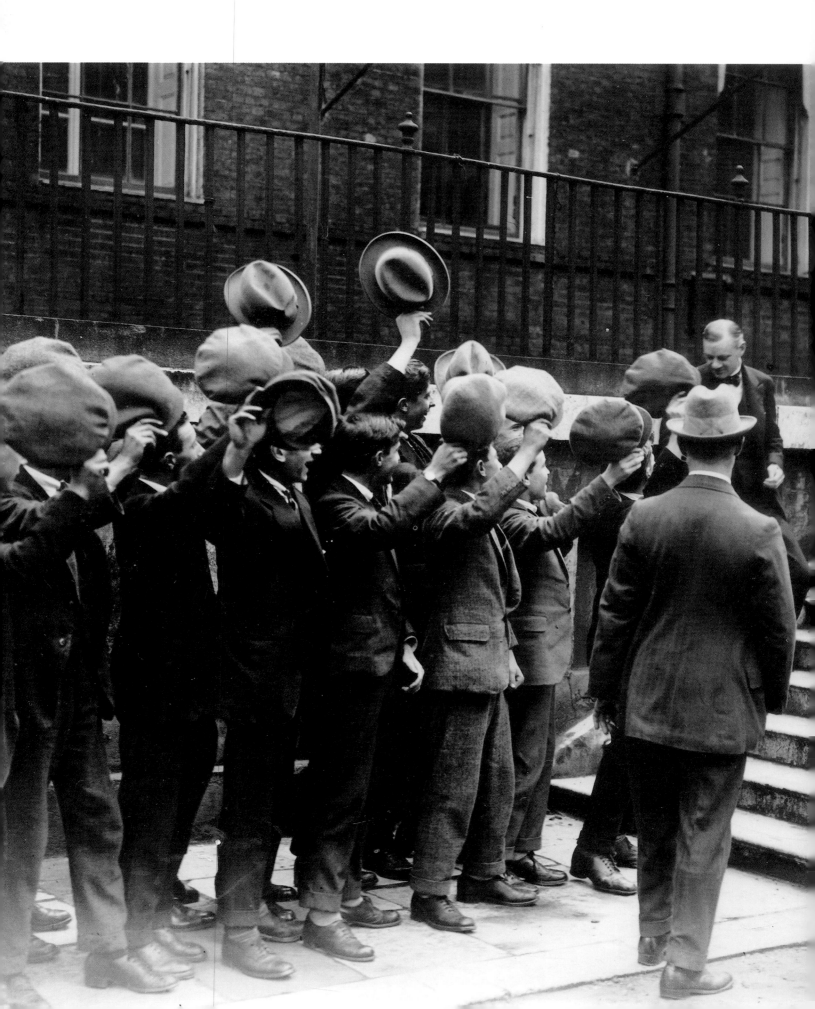

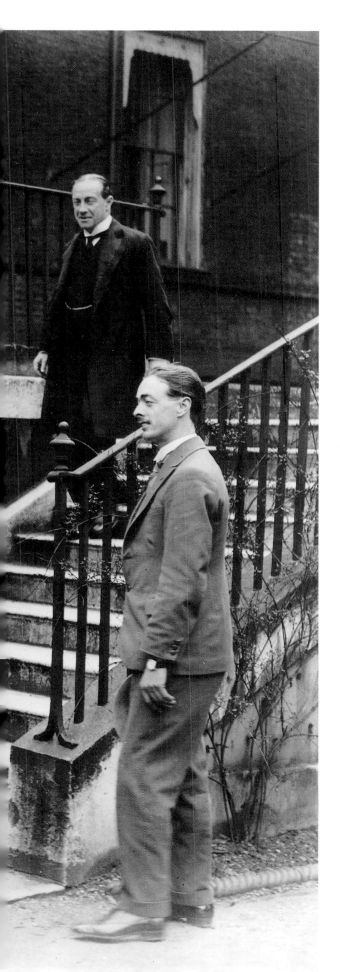

"Little Baldwin" gives up his pigs for No. 10

He claimed that he would have been happier keeping pigs, watching cricket or smoking his pipe with a quiet pint, but he was to become Prime Minister three times.

Here Conservative Prime Minister Stanley Baldwin is greeted by a group of workers on an educational tour of London. After almost ten years languishing in a safe Conservative seat at Bewdley, Worcestershire, which he inherited from his father, Baldwin's political career took an upward turn in 1917. Backed by Andrew Bonar Law, an old friend of his father's, Baldwin became a parliamentary private secretary, and six years later, after Bonar Law's resignation due to ill health, Prime Minister. He was to hold the office in 1923, from 1924 to 1929, and from 1935 to 1937. His appointment surprised many of his contemporaries, who regarded Baldwin as an uncharismatic figure. When speaking, he used notes and would turn pale and break out in a sweat.

Lloyd George, in particular, was wont to dismiss him as "Little Baldwin". Yet it was Baldwin's speech at the Carlton Club in 1922 which helped crush Lloyd George's coalition. "A dynamic force is a terrible thing," Baldwin said, "It may crush you but it is not necessarily right."

Before his appointment by Bonar Law, Baldwin had been on the verge of giving up politics and retiring to the country. A week before he was asked to form a government, Baldwin characteristically declared his ambition "to lead a decent life, and to keep pigs." Although he was later generally vilified for his slowness in rearming before the Second World War, Baldwin's honesty and "John Bullishness" made him a popular figure with the public.

Also this year...

Prince Albert, Duke of York, marries Lady Elizabeth Bowes Lyon

Adolf Hitler attempts to seize power in Germany in the Munich Putsch

Kemal Ataturk institutes a secularising regime in Turkey

Interpol established

The Matrimonial Causes Bill allows women to divorce unfaithful husbands

Lenin retires from power after a stroke

Bolton Wanderers and West Ham become the first teams to play a cup final at Wembley

Jack Hobbs hits his hundredth 100 in first-class cricket

Plans are announced to make Stratford-upon-Avon a cultural centre

The BBC launches Woman's Hour

The Liquor Act forbids the sale of alcohol to under 18s

Enrique Tirabocchi swims the English Channel in 16 hours and 33 minutes

Deaths: Sarah Bernhardt, French engineer Gustav Eiffel, Andrew Bonar Law, Katherine Mansfield

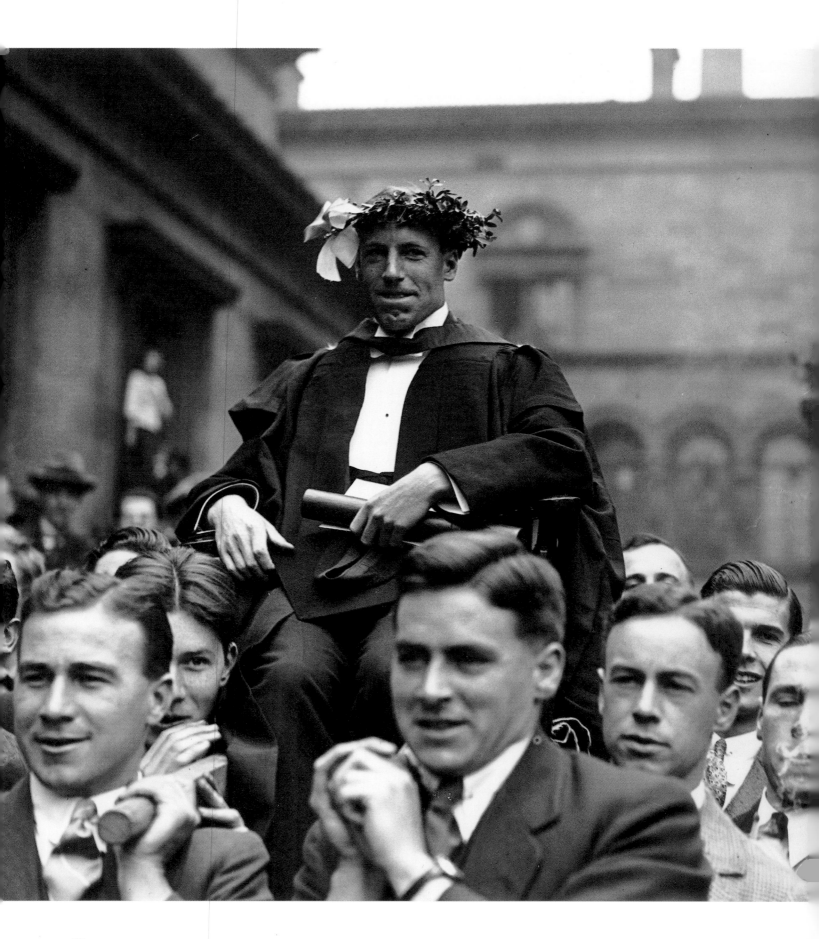

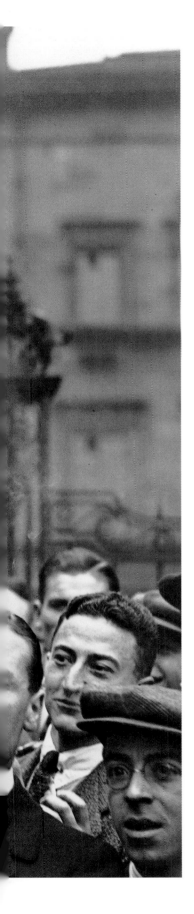

Triumph for the hero of "Chariots of Fire"

Eric Liddell is carried in triumph through Edinburgh University. The athlete returned from the 1924 Paris Olympics with a new Olympic record, having run the 400 metres in 47.6 seconds. Liddell's style of running was unorthodox; a wild sprint with knees lifted high and arms flailing. *The Times* reported: "No one ever looked like catching him. In one, wild minute, what had been the dullest of days was turned into the most memorable that the Olympic Games have ever seen." He also won a bronze medal in the 200 metres at the Paris games and seven Scottish rugby caps. His story was told in the Oscar-winning film *Chariots of Fire*.

Born in 1902 to missionary parents in Tianjin in China, Liddell was to become almost as famous for his religious conviction as for his sporting prowess. It was this that led him to run in the 400 metres at Paris rather than his preferred 100 metres, the heats for which took place on the Sabbath. Instead of competing, Liddell conducted the service and read the sermon at the Scottish church in Paris.

The Church was to guide the remainder of his career: in 1925 Liddell went back to China where he worked as a science teacher and missionary until his death in 1945 from a brain tumour in a Japanese internment camp in Weifang. All Scotland mourned.

Liddell's was not the only notable athletic triumph at the eighth Olympic Games, which were held in Paris for the second time since their relaunch in 1896. A Cambridge law student, Harold Abrahams, won the 100 metres, Paavo Nurmi of Finland won three gold medals in athletics and Johnny Weissmuller, who went on to play Tarzan in Hollywood, won three golds of his own for swimming.

Also this year...

Ramsay MacDonald becomes the first Labour Prime Minister

Tutankhamun's sarcophagus is opened

The BBC begins broadcasting for schools

Metro-Goldwyn Pictures and the Louis B. Mayer Company merge to form MGM

First Winter Olympic Games held, at Chamonix

George Leigh Mallory and Andrew Irvine die on Everest

Gandhi goes on hunger strike

Publication of the Zinoviev letter, allegedly to British Communists calling for revolution, causes political turmoil

Conservatives under Stanley Baldwin come to power

Deaths: Soviet leader Lenin, authors Joseph Conrad and Franz Kafka, composer Giacomo Puccini, architect of the Versailles settlement Woodrow Wilson

Pavlova, an era's prima donna of dance

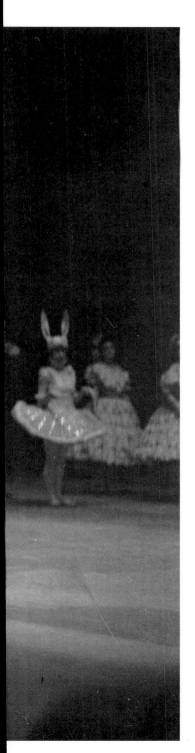

Anna Pavlova, one of the greatest ballerinas the world has known, performs in *The Fairy Doll* at Covent Garden in 1925. Born of humble origins in St Petersburg in 1881, Pavlova set her heart on becoming a ballerina after she was taken to a classical performance as a Christmas treat at the age of eight. Chosen to join the Imperial School of Ballet at St Petersburg when she was ten, Pavlova became prima ballerina in 1906. In 1913 she left the Imperial Ballet and began to spend much of her time touring abroad. Pavlova went on to perform all over the world, taking dance to far-flung places where ballet had never been performed, including Australia and South America. She was an inspiration to thousands, notably the British dancer Sir Frederick Ashton. Soviet officials noted with disdain that she was "the darling of wicked capitalist audiences of Europe and the United States."

Pavlova first performed in London in 1909 at the Palace Theatre, dancing with Nijinsky for the ballet impresario Diaghilev. It was in London that she and Victor Dandré made their home. The couple's marriage was announced in 1924, and had been kept a secret, Pavlova claimed, for 17 years. The swans on the miniature lake at her home in Golders Green were the inspiration for her celebrated performance of Saint-Saëns' *The Dying Swan*. Pavlova's genius was an exacting one: she was said to be prone to histrionics, and it was alleged that she made girls practise until their feet bled and threw wine over those who failed to meet her high standards.

Pavlova died on January 23, 1931, in a hotel in The Hague, four days after catching a cold while on a train from Paris to the Netherlands. One impresario claimed that she had unconsciously performed some of the movements of *The Dying Swan*, which she had performed more than 4,000 times, in her final hours. She was buried in London.

Also this year...

Leon Trotsky begins to lose his position in Soviet leadership following Lenin's death

Cyprus becomes a British colony

First use of insulin for diabetics

Britain returns to the Gold Standard

Skilled jobs in South Africa become exclusive to whites

Hitler's Mein Kampf *published*

Labour Party rejects overtures from Communist Party of Great Britain

George Bernard Shaw wins Nobel Prize for Literature

Deaths: Queen Alexandra, wife of Edward VII, former Chinese president Sun Yat-sen, Lord Curzon, artist John Singer Sargent, H. Rider Haggard

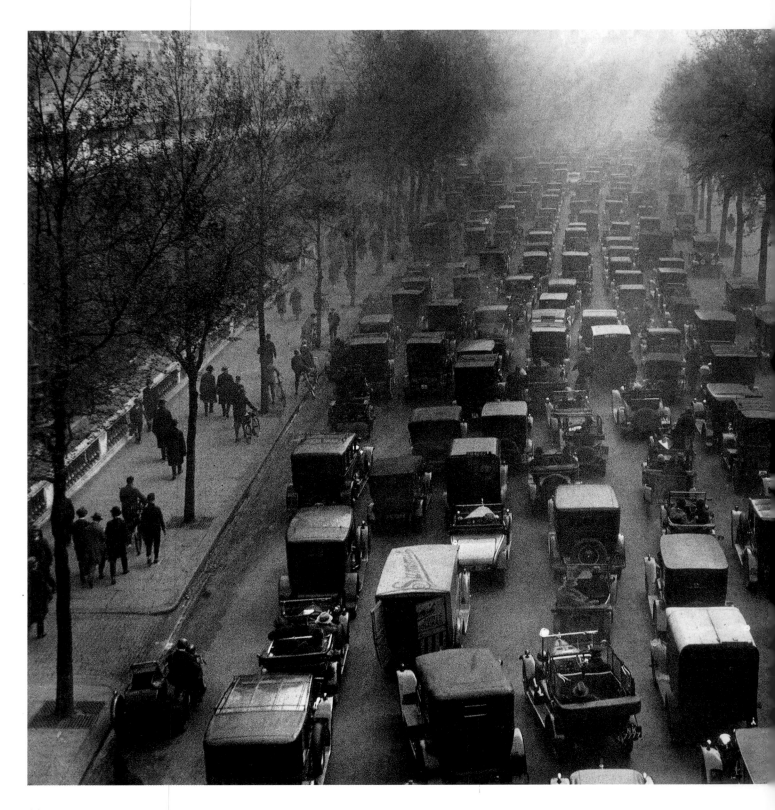

When industrial strife gripped the nation

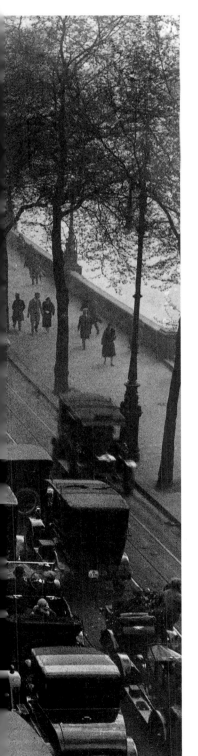

At midnight on May 3, the first and only General Strike that Britain has seen began. Among those to down tools were the transport workers: trains and buses stopped. London's Embankment ground to a halt as motorists took to their cars.

Coal mining incomes had fallen with the decline in exports after Britain returned to the Gold Standard. In April, a Royal Commission had recommended that mine wages be cut. The leader of the Miners Federation of Great Britain, A.J. Cook, urged resistance with the slogan: "Not a penny off the pay, not a minute on the day." Cook told a conference in Clapham: "Let me warn the Government that there is a new mentality in the police, the Army, the Navy, and the Air Force. Ninety-seven per cent of the recruits for the past two years have come from the working classes, and thousands of them miners, who will not shoot against their kith and kin when the order comes, and we shall not be afraid to advise them. This is a war to the death, and it is your death they are after. It is your wages they want."

The miners went on strike on May 1 after the pit owners locked them out. Later that day, when negotiations between the TUC and the government broke down, the TUC, at the request of the miners, called on workers in other industries to come out in support. More than two million did so. Members of the middle classes responded with what Stanley Baldwin, the Prime Minister, later called a "love of freedom and sense of fair play", and drove buses, lorries and trains to ensure that essential supplies got through.

A special edition of the *London Gazette* announced a state of emergency, and Winston Churchill, then the Chancellor, took to editing the *British Gazette*, which published officially approved news. At the BBC, managing director John Reith read a message from the Prime Minister over the air: "Keep steady!" he urged, "Remember that peace on Earth comes to all men of goodwill." Troops were deployed in south Wales, Yorkshire and Scotland. But after nine days, on May 12, the TUC ended the General Strike. The miners' strike went on until November 12, when it ended in failure.

Also this year...

Germany joins the League of Nations

T.E. Lawrence publishes Seven Pillars of Wisdom

A.A. Milne publishes Winnie the Pooh

Agatha Christie disappears for nine days

Robert Goddard produces first rocket powered by liquid fuel

Alan Cobham flies on a 27,000-mile round-trip to Australia

John Logie Baird demonstrates the first practical television system

Deaths: architect Antonio Gaudí, escapologist Harry Houdini, Claude Monet, Rudolf Valentino

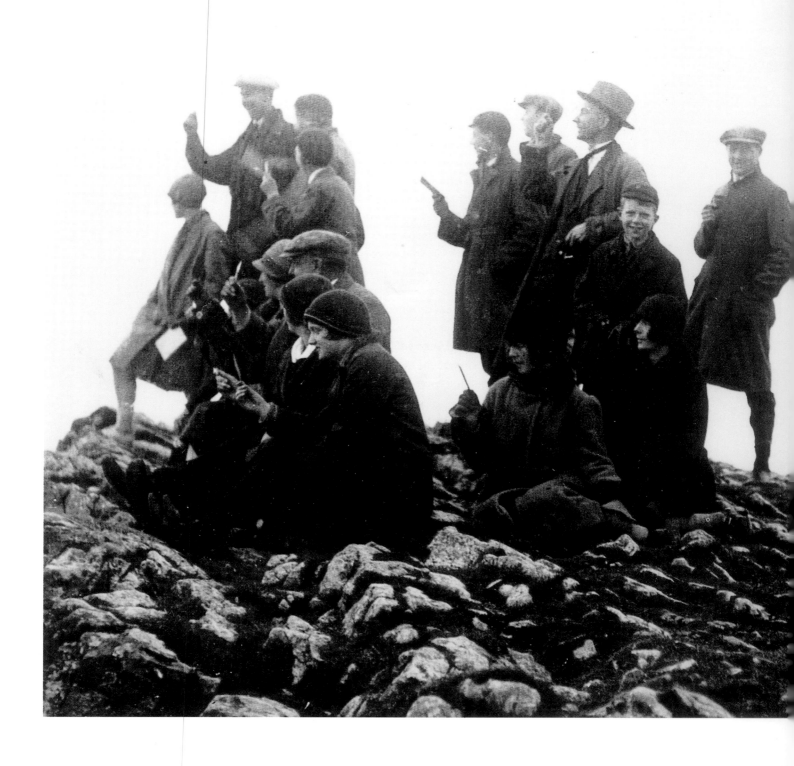

Eclipse enthusiasts defy the bad weather

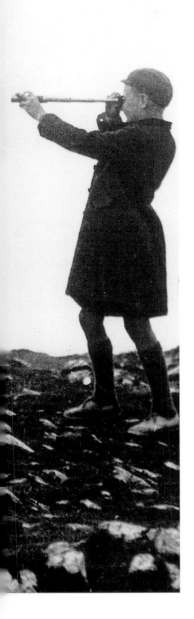

A group turn out at dawn, on June 29, to catch a glimpse of a total eclipse of the Sun, the first visible from mainland Britain this century. The start of the eclipse in Britain was at 5.29am, and totality lasted for 22 to 23 seconds. Starting in north Wales, the corridor of totality passed over Lancashire and the Yorkshire Dales. Special trains were arranged to carry more than three million people – the greatest number of people to travel by train at one time to date – to the best viewing places in Lancashire and Yorkshire. Many prepared for the event by using a candle to smoke a piece of glass, which it was hoped would protect their eyes from the glare of the Sun. The boys in the picture appear to be holding telescopes, which would have damaged their eyes if they had used them to observe the eclipse.

The best view was obtained from Giggleswick, where Ramsay MacDonald, then the Labour leader, was among the fortunate crowd. It was, he said, "the most magnificent and moving spectacle I have ever seen in my life". *The Times* reported that people in Southport and Swanage were able to witness some of the eclipse but those in West Hartlepool and London were "sorely disappointed".

"The state of the weather undoubtedly saved thousands of people in London from early rising," *The Times* reported, "which would have proved useless, for the sound of rain trickling along the gutters at about 5am gave them just the excuse they needed not to get out of bed." But those who did optimistically face the rain – a crowd mainly composed of young women, *The Times* reporter noted – remained cheerful.

Also this year...

The Trades Disputes and Trades Union Act, aimed at curbing the unions, is passed

Storms in Lancashire leave 50 dead and 400 homeless

The Public Morals Committee announces that general access to contraception results in "poorer hereditary stock"

1,000 people a week die from winter flu

Malcolm Campbell reaches world land speed record of 174.22 mph in his car Bluebird

Al Jolson stars in The Jazz Singer, *the first "talkie"*

Captain Charles Lindbergh makes first solo non-stop flight between New York and Paris

The ten-year-old violinist Yehudi Menuhin amazes crowds in Paris

The fashion for short hair produces a big increase in number of hairdressers

Deaths: dancer Isadora Duncan, author Jerome K. Jerome

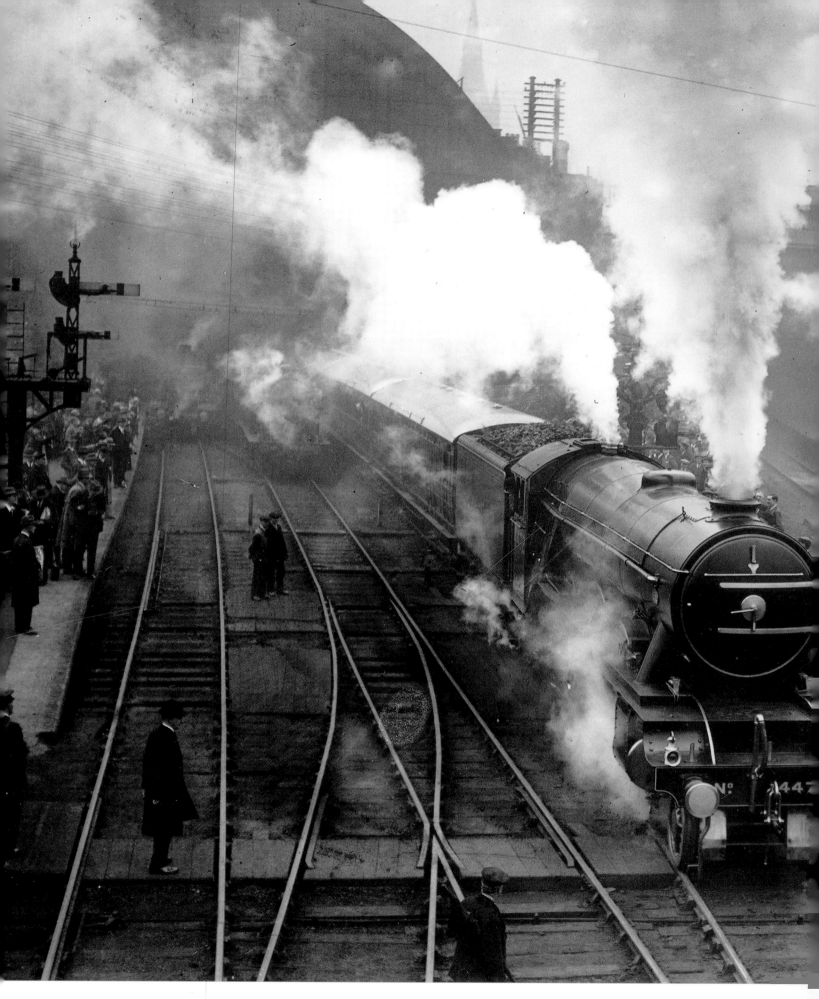

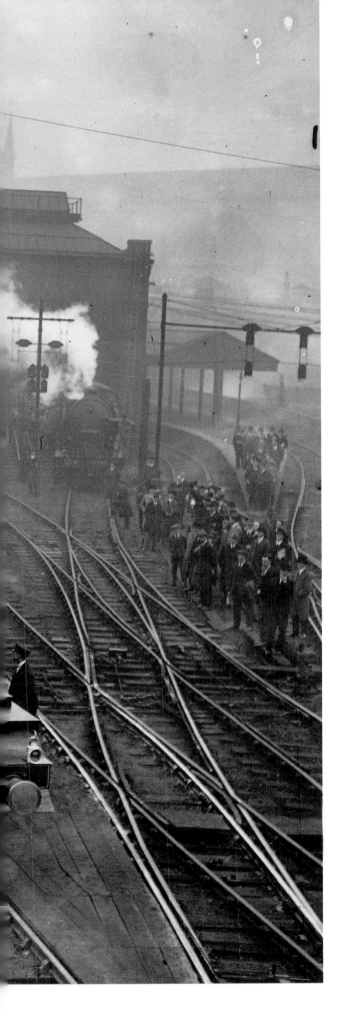

Steaming ahead in the vanguard of engineering

The *Flying Scotsman* leaves King's Cross at the beginning of the first non-stop journey from London to Edinburgh, on May 1, 1928. After a journey of 392 miles, at an average speed of 50 mph, the train completed the longest non-stop run in the world in eight hours and three minutes, arriving at Edinburgh Waverley ahead of schedule.

For those who travelled first-class, the journey aboard the *Flying Scotsman* would have been luxurious. Passengers could dine in the Louis XVI style dining car or take advantage of the hairdressing salon or "ladies' retiring room". Third-class travel would not have been quite so glamorous.

Designed by Sir Nigel Gresley, locomotive No. 4472 was built in Doncaster by the London and North Eastern Railway in 1923 at a cost of about £8,000, and put on display at the British Empire Exhibitions in 1924 and 1925 as an example of the best in British engineering. On November 30, 1934, on a test run between Leeds and London, *Flying Scotsman* proved its worth again by becoming the first locomotive to reach 100mph.

The locomotive was withdrawn from service in Britain in 1963, and passed into private hands. It toured America from 1969 to 1972. In 1988 it played a role in Australia's bicentennial celebrations, setting a world record for a non-stop run by a steam locomotive by hauling a train 422 miles from Parkes to Broken Hill in New South Wales. By 1996, *Flying Scotsman* was in pieces at a depot in London. By July 1999, a restored *Flying Scotsman* was again running passenger services.

Also this year...

Stalin exiles Trotsky and announces the Soviet Union's first Five Year Plan

The voting age for women in Britain is reduced from 30 to 21

In Paris, a number of major nations, including Britain, sign the Kellogg-Briand Pact renouncing war

Four people drown when the Thames floods parts of London

Alexander Fleming discovers penicillin

The Flying Doctor service starts in Australia

Amelia Earhart becomes the first woman to fly the Atlantic

The Morris Minor car goes on the market

Walt Disney introduces Mickey Mouse

The first £1 and 10-shilling notes are brought into circulation

Hyde Park Corner is declared the world's busiest junction

Deaths: Lord Asquith, prime minister 1908-16, suffragette Emmeline Pankhurst, novelist and poet Thomas Hardy, actress Ellen Terry, composer Leos Janácek, Field Marshal Lord Haig, explorer Roald Amundsen

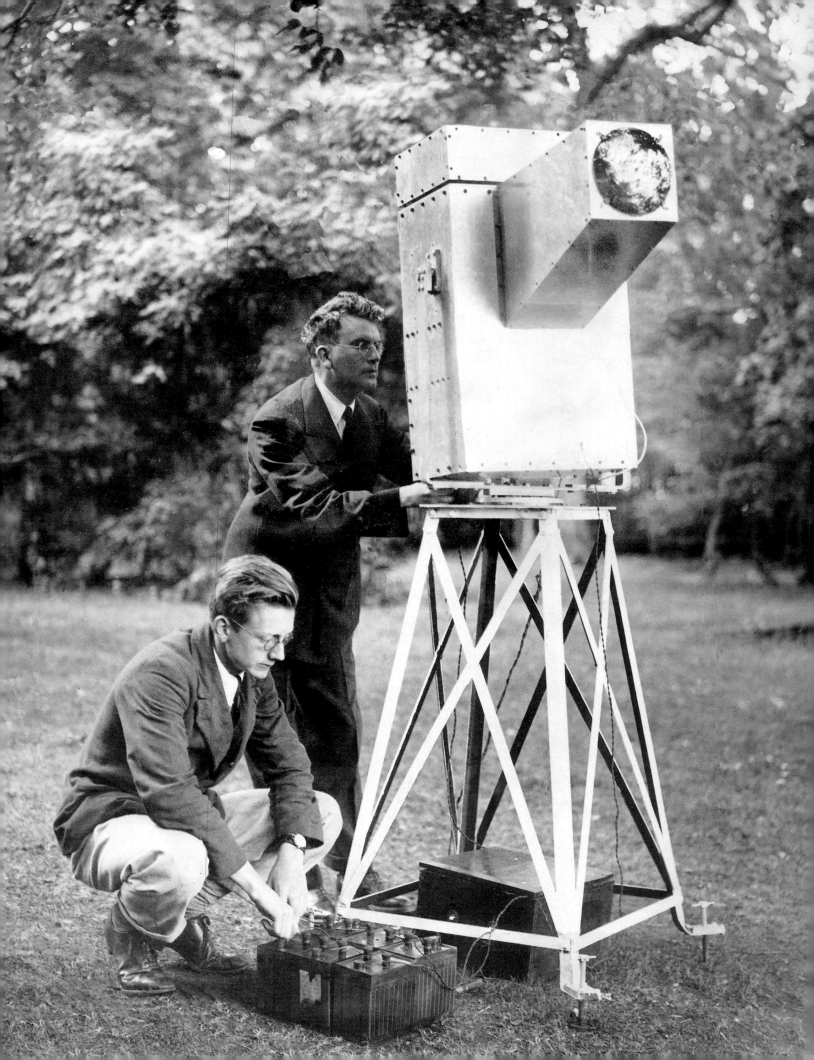

Inventor who overcame poverty

The man who pioneered television, John Logie Baird, demonstrates his latest invention, the noctovisor, with an assistant at Box Hill, Surrey, in 1929. The noctovisor could pick up distant light rays, even through fog, and would, it was hoped, be useful for the military and in navigation.

Baird's enterprises had included a jam factory and soap-making, but it was with television that he made history. The first television, created on a washstand in the inventor's bedroom, was eventually sold for £2 to pay the rent. The impoverished Baird, who suffered persistent ill-health, constructed his early television sets from tea chests, biscuit boxes, hat boxes, scrap timber, cardboard and darning needles, the whole stuck together with glue and sealing wax.

On October 2, 1925, William Taynton – an office boy who was visiting the house in Frith Street, Soho, where Baird rented rooms – became the first person to be seen on television. Baird's first public demonstration of his invention was given to the Royal Institution on January 26, 1926. Though crude, Baird's apparatus allowed light and shade and some detail to be shown. By 1928 Baird was making regular transmissions and was developing colour television. In the event, however, his machine, based on a complex and inherently unreliable mechanical process, was discarded by broadcasters in favour of an electronic system developed by RCA in America. But Baird had at least demonstrated the potential of television.

The inventor made little money from his work – when he died in 1946 he left his widow and children only £7,370. He had, his widow claimed, made more from inventing feet-warming socks than from television.

Also this year...

Wall Street crashes

Eamon de Valera, leader of Fianna Fail, is arrested on entering Northern Ireland

Aristide Briand, the French Prime Minister, proposes a united Europe

The RAF makes first non-stop flight from Britain to India

The Academy of Motion Picture Arts and Sciences holds its first award ceremony

Salvador Dalí has his first exhibition in Paris.

Deaths: The Russian ballet impresario Serge Diaghilev, the actress Lillie Langtry, lawman of the Wild West Wyatt Earp, French politician Georges Clemenceau

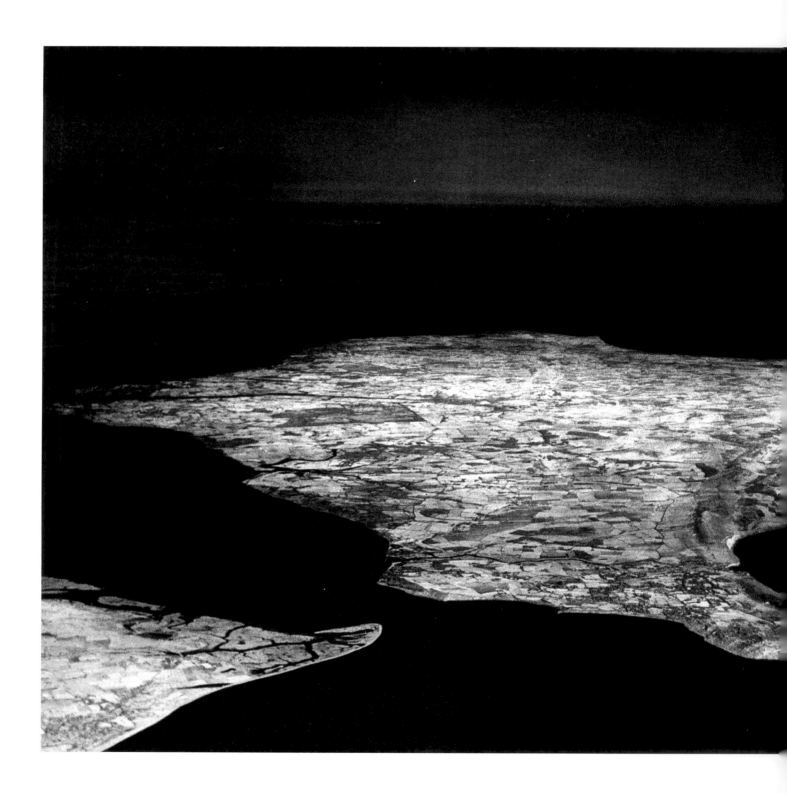

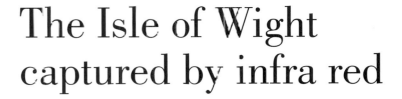

The Isle of Wight captured by infra red

This picture of the Isle of Wight, taken in 1930 from 18,000 feet, is one of the earliest examples of infra-red photography. Beachy Head is to the left and the Kent coast in the distance.

Infra-red photography uses film that is sensitive to both visible light and to longer length infra-red radiation waves. Infra-red plates enabled the photographer who took this picture, U.V. Bogaerde, to obtain a hitherto elusive level of clarity, cutting through haze and mist.

Friedrich Wilhelm Herschel is credited with discovering the infra-red spectrum, which operates between visible light and radar, in 1800. Although it is invisible to the naked eye, its warmth can be felt. Infra-red techniques have since been used for an eclectic variety of purposes: to locate military targets, accident survivors and water sources; to restore paintings; and to see animals more clearly on night safaris.

U.V Bogaerde, a pioneering photographer and father of actor Dirk Bogarde, was employed by Lord Northcliffe, the proprietor of *The Times*, specifically to experiment with photographic techniques. Bogaerde worked in extreme secrecy in a cage in the basement of *The Times* at Printing House Square in London. When *The Times* carried its first halftone photograph, in 1914, the innovation did not prove popular with all readers. It was only in March 1922, when, under Lord Northcliffe's instruction, a page of photographs prepared by Bogaerde was published, that photographs became an established daily feature.

Also this year...

Pluto is discovered

Unemployment reaches two million

Amy Johnson becomes the first woman to make a solo flight from Britain to Australia

Mahatma Gandhi completes 300-mile protest walk against the Salt Law in India and is later arrested

Frozen peas are put on sale in America

Hyde Park Lido opens for mixed bathing

The Church of England backs birth control

Donald Bradman, on his first tour of England, pulverises England's bowlers

Adolf Hitler's National Socialists come second in German elections

The French begin the Maginot Line as a defence against Germany

48 are killed when the airship R101 crashes in northern France

Highway Code is issued

Deaths: Arthur James Balfour, Sir Henry Segrave, creator of Sherlock Holmes Sir Arthur Conan Doyle

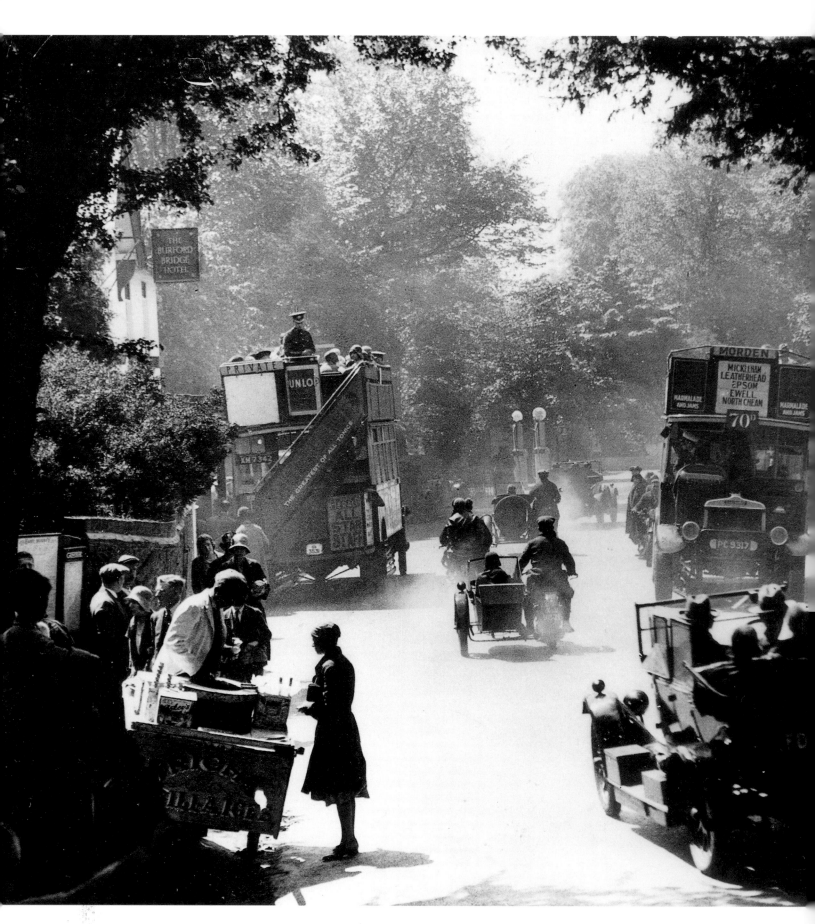

Taking to the road for Bank Holiday break

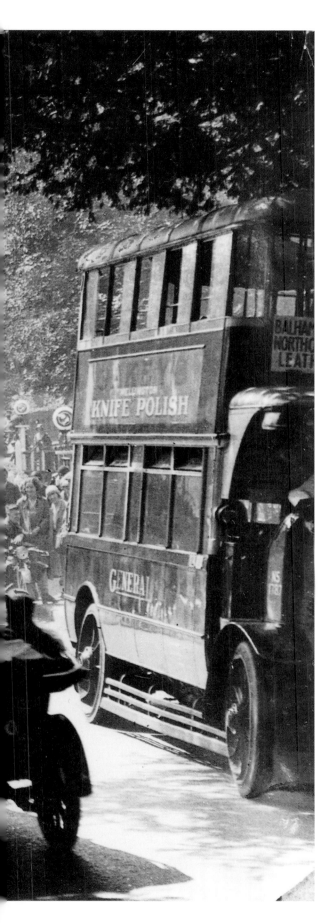

Then, as now, the British spent Bank Holidays on the roads. This picture, taken at Burford Bridge near Dorking in Surrey at Whitsun, shows holiday-makers making their way to spend the day at Box Hill, a grassy hill popular for picnics and with views over the North Downs.

Extra buses were laid on to cater for trippers travelling from Morden, the closest Underground station, to the bus stop nearest to Box Hill. There are still buses running on the 70D route – like the bus on the right of the picture – on summer Sundays between Dorking and Clapham Common via Morden. Richer holidaymakers, meanwhile, crammed into cars. Some travelled in motorcycle sidecars. The glass balls to the left of the road are petrol pumps. After a Budget increase on petrol in April this year, a gallon cost one shilling and fourpence halfpenny.

The Road Traffic Act, passed in 1930, came in to force on January 1, 1931. The Act abolished the 20 mph speed limit for cars and cycles, introduced a specialised traffic police, made third-party insurance compulsory and introduced driving tests for disabled drivers who then had to demonstrate that they were fit to drive. White traffic markers had been introduced in 1925 but it was not until 1931 that plans were made to install traffic lights outside the London area. Signposts were introduced generally in the early 1930s. Before that, drivers were dependent on the system provided by the AA. Help may have been at hand for the drivers pictured above but the pedestrians thronging the roads at Box Hill would have had to keep their wits about them: the first pedestrian crossings were not introduced until 1934.

Also this year...

Wallis Simpson is introduced to the Prince of Wales

New York's Empire State Building is opened

Sir Oswald Mosley forms the New Party

Spain becomes a republic

Unemployment stands at almost three million in Britain, almost five *million in Germany and seven million in the US*

King George V takes a pay cut for the duration of the economic crisis

Britain is forced off the Gold Standard and devalues the pound

Deaths: inventor Thomas Alva Edison, Dame Nellie Melba, ballerina Anna Pavlova

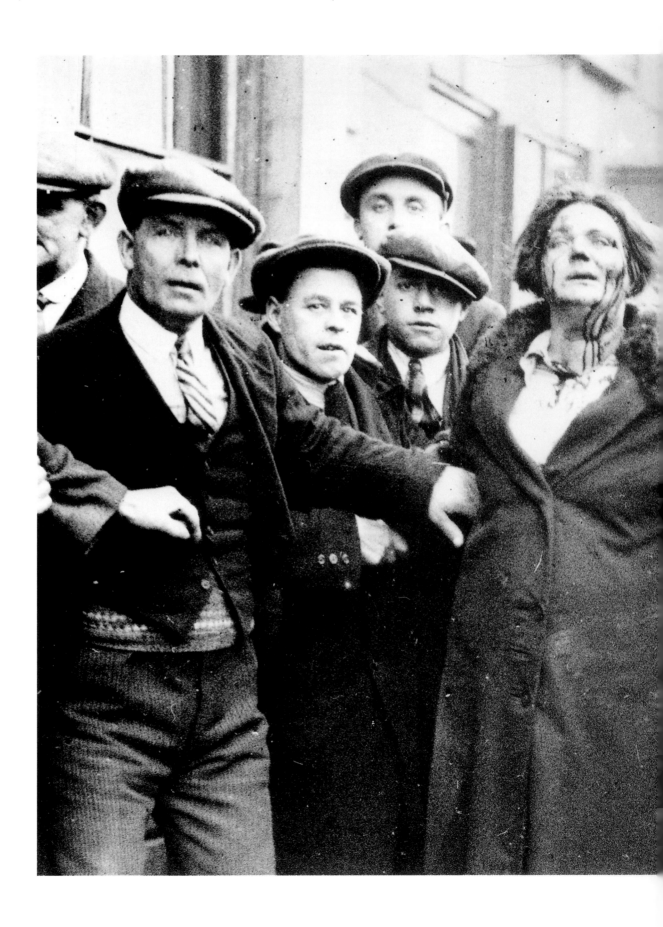

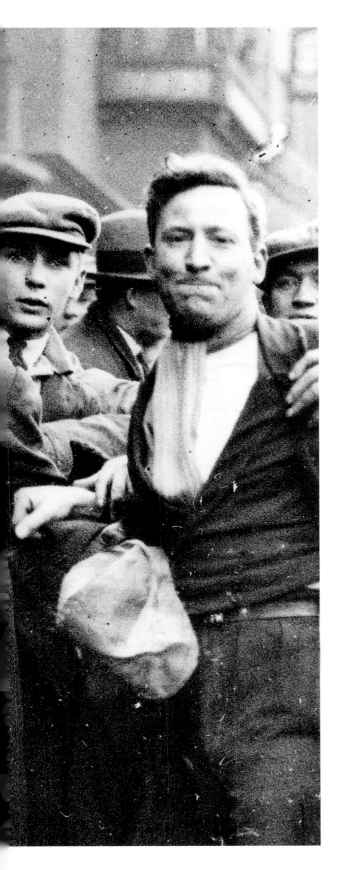

Violence mars protest against the Depression

The pressures of mass unemployment took an ugly turn when demonstrations developed into riots in Bristol on February 23. Violence broke out as a crowd of 6,000 attempted to march from Horsefair in the centre of the city, where Communists had been holding a rally, to Council House to protest against the means-test. Thirty people, probably including the woman pictured here, had to be treated for injuries.

Weekly unemployment benefit had been reduced from October the previous year to 15/3 for men and 13/6 for women; those with dependants were awarded 8 shillings for an adult, and 2 shillings for a child. However, benefit was restricted to six months and for the rest of the year the unemployed were obliged to apply for transitional payments, subject to means-testing. The household means-test, introduced after the economic emergency in 1931, took into account any income within the family, including contributions from relatives and charities, savings and even furniture. By the end of 1932 an estimated 180,000 people had been denied aid because of the means-test.

The people of Bristol were not the only ones to show their frustration this year: hunger marches took place across the country and riots broke out in London when 15,000 marchers and supporters clashed with the police. Three years after the Wall Street Crash, unemployment showed little signs of abating. By September a record one in four British workers was out of work, making a total of almost three million. Unemployment in heavy industry was particularly high: three out of five ship construction workers and two out of five miners were out of work. However, statistics included only those who were signing on for benefits and not the self-employed, married women and agricultural workers.

Also this year...

US unemployment passes eight million

Hitler becomes a German citizen

American Forrest Mars creates the Mars Bar

Oswald Mosley founds British Union of Fascists

Eamon de Valera and the Fianna Fail Party lead new Irish Parliament

Lambeth Bridge is opened

John Galsworthy, author of The Forsyte Saga, wins the Nobel Prize for Literature

The building of Battersea Power Station is begun

Deaths: French President Paul Doumer assassinated, French politician Aristide Briand, US inventor George Eastman

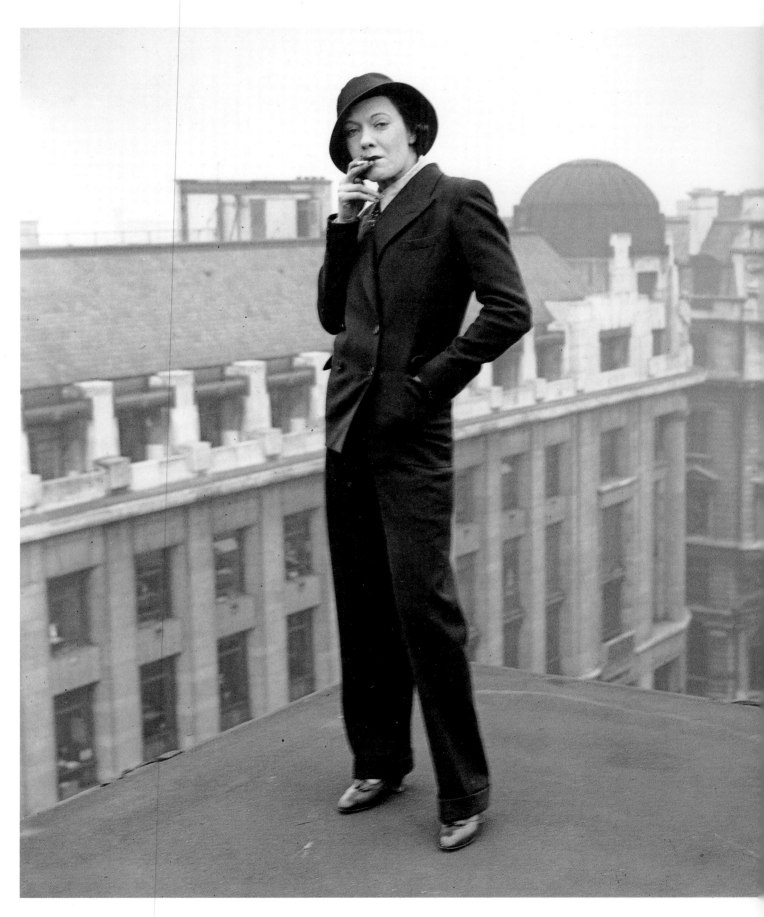

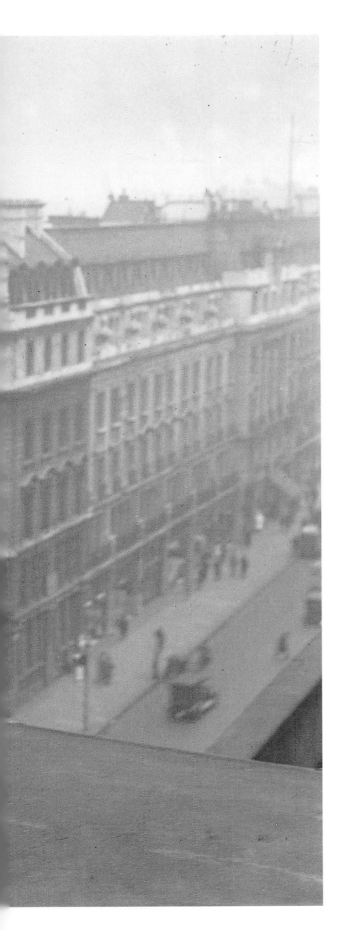

Height of style with a dash of Dietrich

A model sports the new Dietrich-inspired fashion on the rooftop of Nicholl's shop on Regent Street, London, where the outfit was for sale. Amelia Bloomer's attempts to introduce trousers for women in the late 1890s had largely ended in derision and failure. With the memorable exception of Coco Chanel, most women wore trousers only within the sporting arena. However, when Marlene Dietrich, the enigmatic German film actress, took to wearing men's clothes in public, she set a trend. Like the model pictured here, Dietrich chose to wear a suit and a tie – which generally matched her lipstick and her nail polish – topped by a slanted hat.

The fashion, nicknamed "Dietrickery", may have proved popular with female fans but it took a brave woman to adopt it in public. Like most new fashions, the actress's masculine garb was a shock to many. Fashionable French women needed even more nerve than their British counterparts: in Paris a woman was liable to be arrested if she wore men's clothes in public. When Dietrich visited the French capital in 1932, her fashion sense nearly led to the chief of police having her deported. Dietrich's attire, it was argued, would set a bad example and could lead the weak astray. It was not until after the Second World War that women began to wear trousers regularly. By the 1960s women were buying more trousers than skirts.

Also this year...

Hitler becomes German Chancellor and bans all opposition parties

The Nazis open first concentration camp at Dachau

Japan and Germany leave the League of Nations

England win the Ashes in the controversial Bodyline Test series in Australia

Four Britons become the first to fly over Everest

Electric advertisements are unveiled in Piccadilly Circus

UK bans Soviet imports

Lyons opens its first Corner House, which can feed 2,000 diners at a time

Zippo lighter is introduced

George Orwell publishes Down and Out in Paris and London

Communists attempt to seize power in Spain

Deaths: US president Calvin Coolidge, British engineer Sir Frederick Royce

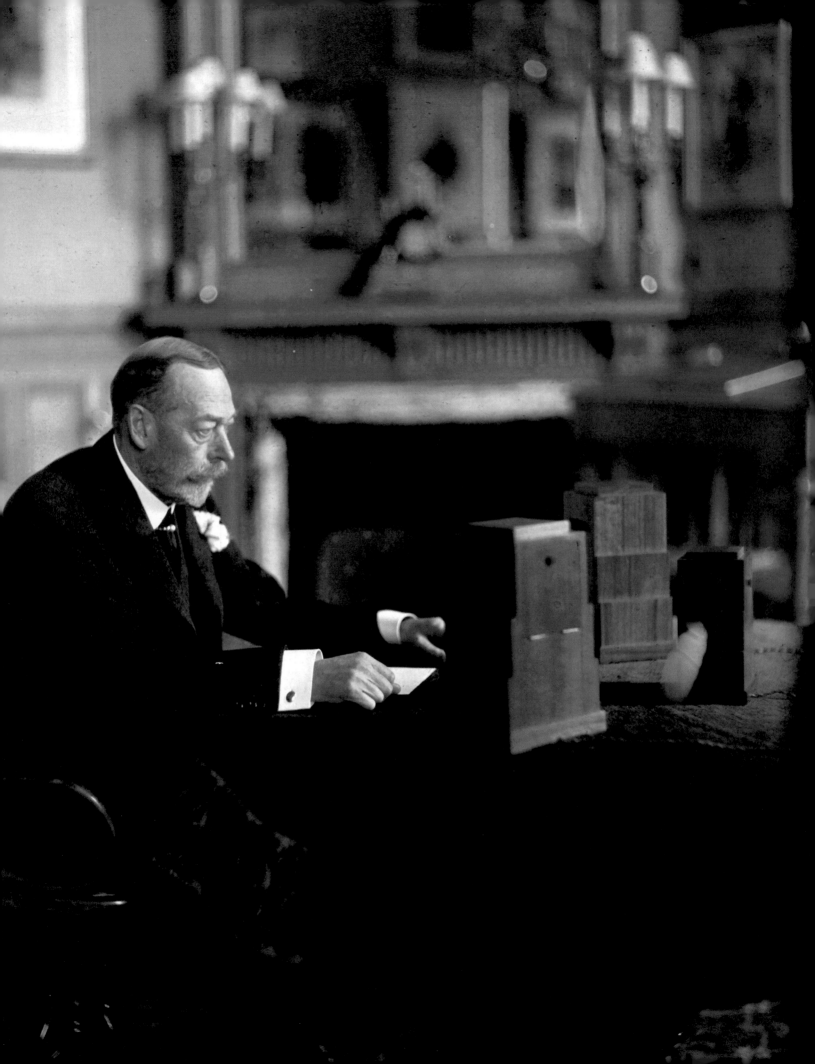

Perfect enunciation as the King broadcasts

A rare early colour photograph of King George V broadcasting his 1934 Christmas message from his residence at Sandringham. The wooden boxes you can see in front of the King were designed to hide two microphones and a red cue light. The tablecloth was used to help lessen the echo.

Two years earlier, George V had become the first British monarch to harness modern technology and speak to his subjects at home and across the empire on the radio. The King kept the broadcast brief but did not underestimate the significance of the occasion. At 3.05 pm he announced: "Through one of the marvels of modern science, I am enabled, this Christmas Day, to speak to all my peoples throughout the Empire. I take it as a good omen that wireless should have reached its present perfection at a time when the Empire has been linked in closer union."

The Times lauded the King's pronunciation, "the perfect and unforced enunciation set the standard for the speaking of the King's English." The speech was "for many millions the outstanding event of Christmas Day. Everywhere throughout the Empire members of the British family gathered together, suspending their merrymaking or their work … to listen to the voice of the head of the family speaking from his own home." Twenty-three years after her grandfather's broadcast, Queen Elizabeth II became the first sovereign to broadcast the royal Christmas message on television.

Also this year...

Road signs are standardised

Female competitors are permitted to wear shorts at Wimbledon, where Britons Fred Perry and Dorothy Round win the men's and women's singles

Pedestrian crossings are introduced in London

262 miners are killed at Gresford Mine, near Wrexham

Bonny Parker and Clyde Barrow are shot

Nazis assassinate the Austrian Chancellor Englebert Dollfuss

Cunard launches the Queen Mary

Deaths: composers Sir Edward William Elgar and Gustav Holst, Marie Curie, Field Marshal Paul von Hindenburg

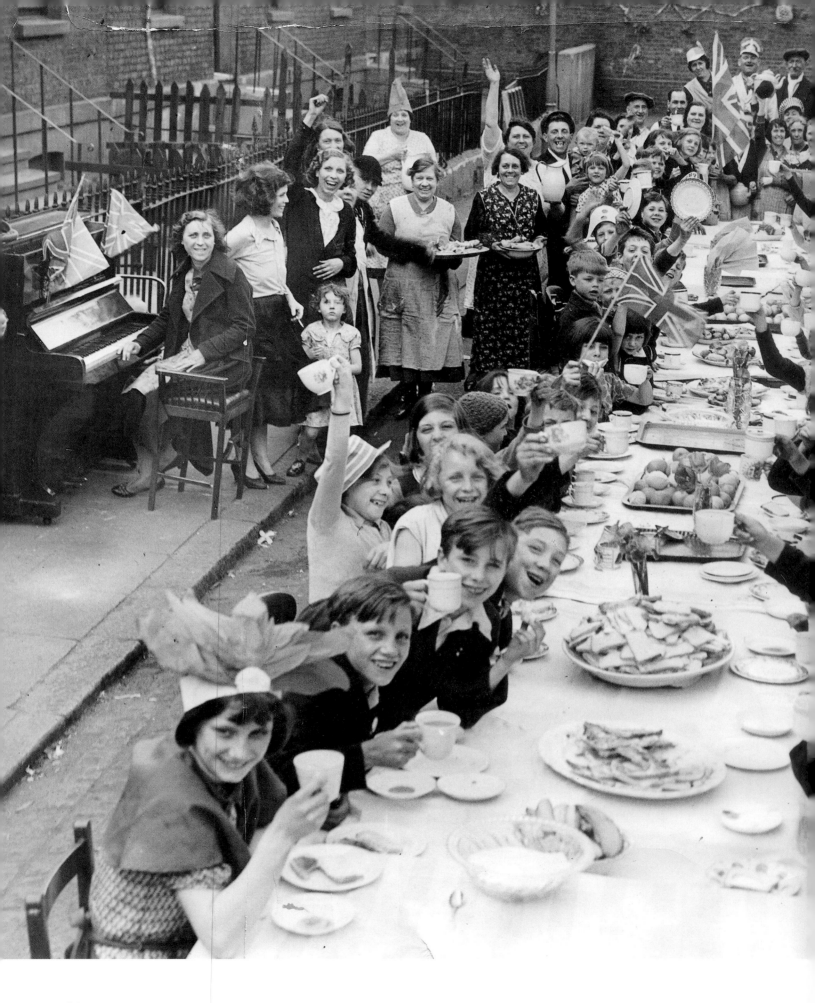

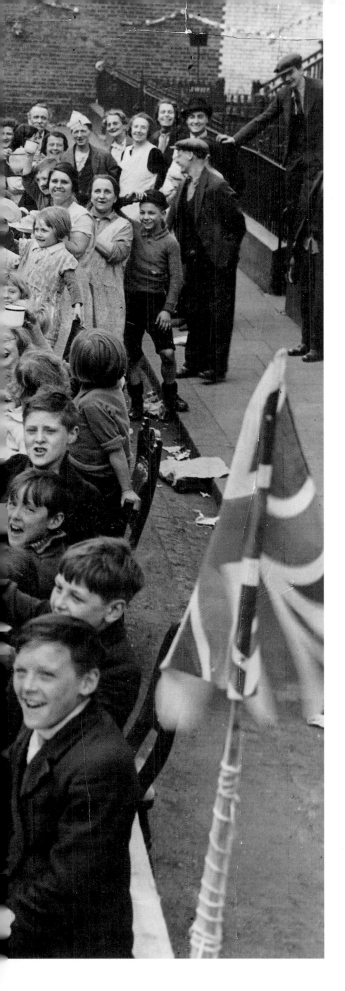

Children have fun on day of circumstance

These children in London, like thousands of others across the country, had a day to remember as they enjoyed a street party to celebrate George V's silver jubilee. People travelled in their thousands to London to witness the celebrations. Despite the heat, they were not disappointed: the King and Emperor marked his jubilee with suitable pomp and ceremony.

By 6am on Monday, May 6, the crowds were already gathered in force outside Buckingham Palace and along the route of the royal procession from Buckingham Palace to St Paul's, where a service of thanksgiving was held. The crowds along the Strand were 10 deep. Where there was no room to stand many took to rooftops and balconies, others climbed lamp posts, statues and trees. Over 7,000 people fainted in the heat. Nonetheless, as *The Times* reported, the crowd waited "with the good-humour and patience which characterize British people on such occasions". Those who could not see were resourceful: *The Times*'s reporter noted that "the women in the crowd produced the mirrors from their vanity bags, turned their backs onto the route, and used them as periscopes." At Temple Bar, the crowd burst into a spontaneous rendition of *For He's a Jolly Good Fellow*.

On their return from St Paul's, the Royal Family greeted the crowds from the balcony of Buckingham Palace. Looking down at the welcoming thousands with the amazement, the King said, "This is the greatest number of people I have ever seen in my life." For many, the highlight was the young Princesses. Dressed in pink and waving daintily, Princess Margaret was a particular favourite. A footman placed her on a stool on the balcony so that she could acknowledge the crowds. She remained there, still waving, after the rest of the Royal Family had retreated.

Also this year...

Cats Eyes introduced to Britain's roads

Italy invades Abyssinia

Mao Tse Tung completes the Long March

Stanley Baldwin becomes Prime Minister

RADAR first tested

Clement Attlee becomes leader of the Labour party

Fred Perry wins men's singles championship at Wimbledon

Hitler forbids German citizenship for German Jews

Anglo-German naval accord facilitates German naval rearmament

Sir Malcolm Campbell sets a new land-speed world record of 301 mph

Penguin 6d paperbacks launched

Deaths: French car manufacturer André Citroën, Alfred Dreyfus, T.E. Lawrence (Lawrence of Arabia), Polish soldier and statesman Jozef Pilsudski

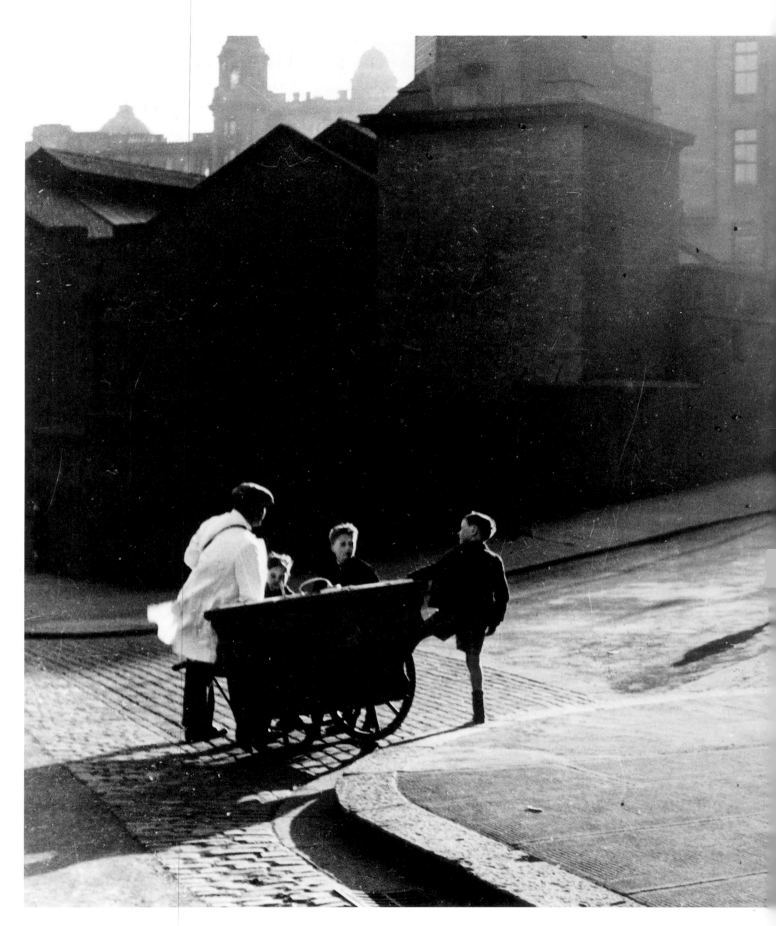

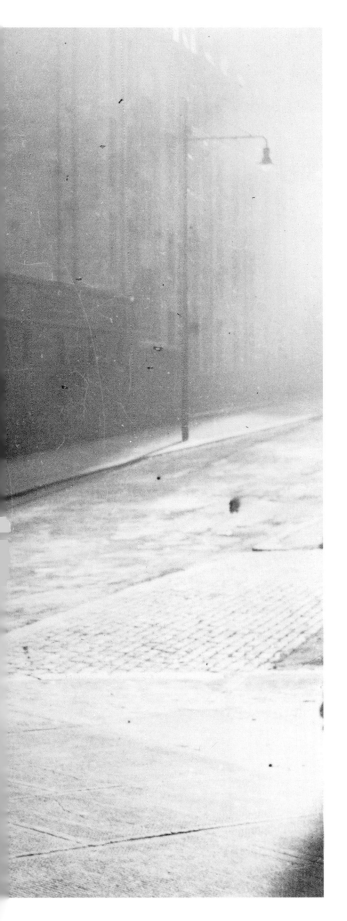

A taste of Italy on the streets of Glasgow

Boys buy Gizzi ice cream on a street corner in Glasgow. The man selling it was most likely Italian. Ice cream was just one of the specialities that Italian immigrants to Scotland made their own.

Almost ten million Italians left their homeland in the 60 years after 1850. The vast majority, almost six million, went to America. But a handful found their way to Scotland. By 1931 there were 5,216 Scots of Italian birth. The earliest of these immigrants were mostly peasants, forced off their lands by population growth and the sharecropping system, which saw farms divided equally among each member of succeeding generations to the point where they could no longer support those who worked them. The majority of these early Italian immigrants came from Toscana in the north of the country or Lazio in the south.

Making and selling ice cream became a livelihood for many Italians in Scotland. To begin with, most had no more than the kind of carts pictured here, set up at park gates and on street corners. The more successful were later able to open shops. The Scottish architect Jack Coia, who died in 1981, was the son of a Glasgow café-owner famous for his ice cream.

The majority of Italian Scots, or Italo-Scozzesi, integrated well. In 1935, the Casa d'Italia was established in Glasgow. This not only promoted Italian language classes and culture, it also provided a place for Italians to meet one another. Nonetheless, Mussolini's expansionist wars at the end of the decade generated suspicion of the Italo-Scozzesi. When Italy subsequently declared war on Britain in June 1940, many were interned as enemy aliens.

Also this year...

Edward VIII abdicates to marry Mrs Simpson

England's rugby team beat the All Blacks for the first time

Hitler launches the Volkswagen

Jesse Owens wins four gold medals at the Berlin Olympics

Pinewood studios are opened

Gatwick airport opens

The first talking television transmission is broadcast

The Spitfire and the Wellington make their maiden flights

The speaking clock is introduced

The Spanish Civil War begins

Fred Perry wins Wimbledon for the third time

Briton Beryl Markham becomes the first woman to fly solo across the Atlantic

Deaths: King George V, Louis Blériot, Maxim Gorky, Rudyard Kipling, A.E Housman, G.K. Chesterton

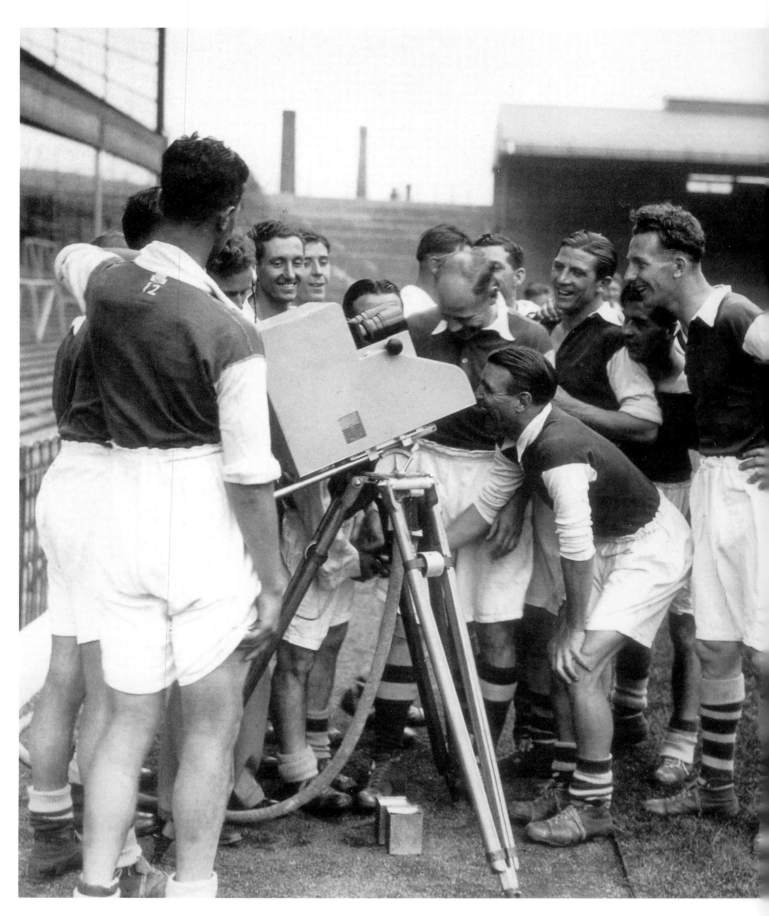

Arsenal score as early TV football stars

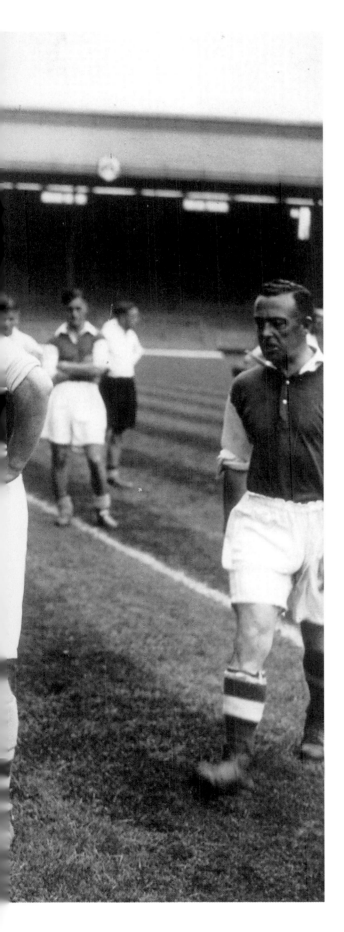

Players of the Arsenal football team inspect a television camera at Highbury. Football in the 1930s underwent an enormous surge of popularity and it was only natural that it should be an early subject for television. The first match to be televised, though only partly, was the 1937 FA Cup final, between Sunderland and Preston (Sunderland won 3-1). But it was not until the following year's FA Cup final, between Preston and Huddersfield, which saw Preston squeak by 1-0, that a match was televised in its entirety.

For most people, football in the 1930s meant only one team: Arsenal. The club dominated the game just as much as Manchester United dominated it in the 1990s. Arsenal won the old First Division five times in the 1930s, in the process becoming only the second team to win it three times in a row, between 1933 and 1935. They also won the FA Cup twice, in 1930 and 1936. Under their influence of their remarkable manager, Herbert Chapman, Arsenal were not only tactically far in advance of their rivals, they were vastly more professional, too. Modern medical equipment and training routines arrived at Highbury long before they had been considered elsewhere. Even shirt numbers were pioneered by them. But Arsenal – "lucky Arsenal" or "boring Arsenal" to many – were never popular away from Highbury. The vast crowds they drew came as much in the hope of seeing the team beaten as to applaud them. When they were beaten by lowly Walsall in the third round of the FA Cup in 1933, the whole country celebrated.

Not even football could escape the growing sense of crisis as the 1930s came to a close. When England played Germany in Berlin in 1938, winning 6-3, the team reluctantly performed a Nazi salute before the game. A year later, the new Arsenal manager, George Allison, addressed the crowd before Arsenal's game with Chelsea on "moral rearmament through sport".

Also this year...

George VI is crowned; the BBC makes its first outside broadcast of the ceremony

Neville Chamberlain replaces Stanley Baldwin as prime minister

The Duke of Windsor marries Wallis Simpson in France

Britain bans volunteers from fighting in Spain

The threepenny bit is introduced

Sir Malcolm Campbell sets a new world water-speed record of 129 mph

Full-scale war breaks out between China and Japan

J.R.R. Tolkien publishes The Hobbit

First feature-length cartoon, Snow White and the Seven Dwarfs, *is produced by Walt Disney*

Deaths: Ramsay MacDonald, John D. Rockefeller, Baron Pierre de Coubertin, Sir James Barrie, George Gershwin, Guglielmo Marconi

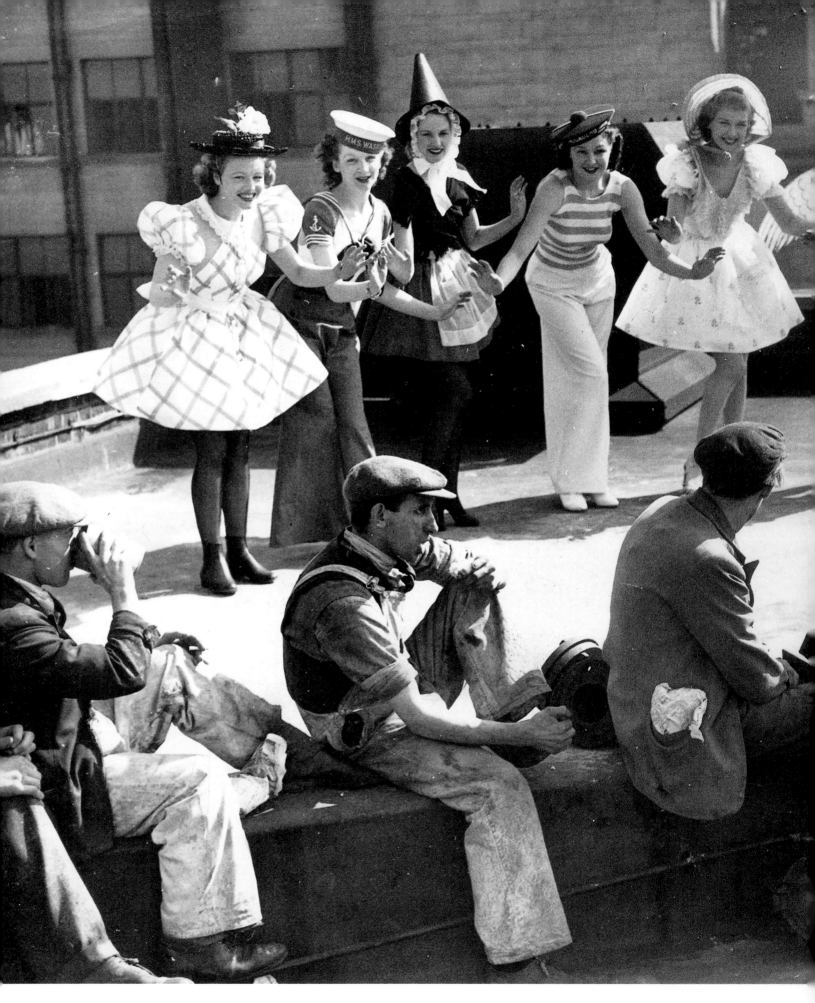

90

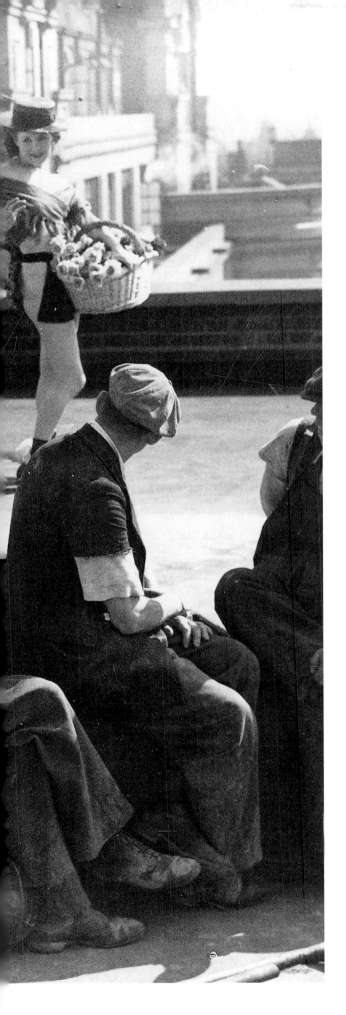

Dancing as the war clouds gather

Dancers from the Trocadero Theatre rehearse on the roof to the evident amusement of workmen taking a tea break. Entertainment between the wars divided sharply into "highbrow" and "popular". These performers were definitely of the popular variety.

The opening in 1932 of the Shakespeare Memorial Theatre in Stratford-upon-Avon established a permanent venue for the Shakespearean repertoire. Meanwhile, comedy and cabaret, similar no doubt in style to that of the Trocadero girls' performance, proved enduringly popular, as did the work of playwrights such as Bernard Shaw and Noel Coward. Musical productions by Irving Berlin, Cole Porter and the Gershwins were warmly received in London and New York. Repertory theatre was also going strong. The first company was formed in 1908 and by the late 1940s there were over 200 repertory companies. Similarly, amateur dramatics flourished.

Alongside the theatre, the cinema also offered growing opportunities for actors. Then, as now, Hollywood dominated but many Britons had managed to establish themselves on both sides of the Atlantic. Charlie Chaplin's fame had been assured for many years. But by the 1930s Britons such as Charles Laughton, Laurence Olivier, Vivien Leigh and Cary Grant had become icons of the silver screen around the world.

Television offered few openings for actors. In 1938, the BBC transmitted for only 90 minutes on weekdays and an hour on Sundays. The first film shown on the BBC, *Man of the Moment*, was transmitted this year, as was the Corporation's first game show, *Spelling Bee*. The embryonic television service was not to last much longer. On the outbreak of hostilities in 1939, it was shut down.

Also this year...

Anthony Eden resigns as Foreign Secretary in protest at Chamberlain's appeasement policies

Anschluss – Germany annexes Austria

Czechoslovakia is dismembered at the Munich conference, after which Neville Chamberlain promises "peace in our time"

Japan withdraws from the League of Nations

The Grand Fascist Council in Italy passes anti-semitic legislation

Kristallnacht – Jewish houses and business across Germany are attacked

Hungarians Ladisla and Georg Biro patent the ball-point pen

Deaths: director Konstantin Stanislavsky, father of modern Turkey Mustafa Kemal Ataturk, Russian politician Nikolai Bukharin

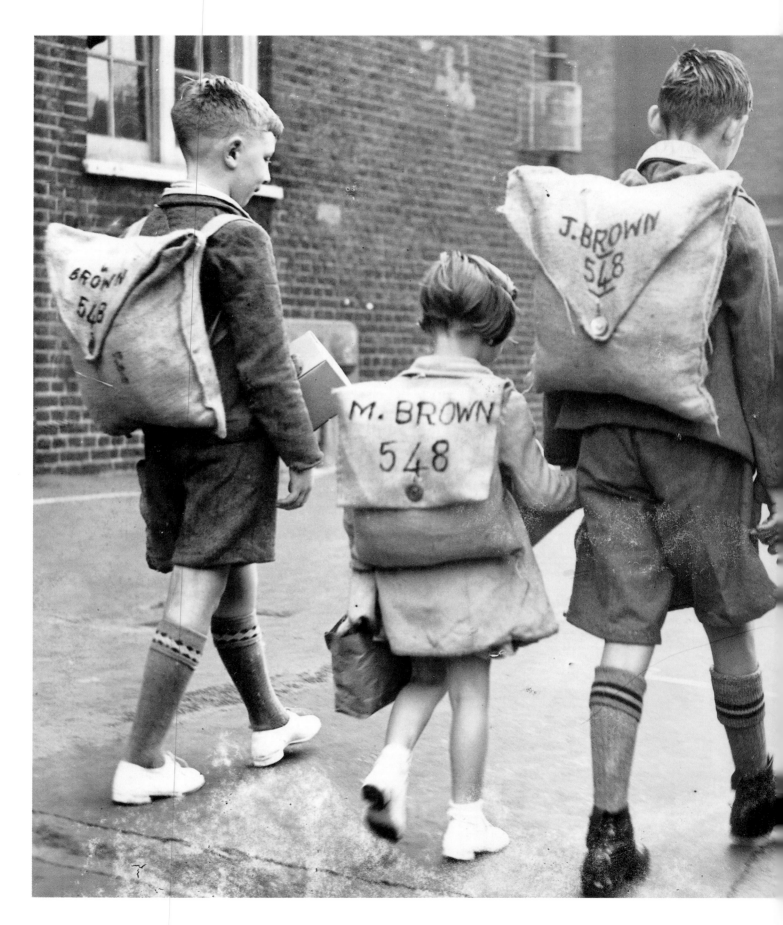

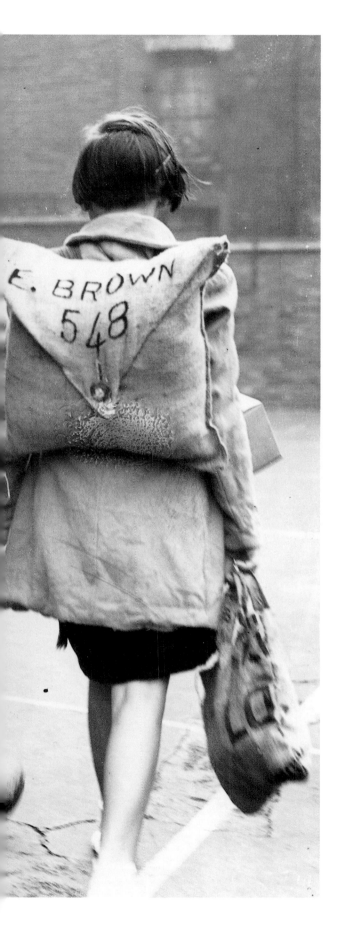

The Browns join the great migration

The Brown children, labelled with their names and the number of their school, are ready to be evacuated from London at the outbreak of the war. The government, believing that modern bombers would devastate cities in a way never seen before, had estimated that up to two million children would be killed in air-raids against cities across the country. Fearing that the morale of the nation could not withstand so great a loss, it organised one of the largest migrations in British history. Though evacuation was voluntary, the pressure to send children away was great and over a million children were evacuated in just three days.

Operation Pied Piper began at 7.30 on the morning of September 1, two days before war was declared. City children, some with their mothers, gathered at their schools ready to be taken to the country for safety. Parents were instructed to provide their children with spare clothing, a toothbrush, a comb, a handkerchief, their gas masks – E. Brown's gas-mask box is just visible to her right – and enough food for the day. Some were to be gone for five years.

Billeting was compulsory, although foster parents were allowed to choose who they would take in. An effort was made to keep siblings together, though it may well have been difficult to find someone prepared to take all four Brown children pictured here. Despite the huge scale of the operation, all the evacuees were billeted within three days. The government paid those who took in children 10/5 a week for the first child and 8/6 for each additional child.

Country foster parents were often shocked by the poverty of their new charges, many of whom were filthy, covered with lice and unschooled in even elementary hygiene. Conversely, many evacuees were astounded by what they found. One child is credited with writing: "they call this 'spring', mum, and they have one down here every year."

Also this year...

German troops overrun Czechoslovakia

Fall of Madrid – Nationalists triumph in Spanish Civil War

Italy invades Albania

George VI becomes first British monarch to visit the United States

Nazi-Soviet Pact

German invasion of Poland; Britain and France declare war

Soviet invasion of Baltic states and eastern Poland

Rationing of meat and sugar is introduced

Pan Am launches first scheduled passenger flights across the Atlantic

German physicist Otto Hahn splits the atom

Gone With the Wind opens

Deaths: W.B. Yeats, Sigmund Freud, Pope Pius XI, US aircraft designer Anthony Fokker

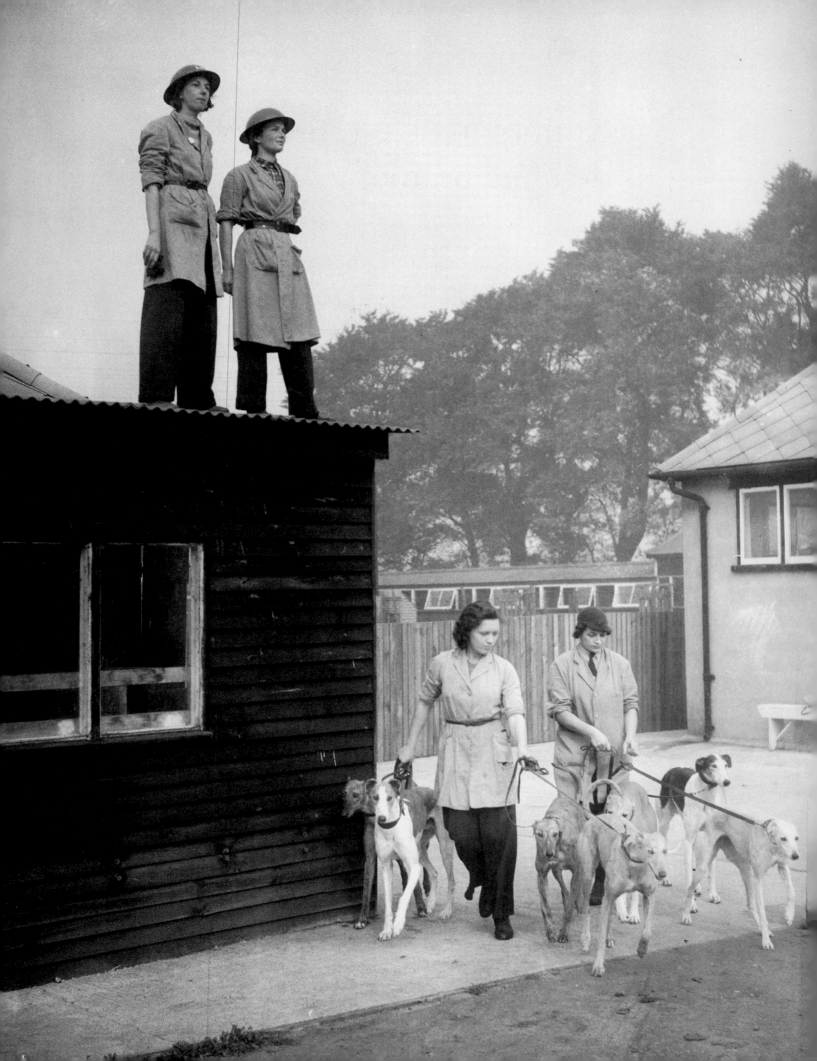

Kennel maids in defiant defence on roof tops

Even kennel maids had a part to play in the defence of Britain as the German threat grew. These women at a kennels in Sunbury-on-Thames were all members of an Air Raid Protection, or ARP, group. The two women on the roof were spotters, looking out for German aircraft. For the women on the ground, like so many others in the country, everyday duties still had to be slotted in.

Since the fall of France in May and the retreat from Dunkirk, the ARP, like the Local Defence Volunteers, re-named the Home Guard by Churchill in July this year, prepared themselves against the daily fear of invasion. The War Minister, Anthony Eden, had called on all men "not presently engaged in military service between the ages of 17 and 65 to come forward and offer their services". Within a month, 750,000 men had enrolled in the first citizen's army raised in Britain since 1803, bringing with them an assortment of weapons: old rifles, swords, even carving knives. Churchill, Prime Minister since May 10 in place of the hapless Neville Chamberlain, ringingly declared in June: "We shall defend our island, whatever the cost may be, we shall fight on the beaches, we shall fight on the landing ground, we shall fight in the fields and in the streets, we shall fight in the hills, we shall never surrender."

On June 24, as Hitler's plans for an invasion took form, German troops were issued with English phrasebooks. On August 25, the first German bombs fell on London.

Also this year...

The Thames freezes for the first time since 1888

Rationing is introduced

Denmark and Norway are overrun by Germany followed by Belgium, Holland and France

300,000 British troops evacuated from Dunkirk

Marshal Pétain becomes head of Vichy French state

The Duke of Windsor is appointed Governor of the Bahamas

The RAF overcomes the Luftwaffe in the Battle of Britain

Franklin Roosevelt wins a third term as President of the United States

Colonel Sanders perfects his recipe for fried chicken

Graham Greene's The Power and the Glory published

Walt Disney releases Pinocchio and Fantasia

Deaths: actress Mrs Patrick Campbell, Neville Chamberlain, Leon Trotsky, F. Scott Fitzgerald, Paul Klee, US car manufacturer Walter P. Chrysler

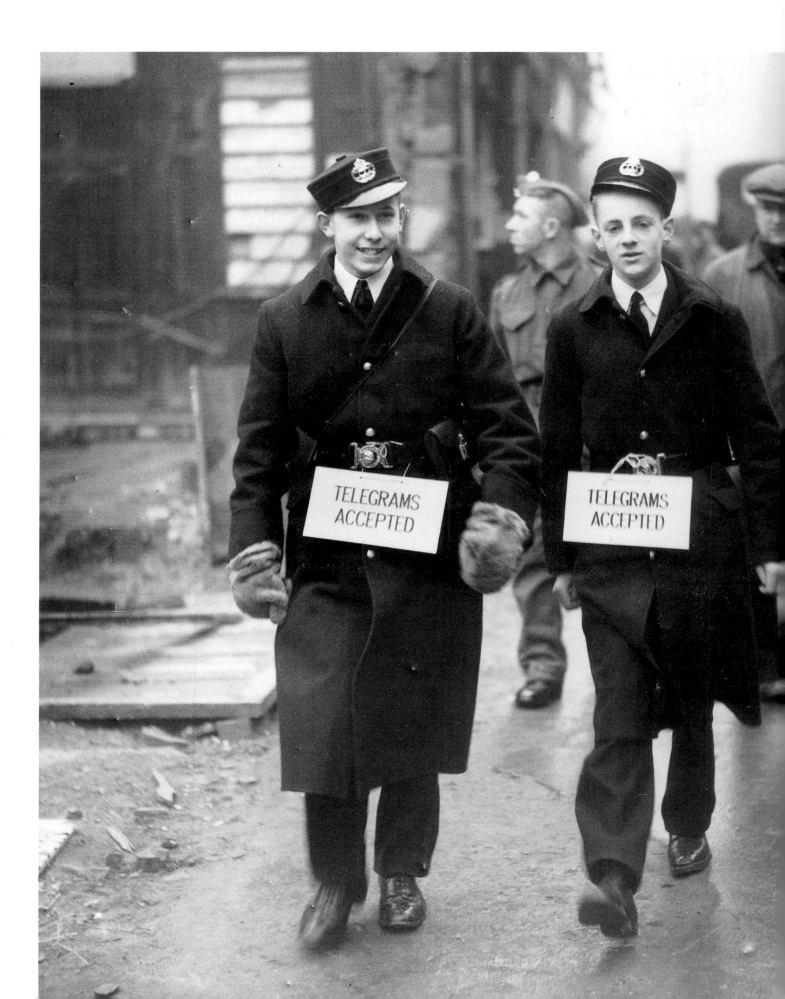

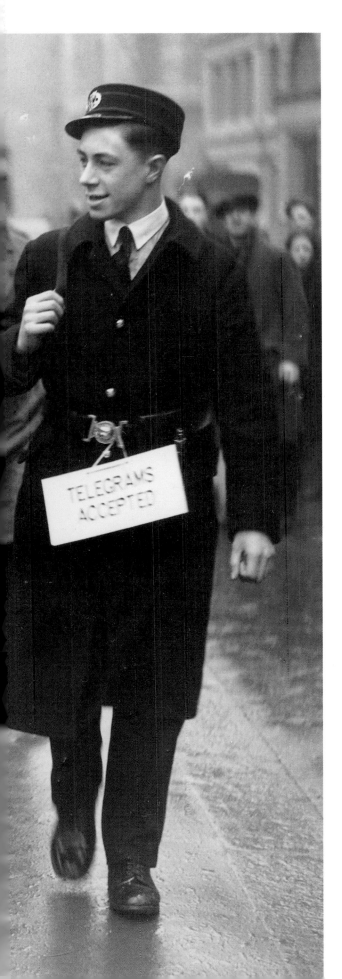

Sending the bad news ... and the good

By January 1941, when the photograph of these telegraph boys was taken, Britain's cities had been under almost continuous attack by the Luftwaffe since early September the previous year. The Blitz was launched – ostensibly in retaliation for British raids on Berlin – on September 7, 1940, when 405 people were killed in a German attack on the East End. Five days later, Buckingham Palace itself was hit, prompting Queen Elizabeth's celebrated comment: "Now I can look the East End in the face." The raids continued almost nightly until May 10, 1941. In March 1941 alone, 4,259 civilians were killed, among them 598 children.

Despite the destruction, a semblance of normality was maintained. Among the wreckage, signs were put up announcing "Business As Usual". Many companies had their offices destroyed and were forced to set up temporary premises in the streets.

It was in response to this bomb damage that the GPO set up a "Wirewalkers" service that employed boys, wearing signs like these, to walk around the City of London as roving post offices from which telegrams could be sent. The GPO also planned to set up telephones in undamaged buildings, though there was of course no certainty that they would remain undamaged.

Telegraph boys may have been a welcome sight in the City. Elsewhere, they were regarded with horror. Telegrams were the normal means by families were notified of the missing or dead.

Also this year...

Rudolf Hess lands in Scotland on a bizarre personal peace mission

The Royal Navy sinks the Bismarck

Yugoslavia and Greece are invaded by Germany; Hitler then launches his crusade against the Soviet Union, Operation Barbarossa – three million German troops attack on a front 1,000 miles long

"Utility" clothing and furniture introduced

Churchill and Roosevelt meet in Newfoundland

Iran is invaded by Britain and the Soviet Union

Pearl Harbor is attacked by Japan, Britain and the United Sates declare war on Japan, Germany and Italy declare war on the USA

Japan invades Malaya

Single women in Britain between 20 and 30 are called up

Citizen Kane is released

Deaths: James Joyce, Virginia Woolf, Lord Baden-Powell, Amy Johnson

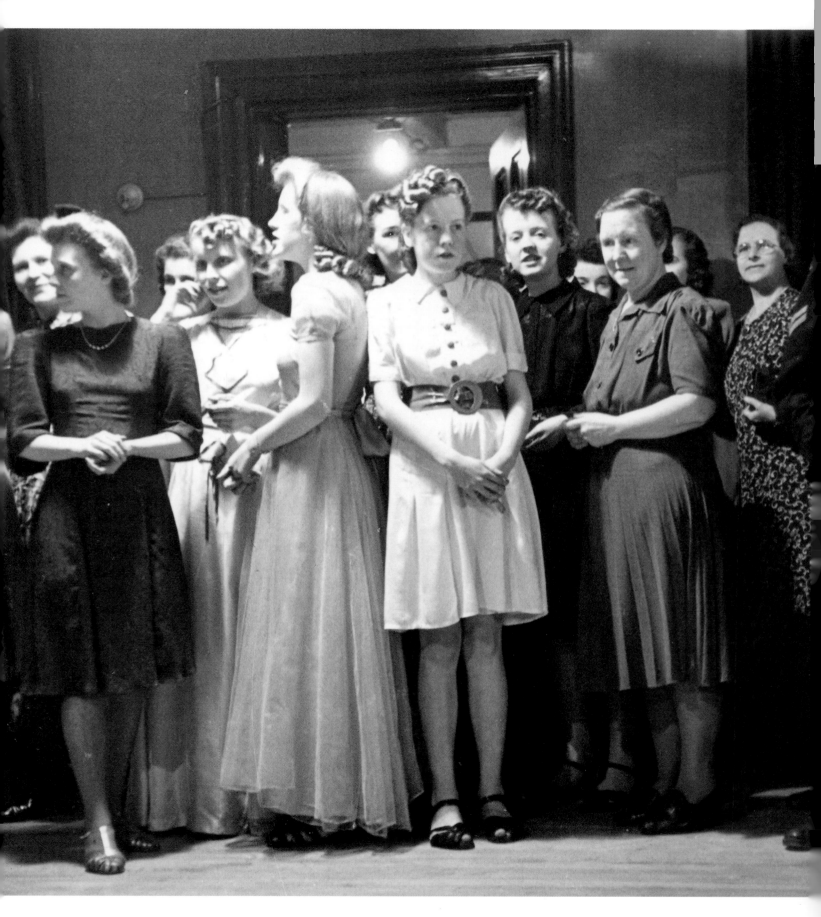

Waiting for the Yanks to be over here

With so many men called up to fight, these women would have waited some time to be asked to dance. However, life was about to get considerably more exciting when the Americans arrived. From 1942, over one and a half million American troops – nicknamed GIs after the General Issue stamp on their uniforms – began to flood into Britain.

So many young men needed a great deal to divert them and dances were held with increasing frequency across the country. For many British women, the combination of dashing Americans in uniform with seemingly limitless supplies of nylons, chocolate and cigarettes and the knowledge that tomorrow might bring only death proved an irresistible combination. An estimated 75,000 women were to leave Britain as GI brides while around a third of all births during the war were illegitimate.

Looking the part was always a struggle. Clothes rationing had been introduced in 1941 while in 1942 the government laid down maximum prices for clothes. The Board of Trade permitted a limited number of styles to be produced and only from specified cloths. Embroidery on underwear and nightgowns was forbidden, for example. Civilians were encouraged to make do and mend – the women pictured here would have had to get a lot of wear out of their dresses.

Cosmetics were in equally short supply and led to many improvisations: soot for eyeliner; beetroot juice for rouge and lipstick. Stockings could be imitated by painting legs with gravy browning and drawing a line down the back of the calf as a seam. Bare legs were akin to patriotism.

Washing was another area where sacrifices were demanded. Soap was rationed to a bar a month, while people were encouraged to take fewer and shallower baths – no more than five inches of hot water– and to share bath water.

Also this year...

The Final Solution is agreed upon at the Wannsee Conference

Vidkun Quisling is appointed head of Norway's puppet government

Singapore falls to Japan – 70,000 Allied troops are captured

Oxford Committee for Famine Relief (later "Oxfam") founded

The people of Malta are awarded the George Cross for their fortitude in withstanding the German bombardment of their island

Japan's advance in the Pacific is halted by the US at the Battle of Midway

Germany's advance in North Africa is halted by the British at El Alamein; Anglo-American landings take place in Morocco and Algeria

The German advance in the Soviet Union is halted in the frozen horrors of Stalingrad

Vera Lynn's We'll Meet Again *is a hit*

Deaths: John Barrymore, Walter Sickert, the Duke of Kent

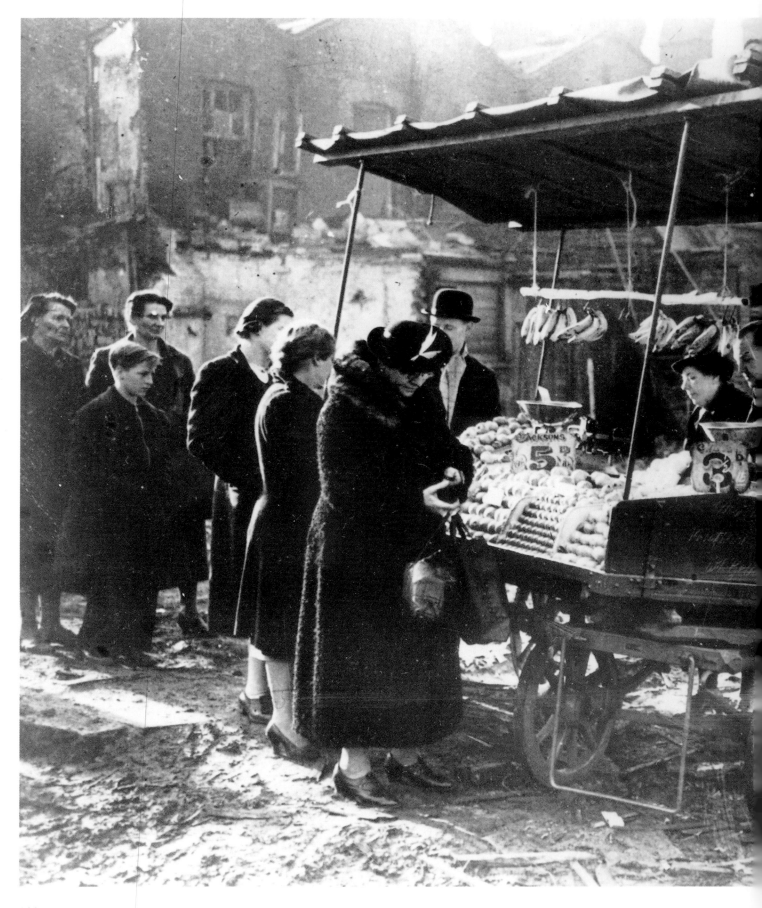

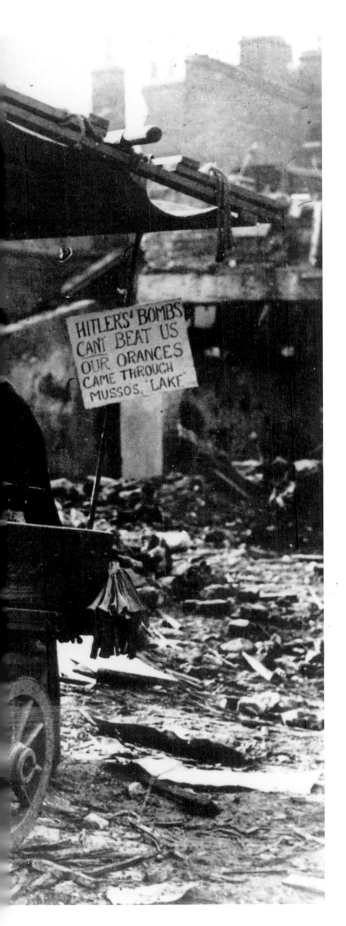

On sale as usual ... the fruits from Musso's lake

The sign on this make-shift market stall was defiant, but oranges and bananas were rarities worth queuing for during the war. This cargo may have made it across "Musso's lake" – the Mediterranean – but many others did not. Rationing was introduced in January 1940, for butter, bacon and sugar. It was to continue in one form or another as late as July 3, 1954. By 1942, the icing of cakes had been banned and many couples celebrated their wedding day with a cardboard replica cake. Restricted foods could be bought only with ration books – children under five had green books, older children blue books and adults white books – and every household was obliged to register at local shops. Hotel guests had to hand over their ration books to the management for the duration of their stay. Anyone caught buying food on the black market was liable to a fine.

Allotted amounts changed frequently, but the basic weekly provision per person was four ounces of bacon or ham, margarine and cooking fat, two ounces of butter, cheese and tea, eight ounces of sugar, three pints of milk, one egg and 6d-worth of meat. A tin of condensed milk, one pound of preserves, 12 ounces of sweets and the powder equivalent of 12 eggs were allowed every four weeks. Offal and kippers were not rationed but were still difficult to come by. Faced with such meagre rations and inspired by the likes of *The Victory Cookbook*, enterprising cooks came up with such delights as Patriotic Pudding, Blitz Broth and Spam Ooh La La.

Also this year...

The German army at Stalingrad surrenders

8th Army enters Tunisia

Warsaw Ghetto uprising begins

German forces in North Africa surrender

Soviet Union defeats Germans at Kursk, the largest tank battle in history

US and British troops land in Italy; Mussolini resigns – Italy signs armistice

PAYE introduced

Heaviest Allied air-raid of the war

so far opens the Battle of Berlin

Tehran Conference

Church bellringing is reinstated and sign posts in rural areas are re-erected

Part-time war work is made for compulsory for British women between 18 and 45

Deaths: Beatrix Potter, Jean Moulin (resistance leader executed by the Nazis), Sergei Rachmaninov, Polish leader Wladislaw Sikorski, Fats Weller

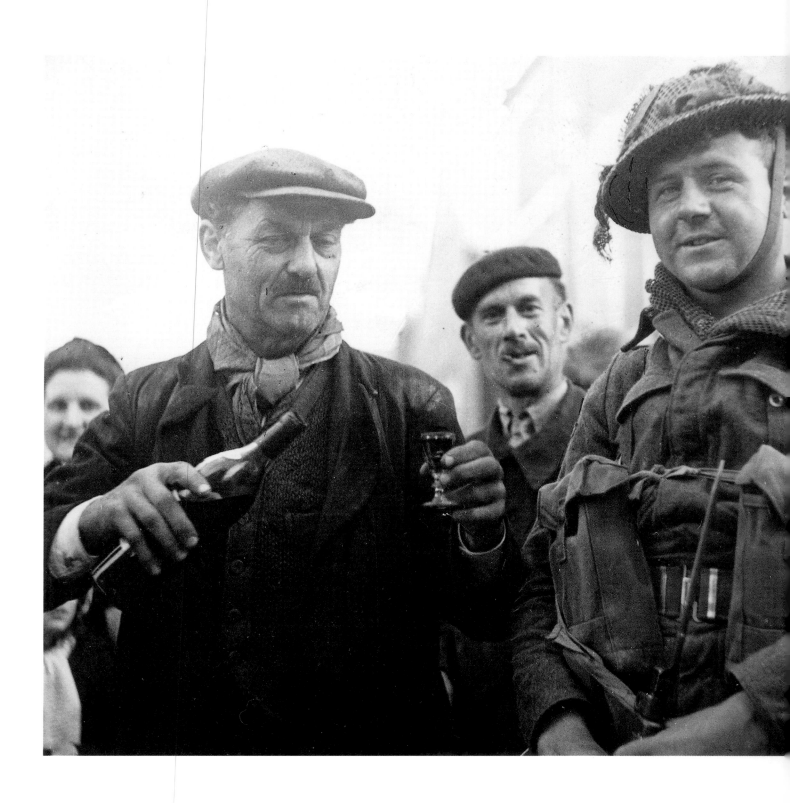

A toast to D-Day's conquering heroes

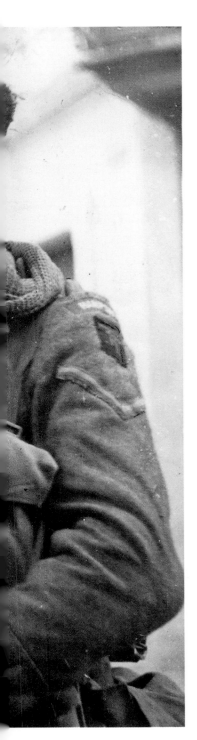

A soldier of the Hampshire Regiment is welcomed to Normandy with a glass of wine – or perhaps the local speciality, calvados – after the D-Day landings of June 6. He was one of the 176,000 Allied troops who took part in the landings, codenamed Operation Overlord, the largest amphibious assault ever launched.

The critical issue was to keep the destination of the landings secret from the Germans, so stretching their forces along the entire coast rather than concentrated at the invasion point. Against all reasonable expectation, the deception plan – Operation Bodyguard – succeeded in persuading Hitler that the major target was the Pas de Calais. Only 14 of the 58 German divisions in France were deployed against the Normandy beaches. It was also imperative to use Allied air superiority to neutralize the German air force and to disrupt German communications in northern France to prevent German reinforcements being moved to Normandy. On D-Day itself, 12,000 Allied aircraft confronted a mere 170 German aircraft. It would take weeks for German reinforcements to be moved to the front in effective numbers.

On the night of June 5, paratroops were sent in to secure the flanks of the invasion areas and establish initial positions. At dawn the next morning, the invasion fleet itself arrived: over 7,000 ships of all sizes. They landed five divisions on five landing beaches: Gold, Juno, Sword, Omaha and Utah. Despite fierce fighting, especially at Omaha beach, all the beach heads were secured by June 6. By June 11, secure positions inland had been established.

Progress thereafter was slow. Marshy ground, thick hedgerows and determined German defence prevented a breakout and threatened to re-create the trench stalemate of the First World War. It was not until July 25 that the decisive thrust could be made. By late August, the Allies were across the Seine and by September stood on the German frontier.

Also this year...

Eisenhower made Supreme Commander Allied Expeditionary Forces

First major Allied daylight air-raids on Berlin

Allied armies enter Rome

Von Stauffenberg's plot to blow up Hitler fails

Paris liberated

Soviet forces cross into Prussia

First US bombing raids on Japanese mainland

Allied invasion force at Arnhem defeated

Battle of the Bulge – German counter-attack in western Europe is repulsed

Deaths: Glenn Miller, Erwin Rommel (through suicide), Sir Edwin Lutyens, William Heath Robinson, Sir Henry Wood

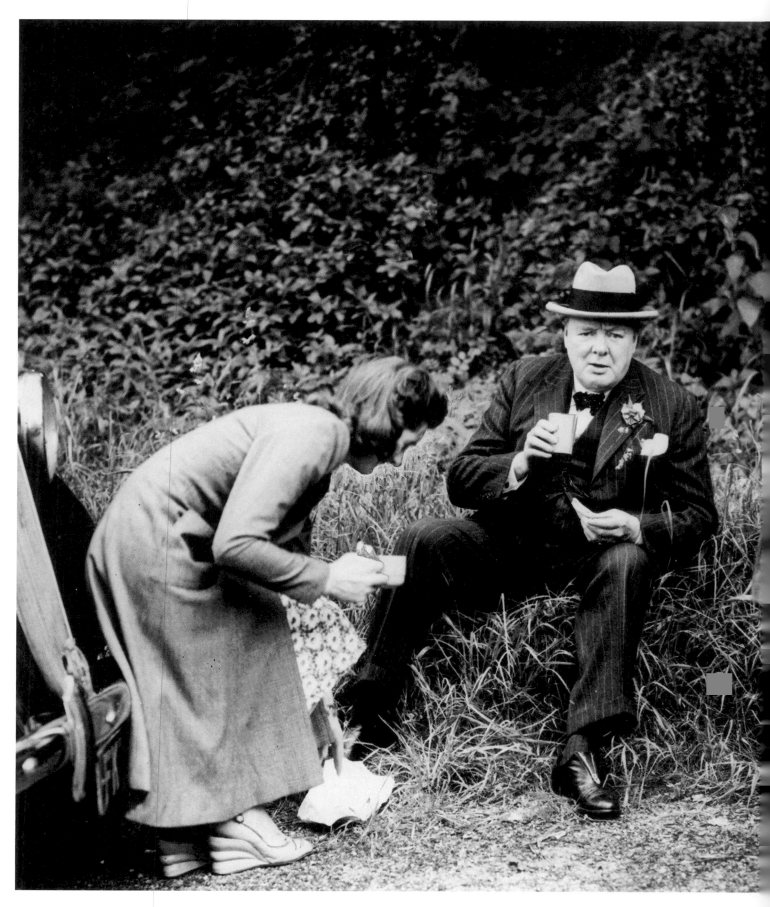

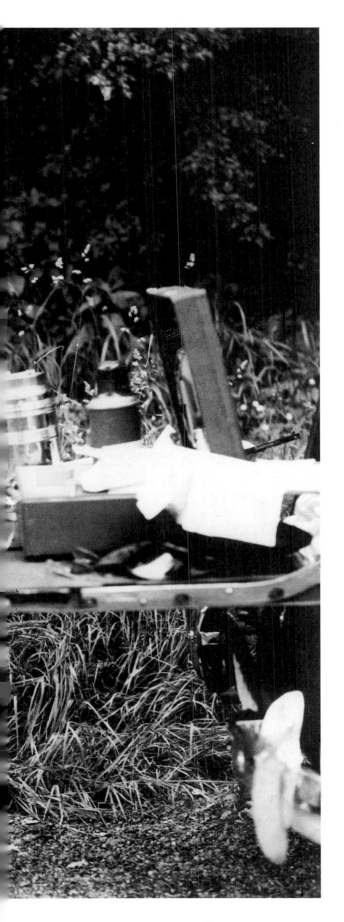

Brief respite on the campaign trail

The Prime Minister, Winston Churchill, stops for a roadside picnic with his daughter, Sarah, on June 25 during the campaigning for the 1945 general election. Churchill had been Prime Minister of the wartime coalition government since May 1940, when Neville Chamberlain had resigned in his favour. When this photograph was taken, just after the end of the war in Europe, he was hoping to lead the Conservative Party to victory.

The picture was taken on the first day of gruelling four-day election tour, which included visits to Manchester, Crewe, Leeds, Bradford, Preston, Glasgow and Edinburgh. On some days he addressed 10 different meetings; on June 26, he spoke in 11 different cities. Wartime co-operation between the parties played no part in the election. Churchill was scathing about his Labour opponents, asserting that: "they could not allow free, sharp or violently worded expressions of discontent" and would "have to fall back on some form of Gestapo".

Despite incidents such as that in Tooting Bec, south London, in early July when a squib was thrown at him and only narrowly missed exploding in his face, Churchill's own popularity as a wartime leader was never in doubt. But the country was much less enthusiastic about him as a peacetime Prime Minister, preferring the Labour Party's vision of a new, post-war Britain with a welfare state at its heart. Though the election was held on July 5, it took three weeks for the votes of three million servicemen and women overseas to be counted and the results were announced only on July 26. The Labour Party under Clement Attlee had won a landslide victory, winning 393 seats to the Conservatives' 213. The "New Jerusalem" was at hand.

Also this year...

US 7th Army reaches the Siegfried Line

US Marines land on Iwo Jima; last V2 lands in Britain

Soviets enter Berlin

Death of Roosevelt, Harry Truman becomes US president

US and Soviet forces meet at Torgau

Hitler kills himself – Germany surrenders

1,000 bomber raid on Japanese mainland

Potsdam conference on the future of Europe

Atomic bombs dropped on Hiroshima and Nagasaki – Japan surrenders

Nuremberg trials begin

RAF Gloster Meteor sets a new world-record speed of 616 mph

The UN, IMF and World Bank are all established

Dock workers strike for a national minimum wage

Deaths: David Lloyd George, Vidkun Quisling, Josef Goebbels and Heinrich Himmler (by suicide), Benito Mussolini

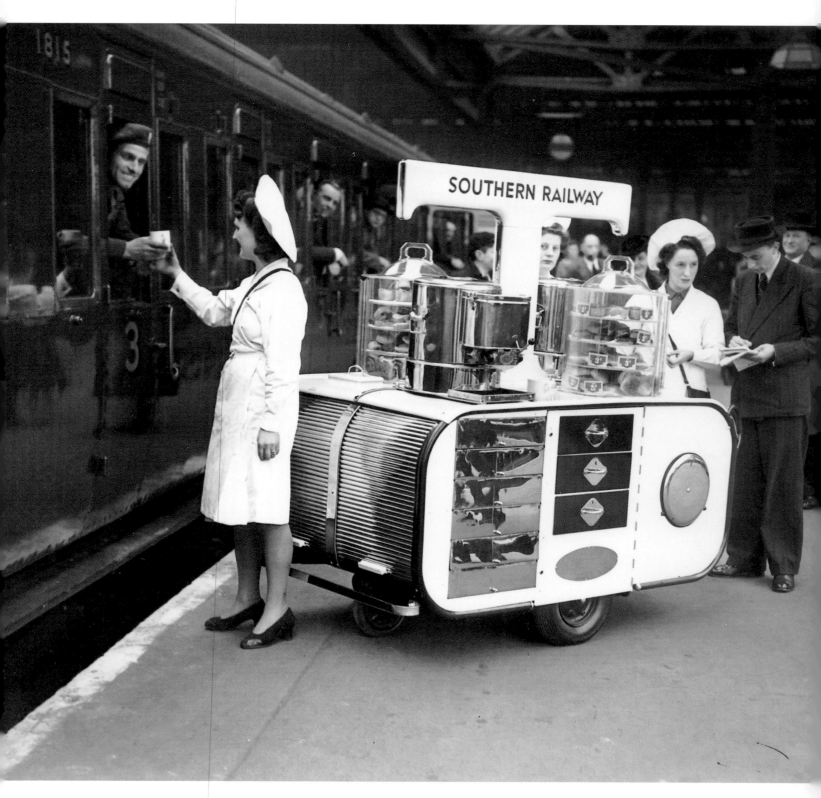

Brief encounter as rail runs out of steam

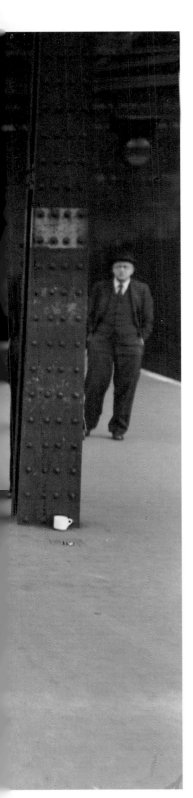

These passengers waiting for their train to leave Waterloo Station were among the first to sample the delights of the new tea trolley introduced by the privately owned Southern Railway. During the war and the years of rationing which followed, catering on the railways was limited. But this trolley, six feet long and three-and-a-half feet wide and with four three-gallon containers, could offer up to 300 cups of tea. It was designed so that customers could be served from either side. Other features included a specially sprung and covered cake rack and two ice-cream containers. Finished in shiny stainless steel and enamel, the trolley, fortunately for the women operating it, was electrically driven. It was designed by Southern Railway and the Empire Tea Bureau and was one of 12 such trolleys used on the network.

Refreshments, the increasing electrification of the railways, which made travel cleaner and quicker, and the success of the film *Brief Encounter*, released the previous year, may have given train travel an added allure. But the golden age of rail was coming to a close. Fares went up this year and the rumblings of future competition could be heard: the first civilian flights took off from the newly opened Heathrow, into which the government planned to invest a further £20 million, and a new airline, British European Airways, was launched.

The days of the Southern Railway – which covered much of the south of England – and of the other railway companies were also numbered. In December this year, the Labour government pushed through the nationalisation of the railways.

Also this year...

The United Nations holds its first session

A recipe for squirrel pie is put forward by the Food Ministry

The government announces grants for university students

The jitterbug starts a new dance craze

Television broadcasts are reintroduced

The Football League restarts

The Chinese civil war begins

Deaths: John Maynard Keynes, John Logie Baird, Gertrude Stein, H.G.Wells, Hermann Goering, W.C. Fields

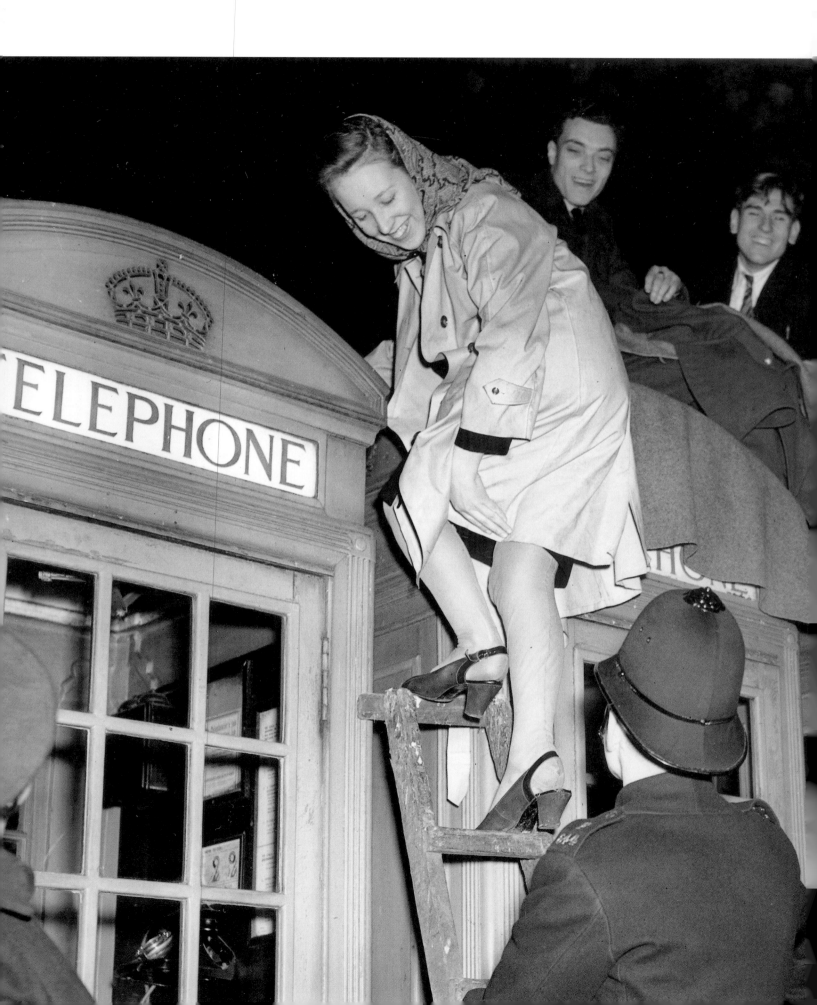

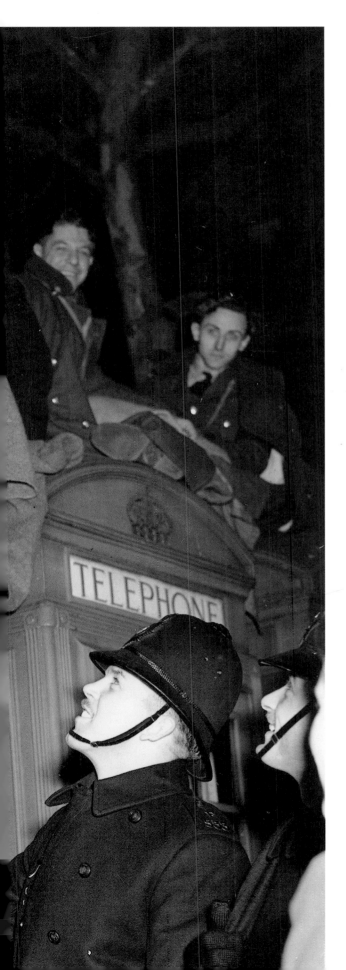

Showing a leg for a glimpse of royalty

In November 1947, Princess Elizabeth married Lieutenant Philip Mountbatten at Westminster Abbey. Those without invitations were forced to make their own arrangements to catch a glimpse of the festivities. This woman may have been persuaded to come down from her vantage spot by a policemen, but others – equally inventive – were more successful. Many of the crowd, in places 50 deep, had braved the autumn weather and camped out overnight.

The long-awaited engagement between the couple was announced on July 9 this year. They had met at various royal engagements before the war but their first significant meeting is said to have been during a visit by the Royal Family to Dartmouth Naval College, where the dashing Philip was a cadet, in July 1939. He was 19, she only 14. They played croquet and then had tea on the royal yacht. Afterwards, the princess is said to have declared that she had just met the man she would marry.

Those among the 2,500 congregation at the Abbey were reported to have been impressed by the simplicity of the ceremony. The couple and their guests then returned for a wedding breakfast at Buckingham Palace, where they cut a 500lb cake. Despite the government's plea that British women should resist emulating Christian Dior's "irresponsibly frivolous" New Look in the interests of the national clothing shortage, the Princess was granted 100 extra coupons for her wedding dress, which was embroidered with beads and pearls. The same privilege did not extend to her trousseau, and the Princess was obliged to go on her honeymoon without one. The honeymoon was at Broadlands in Hampshire, the country house of Lord Mountbatten, Prince Philip's uncle, the man generally thought responsible for engineering the Dartmouth meeting.

Also this year...

Coal mines are nationalised

Indian independence leads to the partition of the sub-continent and huge loss of life

Britain paralysed by fuel shortages and temperatures as low as -16 F

Partition plan for Palestine approved by the UN

Belgium, the Netherlands and Luxembourg establish the Benelux customs union

US airforce pilot Chuck Yeager breaks the sound barrier

Suspected communists put on trial in America

Deaths: Al Capone, Henry Ford, Stanley Baldwin

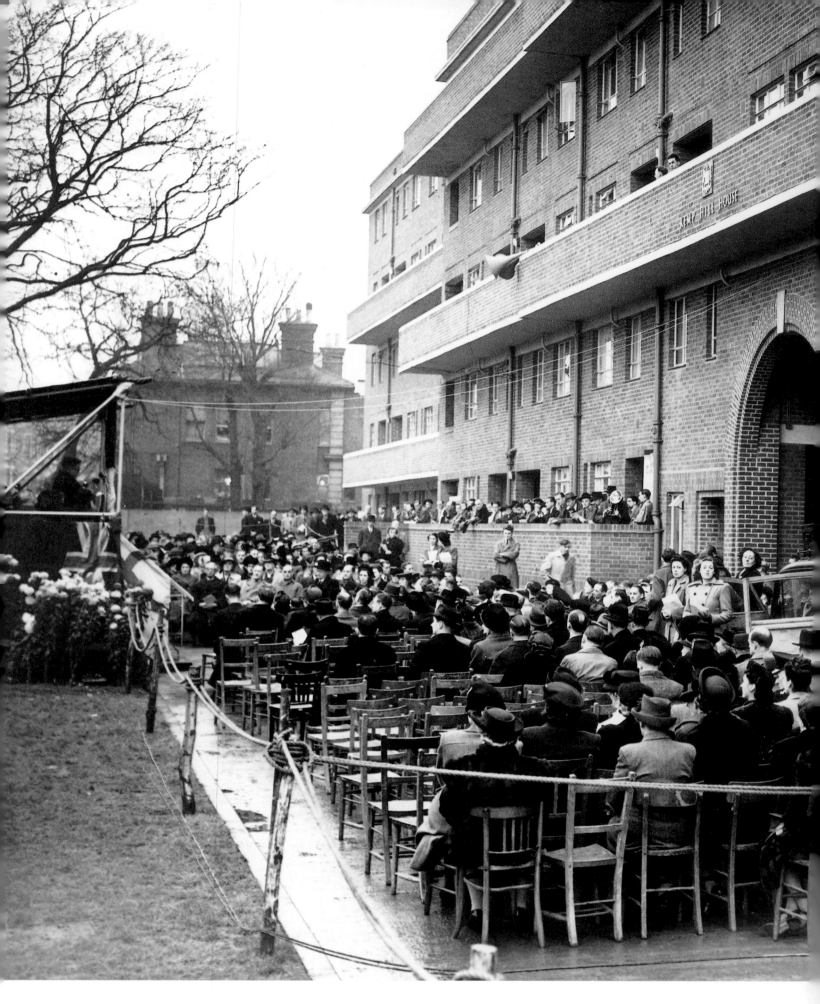

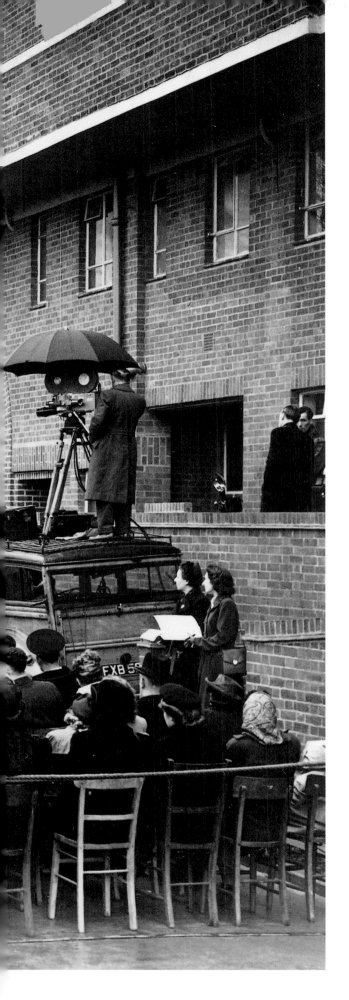

New homes fit for Britain's "mothers"

The right honourable Herbert Morrison, MP for Lewisham East and leader of the Commons, opens the first council flats at Hether Grove, part of Lewisham's proposed Ladywell Park Estate, on Friday, December 3. Mr Morrison thanked those who had worked on the flats: "If you've done a right job, the best reward you can have is from 'Mother' – the women who are going to live here and make homes here for their families. Remember houses and flats are not homes until they are lived in. All who are engaged in domestic building should look ahead, for the job they are doing is not a mere job. It has a social purpose. If it is done efficiently, it is, in however small a way, raising standards. If the builder can take pride in his work, the women who use the finished building will take a pride in theirs."

Some of these women made up the crowd of 500 who were present for the ceremony. The Blitz had not completely flattened London, but it had destroyed many homes – including those on the ground that these flats had been built on – and many were forced to live in cramped and unsuitable accommodation or with relatives.

The entire Ladywell Park Estate was to consist of 156 flats and maisonettes within four blocks. The council intended that the estate would be entirely self-contained, even offering an open air theatre and swimming pool. Hether Grove itself had four maisonettes and 10 flats. Tenants were worried that rents, starting at 23 shillings a week, were high but considered that the modern conveniences, particularly the communal laundry room, which each family was permitted to use once a week, would make them worth while.

The original Ladywell Park Estate plans never materialised. The estate, which came to be known as the Hether Grove Estate, has since been demolished.

Also this year...

Mahatma Gandhi assassinated

Electricity industry nationalised

John A. Costello heads Ireland's first coalition government

State of Israel proclaimed

US Congress approves Marshall Aid programme

Britain sees biggest baby boom for over 20 years

World Health Organisation formed

Russian blockade around Berlin; RAF airlifts to the city begin

R.C. Brock pioneers open-heart surgery at Guys Hospital, London

National Health Service introduced

Olympics held in London

Prince Charles born

T.S. Eliot wins Nobel Prize for literature

Professor Kinsey publishes Sexual Behaviour of the Human Male

Deaths: Orville Wright, Sergei Eisenstein, "Babe" Ruth, Muhammad Ali Jinnah

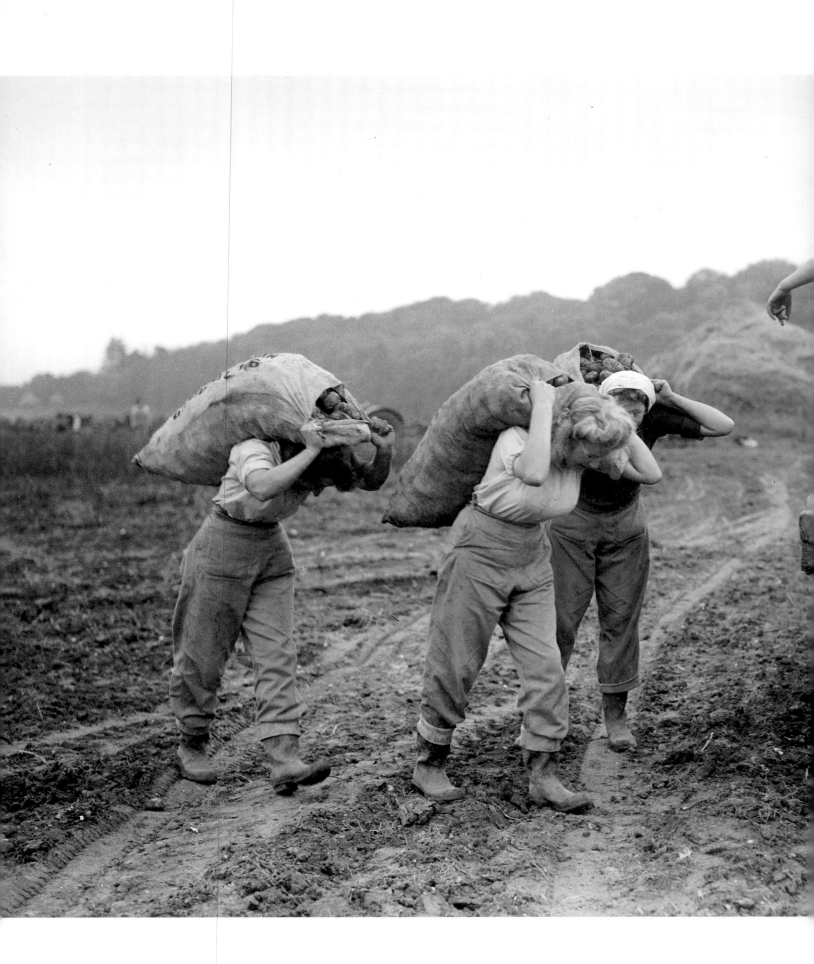

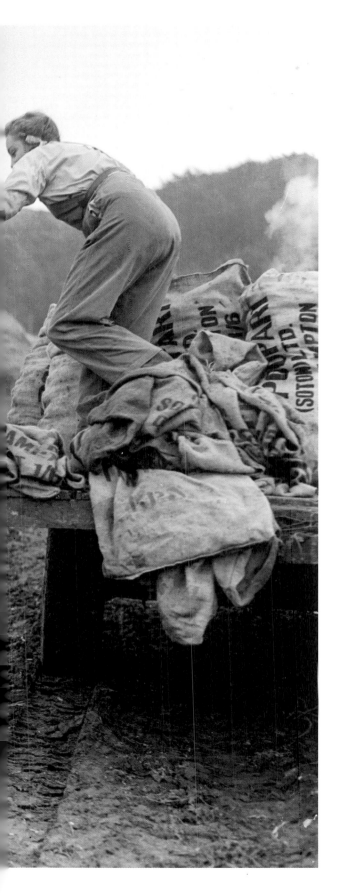

Land Girls continue the battle in the fields

The war may have been won, but the country still had to fight hard to feed itself. The Women's Land Army continued to battle in the fields to keep the nation from starving.

Formed in June 1939, the Women's Land Army became ever more important as the war continued when most able men were fighting abroad or engaged on other vital war work, and food convoys could often not get past the German U-boats. More than 10,000 Land Girls – as the volunteers were commonly called – went to do what had previously been regarded as exclusively male jobs. Many had no previous experience of being on a farm. Some volunteers were given training, but many were expected to learn on the job.

Their duties included driving tractors, pruning, weeding, milking cows, planting, harvesting, cleaning pigs' sties and cow sheds and reclaiming land. They even caught rats and heaved hundredweight bales, like the girls pictured here. It was not unusual to work a 14-hour day. The countryside was as unused to women workers as the women were to the work: although many were warmly welcomed and looked after, just as many were the objects of derision.

When the war ended, those who had volunteered were demobbed on a first-to-join-first-to-leave basis. Release certificates instructed members to return their uniform at their own expense, although the women were allowed to keep their shoes and great coat on the condition they dye it from brown to navy blue. Each woman was allocated six clothing coupons, enough to buy a hat, a tie and some knickers. Having been enrolled as the fourth line of defence, many Land Girls were bitter at the lack of recognition they received. The Women's Land Army was finally disbanded in 1950.

Also this year...

Tate Gallery fully reopens

Clothes rationing ends

Republic of Ireland proclaimed

National Parks Act passed

Berlin blockade ends

NATO established

Gas industry nationalised

George Orwell's 1984 published

De Havilland Comet airliner makes maiden flight

Lord Boyd-Orr, former director of United Nations Food and Agricultural Organisation, wins Nobel Peace Prize

Mao Tse Tung proclaims the People's Republic of China

German Democratic Republic established.

Deaths: Margaret Mitchell, author of Gone With the Wind, composer Richard Strauss, comedian Tommy Handley

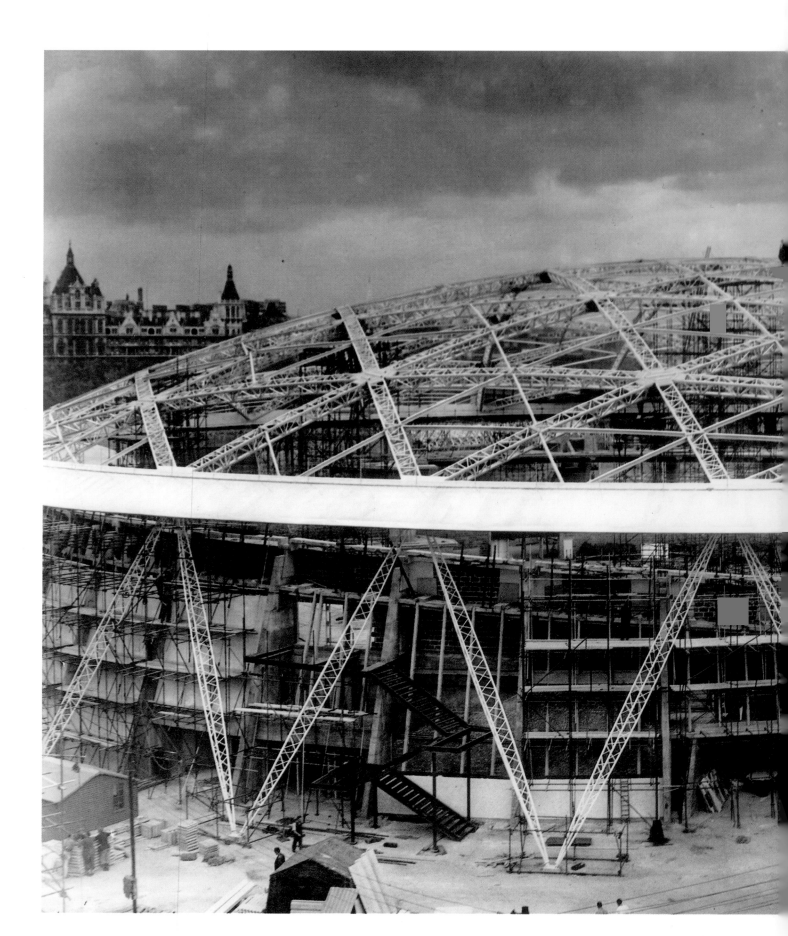

The other Dome ... a "tonic to the nation"

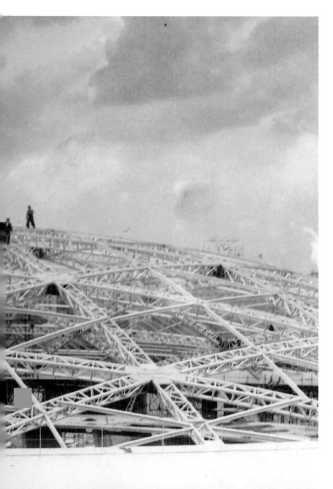

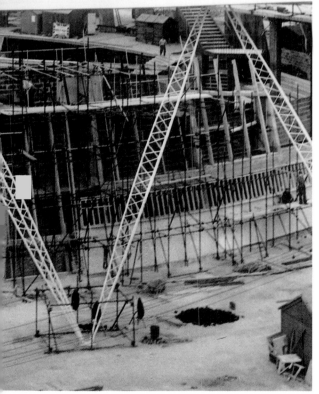

The Dome of Discovery, seen here under construction in 1950 on London's South Bank, was, at 365 feet in diameter, the largest dome in the world. Designed by Ralph Tubbs, it heralded a new era in British architecture. The Dome was built as part of the 1951 Festival of Britain, a nationwide celebration intended as a "tonic to the nation". There were two sites in London, the Festival Pleasure Gardens in Battersea and the South Bank, where the Dome, the 300-foot cigar-shaped Skylon, the Royal Festival Hall and a dozen or so themed pavilions were built.

The idea for the Festival came from the Royal Society of Arts in 1943. The event itself was organised by Herbert Morrison, the Labour MP, who saw it as an occasion that would mark the centenary of the Great Exhibition and "tell the story of British contributions to world civilisation".

On the South Bank, Hugh Casson, the director of architecture, and his team of over 40 architects and designers transformed 27 acres of bombed wasteland into interlocked spaces and buildings which would symbolise the nation's recovery. The Dome was heralded as "a triumph of technical skill reminiscent of the Crystal Palace 100 years earlier." Inside it were eight sections symbolising the nation's achievements in exploration, on land, at sea, in the sky and in space.

Whatever the portrayal of national prowess represented by the Festival, there were inevitably problems in organising such a large and complex undertaking, not least financial difficulties and labour disputes. Both the chairman and the managing director of the Festival Pleasure Gardens resigned. Noel Coward even wrote a satirical song called *Don't Make Fun of the Fair*. Despite the controversy, the Festival was a resounding success and pulled in eight million visitors. The Dome and the other Festival constructions – with the exception of the Royal Festival Hall – were later dismantled.

Also this year...

America announces plans to build the H-bomb

Britain officially recognises Communist China

England lose 1-0 to the United States in the World Cup

Labour wins general election with reduced majority

Petrol rationing ends

The Korean War breaks out

Chinese invade Tibet

Scottish Nationalists steal Stone of Scone

Bertrand Russell wins Nobel Prize for Literature

The Archers first broadcast

Deaths: George Orwell, George Bernard Shaw, Edgar Rice Burroughs, Al Jolson, South African statesman Jan Smuts

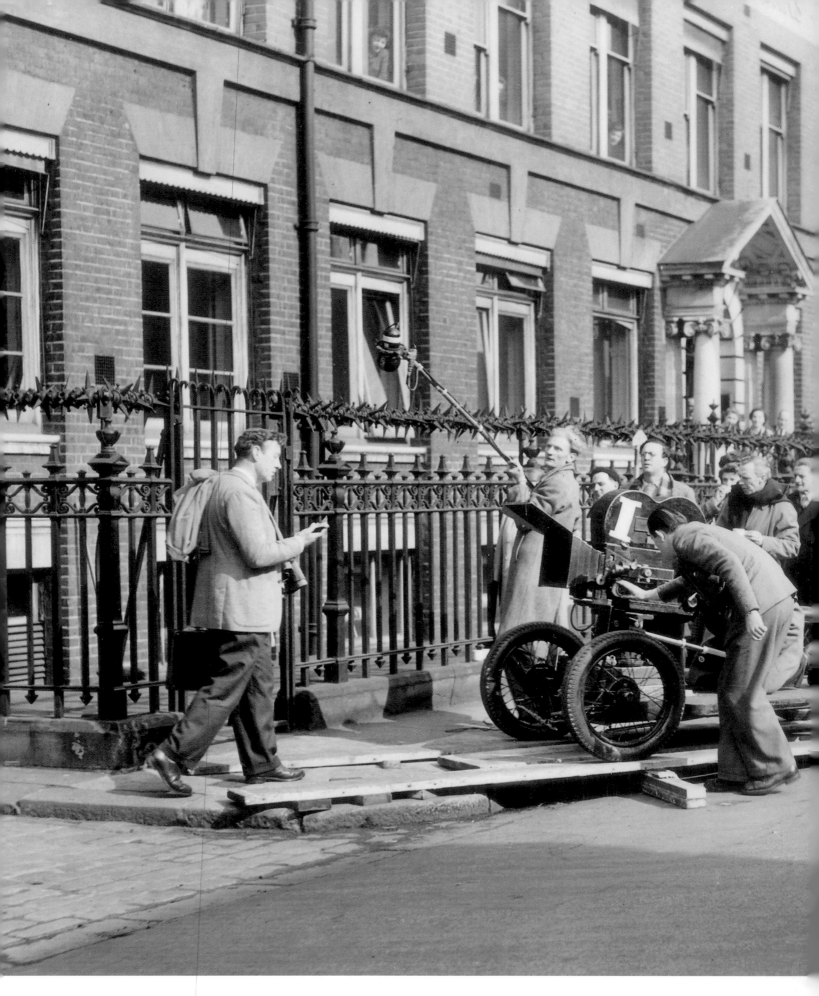

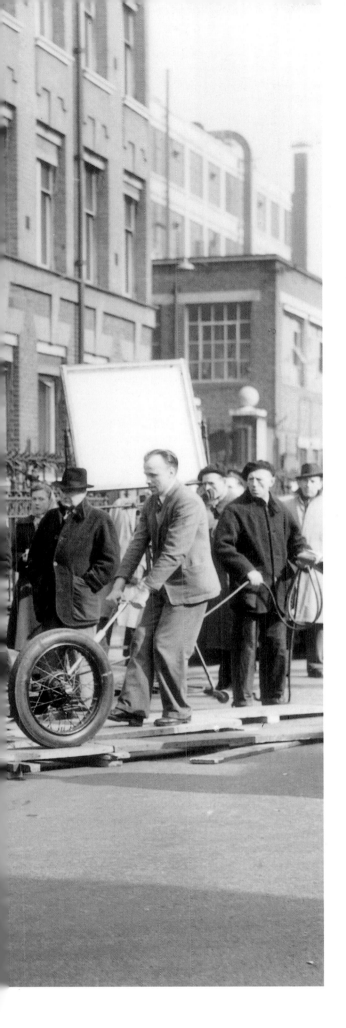

Promoting the virtues of Britain, with a smile

Actors and crew during filming of the last scene of *The Man in the White Suit* on location in London in 1951. The film, which starred Alec Guinness, Joan Greenwood and Cecil Parker, was directed by Alexander Mackendrick, and was one of the many comedies to come out of Ealing Studios, which dominated British cinema in the late forties and early fifties.

Although Ealing's output was by no means restricted to comedy, this was the area where the studio shone. Usually based around working class – and often eccentric – characters, many of whom openly flout the social status quo, the result is self-deprecating humour rather than radical social satire.

The first Ealing comedy, *Hue and Cry*, directed by Charles Crichton, was made in 1947. *Passport to Pimlico*, *Whisky Galore*, *Kind Hearts and Coronets*, *The Man in the White Suit*, *The Titfield Thunderbolt* (again directed by Crichton) and *The Maggie* followed. *The Ladykillers*, the last comedy to be made at Ealing, was shot in 1955.

Ealing was also famous for encouraging new writing talent. T.E.B. Clarke, Robert Hamer, Michael Pertwee and others created comedies that relied on sharp scripts rather than lavish set design. Fostering all this creativity was producer Sir Michael Balcon, who joined Ealing studios – then known as ATP – in 1937. It was Balcon who, influenced by the outbreak of war in 1939, decided that Ealing should be used to promote the virtues of British life. After quarrels with distributors, Ealing Studios were closed down in 1958.

Also this year...

The Festival of Britain opens

Foreign Office diplomats Donald Maclean and Guy Burgess, under suspicion as spies, go missing

"Coloureds" banned from voting in South Africa

Coal and steel industries nationalised

Eamon de Valera returns to power in Ireland

Truce negotiations begin in Korea

Conservatives win general election and Winston Churchill again becomes Prime Minister

King Abdullah of Jordan assassinated in Jerusalem

British civilians evacuated from Egypt

Deaths: novelist André Gide, Ferdinand Porsche, Ivor Novello, Ernest Bevin, Philippe Pétain, Ludwig Wittgenstein, William Randolph Hearst

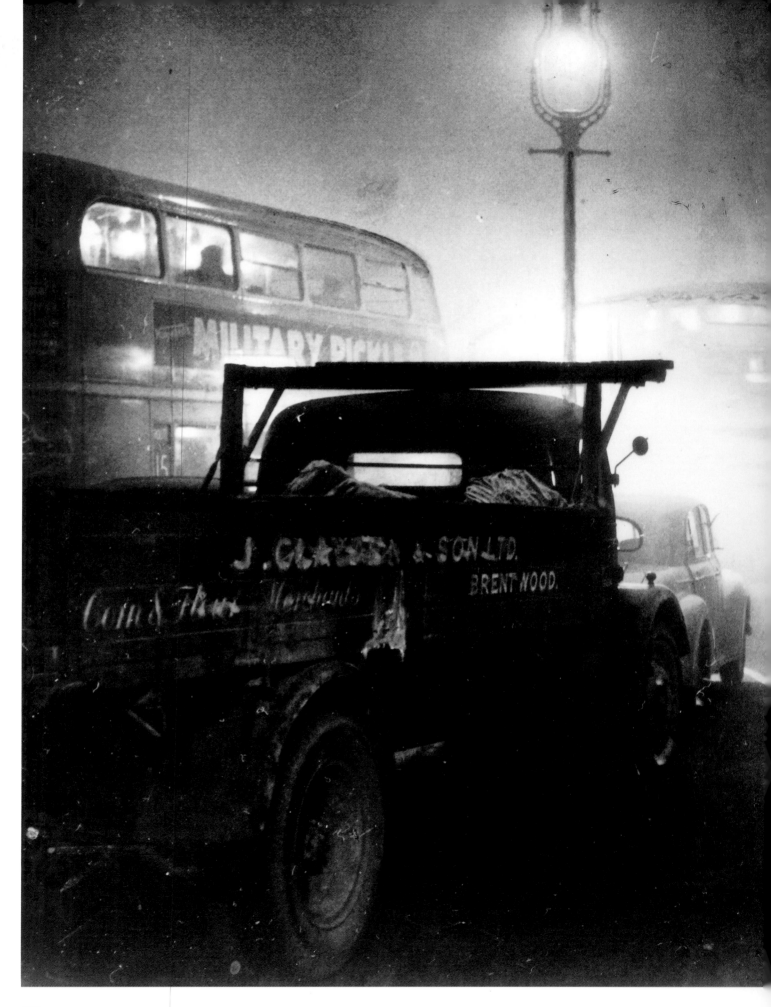

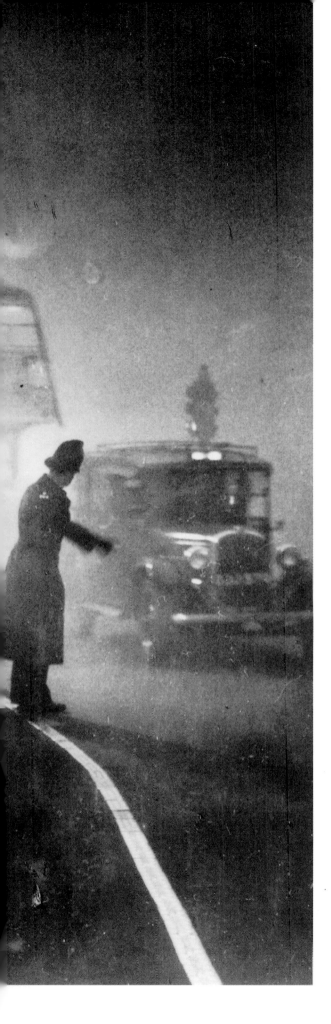

Grinding to a halt in a pea souper

To Londoners, and those living in the suburbs, smog or "pea soupers" were a part of life. Yet the four-day fog that descended on December 4 this year was the worst in living memory. The Automobile Association reported that visibility on roads in central London was, at most, five yards and transport all but came to a standstill. A few buses struggled on using flares or following a man who walked ahead holding a light. There were several train collisions because drivers could not see signal lights, though most trains – and flights – were cancelled. River traffic was also halted.

Some motorists did venture out and inevitably accidents occurred: in Rochester Way, Eltham, there was a pile-up after a car slowed down at the bottom of a hill and was hit by 19 cars which could not stop because the road was icy. Fortunately, no-one was seriously injured. A number of drivers abandoned their cars rather than continue.

Most sports events were cancelled: Wembley Stadium was forced to call off a match for the first time since it was opened. A performance of *La Traviata* at Sadlers Wells was abandoned after the first act as the audience could no longer see the stage. There was a flood of calls to the RSPB to deal with disoriented birds that had crash-landed. Scotland Yard also received an increased number of calls as thieves took advantage of the cover afforded by poor visibility.

The government estimated there were at least 3,000 smog-related deaths, most due to heart and respiratory diseases made worse by the poor air conditions. Later, unofficial, estimates put the death toll at 12,000. Some help was provided for sufferers when smog masks were made available on the NHS in 1953. Though measures such as the 1956 Clean Air Act helped alleviate the worst effects of London's fogs, even as late in 1962 a further smog killed 750.

Also this year...

George VI dies

17 Britons killed in Cairo riots

Identity cards abolished

Britain explodes its first atom bomb

British Standards Institution Kite Mark introduced

The Diary of Anne Frank published in English

Last tram removed from London

Helsinki hosts Olympic Games

First juvenile detention centre opens

Tea rationing ends

112 die in Harrow train disaster

America tests the first H-bomb

Britain's first pop singles chart published

Agatha Christie's The Mousetrap opens

Deaths: Sir Stafford Cripps, educationalist Maria Montessori, Eva Peron, former Israeli president Chaim Weizmann

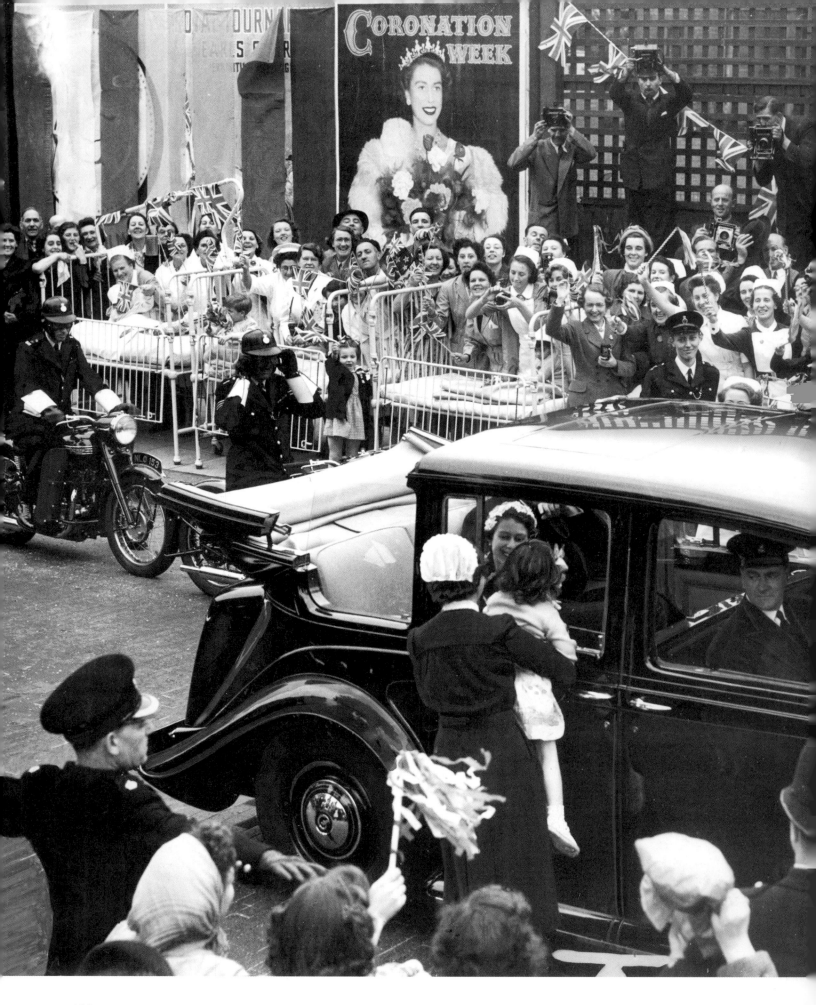

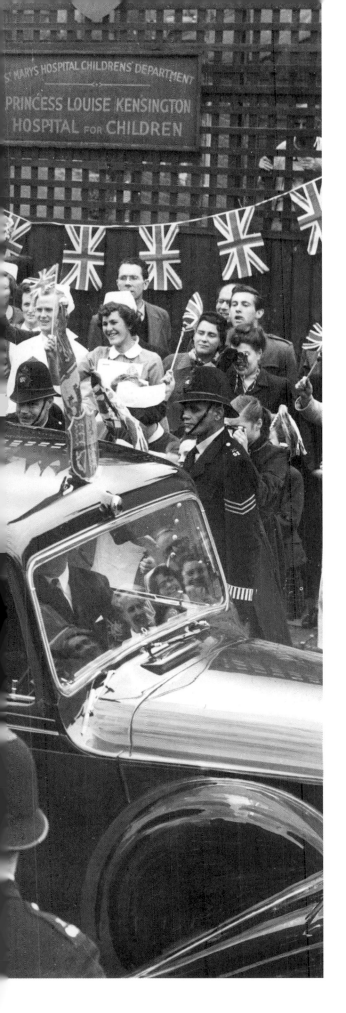

A bouquet for the new Queen Elizabeth

The crowds cheered as Pat O'Brian, a four-year-old patient at the Princess Louise Kensington Hospital for Children in northwest London, was lifted up to give a bouquet to the newly crowned Queen Elizabeth II. Other patients were wheeled out in their beds to welcome the Queen and Prince Philip.

The Queen made many public appearances in the week following her coronation. This photograph was taken on one of her drives through London; she was also seen at The Derby at Epsom, and a variety of state functions and Commonwealth parades. She went on to inspect the fleet at Spithead and to visit Scotland, Northern Ireland and Wales.

The Queen had heard of her father's death, and her accession to the throne, while she was on safari in Kenya in February the previous year. However, it was not until June 2 this year that the Queen was crowned. The ceremony, at Westminster Abbey, was shown live on television across the nation, in the process becoming one of the first major television outside broadcasts. It was also later shown around the world.

The Coronation generated immense fervour and neither the advances of modern technology nor the unseasonably cold and wet weather stopped the crowds from gathering in London. *The Times* reported: "It was a cosmopolitan crowd. Opposite the Cenotaph an American announced proudly that he had hitch-hiked all the way from San Francisco. With equal pride her neighbour claimed 50 years in Walthamstow In the Mall sailors from Ceylon looked for a last-minute place. Some Canadians bivouacked in the Haymarket. A Rhodesian settled down beside them."

Technology was not the only indicator that the Royals had embraced the 20th century – for the first time the Royal Family did not have enough professional coach-men in their employ to cope with the occasion. The Queen and her entourage had to accept the services of country squires and millionaire businessmen who volunteered to make up the shortfall.

Also this year...

Rationing of sweets and sugar ends

Steel and road transport industries denationalised

128 die when car ferry sinks off Irish coast

England win the Ashes back from Australia after 20 years

Floods in eastern England leave at least 280 dead

John Christie sentenced to death for three murders

British POWs return from Korea

Edmund Hillary and Sherpa Tensing conquer Everest

Deaths: Hilaire Belloc, Sergei Prokofiev, Hank Williams, Joseph Stalin, Queen Mary, Dylan Thomas

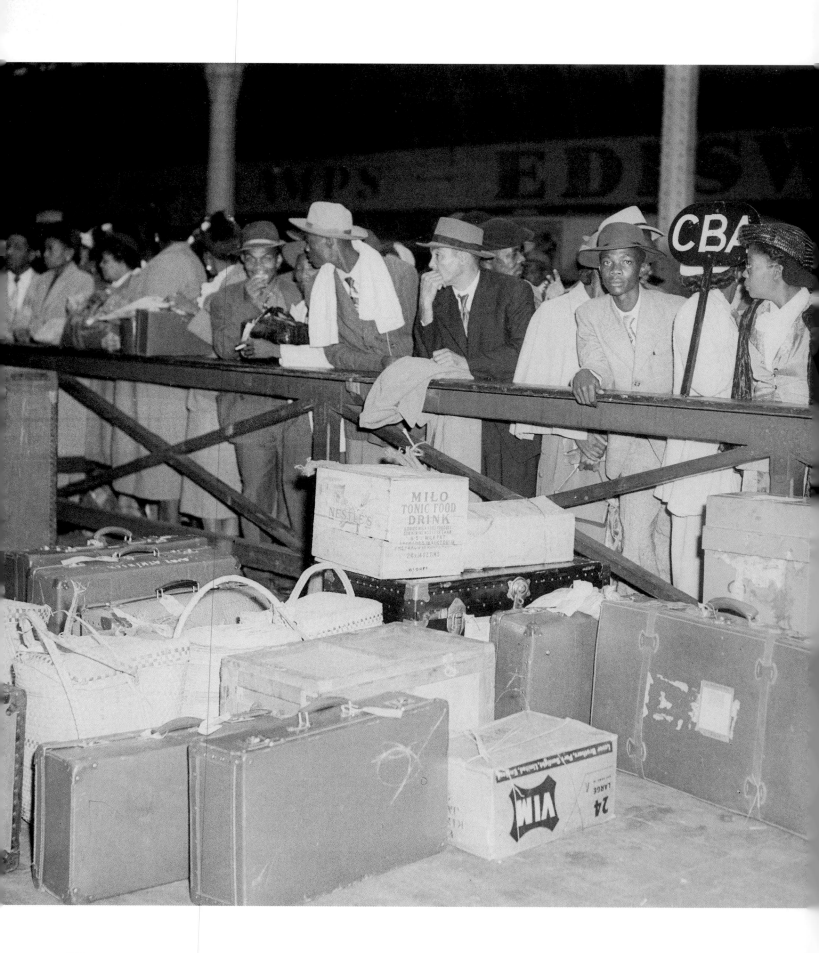

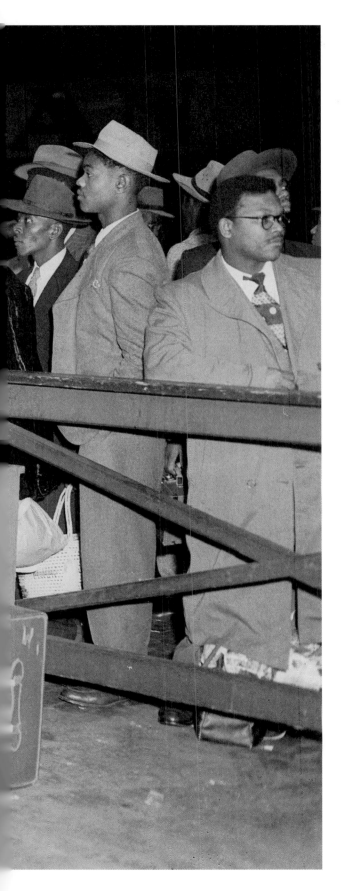

Arriving with hopes soon to be dashed

Having raised £82 to pay for their fare and after 20 days at sea, Jamaican immigrants arrive at London's Victoria Station. By 1971 the number of Caribbean-born inhabitants of Britain was over 300,000.

Some of the first immigrants were welcomed by brass bands, but the dream of a new life turned sour for many. Attracted by the offer of jobs from British companies, particularly in public transport, the reality they found was often one of racial discrimination, low wages and, in many cases, unemployment. Some firms refused to employ non-white workers; at a number of firms that did employ immigrants, white workers went on strike in protest.

The majority of West Indian immigrants moved into the inner-cities, areas that were already fraught with social tensions caused by poverty and poor housing. In 1958, riots broke out in Notting Hill, west London, when gangs of white youths began taunting immigrants.

A second influx of immigrants – more than 50,000 a year from Pakistan and India – was to arrive in Britain in the sixties. In a bid to hold down numbers, the first Immigration Act, which restricted entry to those who held employment vouchers, was introduced in 1962.

Maverick politician Enoch Powell ignited further controversy when he made a speech in Birmingham in 1968 in which he claimed that the government's immigration policy was akin to the nation "busily… heaping up its own funeral pyre." Gallup poll figures released shortly afterwards suggested that 74 per cent of the nation agreed with him.

In an effort to respond to increasing racial harassment the government made discrimination in employment, housing and some financial sectors illegal. The Race Relations Act, passed in 1976, extended the ban and established the Commission for Racial Equality. Ethnic minorities made up around 5.5 per cent of the British population at the 1991 census.

Also this year...

56 die in two Comet jet crashes

Roger Bannister runs the first sub-four minute mile

West Germany beat Hungary 3-2 in the World Cup Final

Chris Chataway sets new world record for 5,000 meters of 13 minutes and 15.6 seconds

Independent Television Authority

established

William Golding's Lord of the Flies *and J.R.R. Tolkien's* Lord of the Rings *published*

Final end of food rationing

Over 51,000 dock workers go on month's strike

Deaths: Henri Matisse, Alan Turing, Lionel Barrymore

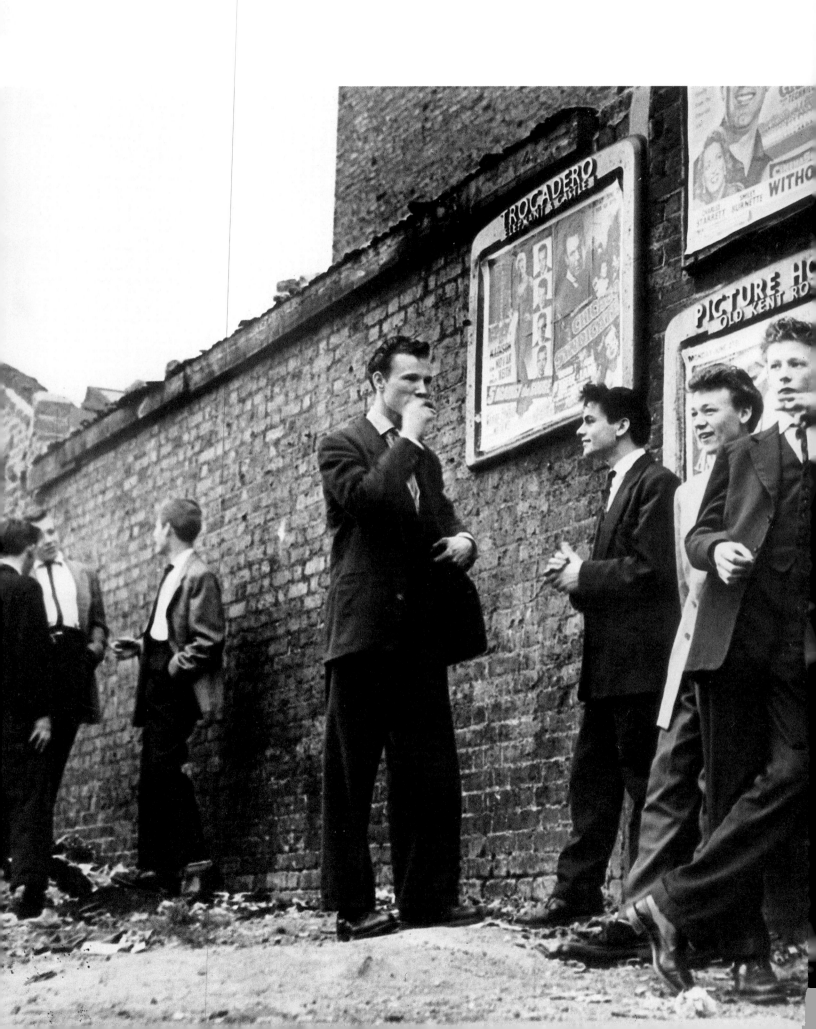

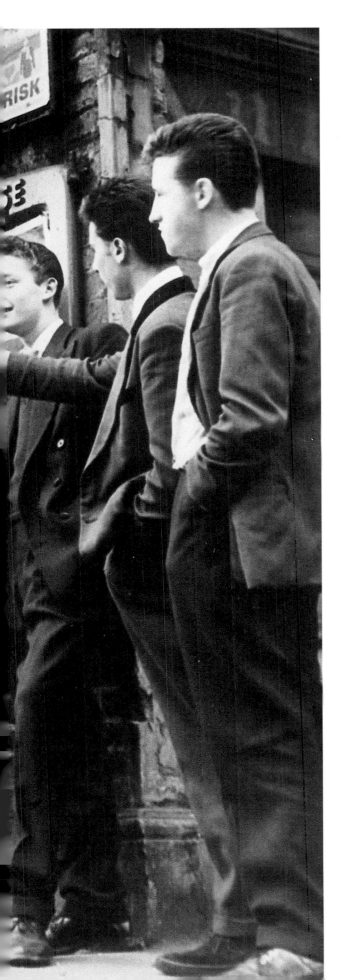

A world of winkle-pickers and drain pipes

Teddy Boys, like this group pictured in south London, were the first teenagers to master the art of hanging around and looking tough. The name "Edwardians" was originally given to aristocratic men who revived the Edwardian dandy look in the late forties. It was later copied by working-class youths, who made it their own. The boys pictured have made a rather half-hearted attempt at the whole ensemble, which consisted of a brightly coloured and velvet-trimmed frockcoat, ornamental waistcoats, drainpipe trousers and a Slim-Jim Western-style tie. Shoes could vary – Teds might wear shiny lace-ups, thick-soled brothel creepers or winkle-pickers.

Hair was important. Teds were the first to sport a style that radically differed from the norm – and basically consisted of variations on the quiff. Aspirant Teddy Boys could choose between a DA (duck's arse), or, towards the late fifties, the elephant trunk – a large and long quiff swept forward over the face. Both styles required heavy amounts of grease. Sideburns were also a source of pride.

The first British teen cult was looked on as trouble. The press carried stories of gang violence and anti-social behaviour. One miscreant, arrested for damaging a greenhouse, was reported as explaining "It's just rock 'n 'roll." Rock 'n' roll didn't really hit the Teddy Boys – or Britain – until 1956, but it was this that would take much of the Teds' teen rebellion into the mainstream.

Also this year...

Churchill resigns as Prime Minster; Anthony Eden leads Conservatives to win general election

Clement Attlee resigns as Labour leader

Christian Dior launches the A-line skirt

Ruth Ellis becomes the last woman in Britain to be hanged

No national newspapers are printed during month-long printers strike

State of Emergency declared after

60,000 dockers go on strike

HMS Ark Royal completed

Warsaw Pact established

ITV opens as Britain's first commercial television station

Princess Margaret decides against marrying Captain Peter Townsend

Cardiff made capital of Wales

Deaths: Albert Einstein, Alexander Fleming, Thomas Mann, James Dean

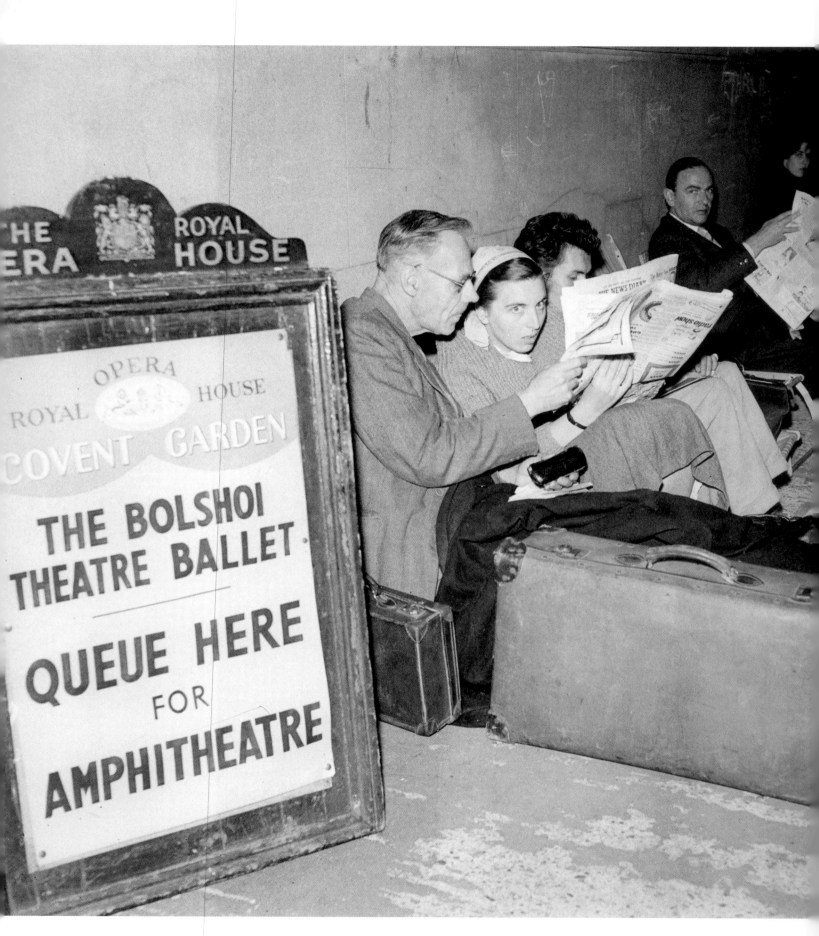

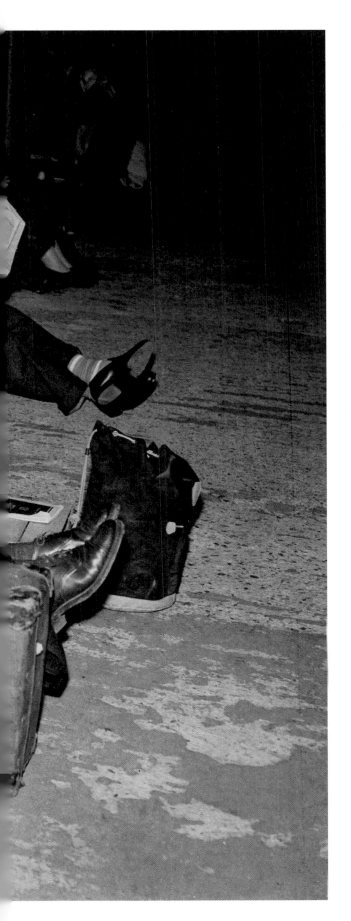

Queuing for a ticket to the Bolshoi

Customers at the front of the queue for tickets to see the Bolshoi Theatre Ballet at the Royal Opera House, Covent Garden. The queue, for the first London performance on Monday, October 3, had begun to form the previous Friday evening.

The Bolshoi's visit, part of an exchange with the Sadler's Wells Ballet Company, took place after much speculation and diplomatic manoeuvring. The dancers threatened not to come for fear of "provocation" – Russian athlete Nina Ponomareva had been arrested for stealing five hats from a shop in London's Oxford Street earlier that year. The implication seemed to be that the Bolshoi would be allowed to travel to Britain only if the charges against Ponomareva were dropped. However, the Bolshoi did come and, despite rumours to the contrary, prima ballerina Galina Ulanova was with them.

For the most part, the British audiences and critics were enraptured. The feeling was mutual – Ulanova praised her British audiences in a telephone interview: "We were amazed both by the attention and the concentration with which they watched the performance, and by some kind of an astonishingly crystal-clear silence that reigned in the theatre. Performances before such a sensitive and appreciative audience give a great creative joy."

Rumours that the Bolshoi's visit had been cut short by Moscow were dismissed by a Royal Opera House spokesman, who explained "It is merely that air transport has become available sooner than was expected."

Also this year...

More British troops sent into Cyprus	*Elvis Presley has first hit with* Heartbreak Hotel
Premium Bonds introduced	
Grace Kelly marries Prince Rainier of Monaco	*Suez Crisis begins; British forced to withdraw as UN troops called in*
Krushchev makes official visit to Britain	*Hungarian revolt violently repressed by Soviets*
Third-class carriages abolished on British Rail	*Olympics held in Melbourne*
Transatlantic telephone service inaugurated	*Deaths: A.A Milne, Sir Alexander Korda, Sir Max Beerbohm, Jackson Pollock, Bertold Brecht, Alfred Kinsey, Bela Lugosi*
Clean Air Act passed	

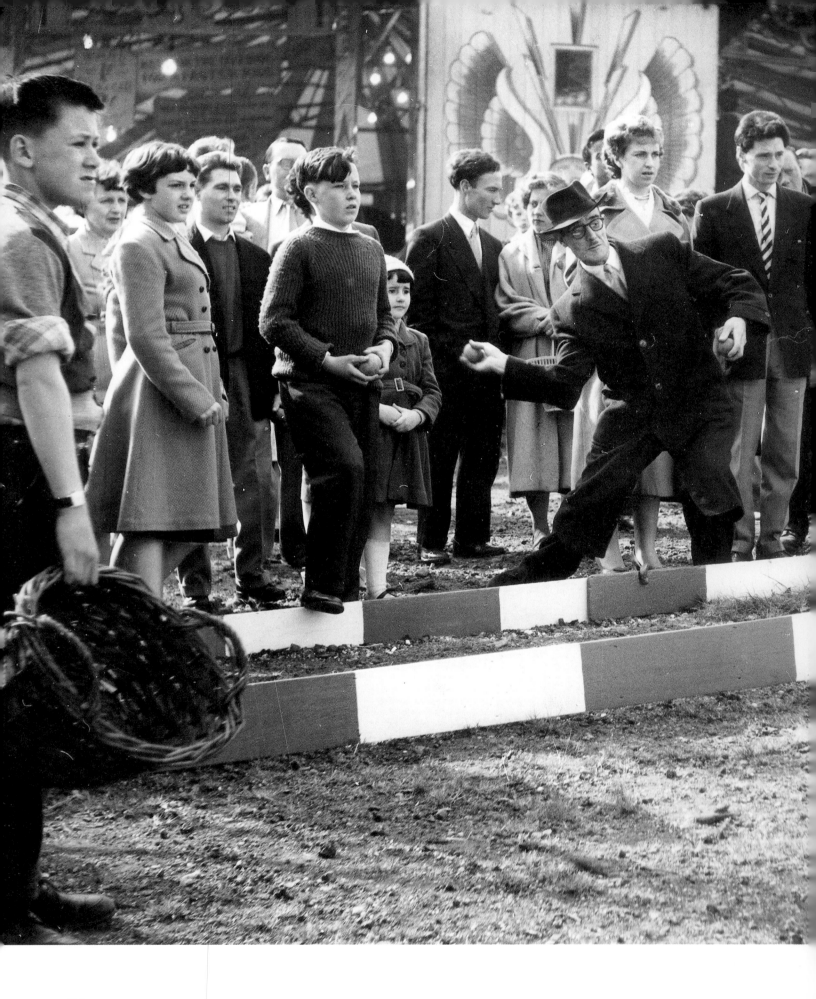

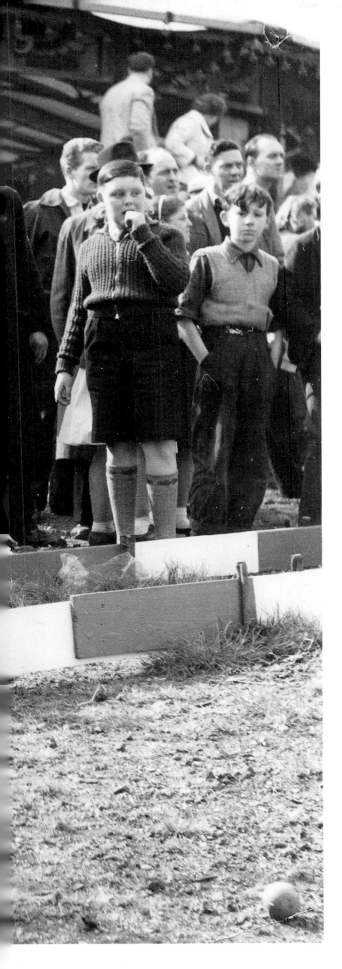

Fifties family fun: coconut shies and circuses

It was hard to beat the fun at the fair – well, there simply wasn't much competition. There were only three stations to listen to on the radio and two (black-and-white) TV channels, and these did not broadcast all day. The fair epitomised the idea of wholesome family entertainment – so much so, that one had been introduced to London's Soho in 1955 in an attempt to clean up the area. There were few attractions greater than the coconut shy. The object was to win the coconut by knocking it off its perch. To judge by the expressions of the crowd, it could be nail-biting action. There were simple pleasures such as darts, skittles, test your strength and Housey Housey – the forerunner of Bingo, played with bottle tops.

An even bigger treat was the circus: audiences could gasp at trapeze artists, roar at the clowns and be amazed as an elephant played the mouth organ, a bear rode a motorcycle, sea lions juggled and dogs jumped through hoops. A few big towns had permanent circus venues offering up to three performances daily during the Christmas and summer seasons, but most of the country had to wait for the visits of touring troupes, which sometimes stayed in each town for as little as three days.

But the lure of the fair and the circus was steadily being overtaken by television: ITV first broadcast in 1955, while BBC 2 was to follow in 1964.

Also this year...

Sir Anthony Eden resigns due to ill health; Harold Macmillan becomes Prime Minister

Royal Ballet created

22 die in plane crash at Manchester Airport

Treaty of Rome establishes the European Economic Community

Wolfenden report recommends decriminalisation of homosexuality

Church of England allows divorcees to remarry with bishop's permission

Althea Gibson becomes first black woman to win Wimbledon

Ghana and Malaya become independent

Russians launch first satellite (Sputnik 1) and first dog in space (on Sputnik 2)

The United Kingdom tests its first H-bomb

The Sky at Night first broadcast

Jack Kerouac's On the Road published

Nuclear civil defence manual published

Women admitted to House of Lords

Queen makes first televised Christmas broadcast

Deaths: Humphrey Bogart, Dorothy Sayers, Senator Joseph McCarthy, Jean Sibelius, Oliver Hardy, Christian Dior

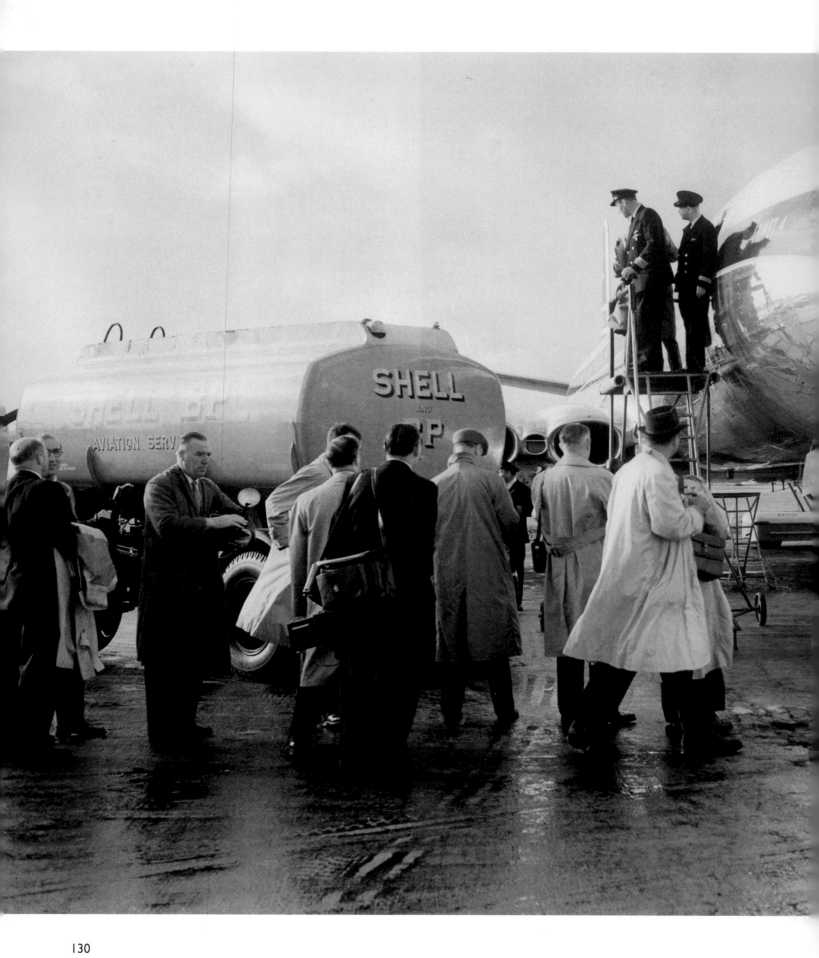

Comet crashes to Earth in jet supremacy race

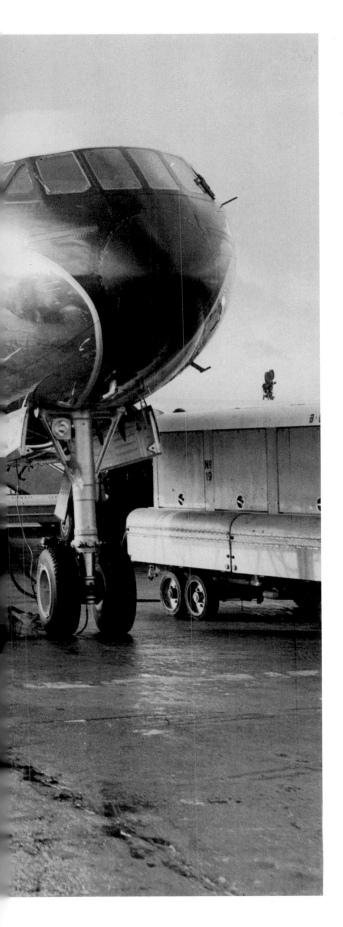

Press photographers wait to record the flight of a De Havilland Comet at Heathrow Airport in 1958. After the Second World War, air travel rapidly began to supplant travel by sea for long-distance journeys. Airplanes became larger, faster and significantly more comfortable, especially with the introduction of pressurised cabins. The biggest breakthrough was the introduction of jet engines.

The De Havilland Comet, the first commercial jet airliner, was used by the British Overseas Airways Corporation – later to form part of British Airways – from 1952. Its safety record, however, was far from good: in April 1954 the government ordered that all seven BOAC Comets be grounded after one crashed into the Mediterranean, killing 21. This was the third Comet to crash in a year: 35 passengers and crew died in a crash, also in the Mediterranean, in January 1954, while 43 had died when a Comet crashed near Calcutta in May 1953. An inquiry carried out by the Royal Aircraft Establishment at Farnborough attributed the disasters to metal fatigue.

The American-designed Boeing 707, which could carry more passengers and was generally considered more reliable, made its first commercial flight in 1958, and rapidly supplanted the Comet.

In May 1945, the government had decided that Heathrow should become London's main airport. It was to be called London Airport, as it was considered that non-English speakers would find Heathrow too difficult to pronounce. The first terminal was built in 1951. Checking-in originally involved weighing the passengers as well as their luggage. By the mid-fifties London Airport was handling three million passengers a year. By 1997, despite the growth of Gatwick, Stansted and Luton airports, it would be 58 million.

Also this year...

Eight Manchester United footballers amongst 23 passengers and crew killed in Munich plane crash

Last debutantes presented to the Queen

Campaign for Nuclear Disarmament formed

Church of England backs family planning

Prince Charles becomes the Prince of Wales

Stereophonic recording introduced

First Life Peers created

Double yellow lines and parking meters introduced

Blue Peter first broadcast

Race riots in west London

Boris Pasternak publishes Doctor Zhivago

Pope John XXIII enthroned

First motorway opened

Frederick Sanger awarded Nobel Prize for Chemistry

Deaths: Pope Pius XII, Ralph Vaughan Williams, Christabel Pankhurst, Douglas Jardine, Marie Stopes

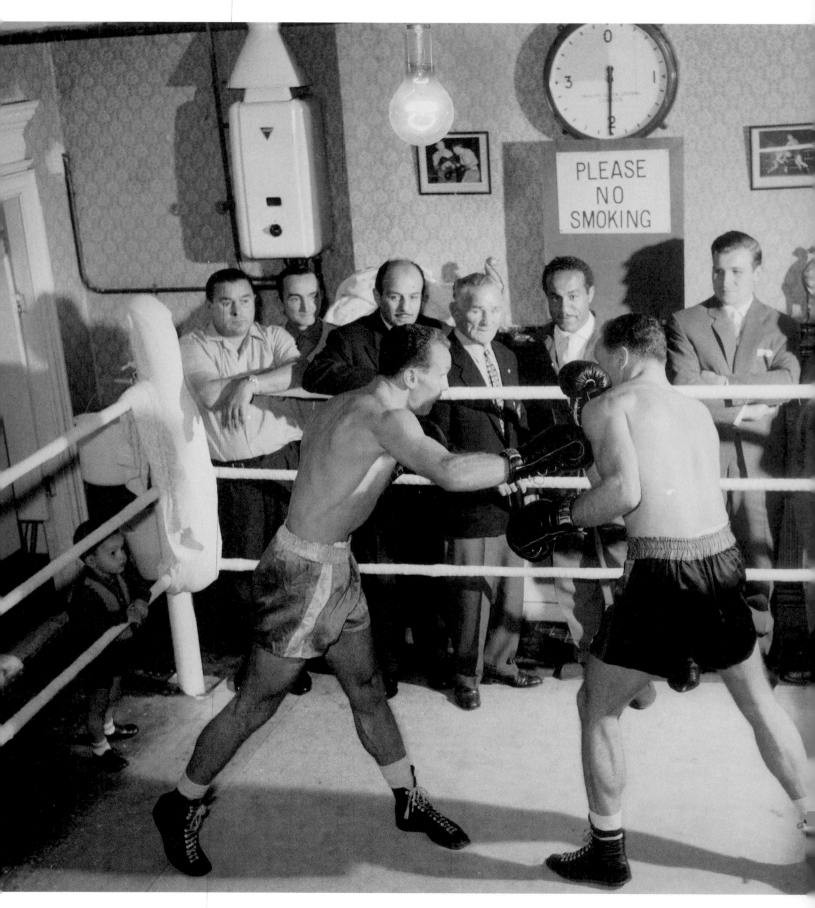

The pub where fighting was encouraged

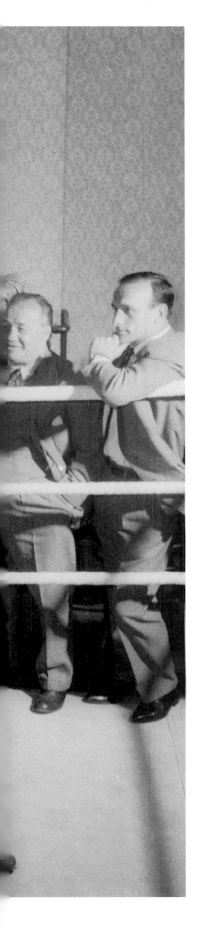

Henry Cooper and his twin brother George (also known as Jim) spar in the ring at the Thomas A' Becket gym. Looking on are some of the leading characters from British boxing of the era, plus, on the far left, light-heavyweight Eddie Wright's two-year-old son. The other figures, from left to right, are: Danny Holland (trainer); Alf Skelton (ex-amateur); Jackie Negal (ex-lightweight); Ted Broadribb, Alex Buxton (ex-light-heavyweight); Georgie Walker; Ernie Javis (ex-flyweight); and the landlord, Joe Lucy.

South Londoner Henry Cooper became the British and Empire heavyweight champion for the first time in 1959, aged 24. He was to hold the British and Commonwealth heavyweight titles until 1970. Cooper's other claim to fame was losing twice to Muhammad Ali – although he did once floor him in a non-title fight in 1963.

The Thomas A' Becket gym, at 32 Old Kent Road, in southeast London, was upstairs from the pub of the same name. The gym was considered to be the best place to train in London. Boxers such as Muhammad Ali, Sugar Ray Robinson, Rocky Marciano and Jack Dempsey all visited.

Alan Minter was honoured with the freedom of the pub when he won the world middleweight championship in 1980. "The atmosphere in there is unbelievable," he said. "It's so small, when there's a crowd pressing round the ring it's like sparring in a phone booth."

Inevitably the fights were not always contained to the upstairs boxing ring: the pub had long been associated with the east London underworld and in 1993, the former world welterweight champion, Lloyd Honeyghan, was attacked with a hammer when he went to watch a fight at the pub.

Despite efforts to keep the pub and gym open, both were closed in 1997.

Also this year...

Fidel Castro takes control of Cuba

British Motor Corporation launches the Mini

European Free Trade Association (EFTA) established with Britain as founder member

Soviet rocket Lunik II crash lands on moon

Conservatives led by Harold Macmillan win general election

Maiden voyage of first working hovercraft

Queen's head first appears on banknotes

Antarctica declared multi-national science reserve

Deaths: Buddy Holly, Frank Lloyd Wright, Mario Lanza, Cecil B. De Mille, Billie Holliday, Sir Jacob Epstein, Errol Flynn, Sir Stanley Spencer

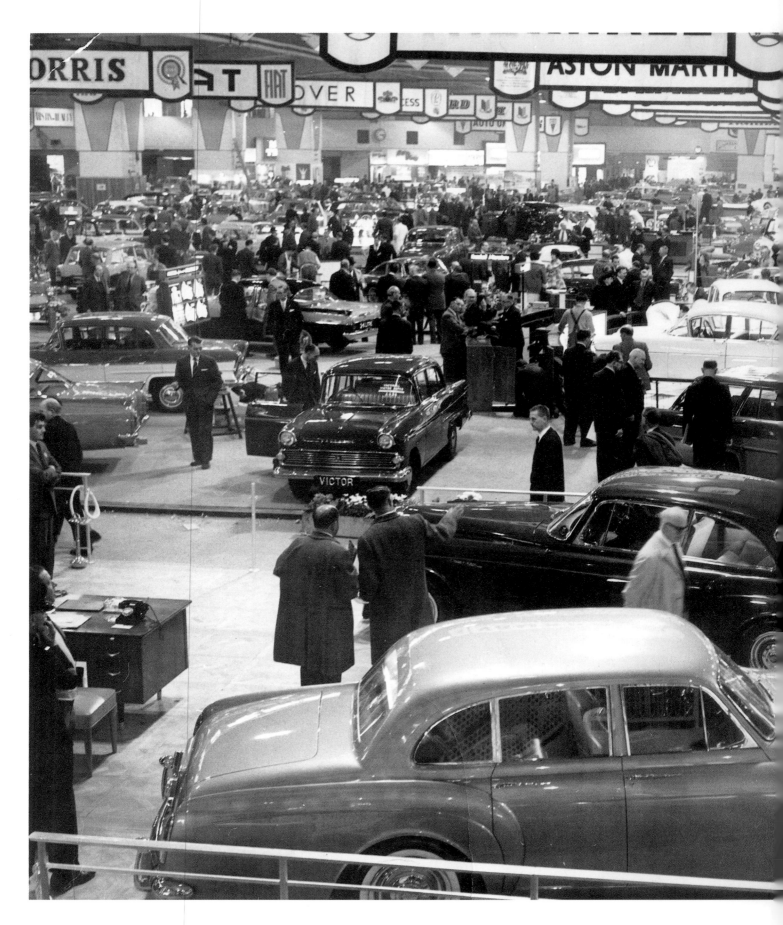

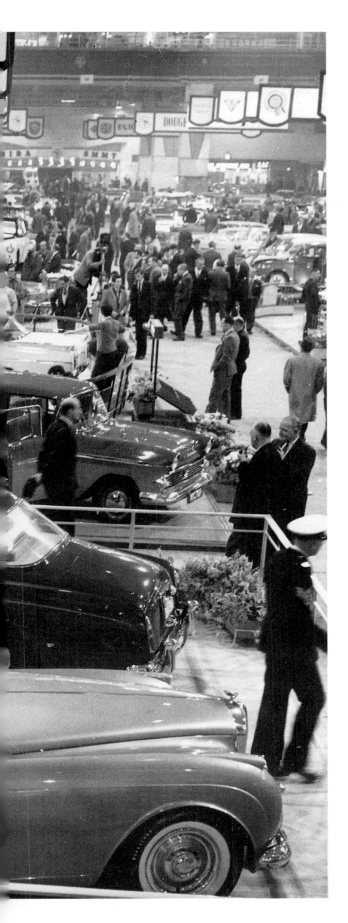

Buying British – when motorists still could

There were 360 cars at London's Motor Show at Earl's Court in 1960, including 35 British makes, 12 American and Canadian models, seven from Germany and six from both France and Italy.

The President of the Board of Trade, Reginald Maudling, opened the show on Wednesday, October 19. He lauded the British motor industry's doubled production rate since 1950, but admitted that export numbers had almost halved. Strikes at BMC factories, most of which had ended that day, also cast a shadow. This slump was reflected in the number of people attending the Motor Show – ticket sales on the first day were down 25 per cent on the previous year, which had been notable for the number of new models. This year's show could not hope to offer a comparable selection, but it did have new American "compact" cars and several new estate versions of existing models.

The British Motor Corporation's new 850 version of the Austin A55 was on show, as was the Morris Consul. Ford's Zephyr and Zodiac models boasted front disc breaks. The previous week Rootes announced a new Humber Super Snipe with four headlights, while its Humber Hawk also had disc breaks among a series of improvements. Standard Triumph International offered the Vanguard Luxury Six, a development on the Vanguard Vignale Saloon, that had a two-litre six-cylinder engine and a maximum speed of 80 mph. The 1960 Motor Show could also claim to be the first since the war where motorists could buy a car "off the shelf" without joining a waiting list.

Also this year...

Prince Andrew born

Princess Margaret marries Anthony Armstrong-Jones

£1 note goes into circulation

Francis Chichester's 40-day solo Atlantic crossing sets record

Alfred Hitchcock produces Psycho

Gary Powers shot down in U-2 spy plane

Harold Macmillan makes "Wind of Change" speech in Cape Town

UN forces arrive in Congo

Nigeria becomes independent

Doc Marten boots launched

Coronation Street first broadcast on ITV

South African police shoot 69 dead in Sharpeville massacre

Olympics held in Rome

First British nuclear submarine, HMS Dreadnought, launched

D.H. Lawrence's Lady Chatterley's Lover published after 30-year ban

J.F. Kennedy is elected US President

Last National Servicemen called up

Theodore Maiman develops the laser

Royal Shakespeare Company formed

Deaths: Albert Camus, Nevil Shute, Boris Pasternak, Nye Bevan, Sylvia Pankhurst, Clark Gable

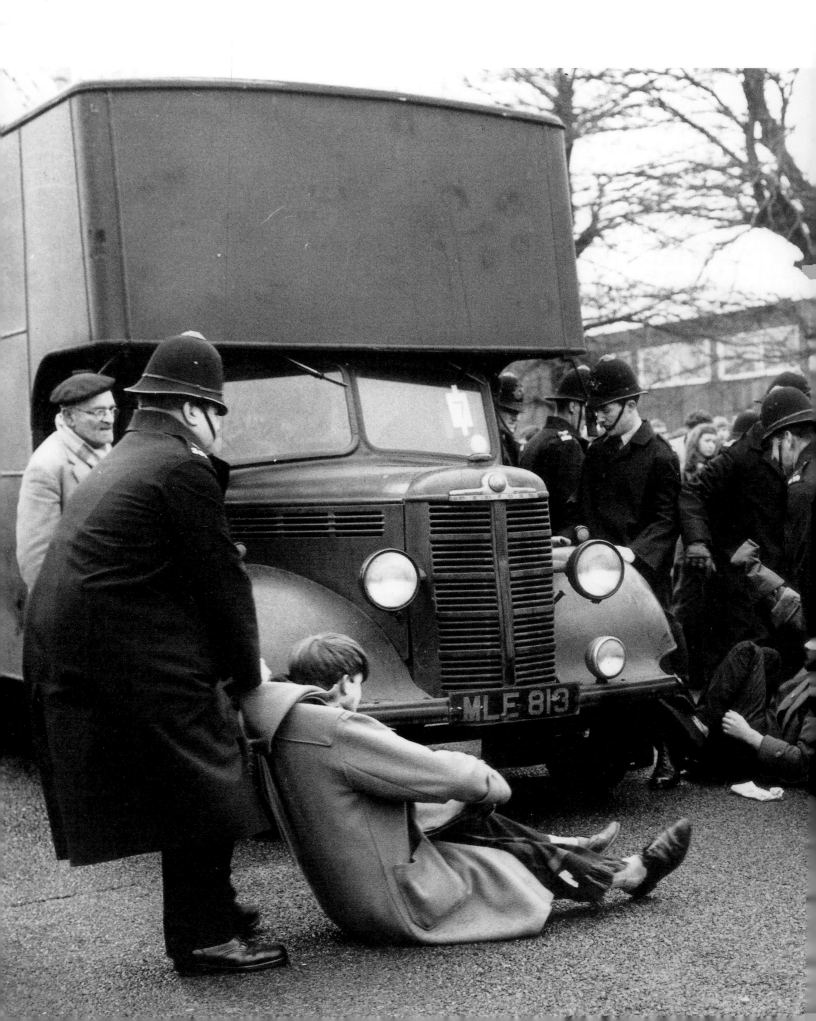

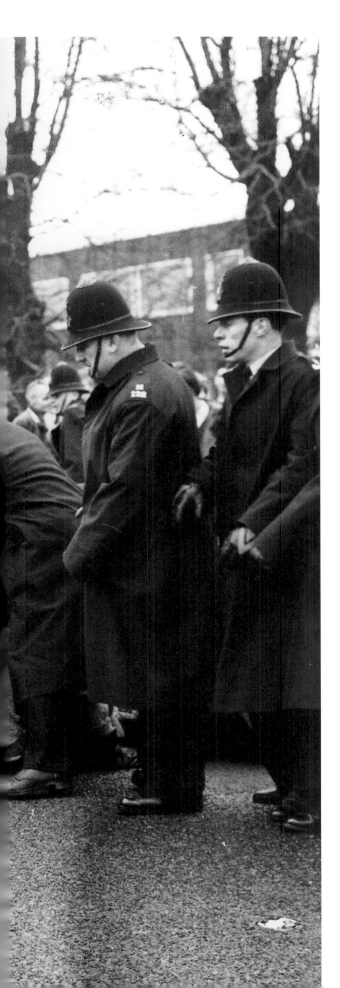

Police ban the bomb protestors

Police haul demonstrators away from a van outside the United States Air Force headquarters, at Ruislip in Middlesex. The demonstration was organised by the Committee of 100 – an offshoot of the Campaign for Nuclear Disarmament (CND) – which had staged a sit-in when police attempted to prevent their ban-the-bomb demonstration.

CND, founded by philosopher Bertrand Russell and the Canon of St Paul's Cathedral, John Collins, was originally set up in 1958 to oppose British development of the H-bomb. By 1960 there was a split between those who espoused lawful protest and those who believed in non-violent direct action – which mainly involved causing obstructions through sit-down protests. Many of the exponents of direct action joined the Committee of 100, which included such high-profile members as the writers John Osborne, Doris Lessing and Hugh MacDiarmid.

In September 1961, a group of over 12,000 Committee supporters took part in a protest at Trafalgar Square; 1,300 were arrested. Shortly afterwards police raided the Committee's London offices and more arrests were made. After this the group lost some of its impetus. It was finally disbanded in 1968.

CND's remit was to grow over the following decades to include campaigning for the unilateral abandonment of nuclear weapons and bases, and a global ban on nuclear, chemical and biological armaments.

Also this year...

Thousands flee to West Berlin as the Berlin Wall is erected

Russian Yuri Gagarin becomes first man in space

First oral contraceptive pill on sale

Walt Disney's 101 Dalmatians on general release

Former diplomat George Blake jailed for 42 years for spying

Anthony Wedgwood Benn prevented from taking up House of Commons seat because of his peerage

Coup by army rebels in Algeria against French government collapses

Dr Ramsey becomes the 100th Archbishop of Canterbury

The Beatles make first appearance at Liverpool's Cavern Club

Rudolf Nureyev defects from Soviet Union

British Terry Downes becomes world middleweight champion

Britain applies to enter Common Market

Chemists Francis Crick and Sydney Brenner determine structure of DNA

Deaths: Sir Thomas Beecham, George Formby, Gary Cooper, Carl Gustav Jung, Ernest Hemingway, Augustus John

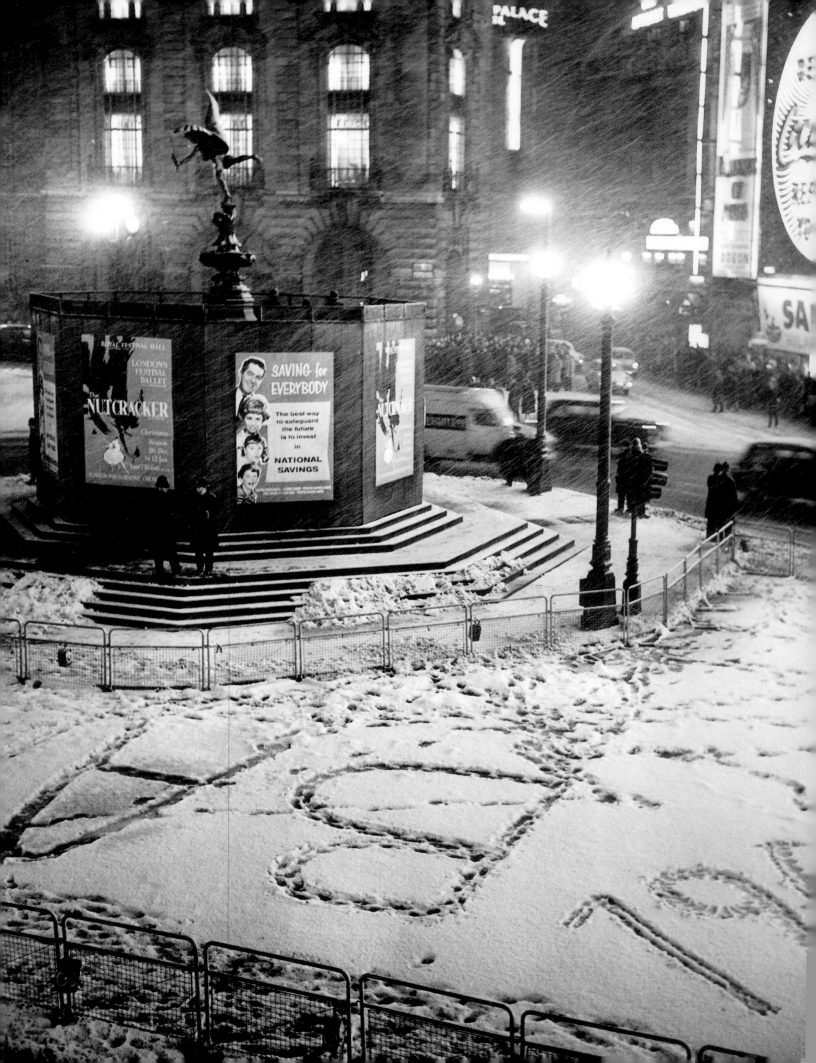

Heavy snow puts New Year celebrations on ice

Revellers celebrate an uncharacteristically subdued New Year's Eve in the snow at Piccadilly Circus in London. The capital – and much of the rest of the country – was experiencing the heaviest winter since 1947. Many villages were cut off as roads became impassable. Only Cornwall, the eastern districts of Norfolk and Suffolk and parts of Lincolnshire escaped the snow and ice.

The cold spell even slowed down Big Ben's clock. Snow lodged on its north face led to its striking 10 minutes late. Engineers solved the problem by melting the accumulating heap of ice.

Only the hardiest made it to London's traditional festive locales. *The Times* reported: "In Piccadilly the barricades round Eros were not needed. The pedestrians kept moving. There it was the quietest New Year's Eve for many years." Several thousand ventured onto Trafalgar Square, but it, too, was quieter than usual. However, according to *The Times*, the weather did not dampen the crowd's spirits: "Constables dodged snowballs hurled from the balcony on the National Gallery side of the square. Carnival hats were worn."

The snow may not have stopped the party, but trying to get home in the ensuing chaos may have brought festivities to an abrupt end. Trains and buses were severely delayed, and 20 of London Transport's special New Year's Eve services had to be cancelled.

The weather also put a stop to many traditional Hogmanay rituals in Scotland. In most rural areas would-be revellers were forced to stay indoors, and only the most determined tall dark strangers went on with their traditional task of first footing.

Also this year...

Sunday Times *colour supplement launched*

James Hanratty sentenced to death after longest murder trial in the nation's legal history

Launch of Telstar *satellite enables live television pictures to be transmitted across the Atlantic*

Graham Hill wins world Grand Prix championship

Private Eye *first published*

Algeria becomes independent

First James Bond film, Dr No, *opens*

Coventry Cathedral consecrated

John Glenn becomes first American to orbit the earth

Harold Macmillan sacks seven cabinet members ("Night of the Long Knives")

Khrushchev and Kennedy back down over Cuban crisis

Amnesty International created

Anthony Burgess' A Clockwork Orange *is published*

Second Vatican Council opens

Deaths: Vita Sackville-West, John Christie, William Faulkner, Marilyn Monroe, Herman Hesse, e.e. cummings

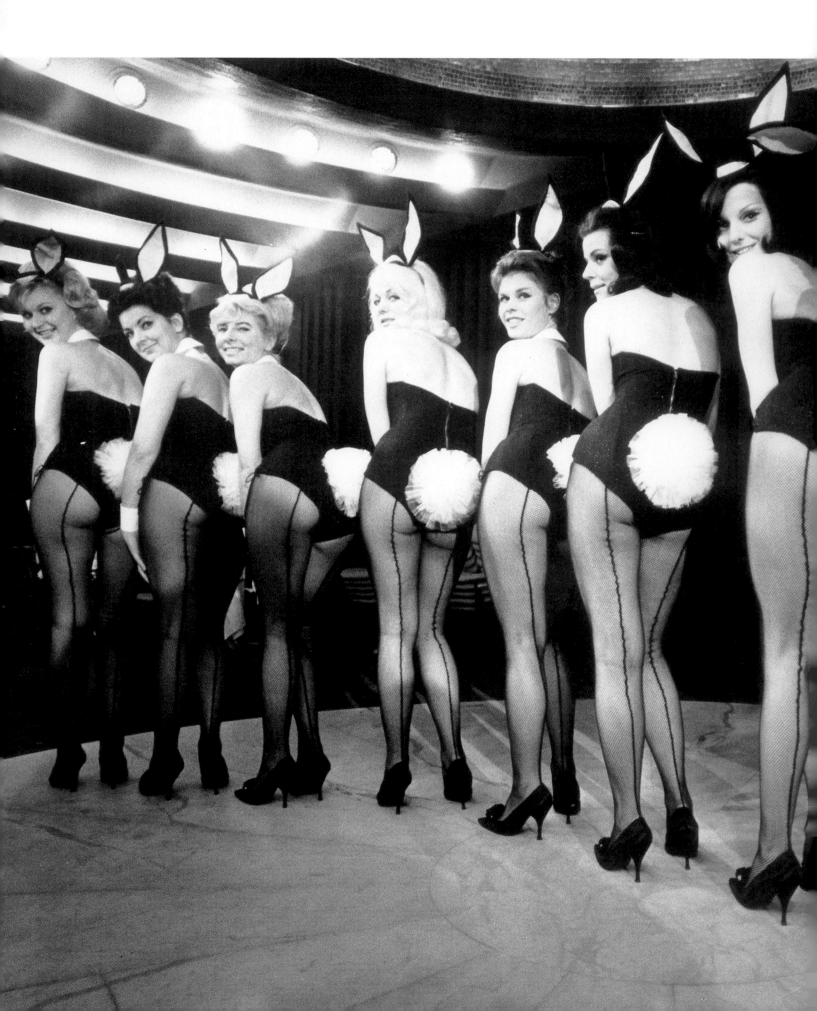

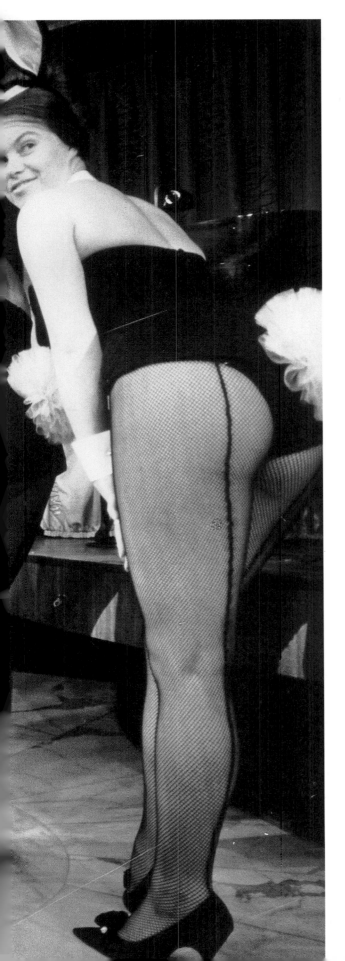

Going to work in swimsuit, ears and tail

Their working uniform was a swimsuit, a fluffy tail, pointy ears and spiky stilettos. These bunny girls, working at the Bal Tabarin Club in London, were wearing a look that would come to epitomise a certain sixties pseudo-glamour. The bunny girl was more generally associated with the clubs owned by millionaire Hugh Hefner's Playboy empire. Other than gambling, Playboy bunnies were one of the main draws of the Playboy Club in Park Lane, which opened in 1966. Girls aged between 18 and 25 were eligible for the job, providing that they looked the part and had a basic grasp of maths. Applicants were informed: "You must possess a charming personality, intelligence, have an attractive appearance and posture with a good figure." Once employed the girls were expected to follow strict rules about costume, make-up and weight. Each girl was checked by a "Bunny Mother" before she went to work.

Through their work the girls met a large number of celebrities, but until 1975 they were banned from giving their real names or going out with customers. Some, like Lauren Hutton, Sally Field and Deborah Harry, who worked in American Playboy Clubs, went on to stardom.

Always considered risqué, in the eighties the London Playboy Club was hit by scandal. The club was stripped of its gambling license in October 1981. Months later, Abdul Khawaja, one of the club's owners, was forced to flee the country. Khawaja owed over £1 million in taxes, and was wanted by the police in connection with the murder of former bunny girl Eve Stratford and allegations that he had been procuring girls for clients.

Also this year...

Kim Philby, suspected spy, disappears

Over 2,000 rail stations to close after Beeching Report

Profumo scandal shakes Macmillan government; Christine Keeler jailed

De Gaulle vetos British Common Market membership

Peerage Bill allows peers to renounce titles

Mailbags worth over £1 million pounds stolen in the Great Train Robbery

Hot-line installed between the White House and the Kremlin

Dr Who *first broadcast*

Rachel Carson's Silent Spring *marks start of environmental movement*

Kenya becomes independent

Valentina Tereshkova becomes first woman in space

Lawrence of Arabia *wins seven Oscars*

Martin Luther King speaks to over 200,000 in Washington

Harold Macmillan resigns; Lord Home appointed Prime Minister

J.F. Kennedy assassinated; his killer, Lee Harvey Oswald, also assassinated

Deaths: Hugh Gaitskell, C.S. Lewis, Sylvia Plath, Edith Piaf, Lord Beveridge, William Carlos Williams, Pope John XXIII, Aldous Huxley

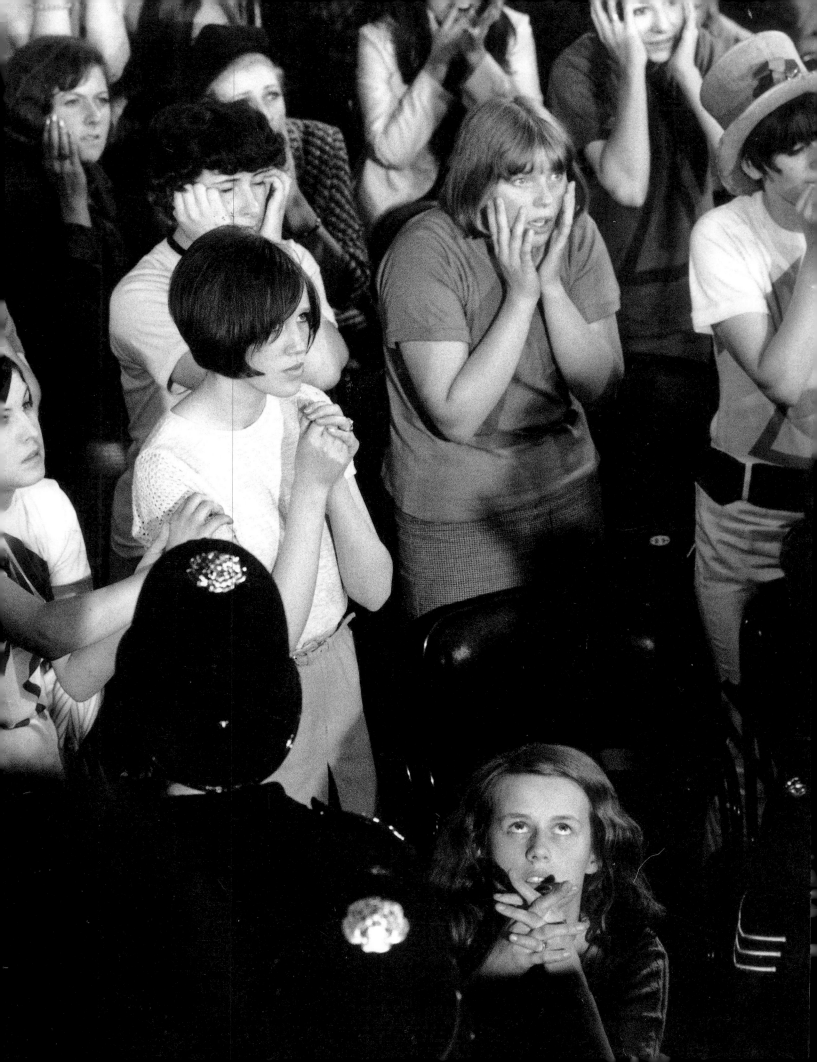

We love you, yeah, yeah, yeah

They screamed, they wept, they fainted – and all for four boys who had funny haircuts, funny suits and came from Liverpool. In 1964 John, Paul, George and Ringo, otherwise known as the "fab four", the "mop tops" or The Beatles, were named Britain's top tourist attraction in a BBC survey.

The name, John Lennon explained, came "to us in a vision. A man descended unto us astride a flaming pie and spake these words unto us, saying 'From this day on you are The Beatles with an A.' Thus it did come to pass thus."

The band's first single, *Love Me Do*, was released to moderate success. Their follow-up single, *Please Please Me*, only went to number two in the British charts, but it sent teenagers over the brink of hysteria. America proved equally susceptible: *She Loves You* went to number one in America as well as in Britain, and the band's appearance on the Ed Sullivan show in 1964 attracted an audience of 73 million. By March 1964, The Beatles had become the first band to hold the top five places in the American charts.

The Beatles were to dominate the pop world for almost a decade. The influence of their music, perhaps above all the mould-breaking album *Sgt. Pepper's Lonely Hearts Club Band*, which took 700 hours to record, was to endure long after Paul McCartney obtained a court injunction to split The Beatles in 1970. The former members of The Beatles pursued solo careers. John Lennon was assassinated in 1980.

Also this year...

12 men found guilty of Great Train Robbery

Prince Edward born

Pirate Radio Caroline broadcasts from North Sea

Congo crisis erupts

China explodes an atomic bomb

Krushchev deposed as Soviet leader by Brezhnev and Kosygin

UK sends in reinforcements to stop intercommunal violence in Cyprus

Nelson Mandela sentenced to life imprisonment in South Africa

Forth Road Bridge opened

The Sun first published as successor to The Daily Herald

Labour under Harold Wilson wins narrow majority in general election

Briton Dorothy Hodgkin wins Nobel Prize for Chemistry

IBM produces first practical word processor

Olympic games held in Tokyo

Top of the Pops first broadcast

MPs vote to abolish capital punishment

Deaths: Lord Beaverbrook, Ian Fleming, Jawarharlal Nehru, Herbert Hoover, Douglas MacArthur, Cole Porter, Edith Sitwell

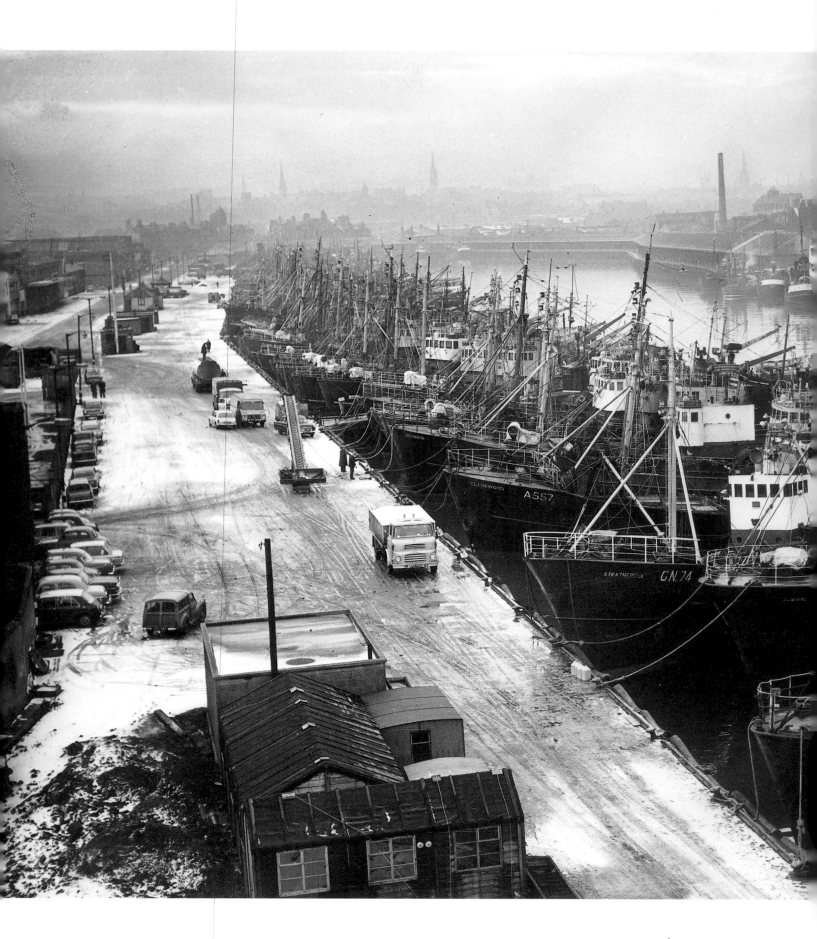

Another berthed day as trawler dispute drags on

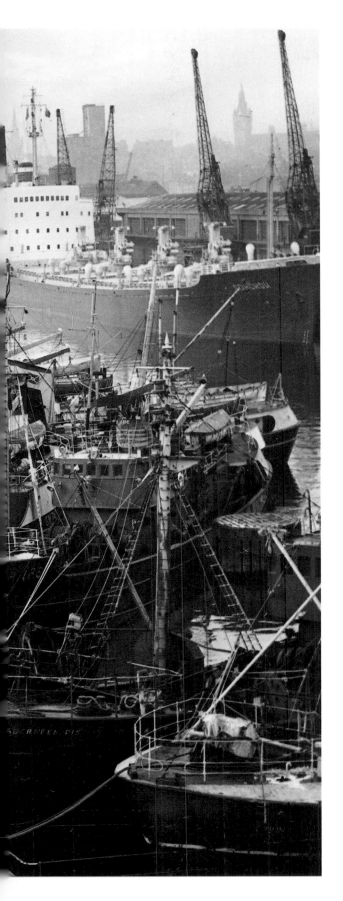

Up to 120 trawlers lie idle in their berths at Aberdeen. The dispute started on January 4, when skippers and mates decided to stay in port until the Aberdeen Fishing Vessel Owners Association negotiated about local employment agreements. The Owners Association refused to do so until the trawlers put to sea.

Most of the skippers had refused to re-sign contracts which had expired on the previous New Year's Eve in protest against a local practice that required skippers to have a letter of clearance from their old employer before starting a new job. The mates, who were supposed to re-sign at the same time as the skippers, also refused. They wanted to end another local practice that held mates responsible for supervising the landing of fish and the transfers of trawlers to mooring berths, which they did not have to do in other ports. They also complained about having to pay crew members who helped store the fish out of their own pockets, which, some mates claimed, could cost up to £3,100 a year.

A spokesman for both skippers and mates, Mr J. M. Crockett, claimed the existing employment agreement was "oppressive and against the principle of natural justice. It is like the professional football players' retain and transfer agreement – without the big transfers fees." Meanwhile the owners were losing a lot of money – an estimated 66 tons of fish a day, worth more than £325,000. Twenty of the 140 Aberdeen trawlers were at sea, but it was expected they, too, would join the dispute on their return.

Also this year...

The Kray brothers cleared of running a protection racket

Cigarette adverts banned from television

American troops sent to Vietnam

Race riots in Los Angeles

Soviet cosmonaut Alexei Leonev becomes first man to "walk" in space

Rhodesia declares UDI

Capital gains tax introduced

Edward Heath becomes Conservative leader

Judge Elizabeth Lane becomes nation's first female high court judge

Ian Brady and Myra Hindley charged with Moors murders

Beatles awarded MBE

Mary Whitehouse creates National Viewers and Listeners' Association

Capital punishment abolished

70 mph speed limit introduced on motorways

13 die in North Sea oil rig disaster

Queen dedicates Runnymede to memory of JFK

Deaths: Winston Churchill, T.S. Eliot, Stan Laurel, Herbert Morrison, Le Corbusier, Richard Dimbleby, Somerset Maugham

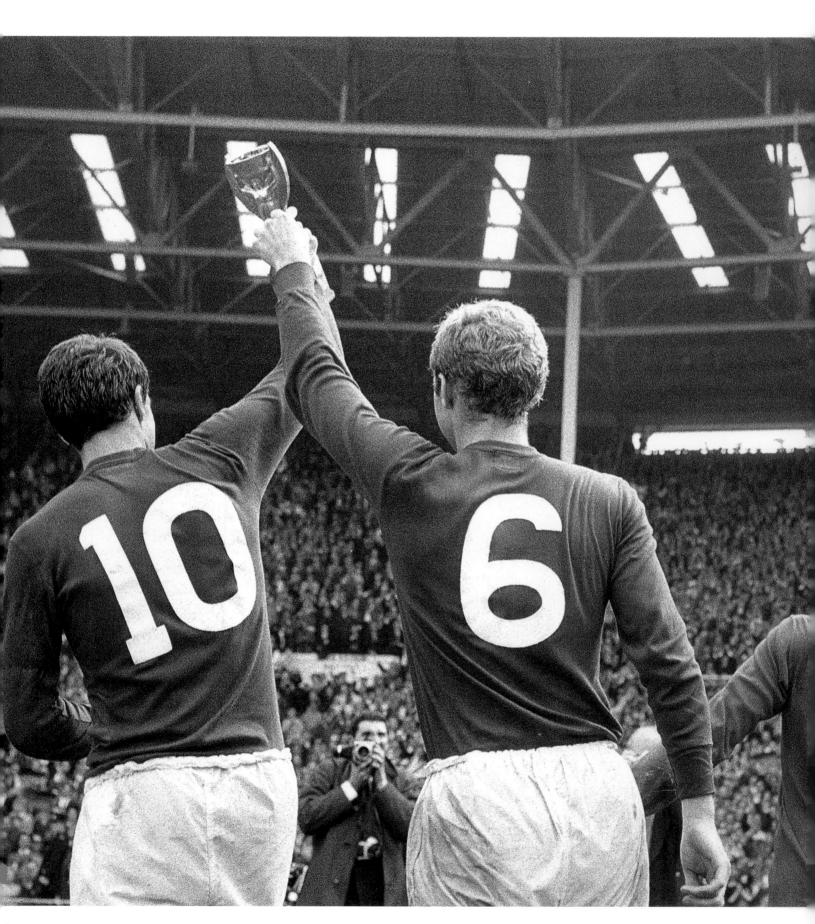

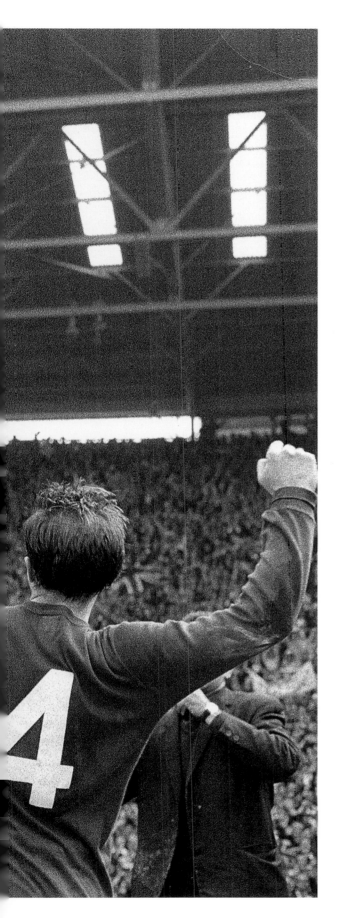

England expects … and wins World Cup glory

Bobby Moore (No.6) and Geoff Hurst (No.10) raise the World Cup and, together with Nobby Stiles, share their triumph with the crowd. 93,000 saw England win the 1966 World Cup at Wembley Stadium. A further 400 million around the world watched it on television.

For those who were at Wembley, *The Times*'s football correspondent reported, "the atmosphere was electric It fairly crackled. The terracing was a sea of waving flags, the standards of two nations; the noise was a wall of sound that drowned the flutterings of one's heart. High in the stands there came the beating of a drum, a deep, pulsating thud, almost tribal."

In a game supporters would remember for decades, captain Bobby Moore led England to imperishable triumph. Behind the team was the enigmatic figure of Alf Ramsey, the team's manager, the ultimate architect of victory and soon to be knighted. The match was intensely dramatic. With only seconds left, England led 2-1. Remarkably, the Germans then equalised. In extra time, England took the lead again when Geoff Hurst scored one of the World Cup's most controversial goals. Die-hard Germans – and Scots – still maintain the ball never crossed the line But in the event, it hardly mattered. At the very death, Hurst scored an emphatic fourth to give him his hat-trick and England the World Cup.

There had nearly been no cup to win – the Jules Rimet trophy was stolen from the Football Association while on display at Westminster Central Hall in March. However, Londoner David Corbett saved the day when his dog Pickles found the trophy wrapped in newspaper on a walk a week later.

Also this year…

Archbishop of Canterbury and Pope have first official meeting for 400 years

Labour wins general election led under Harold Wilson

Brezhnev becomes Soviet leader

Double agent George Blake escapes from Wormwood Scrubs

France withdraws its forces from NATO

State of Emergency declared during seamen's strike

Ian Brady and Myra Hindley convicted of Moors murders

First British credit card introduced by Barclay's Bank

Gwynfor Evans becomes first Welsh Nationalist MP after Carmarthen by-election

British Board of Film Classification set up

116 children and 28 adults die when slag heap buries school in Aberfan

Time magazine declares London is swinging

Deaths: Buster Keaton, Evelyn Waugh, Walt Disney, Montgomery Clift, comedian Lenny Bruce

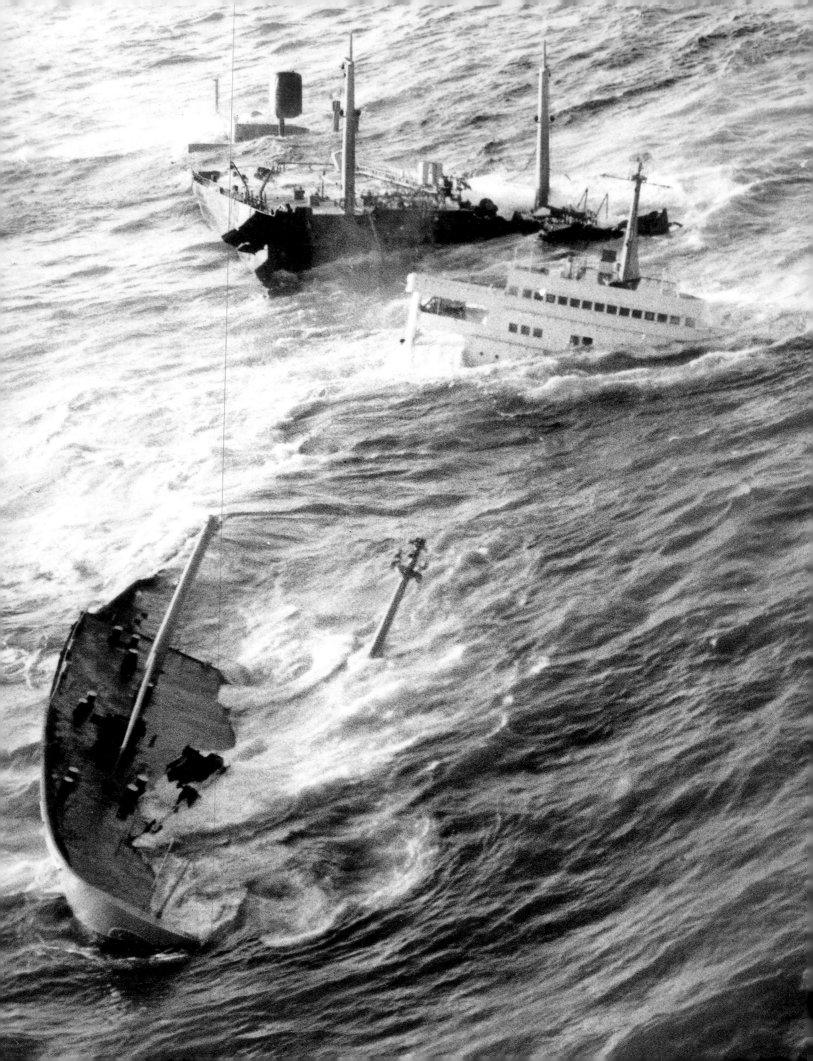

Ten days to tame the *Torrey Canyon*

Between 8.45 and 9.05 on the morning of Saturday, March 18, the *Torrey Canyon*, owned by US company Union Oil, hit the Seven Stones reef off the coast of Cornwall, ripping her hull open. The 61,000-ton tanker was carrying 118,000 tons of oil.

A Dutch deep-sea tug answered the tanker's distress call. It was agreed that the tug would attempt to salvage the tanker. Detergent spray guns were used to try to disperse escaping oil, but to little avail. On Tuesday one of the salvage team was killed in an engine room explosion. The captain and remaining three officers were evacuated from the *Torrey Canyon*.

By Wednesday, March 22, an estimated 25,000 to 30,000 tons of oil had spilled into the sea. Two days later the wind changed, blowing the spillage directly onto the coast. The salvage attempt was abandoned on Sunday, March 26. The next day, the tanker broke into three pieces. It was only on Tuesday, March 28, that the government implemented its plan to bomb the tanker: 1,000-pound incendiary bombs and 1,200 gallons of napalm were dropped to keep the tanker ablaze.

The government was criticised for its slowness to respond, failure to take expert advice – which suggested that setting fire to the tanker would have been more effective than bombing it – and its apparent vagueness about the ownership of the wreckage under international law. Mr Foley, Under Secretary for Defence, riposted by asserting: "Given the extra oil now floating off Cornwall, all the men and the equipment in the world could not deal with this problem. It is a problem no country has had to face before." More than 100 miles of coast were polluted.

Also this year...

Dr Emil Savundra convicted on insurance fraud

Donald Campbell dies trying to set world water-speed record of 300 mph

William Rees-Mogg becomes editor of The Times

Israel victorious in the Six Day War

Americans protest against Vietnam war

The Colonels seize power in Greece

British application to join Common Market vetoed by de Gaulle

ITV launches News at Ten

QE2 launched

Sandie Shaw wins Eurovision song contest

Sir Francis Chichester completes solo round-the-world yacht voyage

BBC Radio One begins broadcasting

Abortion legalised

Deaths: Konrad Adenauer, John Masefield, Vivien Leigh, René Magritte, Siegfried Sassoon, Joe Orton, Beatles manager Brian Epstein, Clement Attlee, Ernesto "Che" Guevara

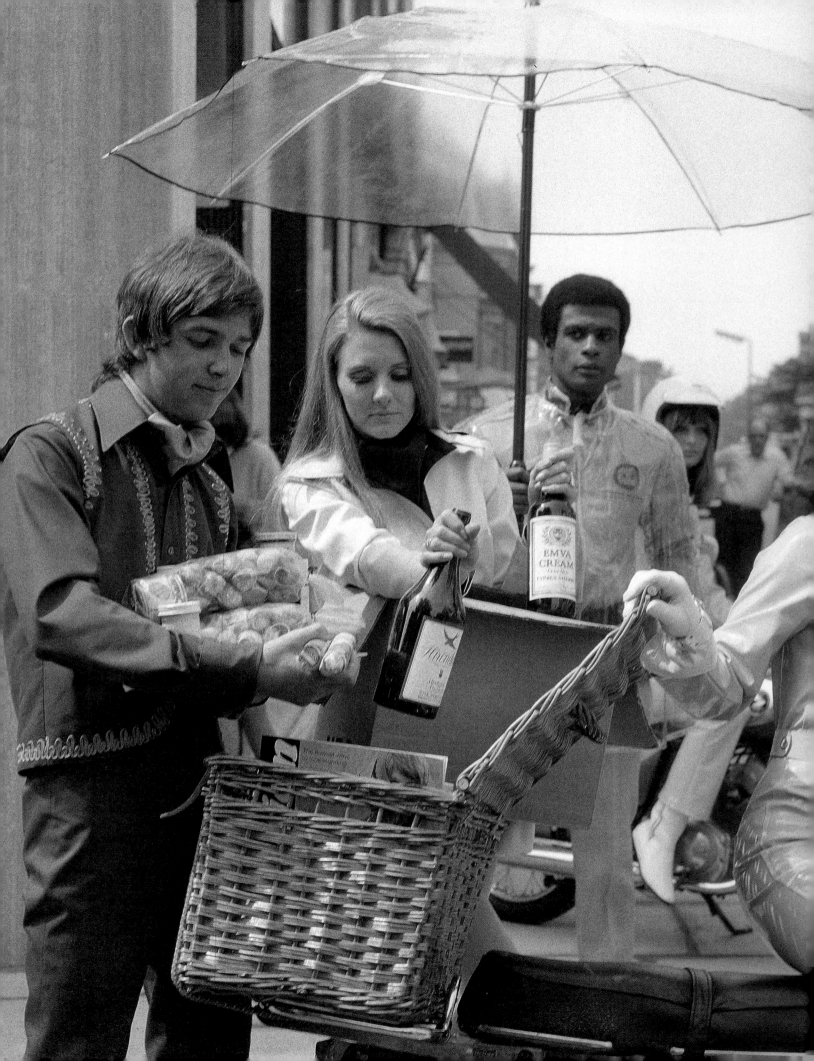

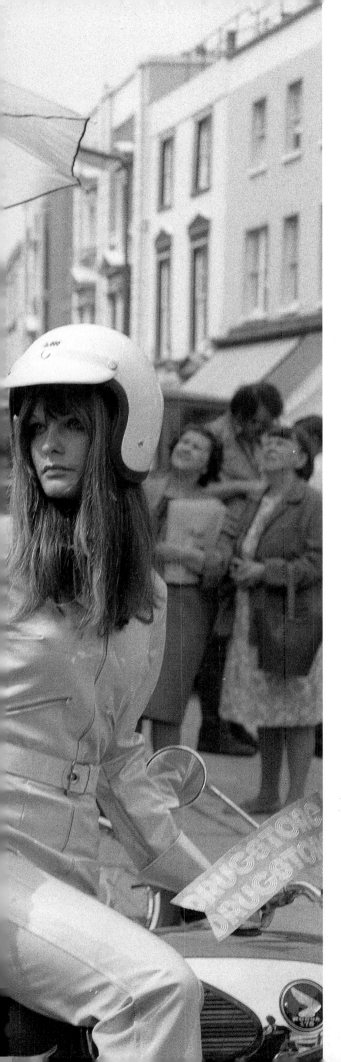

Style on prescription at the Chelsea Drug Store

Hanging out at the Chelsea Drug Store, on the King's Road, London. The Rolling Stones made the shop famous, ("I went down to the Chelsea Drug Store/To get your prescription filled"). But if drugs were the attraction for some, for most it was just a question of being where it was all happening.

In the sixties, nowhere swung quite like London. The capital became the backdrop for a phenomenal burst of creativity: The Beatles and The Rolling Stones dominated the world of popular music; David Bailey and Terry Donovan transformed photography; actors Michael Caine and *Blow-Up* star David Hemmings epitomised the super-cool London lad; models Twiggy and The Shrimp personified "the look". The American actor Dennis Hopper, visiting London in 1966, remembered it as "the most exciting time I'd ever seen or have seen since ... London was dictating fashion, music, everything."

The Chelsea Drug Store held a prime position at the top of the King's Road – number 49 – close to Sloane Square. But it didn't really matter where on the King's Road you were: the whole road was a fashion parade, the place to see and be seen. To those who weren't part of the scene, the beautiful people looked as if there were attending an increasingly outlandish fancy-dress party: mini skirts, Afghan coats, pyjamas, smocks, huge floppy hats, boots or barefoot – almost anything went.

The Chelsea Drug Store has since been replaced by a MacDonald's restaurant.

Also this year...

Cecil Day-Lewis becomes Poet Laureate

Government launches "I'm backing Britain" campaign

Anti-Vietnam war demonstrations lead to violence in London

Martin Luther King is assassinated

Enoch Powell is accused of inciting racial prejudice by his "rivers of blood" speech

Students riot in Paris

Prescription charges re-introduced

Nixon elected US president

First decimal coins introduced in Britain

Manchester United beat Benfica 4-1 to win the European Cup

The Booker Prize established

Prague Spring crushed by Soviet invasion

Epidural technique introduced

Sheila Ann Thorns becomes mother of Britain's first sextuplets

Mexico hosts Olympic Games

11-year-old Mary Bell sentenced to life for manslaughter

American astronauts orbit moon

Deaths: Yuri Gagarin, John Steinbeck, Robert Kennedy, Tony Hancock, Enid Blyton

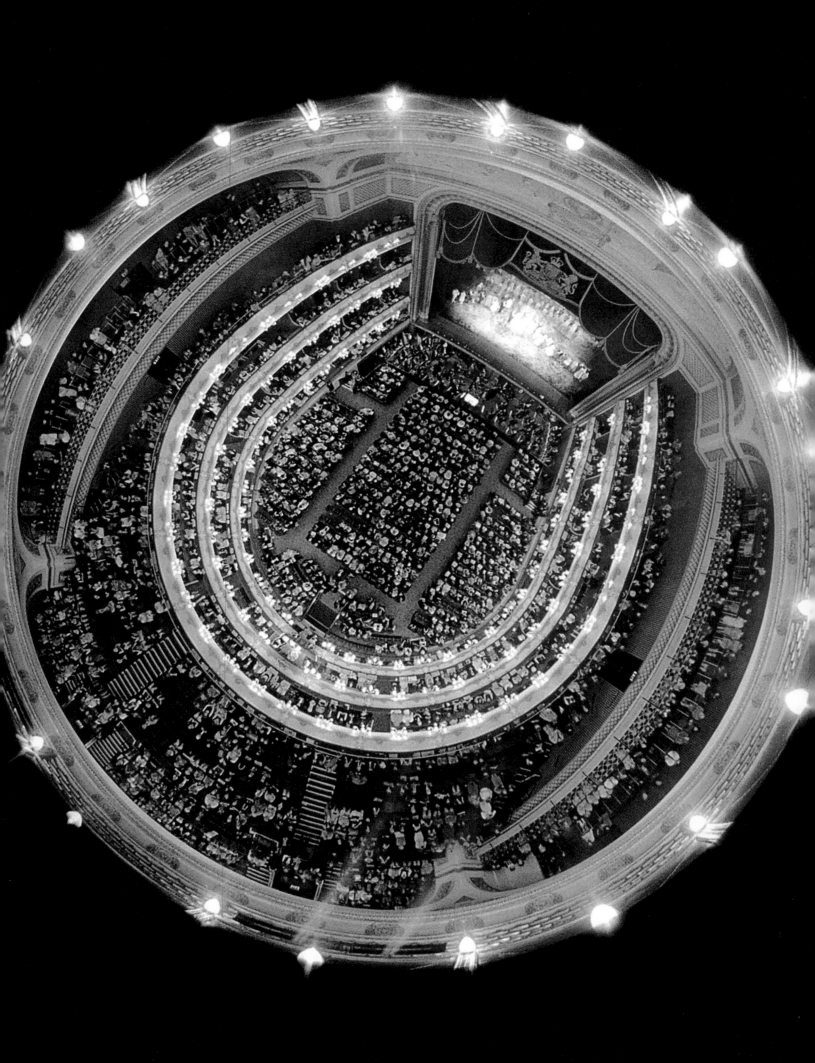

Keeping an eye on Fonteyn and Nureyev

The Royal Gala at the Royal Opera House, Covent Garden, on March 26. This picture was taken with a remote-control Nikon suspended from the roof of the Royal Opera House and using a fish-eye lens.

The distinctive features of the fish-eye lens are a very short focal length, a large, highly curved and protruding front element – which earned the lens its name – and a wide angle of view which, if barrel distortion is possible, can be up to 180 degrees. The result is a distortion of size – objects close to the lens come out very large, and those further away look very small. True fish eyes which can be used for 35 mm – like the one used for this photograph – include more of the scene and produce a circular image. Experimentation with the fish-eye lens was very popular in the late sixties, when the lens was first developed.

The couple that can just be made out standing at the very front of the stage are Margot Fonteyn and Rudolf Nureyev. The picture was taken at curtain call, as they received applause for their world premiere of *Pelleas and Melisande*, a ballet written especially to celebrate Fonteyn's 35th anniversary with the Royal Ballet. Queen Elizabeth was part of the audience.

Nureyev and Fonteyn danced together many times throughout the sixties and seventies. Fonteyn went on to be given the title of *prima ballerina assoluta* by the Royal Ballet in 1979.

Also this year...

Rupert Murdoch buys News of the World *and* The Sun

Yassir Arafat becomes leader of PLO

Kray twins sentenced to life imprisonment

Scientists fertilise human egg in test tube

Voting age reduced to 18

John Lennon and Yoko Ono stage "bed-in" for peace

British troops sent into Northern Ireland following serious unrest

Provisional IRA formed as breakaway from Official IRA

Concorde makes maiden flight at Toulouse

The Woodstock Festival

Robin Knox-Johnson sails solo non-stop around the world

Colonel Gaddafi seizes power in Libya; President de Gaulle resigns

Neil Armstrong becomes first man to walk on moon

Internet established under aegis of US Defense Department

Sharon Tate and four others murdered by Charles Manson "family"

Monty Python's Flying Circus first broadcast on BBC

Deaths: Lord Alexander of Tunis, Jack Kerouac, Rocky Marciano, Boris Karloff, Judy Garland, Ho Chi Minh, Dwight Eisenhower

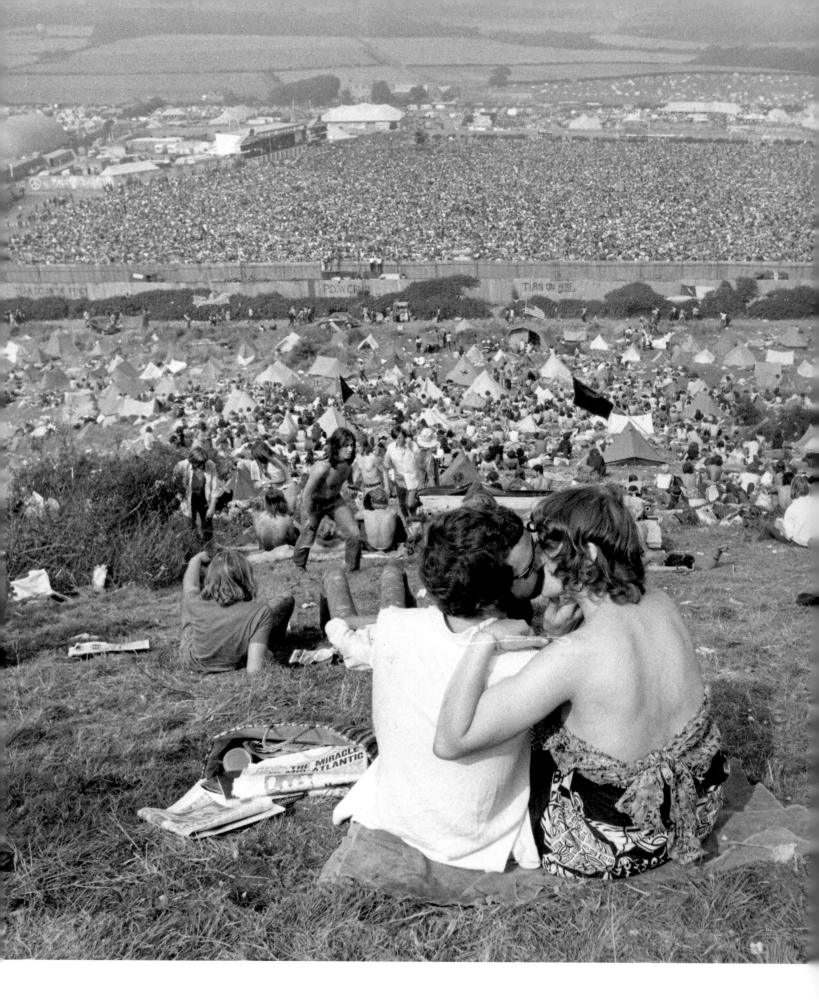

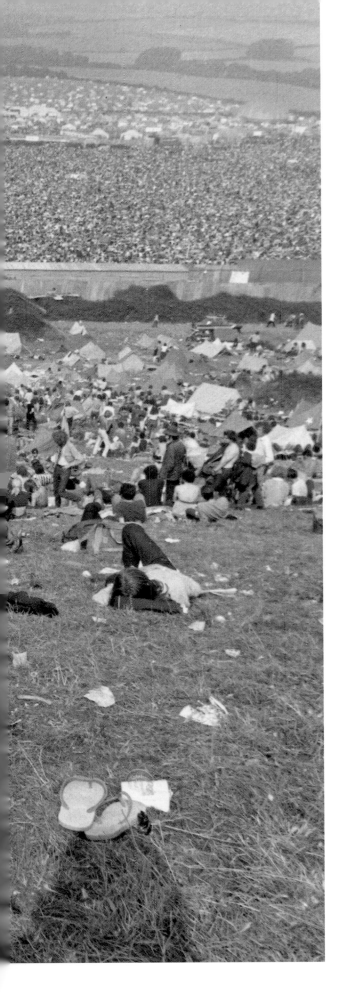

Love and peace rocked by festival fighting

Free love, peace, flowers and acid: the sixties were over, but these hippies weren't giving up, although the Isle of Wight festival, dubbed the British Woodstock, was seen by many as the end of an era.

This was the third Isle of Wight festival. Like the previous two, it was organised by Fiery Creations, also known as the Foulk brothers. It was also the largest – the five-day festival was spread over 1,100 acres at Freshwater and attended by 250,000 people. The line up – Jimi Hendrix (who was to die this year), The Who, The Doors, Joni Mitchell, Free, Jethro Tull and Leonard Cohen – was impressive, but ultimately disappointing: Hendrix and The Doors gave flat performances; Joni Mitchell was booed; and The Who didn't come on until 3am.

Perhaps more memorable was the Battle of Devastation Hill. Arguments broke out between organisers and hippies sitting on the hill behind the festival where they could see and hear for free. Others pulled festival fences down as a symbol of anarchy against the capitalist breadheads, the Foulk brothers. Some blamed the French anarchists, others the White Panthers, the Trotskyists or the Hells Angels – either way the spirit of peace and love was in short supply.

Faced with an enormous clearing-up job and the logistics of getting 250,000 off the island again, the police had another problem on their hands – thousands appealed for help with their fares home. Some had been robbed, but others had simply run out of money. The police had to contact parents to ask them to deposit the required amount at their local police station before the authorities could lend the money to their children.

Also this year...

More than 4,000 die in Hong Kong flu epidemic

Age of majority lowered to 18

First Jumbo jet lands at Heathrow

New English Bible sells out in first day

Crew of Apollo 13 *survive after oxygen tank bursts*

IBM introduces the floppy disk

Germaine Greer publishes The Female Eunuch

Brazil wins the World Cup

The Beatles are legally disbanded

The Conservatives under Edward Heath win general election

Seven Arab terrorists released after sympathisers blow up three airplanes in Jordan

Over eight million days lost to industrial action

Deaths: Bertrand Russell, E.M. Forster, Janis Joplin, Alexander Kerensky, Gamal Abdel Nasser, Viscount Slim, Bertrand Russell, Charles de Gaulle, athlete Lillian Board

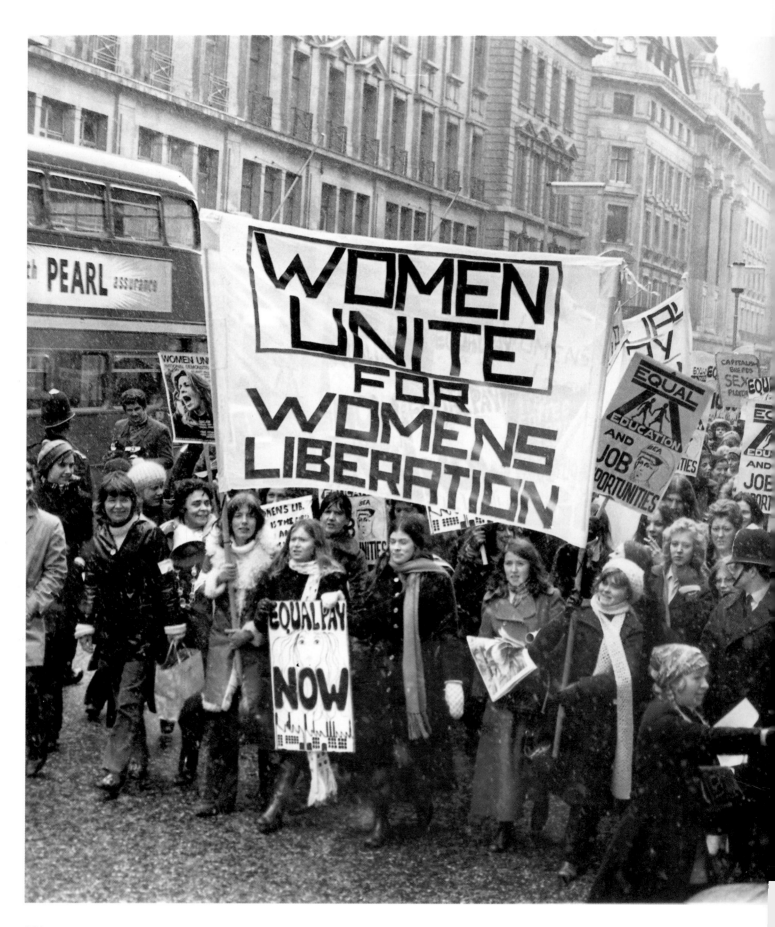

A woman's place is on the march

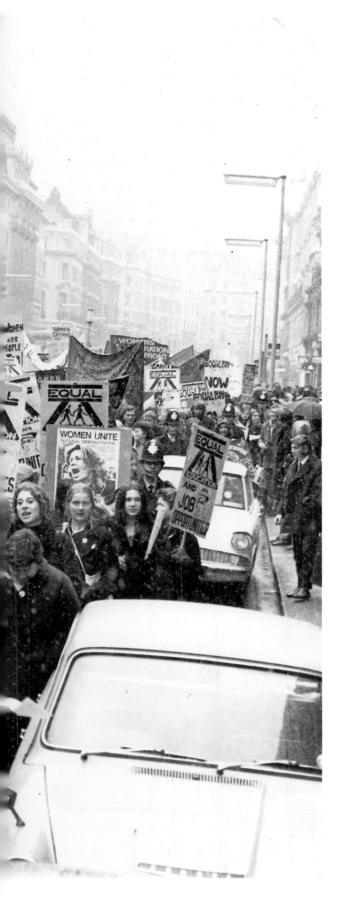

The women's liberation movement – "women's lib" – had come a long way since the Pankhursts and their supporters chained themselves to railings more than 60 years earlier. The Second World War had transformed women's roles in many industries, introducing large numbers of women into the workforce, while the social developments of the sixties – the contraceptive pill, lower infant mortality rates, longer life expectancy and a higher divorce rate – had had an equally dramatic effect. However, many felt that sexual stereotypes persisted nonetheless. An example of this was women's unequal status in regards to education, jobs, pay and benefits. It was for this that the women pictured here were fighting in 1971.

Australian feminist Germaine Greer had done much to draw attention to the women's cause when her book, *The Female Eunuch*, was published in 1970. Greer criticised traditional gender roles within the nuclear family and favoured female empowerment. Her outspokenness and flair for controversy inspired many women to take action.

The protest pictured appears to be peaceful, but not all women's libbers kept within the law. In February 1971, five women were tried for throwing smoke bombs, flour bags and tomatoes at a Miss World competition. Their actions, however, were frequently mocked. When one of the Miss World defendants asked to be excused to go to the lavatory, the judge replied: "I shall allow you to go this time – just remember you are big girls now and should behave as such."

The Sex Discrimination Act and the Equal Pay Act came into force in 1975, entitling women to equal treatment in employment, training and education. Excluded from the acts were pensions, taxes and social security benefits.

Also this year...

Angry Brigade plants series of bombs

66 killed when barriers collapse at Glasgow's Ibrox Park football stadium

Full decimalisation is introduced

Rolls-Royce is declared bankrupt

Immigration Act abolishes Commonwealth workers' automatic right to live in Britain

London Bridge removed to Arizona

Bangladesh splits from Pakistan

105 Soviet officials expelled from Britain for spying

First British soldier killed in Ulster

Greenpeace is established

Intel launches the microprocessor

Manson "family" sentenced to death

Margaret Thatcher, Education Secretary, stops free school milk

Princess Anne is Sportswoman of the Year

Ted Heath skippers Britain to victory in the Admiral's Cup

Queen's allowance is doubled

Deaths: Coco Chanel, Igor Stravinsky, Louis Armstrong, Dean Acheson, Nikita Khrushchev

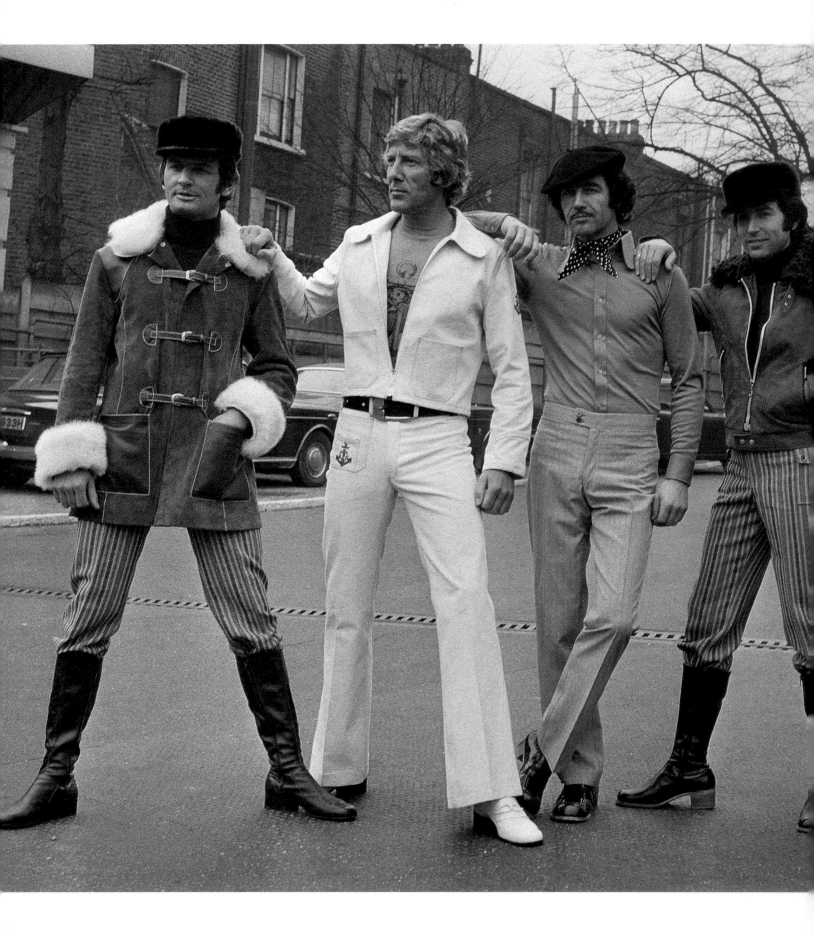

158

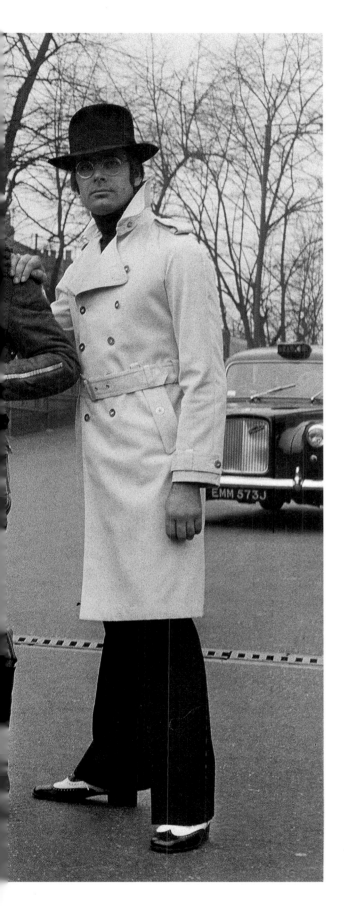

Fashion war claims male victims

Knee boots, big collars (fur trim optional) and a variety of headwear were clearly in for men's fashion in 1972. These men model the latest look for the "Imbex 72" men- and boyswear preview at London's Earl's Court.

British men may have adopted a French look – like the man in the centre, modelling beret and cravat – but on the Continent, leading French designer Yves St Laurent, the man responsible for taking the safari shirt into the fashion mainstream, was creating "Le Lock Anglais". Clothes influenced by the wardrobes of traditional country squires, particularly tweed, proved popular.

But not all men followed the catwalk. From the late sixties many students had taken to wearing clothes that had originally been associated with workers, particularly jeans; some hippies affected a cowboy look, to show empathy with a lifestyle that they saw as being on the edge of civilisation. Skinheads, one of Britain's more violent teen cults, also emerged in the late sixties as a predominantly working-class reaction against hippie culture. Easily identified by their trademark short hair, they wore ankle-length jeans and "bovver" boots.

Many men were influenced by pop stars: Rod Stewart's spiky hair was an example of the shag haircut, a more manicured version of the hippy's flowing locks. Bryan Ferry, lead singer of Roxy Music, set a trend for coloured hair when he dyed his black. David Bowie's glamorous androgynous look, perfected through his incarnation as Ziggy Stardust, was adopted by both sexes. In Glasgow, men who called themselves "poseurs" took this one stage further by dressing in female clothes and wearing make-up – which they insisted proved very popular with women.

Also this year...

Miners' strike begins

Fighting in Northern Ireland prompts British government to reinstate direct rule

"Bloody Sunday" in Londonderry

IRA and British ceasefire

Five Oxford colleges admit women

Watergate scandal erupts in US

President Nixon visits China

Iceland unilaterally extends fishing limits leading to "Cod War" with Britain

First home video-recorders on sale

118 die in Heathrow's worst plane crash to date

Ugandan General Amin expels 50,000 Asians with British passports

11 Israeli athletes are murdered by Arab terrorists at the Munich Olympics

Deaths: Poet laureate Cecil Day-Lewis, the Duke of Windsor, Maurice Chevalier, J. Edgar Hoover, Kwame Nkrumah, Ezra Pound, Dr Louis Leakey, Harry S. Truman

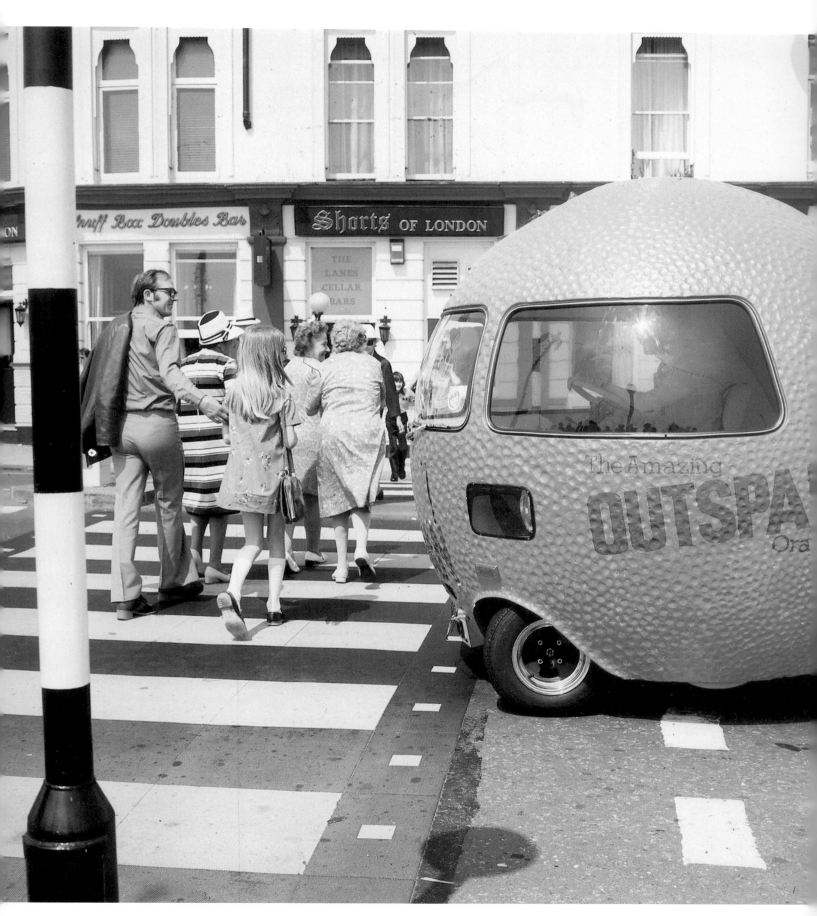

Outspan tries to outflank apartheid

A novel advertising campaign for Outspan oranges: the clockwork orange, no doubt inspired by the book and film of the same name. Outspan, like many South African companies over the following decades, needed all the advertising help it could get. South Africa's apartheid system, introduced from the late forties, meant that black and coloured (or mixed-race) South Africans had substantially fewer rights than their white compatriots. The apartheid system attracted ever-increasing criticism from the international community.

Nelson Mandela, a lawyer and active member of the African National Congress, was sentenced to life for his political activities in 1964. Mandela came to personify the political struggle of South African blacks. He inspired his nation and supporters the world over when speaking at his trial: "During my lifetime I have dedicated myself to this struggle of the African people. I have fought against white domination and I have fought against black domination. I have cherished the ideal of a democratic and free society in which all persons live together in harmony and with equal opportunities. It is an ideal which I hope to live for and to achieve. But if needs be, it is an ideal for which I am prepared to die."

Sanctions – in the form of refusing financial loans, boycotting South African products and excluding them from sporting events – were imposed by many of the most powerful nations in the world. It was partly in response to this shunning of it on the part of the rest of the world that South Africa left the Commonwealth in 1961. In the late 1980s the South African regime began to acknowledge that the country's isolation could be broken only through reform of apartheid. Eventually, in 1990 President F.W. de Klerk authorised Mandela's release. He had served almost 27 years. Nelson Mandela was elected President in South Africa's first free elections in 1994.

Also this year...

Britain joins the EEC

Last US troops leave Vietnam

First women allowed on Stock Exchange floor

Lord Lambton resigns after sex scandal

Watergate hearings begin

First Open University degrees awarded

US space-station Skylab *launched*

School leaving age raised to 16

VAT introduced in Britain

Thalidomide victims awarded compensation

Princess Anne marries Captain Mark Phillips

Yom Kippur War; OPEC increases oil prices by 70 per cent

Three-day week introduced on railways, coal mines and power stations

Protestant and Catholic power-sharing deal agreed in Northern Ireland

Deaths: Salvador Allende, Noel Coward, Pablo Picasso, W.H. Auden, Betty Grable, Nancy Mitford

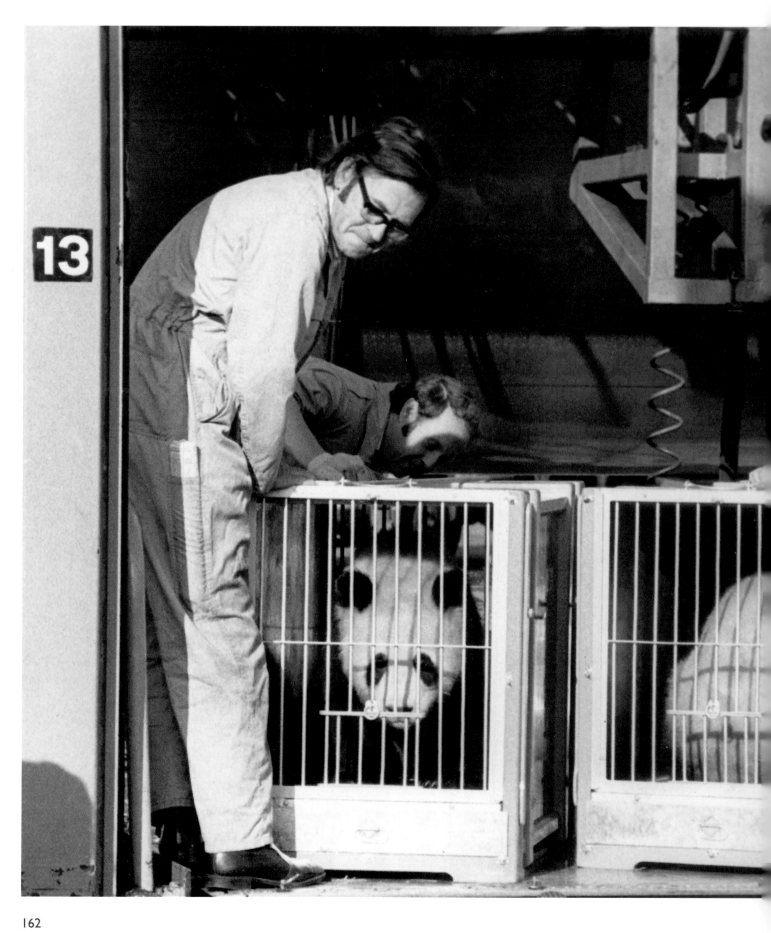

Troubled panda love keeps nation guessing

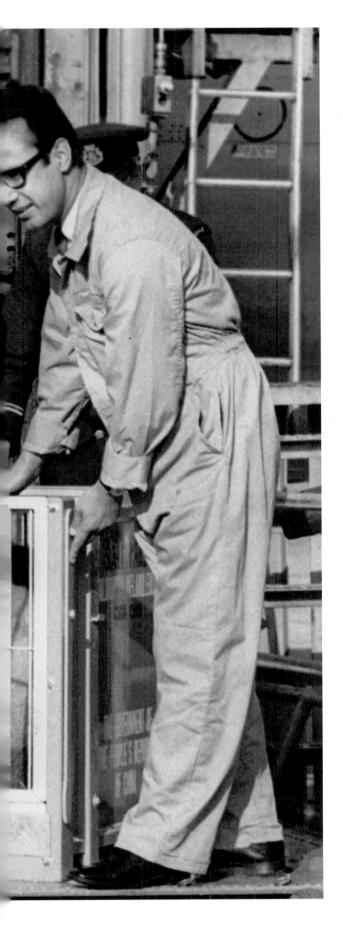

Chia-Chia and Ching-Ching, gifts from the Chinese government to the former Prime Minister Edward Heath and the people of Britain, arrive in the country. The pair, the first Giant Pandas to arrive in Britain, were to live at London Zoo, and their love-life – or the lack of it – was the source of much speculation. For many years the couple were the top attraction at the Zoo.

In 1978 the Giant Pandas reached puberty, and the keepers hoped that the following spring they would produce a cub. Sadly Ching-Ching (meaning "crystal bright") was never well enough to breed and died cubless in 1985. Chia-Chia (meaning "the very best") was moved to Mexico Zoo in 1988, where he fathered two cubs with a panda called Tohul, one through artificial insemination, before he died in 1991. Despite Chia-Chia and Tohul's success, most attempts to breed pandas in captivity have been unsuccessful.

The Giant Panda's natural habitat is the remote mountain forests of western China. Always a rare animal – and once regarded as semi-divine in China because of it – numbers diminished rapidly as many starved due to increasing human development of the forests.

The World Wide Fund for Nature – which uses the panda a part of its emblem – now estimates that there are 1,000 surviving pandas in the wild. Panda reserves have been set up in China and the WWF works with local communities to encourage them to use the land in a way that does not threaten the panda population. The penalty for poaching pandas in China is death, but this has not totally deterred poachers.

Also this year...

Miners' strike prompts Heath to call general election; Labour wins elections in February and October

First Teletext transmissions made by the BBC

West Germany wins the World Cup

Abducted heiress Patty Hearst assists her kidnappers in a bank robbery

Princess Anne escapes kidnap attempt

India tests its first nuclear weapon

21 killed in Birmingham pub bombs

Prevention of Terrorism Act passed

Inflation reaches 19%

Family planning available on NHS

Local government reshuffle

introduces new counties and abolishes Rutland, Cumberland, Huntingdonshire and Westmoreland

British and Irish restaurants fail to win a single Michelin star between them

UK's first McDonalds opens

Ulster power-sharing executive collapses

Turks and Greeks agree to ceasefire in Cyprus after Turkish forces intervene

President Nixon resigns

Lord Lucan disappears after his wife is attacked and their nanny murdered

Deaths: Sam Goldwyn, Georges Pompidou, U Thant, Juan Perón, Georgi Zhukov, Duke Ellington

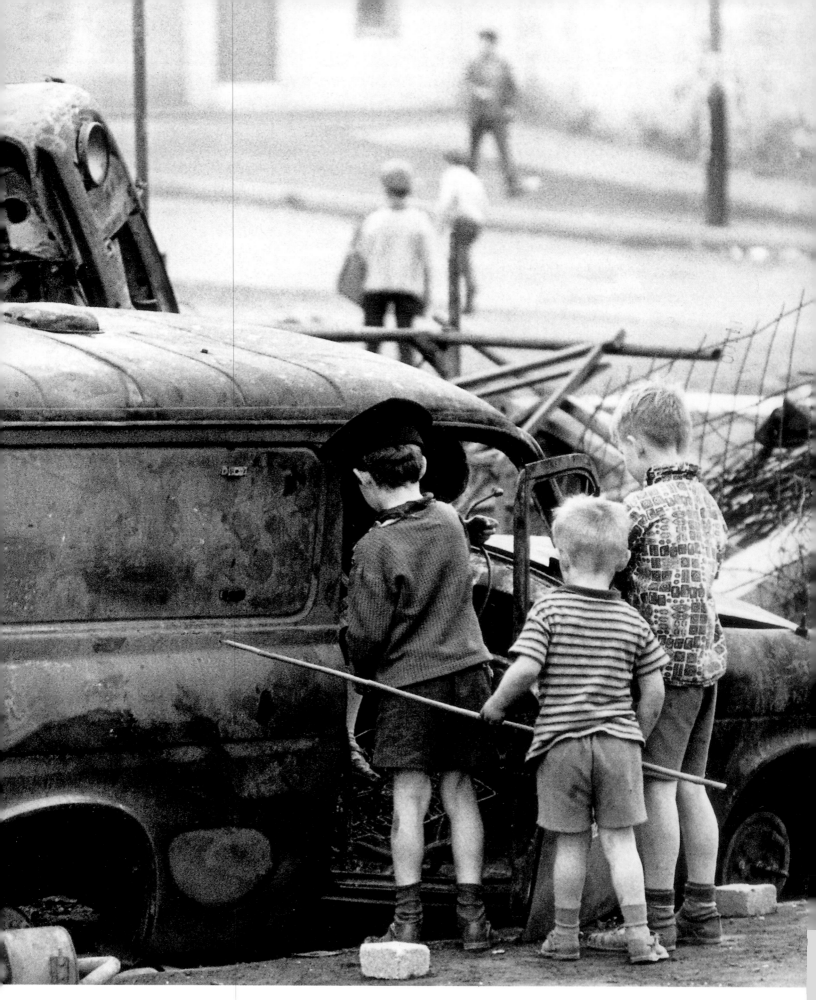

Growing up in a world of bombs and bullets

Boys investigate the burnt-out wreck of a van used to form a barricade in Belfast. There were to be plenty more: on January 16 the IRA called off a truce that had lasted 25 days. Police and troops in northern Ireland immediately stepped up security. Ulster Secretary, Merlyn Rees, declared the British government unmoved: "I will not be influenced by any views which are backed by the bomb and the bullet."

The situation in Northern Ireland had not improved since British troops were first sent in to keep the peace in 1969. Although initially introduced to help protect Catholics – and welcomed – the forces soon came to be resented as a symbol of British authority and became the target of terrorist attacks.

The Troubles deepened still further on January 30, 1972, when British troops opened fire on civil rights protesters in Londonderry, killing 13. The day became known as "Bloody Sunday". Thereafter direct rule was imposed from London, with the exception of a short-lived power-sharing executive in 1974, abandoned after Protestant hard-liners called for a general strike.

Television presenter Ross McWhirter and off-duty policeman Stephen Tibble were two of the many killed as a result of the Troubles in 1975. Tiede Herrema, an industrialist, and Sheila and John Matthews, a middle-aged couple whose Balcombe Street flat was broken into by IRA gunmen fleeing police, were all held hostage by the IRA but released unharmed.

The 25-day truce had been called after two years of intensive violence and bombing campaigns in Ulster on the British mainland. The next cease-fire in Northern Ireland was not to be called until 1994.

Also this year...

Margaret Thatcher becomes Conservative leader

35 die in Moorgate Underground crash

Civil war erupts in Lebanon

Inflation reaches 26.9%

Over one million unemployed

Sex Discrimination Act comes into force

Kidnapped heiress Lesley Whittle killed by Black Panthers

37 countries sign Helsinki Accords

First home computer goes on sale

Cambridge rapist Peter Cook arrested

Cambodia falls to Khmer Rouge

Viet Cong capture Saigon

OPEC oil ministers held hostage by Palestinian terrorists

Majority vote for Common Market in referendum

Russian "Concordski" enters service

North Sea oil pipeline opens

Martina Navratilova defects

Deaths: P.G.Wodehouse, Sir Julian Huxley, Josephine Baker, Haile Selassie, Graham Hill, Barbara Hepworth, Dimitri Shostakovich, Eamon de Valera, Chiang Kai Shek, General Franco

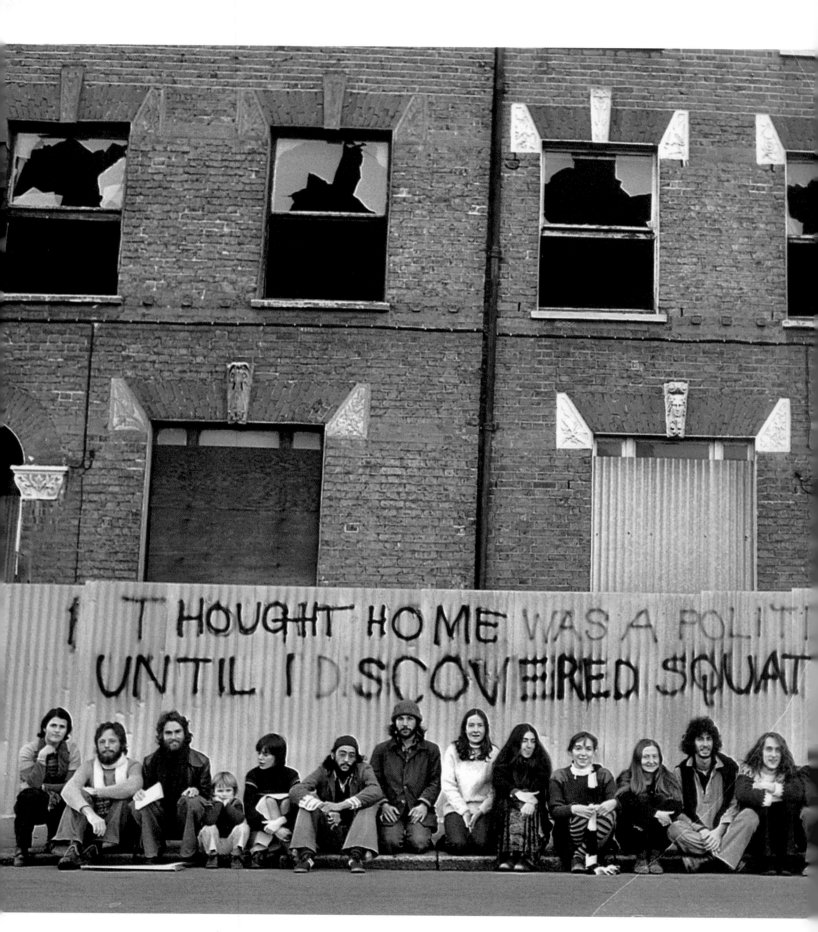

Sex, drugs, rock 'n' roll ... and squatters

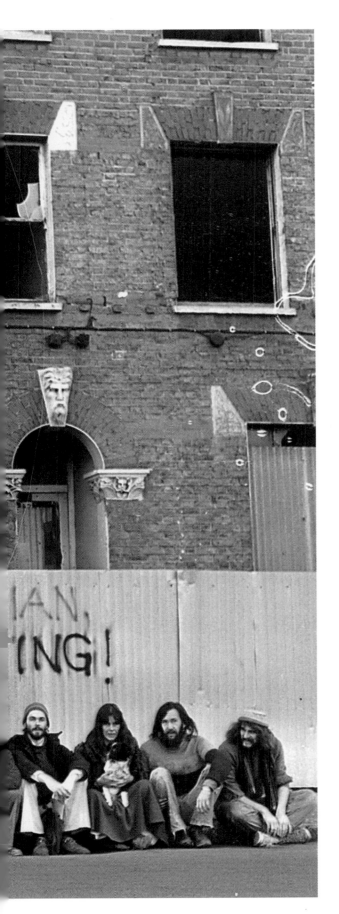

An estimated 30,000 squatters in England and Wales made themselves at home in houses which did not belong to them. The vast majority were to be found in London, where housing shortages were most acute.

Squatting started at the end of the sixties as a politically motivated campaign against homelessness. The squatters' aim was to pressurise local authorities into permitting temporary residence of the vast number of publicly owned buildings that lay empty while awaiting redevelopment. The housing shortage was exacerbated by a decline in the availability of private rented accommodation: in 1966, 26% of households rented from private landlords; by 1977, only 9%.

The early squatters even entered into agreements with local authorities, paid bills and carried out repairs in return for free accommodation. They also left when the authorities brought in the builders or the bulldozers. But by the mid-seventies, squatting had attracted a rather less pliable and, from the authorities' point of view, desirable calibre of resident. Peaceful protest was replaced by marginalised anarchy. Nor were the squatters moving into exclusively abandoned buildings – some were accused of taking long-awaited homes from families.

It could prove difficult to evict squatters. Police were not legally obliged to interfere unless the squatters caused a breach of the peace or criminal damage or could be shown to have used force to enter a property. A court injunction was required for property owners to remove unwanted inhabitants. Even then, force was often required to implement it.

Also this year...

SAS sent into Northern Ireland

Race Relations Act passed

Prime Minister Harold Wilson resigns; James Callaghan becomes Prime Minister

Viking 1 transmits first pictures of surface of Mars

Hijack of Air France aircraft at Entebbe

African nations boycott Montreal Olympics

Britain nears drought after record hours of sunshine

National Theatre opens

Concorde begins transatlantic services

British Leyland is nationalised

Jimmy Carter is elected US president

Britain takes £2.3 billion loan from International Monetary Fund as sterling collapses below $2 for first time

Princess Margaret and Earl of Snowdon separate

Deaths: Agatha Christie, Field Marshal Montgomery, L.S. Lowry, Sir Carol Reed, Fritz Lang, Howard Hughes, Dame Sybil Thorndike, Mao Tse Tung, Benjamin Britten, Sir Mortimer Wheeler, Man Ray

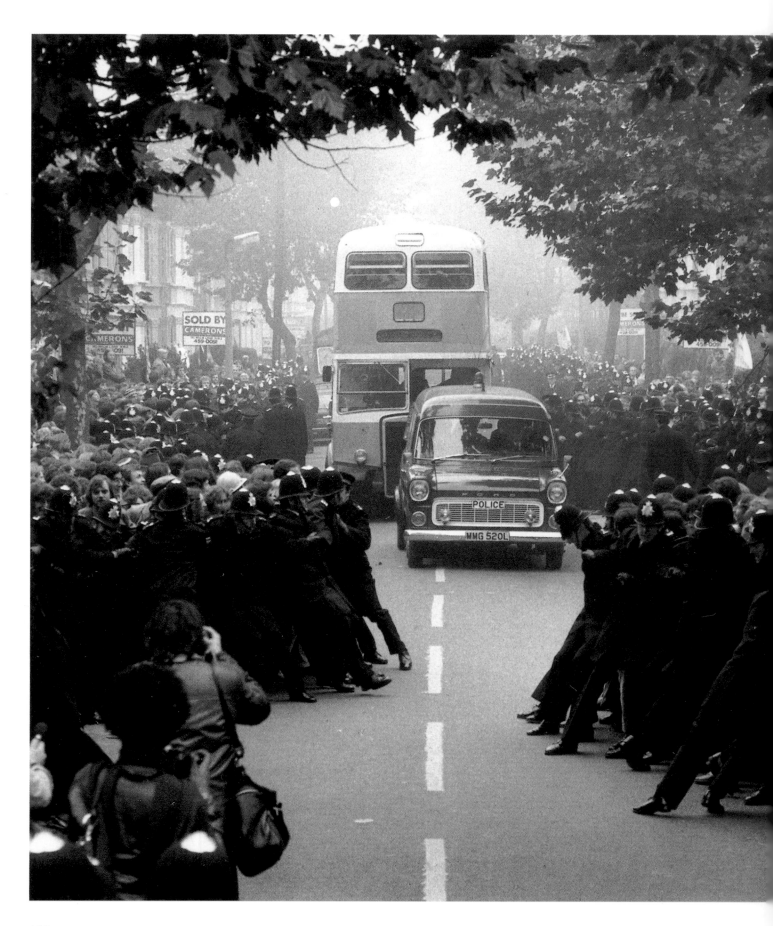

A strike which polarised society

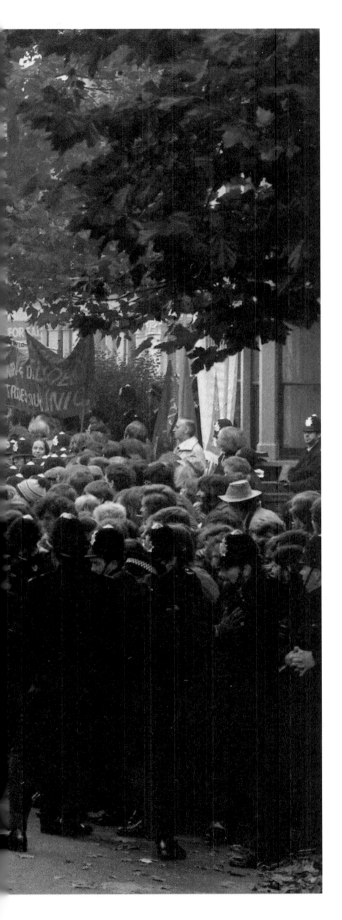

Police restrain demonstrators to allow a bus carrying workers through to the Grunwick photo-processing laboratory in Willesden, north west London, on October 17. Fourteen months of industrial action had started in the summer of 1976 when Grunwick's owner, George Ward, refused to recognise the trade union APEX. In response, around 150 workers – just under half the workforce – went on strike. All of the strikers were sacked.

The strike developed into one of the biggest trade union disputes of the decade, and polarised British society. The unions brought in flying pickets; secondary strikes were held in sympathy. Those against the strike believed that victory for the unions would lead to closed-shop union membership and deal a potentially terminal blow to British industry.

Those who continued to work were harassed: they had milk bottles thrown at them; buses taking them to work had to be fitted with metal grilles; posters were made showing people the demonstrators believed had defied the strike. The police came in for similar attacks. Clashes were frequent and demonstrators taunted the police by dressing up in pig masks and toy police helmets. Both police and pickets were injured. Many arrests were made.

Despite sympathy for the unions from the Labour government, George Ward's right not to recognise the union was upheld in the House of Lords. Ward became a Conservative hero, and the Battle of Grunwick was to influence many of Mrs Thatcher's union reforms.

The dispute was only finally declared over in July 1978.

Also this year...

Roy Jenkins becomes EEC president

Space shuttle makes maiden flight

The Lib-Lab pact keeps minority Labour government in power

Queen Elizabeth's silver jubilee

Red Rum wins third Grand National

574 killed when two jumbos collide in Canary Islands

Bravo oil rig disaster leaves 1,000-square mile oil slick

Freddie Laker starts Skytrain service to New York

Charter 77 movement begins in Czechoslovakia

Star Wars released

Nigel Short becomes youngest ever British chess champion

Virginia Wade becomes Wimbledon women's champion

Amnesty International win Nobel Peace Prize

Betty Williams and Mairead Corrigan, Northern Ireland campaigners belatedly awarded 1976 Prize

Police search for Yorkshire Ripper

Deaths: Sir Anthony Eden, Tony Crosland, Anais Nin, Joan Crawford, Elvis Presley, Maria Callas, Groucho Marx, Marc Bolan, Vladimir Nabokov, Bing Crosby, Charlie Chaplin

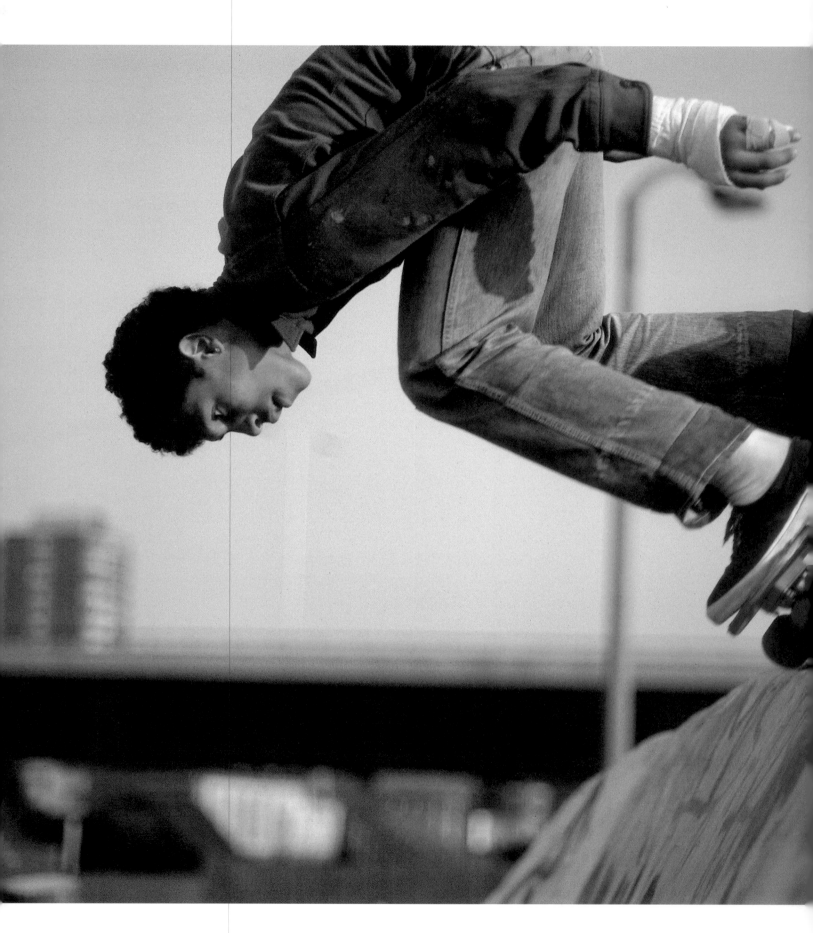

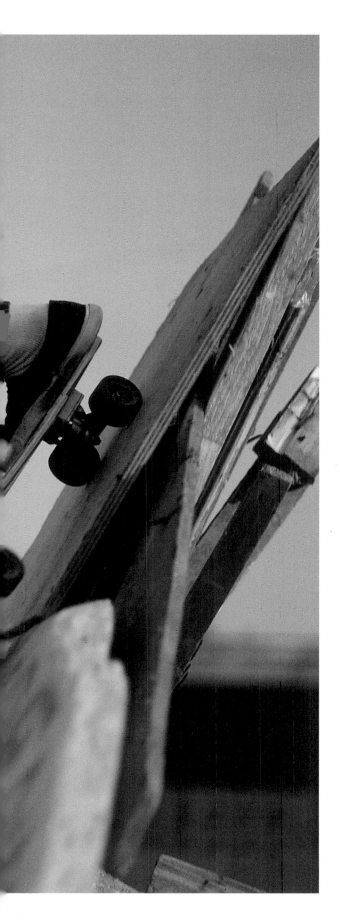

Crazy about kerbies and kick turns

It came, like many a craze before it, from America, and by 1978 Britain's children were in the grips of skateboarding fever. Two-million boards were sold in 1977. When skateparks began to open up across the nation, a stampede of children eager to pay up to 75p for suitable skate territory responded. At its opening in August, 1977, Skate City, in London's docklands, had to turn away 800 disappointed skateboarders. Many took to the streets – and sometimes the roads. The Royal Society for the Prevention of Accidents estimated that skateboarding-related injuries would cost the country £6m in 1978. Enthusiasts were encouraged to don knee and elbow pads and helmets, but even these couldn't always prevent broken bones.

Skateboarding might have been big, but it wasn't new. Boards of varying safety had been around for years. The popularity of surfing led to a renewed interest in boards in general, and eventually to great improvements in skateboard technology, allowing for more manoeuvrability. In 1977, the Ministry of Sport recognised skateboarding as a sport. Sports Minister Denis Howell was even seen to have a go.

It was not only children who welcomed the boards. Entrepreneurs were quick to see that enthusiasts would save up their pennies and buy a more sophisticated – and expensive – version if they thought it would improve their kerbies, kick turns or hang tens. Skate parks were seen as a potential money earner, but enthusiasm ebbed when it became clear that pocket money didn't have as much purchasing power as was originally hoped. With costs of at least £70,000 to establish a park, most needed local authority support to survive – and with few prepared to give it, skateboarding's star began to wane.

Also this year...

Anna Ford becomes ITN's first female newsreader

Italian Prime Minister Aldo Moro kidnapped and murdered

Camp David agreement between Egypt and Israel

Princess Margaret announces her divorce

Live BBC radio coverage of House of Commons shocks listeners

World Health Organisation announces eradication of smallpox

Louise Brown, first test-tube baby, born

Swede Bjorn Borg wins Wimbledon for third time

Pope John Paul II enthroned

Former Liberal leader Jeremy Thorpe charged with conspiracy to murder

Printing of The Times and The Sunday Times suspended due to industrial dispute

Deaths: Pope Paul VI and his successor John Paul I, Golda Meir, Sir Robert Menzies, Jomo Kenyatta

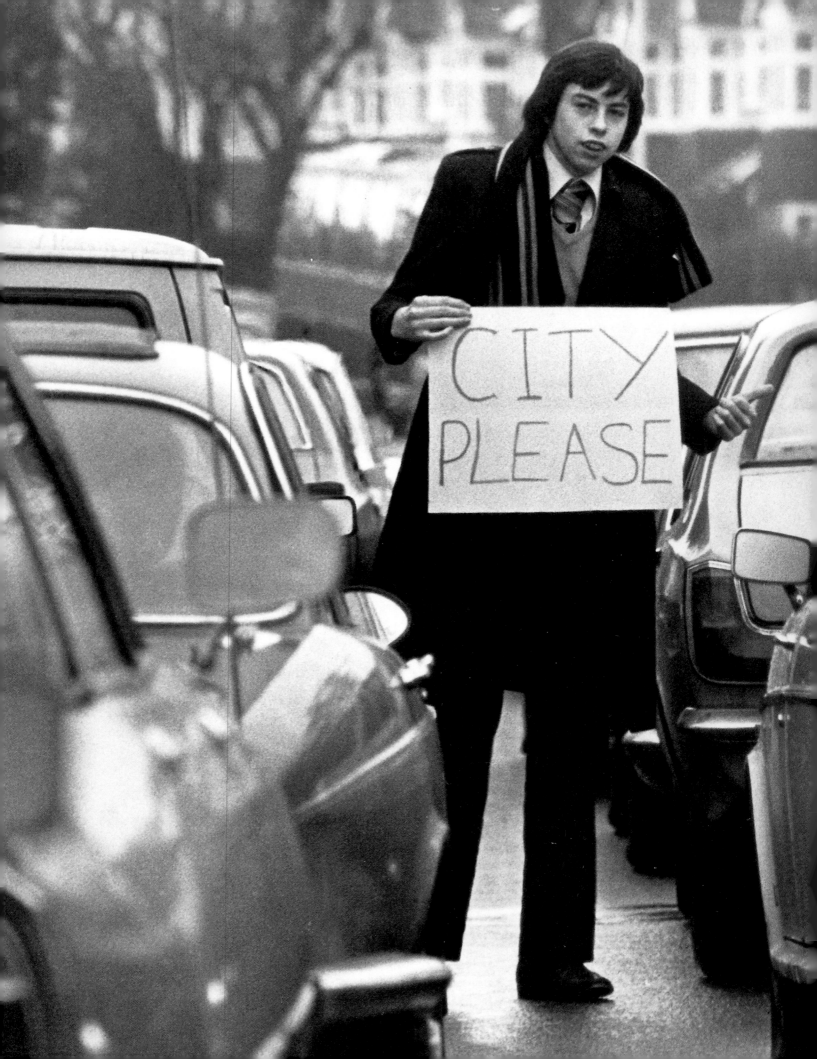

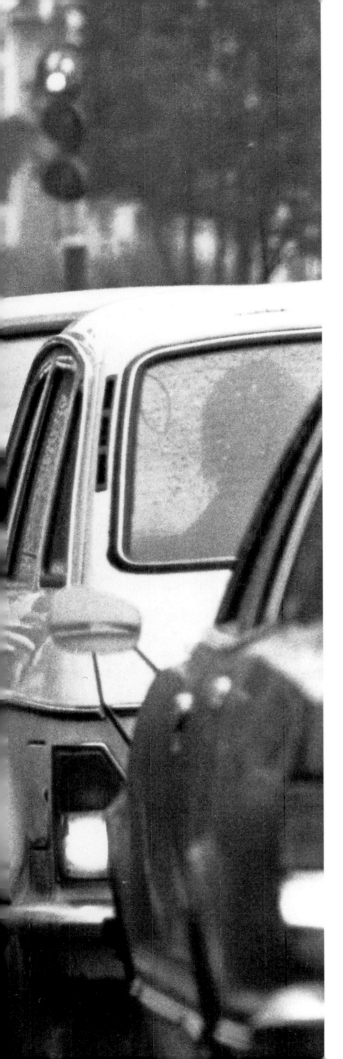

Now is the winter of our discontent ...

A commuter tries to hitch to work during the series of one-day rail strikes that started on January 15, 1979. Dubbed the "Winter of Discontent", the winter of 1978-9 saw Britain paralysed by the worst industrial action since the general strike of 1926.

The strikes were caused by the five per cent limit that the government imposed on pay rises. Throughout 1979 some 29 million working days were lost, as 4.5 million workers went on strike. Hospitals in Birmingham were forced to turn away cancer patients, troops had to be brought in to drive ambulances; rats scavenged in overflowing London dustbins; with temperatures falling to minus 16, over half the nation's schools closed, unable to provide adequate heating due to the striking lorry drivers; in Liverpool the dead were left unburied when gravediggers took industrial action.

James Callaghan, the Labour Prime Minister, astounded reporters when, on his return from an arms summit in Guadeloupe in January this year, he reprimanded them for scare-mongering: "Please don't run your country down by talking of mounting chaos. If you look at it from the outside, you can see you are taking a rather parochial view. I do not feel there is a mounting crisis." Headline writers recast his words as: "Crisis, what crisis?"

In August 1978, a Gallup poll had credited Labour with a four per cent lead. But the nation was tired of industrial strife: on May 3, 1979, the Conservative party won the general election with a 43-seat majority. Margaret Thatcher, the nation's first female Prime Minister, quoting a prayer of St Francis of Assisi, pronounced: "Where there is discord, let there be harmony."

Also this year...

In referenda on devolution, Welsh vote against, but a small majority of Scots vote in favour

Sebastian Coe is first to hold world records for 800 metres, 1,500 metres and the mile simultaneously

Soviet Union invades Afghanistan

The Shah overthrown in Iran

Soviet Union and US sign Strategic Arms Limitation Treaty

Serious accident at Three Mile Island nuclear plant

Peace agreement on Zimbabwe-Rhodesia signed

Brighton opens naturist beach

The Rubik's cube goes on sale

Airey Neave and Lord Mountbatten assassinated by IRA

IBM introduces the modem

25 boats wrecked and 14 people drowned in the Fastnet Race

Nobel Prizes awarded in Medicine to Geoffrey Hounsfield for inventing CAT scan and to Mother Theresa for Peace

Queen's art adviser, Anthony Blunt, revealed as Soviet spy

Deaths: Zulfikar Ali Bhutto, Jean Monnet, Mary Pickford, John Wayne, Lord Mountbatten, Dame Gracie Fields

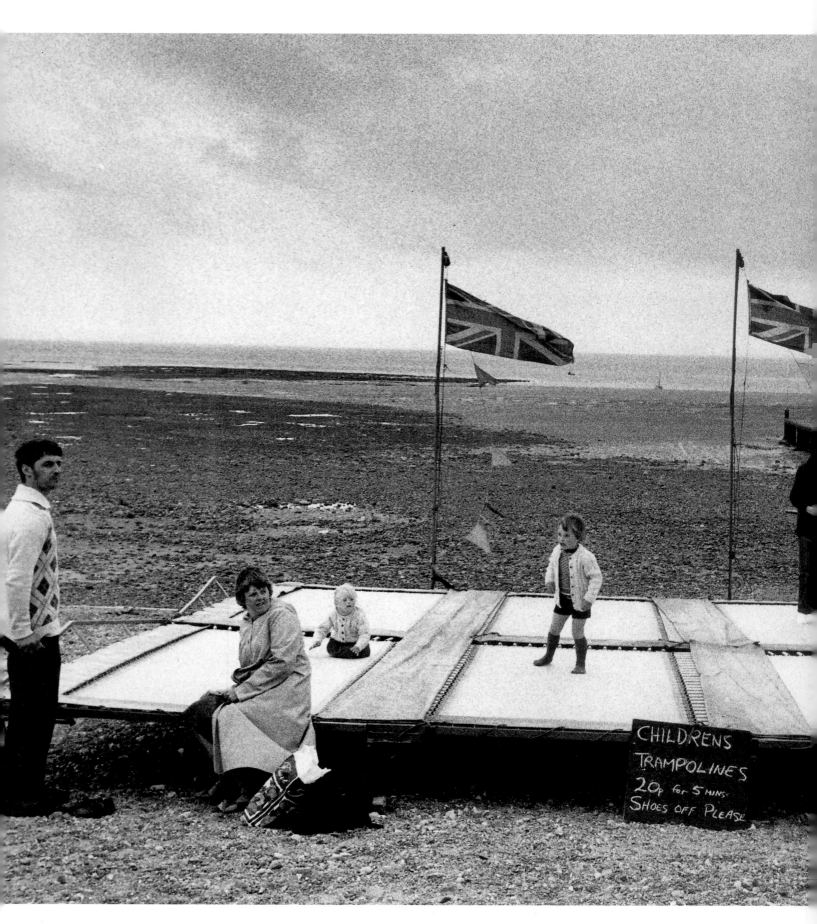

CHILDRENS
TRAMPOLINES
20p for 5 mins.
SHOES OFF PLEASE

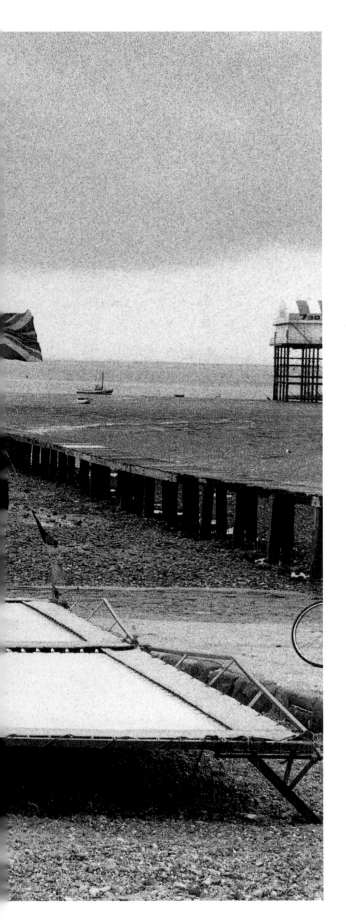

Morecambe: the answer to a package in the sun

Sadly, the sun doesn't always shine at the seaside, as these windswept holiday-makers found out at Morecambe, Lancashire. Travelling to far-flung and exotic locations might have been becoming ever-more popular with the average holidaymaker but for some the British seaside retained its reassuring advantages: a familiar pint and little danger of an upset stomach.

Children's trampolines and bracing walks were not Morecambe's only attractions: a Pontin's holiday camp provided free entertainment, while the marina offered dolphin shows, alligators, turtles and tropical fish. But it wasn't just the seaside that pulled in the crowds: in 1980 the nation's castles and stately homes received 49 million visits.

Yet whatever the appeal of Britain for many holidaymakers, since the seventies the pattern of the traditional British holiday had been changing decisively with an ever-growing number deciding that native sea and sun just wouldn't do. Fashion dictated that acquiring a deep tan – of the sort not often found in Morecambe – was both physically and socially desirable. It was no longer just the very rich who sojourned abroad: an increasingly competitive package-holiday market meant that overseas trips grew more attainable. An estimated five-million Britons had holidays abroad during the summer of 1980 while a further two million went looking for winter sun.

Despite the increasing appeal of long-haul destinations, for most people abroad meant the Mediterranean – and above all Spain, the original home of the package holiday.

Also this year...

North Sea oil platform capsizes killing 123

John Lennon shot dead

Solidarity formed in Poland

Iran-Iraq war begins

Rhodesia, Britain's last African colony, becomes independent Zimbabwe

British Airways privatised

Britain becomes a net exporter of oil

Over two million unemployed

First Sony Walkman on sale in UK

SAS rescue 19 hostages from London's Iranian embassy

Biochemist Frederick Sanger awarded second Nobel Prize

Space probe Voyager *reveals 15th moon of Saturn*

Michael Foot becomes Labour leader

Deaths: Joy Adamson, Cecil Beaton, Alfred Hitchcock, Sir Oswald Mosley, Marshal Tito, Jean-Paul Sartre, Billy Butlin, Henry Miller, Peter Sellers, Steve McQueen, Mae West

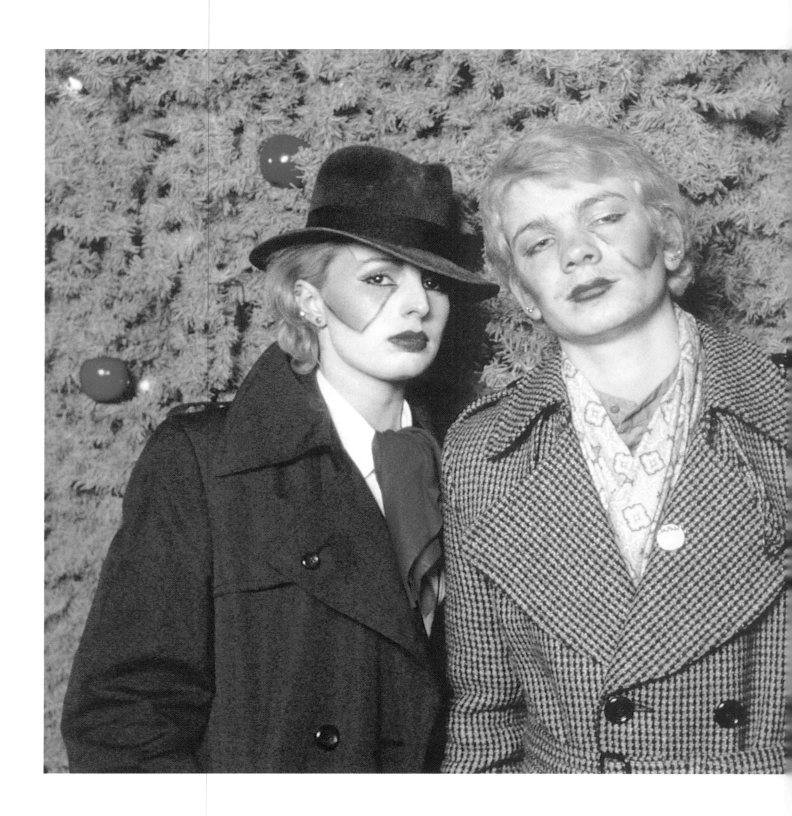

Relax, we're the New Romantics

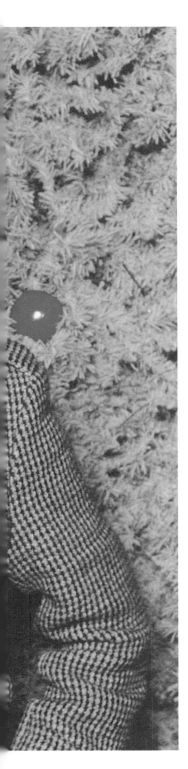

Frilly shirts, pixie boots, fingerless gloves and the obligatory black eye-liner and make-up for boys and girls: the New Romantics looked as if they had been dressed by a theatrical props company.

Also known as "the cult with no name" and "futurism", the New Romantics made up a short-lived movement in the early eighties, which originated as an antidote to punk and relied heavily on style over content. Their image was quasi-medieval, although the highwayman look was also popular. The music, propagated by such bands as Spandau Ballet, Duran Duran, Human League, Adam Ant, Soft Cell and Culture Club, was best defined as white pop rock.

Fey and foppish, the New Romantics – gay or straight – brought homosexual culture into the mainstream. Boy George, lead singer of Culture Club and the most ambiguous gender-bender of them all, was adored for his outspokenness. "I am tri-sexual. I will try anything," he admitted.

Frankie Goes to Hollywood's phenomenal commercial success with three hit singles in a row – including the gay anthem *Relax* – was considered by many, particularly the BBC, to have taken the movement too far.

Boy George's love affair with the media turned sour in 1986 when the tabloids revealed his heroin addiction. Marc Almond, lead singer of Soft Cell, similarly succumbed to drugs. The New Romantics gradually gave way to a more masculine rock revival in the mid-eighties.

Also this year...

Prince Charles marries Lady Diana Spencer

Peter Sutcliffe, the Yorkshire Ripper, charged with murdering 13 women

President Anwar Sadat of Egypt assassinated

Pope John Paul II shot

Michael Foot elected Labour leader; Social Democratic Party formed as breakaway from Labour

Rupert Murdoch buys The Times *and* The Sunday Times

Greece joins the EEC

Iran releases American hostages

Martial law imposed in Poland

AIDS first identified

Ken Livingstone elected leader of the GLC

First IBM PC launched

President Ronald Reagan shot

Death of IRA hunger-striker Bobby Sands

Riots in Brixton and across the country

Over 150,000 protest against Cruise missiles.

Deaths: Bob Marley, General Omar Bradley, Bill Haley, Anwar Sadat, Jessie Matthews, Irish novelist Christy Brown, Natalie Wood

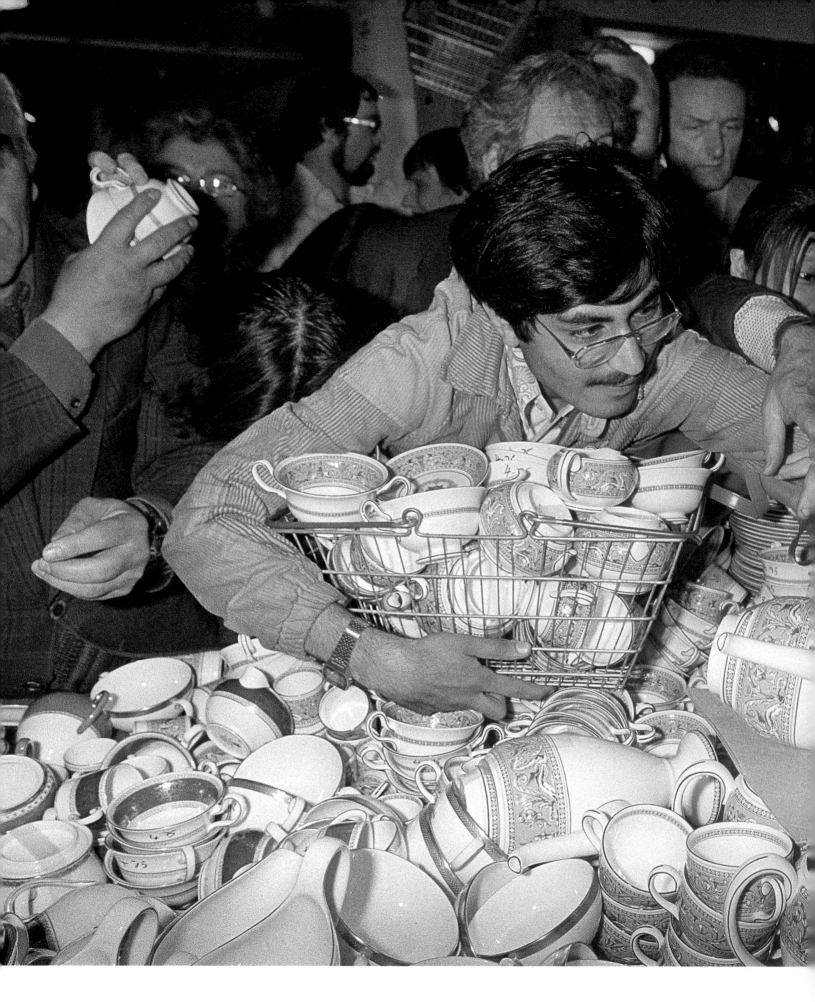

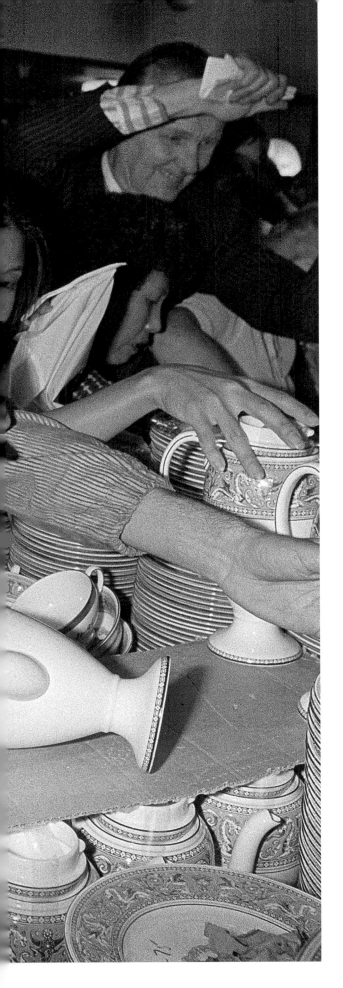

The Battle of Harrods: the fight for china

Bargain hunters needed stamina, determination and sharp elbows to make the most of the Harrods sale – qualities expertly demonstrated by this competitive shopper. London's most famous store, whose owners once boasted that it could provide customers with anything from a pin to an elephant, held its first "winter clearance" sale in 1894. Future sales were to prove enduringly popular, and by 1910 the store was putting on a special train service to bring shoppers to London for the sale. The characteristic green-liveried carrier bags were introduced for the sale in 1935 and have been used ever since.

The shoppers pictured here were not the only ones to stock up on cheap china: every single bit of Wedgewood was cleared out on the first day of the sale this year. It had been feared that a rail strike would prevent shoppers getting to the sale, but 5,000 people turned up and by the end of the day 200,000 sales had been made. From 1988 the sale was given an even more glamorous edge with the introduction of celebrity openings.

But the battle at the counters was nothing compared to the fight for ownership of the store itself. From 1977 "Tiny" Rowland, the chief executive of Lonrho, had been gradually buying into the House of Fraser group, of which Harrods was the flagship store. Lonrho made a bid for the company in 1981 which was blocked by the Monopolies and Mergers Commission. Much to Rowland's fury, the Al Fayed brothers' bid was accepted in 1985.

Harrods' high profile did not always just attract those looking for a bargain. The shop was part of a bombing campaign in 1988 against the House of Fraser group. The Animal Liberation Front claimed responsibility for the bomb, which was part of its campaign against the sale of fur. The IRA also bombed the store at Christmas 1983, killing five people.

Also this year...

Unemployment reaches three million

Mark Thatcher goes missing on Paris to Dakar rally

16 die in IRA Ballykelly pub bombing; IRA bombs in Regent's Park and Hyde Park kill ten

CD players go on sale

Argentina invades the Falklands; Foreign Secretary Lord Carrington resigns; Argentine forces driven off Falklands by British Task Force

First Papal visit to Britain in 450 years

Prince William born

Michael Fagan breaks into the Queen's bedroom

Wreck of the Mary Rose *raised*

Channel 4 launched

30,000 women protest against US Cruise missiles at Greenham Common

Deaths: "Rab" Butler, Henry Fonda, Ingrid Bergman, Sir Douglas Bader, Princess Grace of Monaco, Leonid Brezhnev

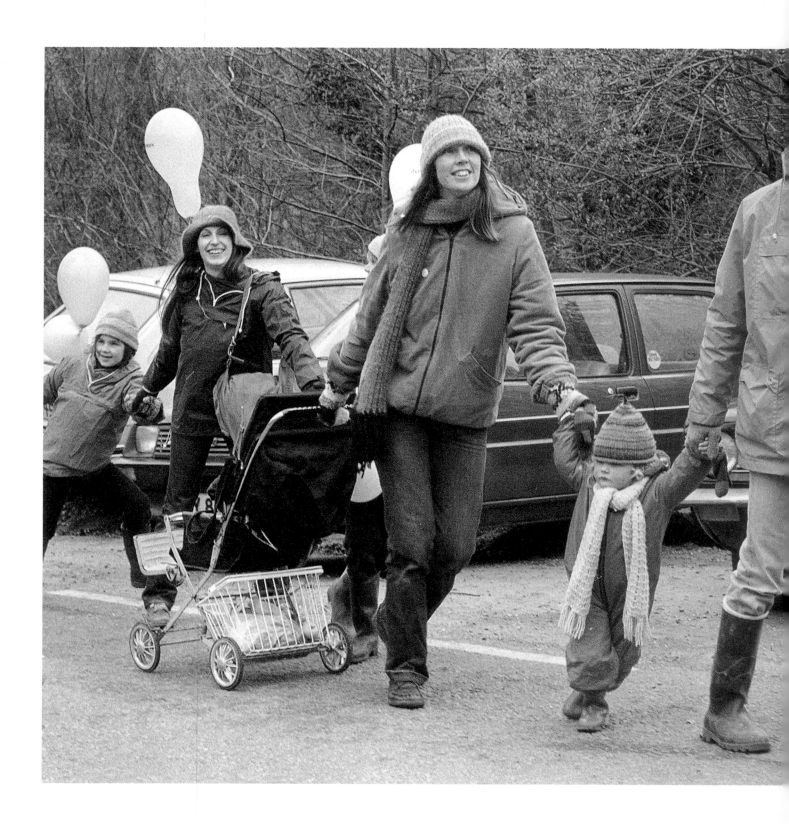

Marching for peace ... or the Kremlin?

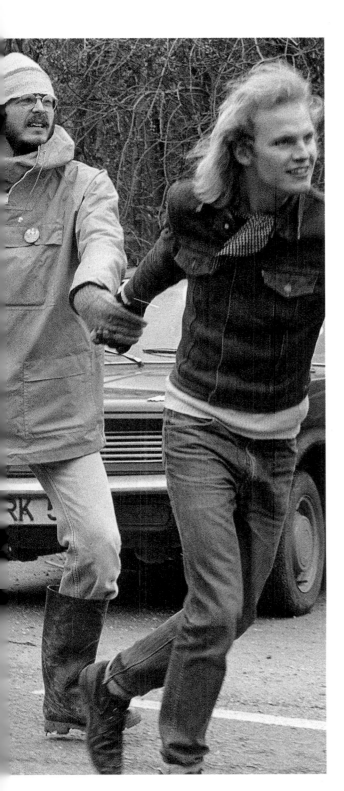

CND supporters link hands at Greenham Common, Berkshire. On April 1, over 40,000 protesters formed a 14-mile human chain between the bases at Greenham, Aldermaston and Burghfield, all of which were to host or produced nuclear weapons. Michael Heseltine, the Defence Secretary, condemned the protest: "Every mile they march, every yard they stretch, they strengthen the Kremlin case."

Greenham Common had become notorious for its peace camp, inspired, like the CND human chain, by plans to station American Cruise missiles there. The majority of demonstrators at the peace camp were women. At the camp's height, in December 1982, 30,000 demonstrators linked hands to form a human chain embracing the base. When the missiles themselves arrived on November 15, 1983, 300 predominantly female protesters were arrested at the House of Commons. Arrests were also made at Greenham Common itself.

The peace camp survived clashes with bailiffs, police and locals and repeated arrests and fines. Equally damaging was public derision. Many at the peace camp saw their battle as being as much on behalf of women as a protest against nuclear weapons. As a result the women were often dismissed as militant – and probably mad – lesbians. The Cruise missiles were removed in 1991; the fence surrounding the air base was pulled down in 1997.

Also this year...

The BBC launches Breakfast Time; ITV launches TV-AM

Wearing of car seat-belts becomes compulsory; wheel clamps introduced

Margaret Thatcher and Conservatives win landslide second general election victory

Dennis Nilsen accused of murdering 17 people

Forged Hitler diaries published

Mass breakout of IRA prisoners from Maze Prison

Thames flood barrier used for the first time

Derby winner Shergar kidnapped

Soviet Union shoots down Korean airliner

£25 million of gold bars stolen in Brinks-Mat robbery

Steve Cram and Daley Thompson victorious at first World Athletics Championships in Helsinki

President Reagan proposes "Star Wars" defence system

US invades Grenada

Cecil Parkinson resigns after Sara Keays scandal

Janet Walton gives birth to sextuplets

Deaths: Tennessee Williams, Sir William Walton, Anthony Blunt, Dame Rebecca West, Lord Clark, Joan Miró, David Niven, Gloria Swanson, Sir Ralph Richardson, Benigno Aquino (assassinated)

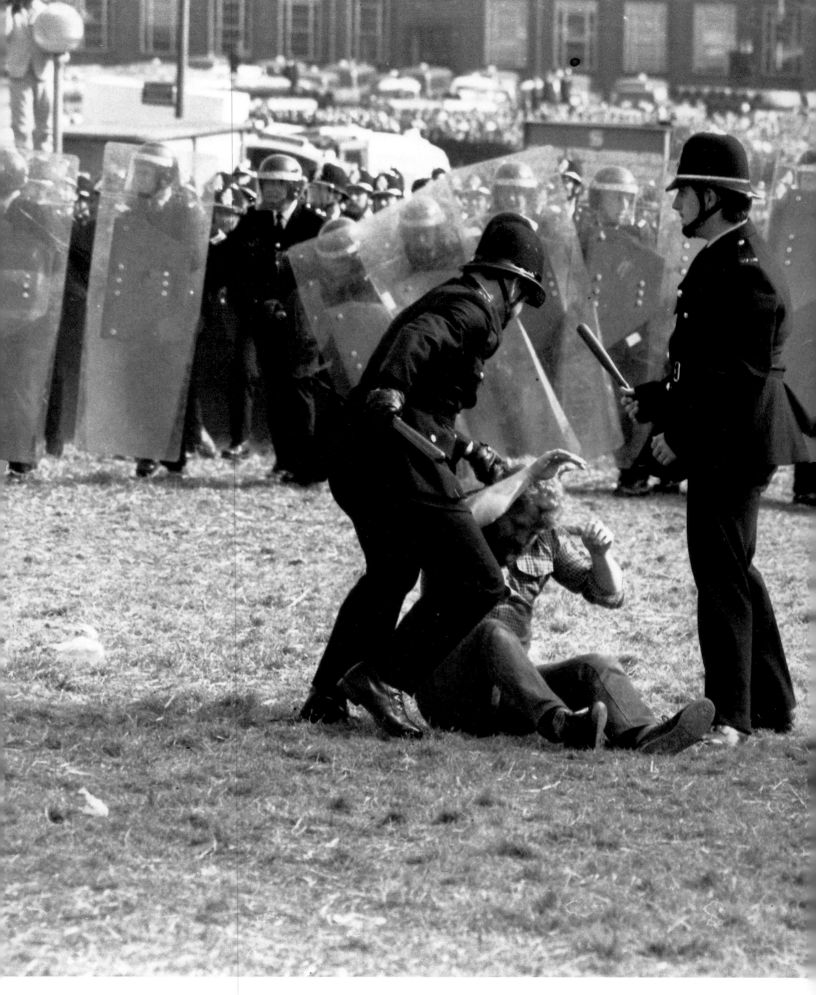

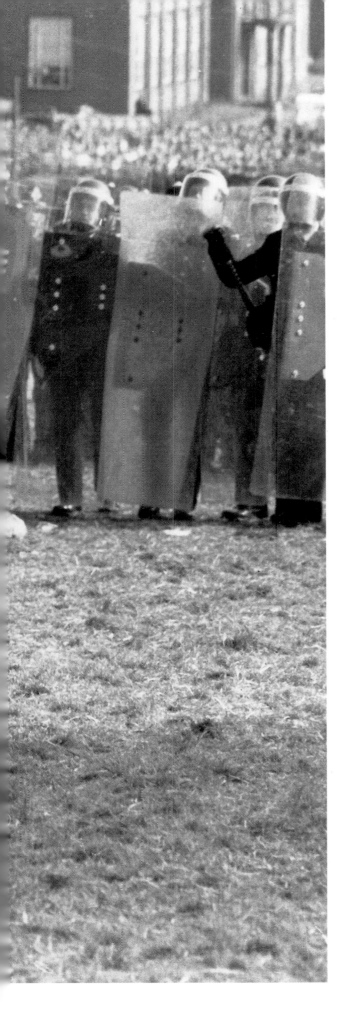

Crushing the spirit of the striking miners

A striking miner suffers rough treatment at the hands of the police as their colleagues, armed with riot shields, look on. The miners' strike, which was to drag on for a year, began on March 12, 1984. Within three days only 21 of the nation's 174 pits were working to full capacity.

The catalyst was a plan by the National Coal Board (NCB) to streamline coal production to suit demand by reducing annual output by four million tons, to close 20 uneconomic pits and to cut 20,000 jobs within 12 months. The National Union of Miners (NUM), led by Arthur Scargill, demanded no pit closures unless the pits affected were classified as exhausted or dangerous and no job losses. The first talks between Scargill and Ian MacGregor, chairman of the NCB, broke down after an hour.

However, the miners were not as unified as Scargill claimed. In April 1984, fearing he would not get the support of the necessary 55 per cent majority, Scargill vetoed a national ballot on continuing the strike. Many miners carried on working in Nottinghamshire, the nation's second largest coalfield. Violence broke out between flying pickets and those who continued to work – a 24-year-old Yorkshire miner was killed during one of these battles. Inevitably, pickets also clashed with police. Scargill earned further opprobrium when he refused to condemn the violence, just as Prime Minister Margaret Thatcher was criticised by the Left for her uncompromising stand.

From November 1984 economic hardship and the government's firm stance forced a steady stream of miners back to work. By February 25, 1985, only 51 per cent of miners remained on strike. With not a single one of its demands met, the NUM voted for a return to work on March 3, 1985.

Also this year...

Ronald Reagan wins second term as US president

British Telecom privatised

Four die in IRA Brighton Conservative Conference bombing

Virus responsible for AIDS identified

Agreement on return of Hong Kong to China signed

WPC Yvonne Fletcher shot dead outside Libyan People's Bureau

Particularly high incidence of childhood leukaemia identified near Sellafield nuclear plant

Konstantin Chernenko becomes Soviet leader

DNA fingerprinting developed

Band Aid release Do They Know it's Christmas?

York Minster hit by lightning

Olympics held in Los Angeles

Prince Harry born

Deaths: Johnny Weissmuller, Tommy Cooper, Marvin Gaye, "Bomber" Harris, Eric Morecambe, Sir John Betjeman, Yuri Andropov, Indira Gandhi, James Mason, J.B. Priestley, Richard Burton

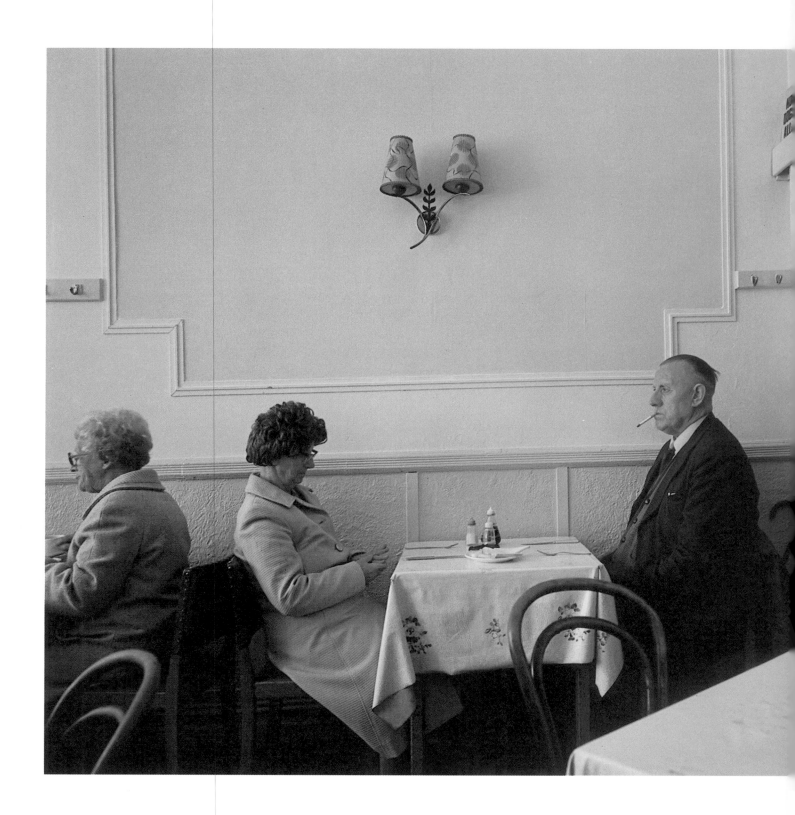

A pause for pensioners in their fight for rights

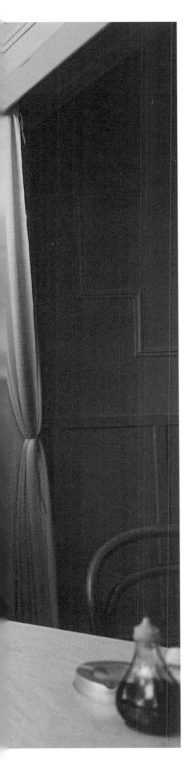

Stopping for a spot of lunch: an elderly couple wait to be served in an old-fashioned restaurant. Not all pensioners were as patient. In October, around 5,000 OAPs forsook their creature comforts and met at Trafalgar Square to protest against the proposal put forward by Norman Fowler, Secretary of State for Social Services, for the abolition of the state earnings-related pension (Serps).

Despite the government's persistence with a wide range of reforms to other social benefits, the pensioners won. It was a small victory. In 1985, the full basic rate pension was £35.80 a week for a single person and £57.30 for a couple. Government support for home helps and home nursing care was widely regarded as inadequate.

Pensioners were to lose out further in the December White Paper on social security – Serps was retained but at half the cost to the government. Financial hardship was not the only problem facing pensioners. The National Council for Careers and their Elderly Dependents warned that Britain was turning into "a nation in which grannies are being left to care at home for other grannies, because there is no one else willing or able to undertake the task." Contemporary estimates predicted that the number of people aged over 75 would rise by at least a third over the next ten years.

Also this year...

Sir Clive Sinclair launches the C5

Sterling falls to record low against dollar ($1.03)

Miners' strike ends

Blood donors screened for AIDS

Gibraltar's frontier with Spain re-opened after 16 years

Microsoft releases Windows

Greenpeace ship Rainbow Warrior *sunk in Auckland harbour*

56 football fans die at Bradford City; 41 Italians and Belgians die when Liverpool football fans riot at Brussel's Heysel stadium; English football teams banned from European competition

Wreck of the Titanic *located*

Bob Geldof's Live Aid concert raises millions for Ethiopia

20,000 die in mud-slide in Colombia

13-year-old Ruth Lawrence wins first at Oxford

25 Soviet spies expelled from Britain

55 killed in Manchester air disaster; 13 killed in M6 crash

PC Blakelock killed in north London riots

Anglo-Irish agreement signed

Deaths: Sir Michael Redgrave, Marc Chagall, Italo Calvino, Roy Plumley, Laura Ashley, Rock Hudson, Orson Welles, Yul Brynner, Konstantin Chernenko, Enver Hoxha, Philip Larkin, Robert Graves

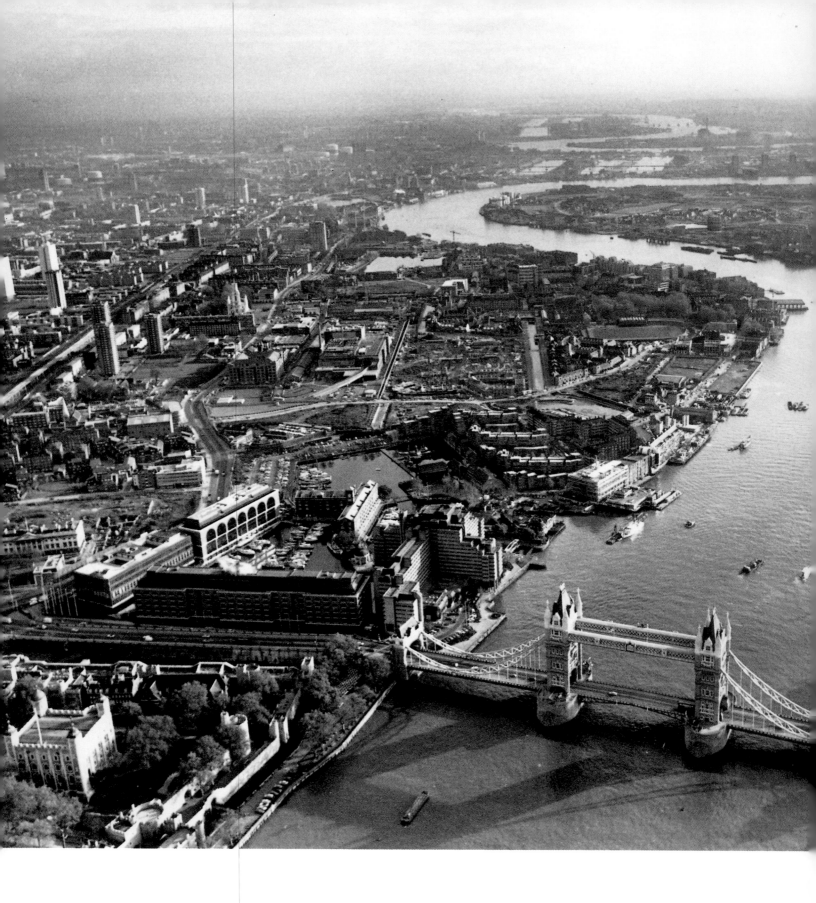

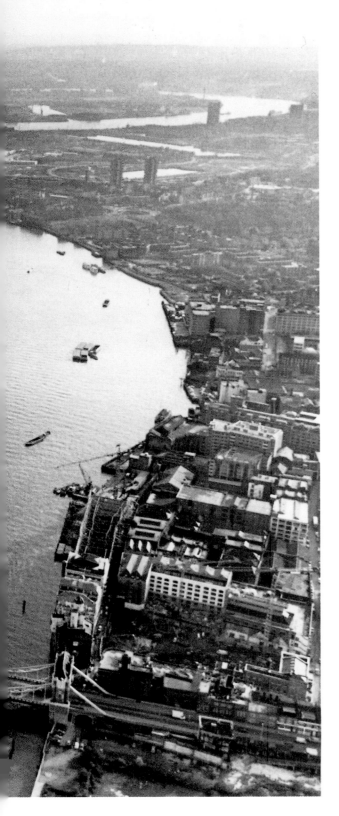

Poised for an explosion of high-rise living

An aerial view of London over the east of the city. Since the Second World War, London had seen an enormous amount of rebuilding and development. But in the eighties the docklands area, which can be seen beyond Tower Bridge, was the major focus for change.

The wharves began to close from the sixties onwards, as a once-thriving shipping industry disintegrated after a series of damaging strikes. The last major docks, the Royal, were closed in 1981. The same year, the government set up the London Docklands Development Corporation (LDDC) in an attempt to bring prosperity to the ailing area.

Initially, the scheme appeared to work. Christopher Benson, chairman of the LDDC, hailed the area in 1985 as "the great water city of the 1990s". Flats, offices and three of the tallest buildings in Europe were planned for Canary Wharf. For those who could afford them, the new dockland developments offered space and breathtaking views along the river. As companies began to move, more people came to work there than in the heyday of the docks, a development which caused bitterness among local people: the majority of jobs went to people outside the area, and locals benefited little from the area's renewal.

In spite of the hype, the expected boom at first failed to materialise, with the company owning Canary Wharf going into administration in 1992. Since then, however, with the extensions of the Jubilee Line (1998) and Docklands Light Railway (first opened 1987) and large new building projects, this is changing fast and some estimate that London's Docklands will house up to ten per cent of the City's office space by 2005.

Also this year...

Spain and Portugal join EC

GLC abolished

"Iran-Contra" scandal in US

Challenger space shuttle explodes

The Royal Yacht Britannia shelters 440 refugees from Aden

Queen is first monarch to visit China

British Gas is privatised

Pickets and police clash at Wapping printing plant

Prince Andrew marries Sarah Ferguson

15,000 evacuated after Chernobyl nuclear reactor disaster

President Marcos is toppled in the Philippines

Westland affair leads to resignations of two cabinet ministers

Suzy Lamplugh reported missing

London stock exchange introduces computerised dealing system

Government launches "Safe Sex" campaign

45 die in Chinook helicopter crash

Deaths: James Cagney, Simone de Beauvoir, Duchess of Windsor, Dame Anna Neagle, Henry Moore, Cary Grant, Harold Macmillan

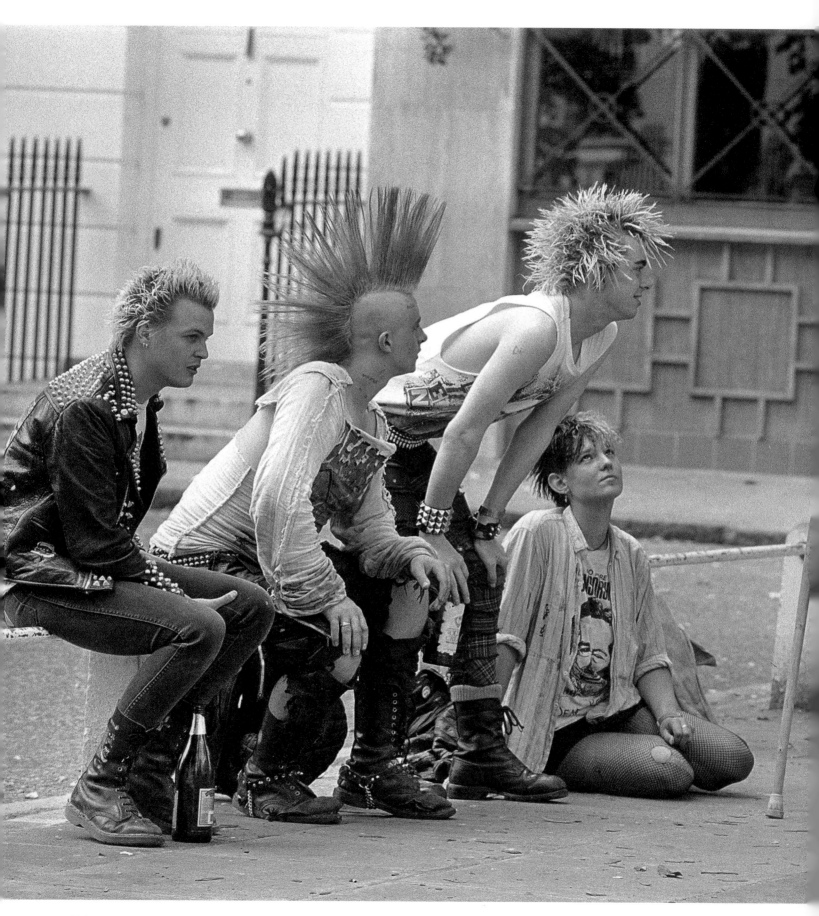

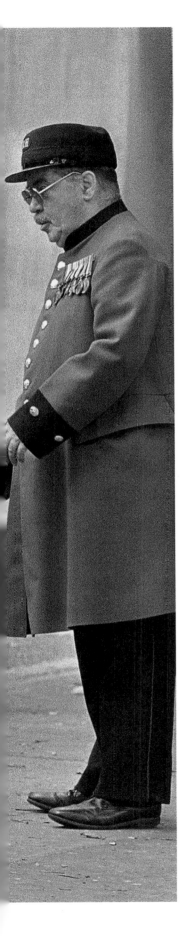

Make my day ... the punk and the pensioner

It might not have been anarchy in the UK, but these punks were keen to shock as many as possible – though this Chelsea Pensioner seems to be taking it all in his stride.

Punk first emerged on the British scene in 1976. The leading lights of the movement were The Sex Pistols, managed by Malcolm McLaren and Vivienne Westwood, who also dictated the look from her shop in the King's Road. It was here that the Sex Pistols' lead singer Johnny Lyndon – renamed Johnny Rotten – auditioned to be the band's lead singer. Their music was typical of the punk genre: energetic, abrupt and very loud.

God Save The Queen, one of the Sex Pistols' biggest hits, which reached number two in the charts and was released to coincide with the Queen's silver jubilee in 1977, was regarded as particularly offensive: "God save the Queen - She's not a human being ... There is no future – in England's dream ..." The look, like the music, was angry: multiple body piercings, black clothing, usually slashed or ripped, studded leather and spiky, luridly coloured hair.

The musical movement was largely over by the end of the seventies, but the image – and the attitude – lived on, influencing mainstream fashion and music. These punks may have been a decade late, but the one second from the left models a convincing trademark mohican cut – shaved on either side with hair spiked like a porcupine down the middle. No doubt he would have agreed with Polly the Loony, 17, unemployed from Finchley, who told *The Sun*: "It's ridiculous that we should get so much abuse just because of the way we look. Don't people realise it takes a highly original mind to look like this?"

Also this year...

Margaret Thatcher and Conservatives win third successive general election victory

Terry Waite kidnapped in Beirut

Ernest Saunders, Guinness chairman, sacked

Cynthia Payne cleared of running a brothel

SOGAT ends picket of Wapping plant

Matthias Rust lands a plane in Red Square

Single European Act comes into force

Over 200 die in Herald of Free Enterprise Zeebrugge ferry disaster

Government promotes anti-AIDS campaign

Michael Ryan kills 16 in Hungerford massacre

Cleveland child abuse inquiry questions 202 children taken into care

Southern England hit by winds of up to 110 miles per hour

Peter Wright's Spycatcher banned in Britain

Stock market crashes on Black Monday

30 die in King's Cross Underground fire

Deaths: Andy Warhol, Liberace, Danny Kaye, Fred Astaire, Rudolf Hess, Jacqueline du Pré

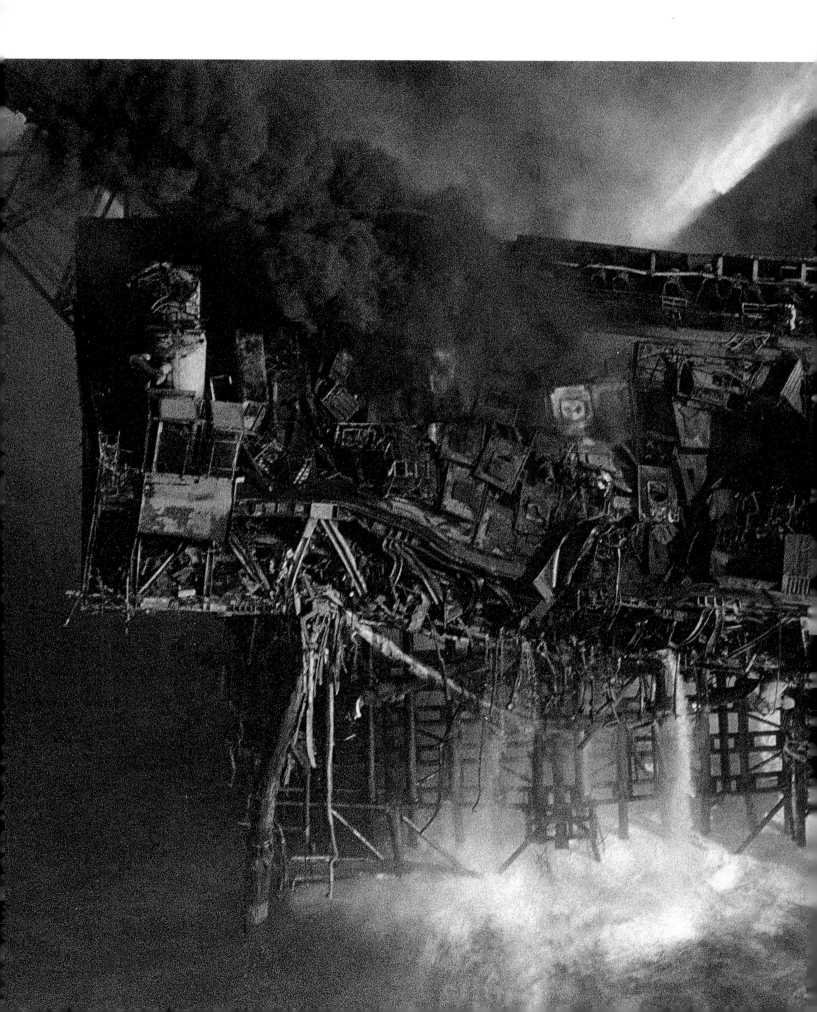

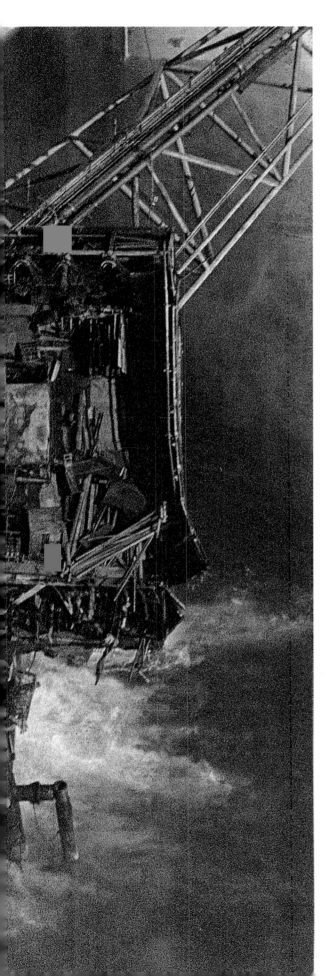

A night of terror in the North Sea

Some were watching a film or playing snooker, others preparing for bed, when explosions on the North Sea oil rig Piper Alpha claimed 167 lives. The Piper Alpha disaster, on July 6 this year, was the worst offshore disaster in the North Sea, and the worst the oil industry has known.

The rig, approximately 100 miles southeast of the Orkneys, was one of the first to be built in the area. It stood in 470 feet of water and towered almost 200 feet above sea level. Before the disaster its 227 workers, working on a two-weeks-on, two-weeks-off rotation, produced an estimated 123,000 barrels of oil a day. Only eight days earlier, Piper Alpha had passed a Department of Energy safety inspection. The rig was equipped with gas, smoke and heat detectors. Occidental, the company who ran Piper Alpha, required all off-shore workers to take part in a two-week fire course and a week's survival training. On the rig, there were regular drills.

Warned only by a screech of escaping gas, which was followed almost immediately by the explosions, few of the men on Piper Alpha stood a chance. Some attempted to jump into the boiling waters below as flames up to 700-feet-high engulfed the platform.

It was believed the disaster was triggered by a leak from the "C Module", which contained the platform's gas compressors, or from the neighbouring gas and oil separation unit, which was below the workers' sleeping quarters. Since the disaster, emergency isolation valves to separate platforms from under-sea pipelines have become mandatory.

Also this year...

Prince Charles narrowly escapes an avalanche in Klosters

Soviet troops begin withdrawal from Afghanistan

GCSE exams introduced

First Red Nose Day

Belfast lynch mob kills two British soldiers

Seoul hosts Olympics; Ben Johnson, 100m gold-medal winner, fails drugs test

Professor Stephen Hawking's A Brief History of Time published

George Bush elected US president

USS Vincennes shoots down Iranian civilian airliner

Ceasefire in Iran-Iraq war

Mikhail Gorbachev becomes President of the USSR

Prince Charles criticises modern architects

259 passengers and 11 on the ground killed as bomb causes PanAm jumbo to crash on Lockerbie

35 die and 113 injured in Clapham Junction rail disaster

Health Minister Edwina Currie, resigns over salmonella scandal

Deaths: Trevor Howard, Sean McBride, Kenneth Williams, Lord Ramsey, Kim Philby, Russell Harty, Christina Onassis, Sir Frederick Ashton

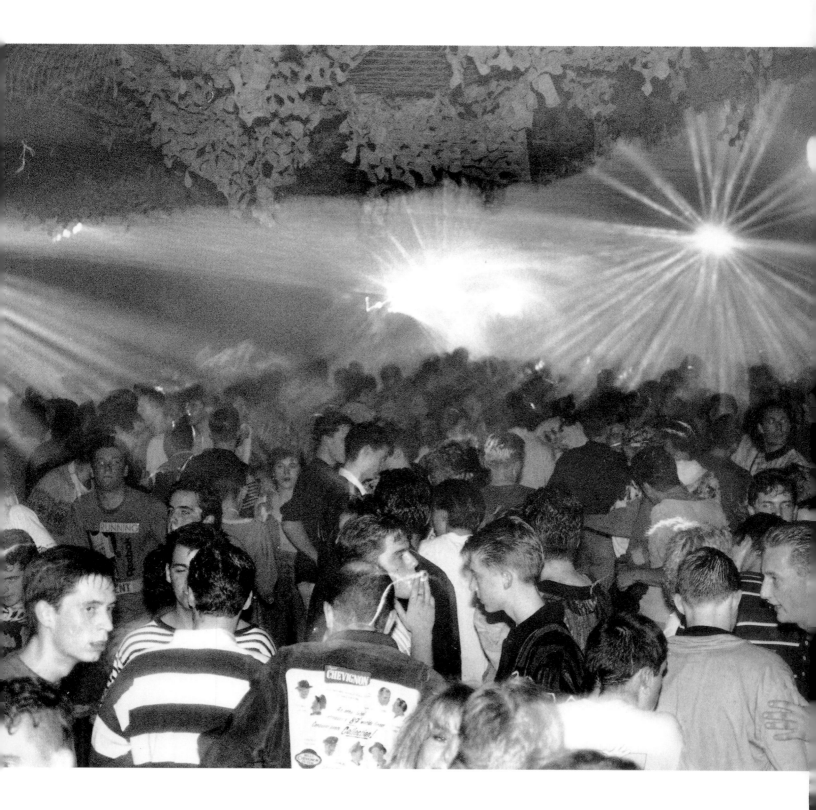

Dancing on with one foot in the rave

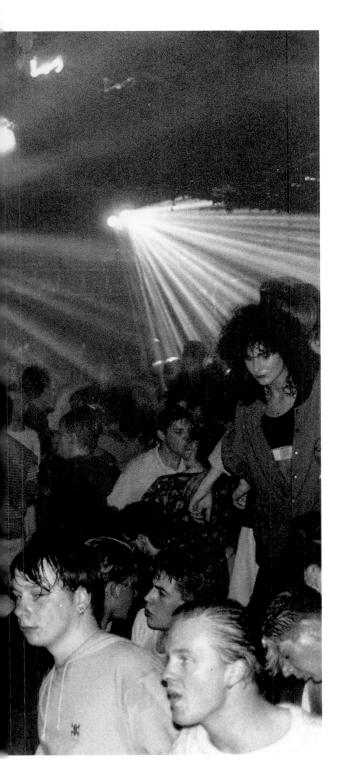

Garage, jungle, drum and bass, techno, house: to the uninitiated possibly an obscure area of DIY, but to an increasing number of ravers styles of music that were beginning to define a way of life. The common denominators of all types of rave music are volume and repetitive beats. Acid House, arguably the first type of rave music, hit Britain in 1986. But the trend really took off after "the second summer of love" in 1988, when unofficial "acid" tents became the centre of attention at the Glastonbury Festival.

Raves sprung up across the country. The larger – and generally illegal – ones were held in fields and attended by hundreds, even thousands, of people. Some were prepared to drive for miles to attend. In order to dodge the police, ravers would often follow directions given out on flyers or congregate in supermarket car parks while awaiting further directions. Early ravers sported pork pie hats, whistles and white gloves. Yet the most common ingredient of a rave is a class A category drug known as Ecstasy which is so prevalent at many rave venues that some no longer bother to sell alcohol.

Colloquially known as "E", Ecstasy is supposed to make the user feel "loved up" – or generally benign to those around. However, the drug is often mixed with stronger drugs such as heroin or animal tranquillisers, sometimes even with washing powder. While some users may feel a sense of euphoric energy, side effects can include paranoia, exhaustion, weight-loss, mental illness and in extreme cases death.

Also this year...

Salman Rushdie's The Satanic Verses *provokes Muslim outrage and a fatwa from Ayatollah Khomeini*

British Midlands plane crash kills 44

Sky TV launched

95 die in Hillsborough disaster

Tiananmen Square massacre shocks world

51 die in Thames when pleasure boat Marchioness *crashes with* Bowbelle

Guildford Four, falsely accused of 1975 IRA pub bombing, released

Ambulance strike in London; Army and RAF ambulances provide cover

House of Commons televised

Water companies privatised

Solidarity achieves landslide victory in Polish elections; Berlin Wall comes down as Communism collapses in East Germany, Hungary, Czechoslovakia and Bulgaria; in Romania, dictator Ceasescu and his wife executed as the regime collapses

US troops invade Panama

Deaths: Salvador Dali, Daphne du Maurier, Andrei Gromyko, Ayatollah Khomeini, Ferdinand Marcos, Laurence Olivier, R.D. Laing, Irving Berlin, Bette Davis, Samuel Beckett, Emperor Hirohito of Japan

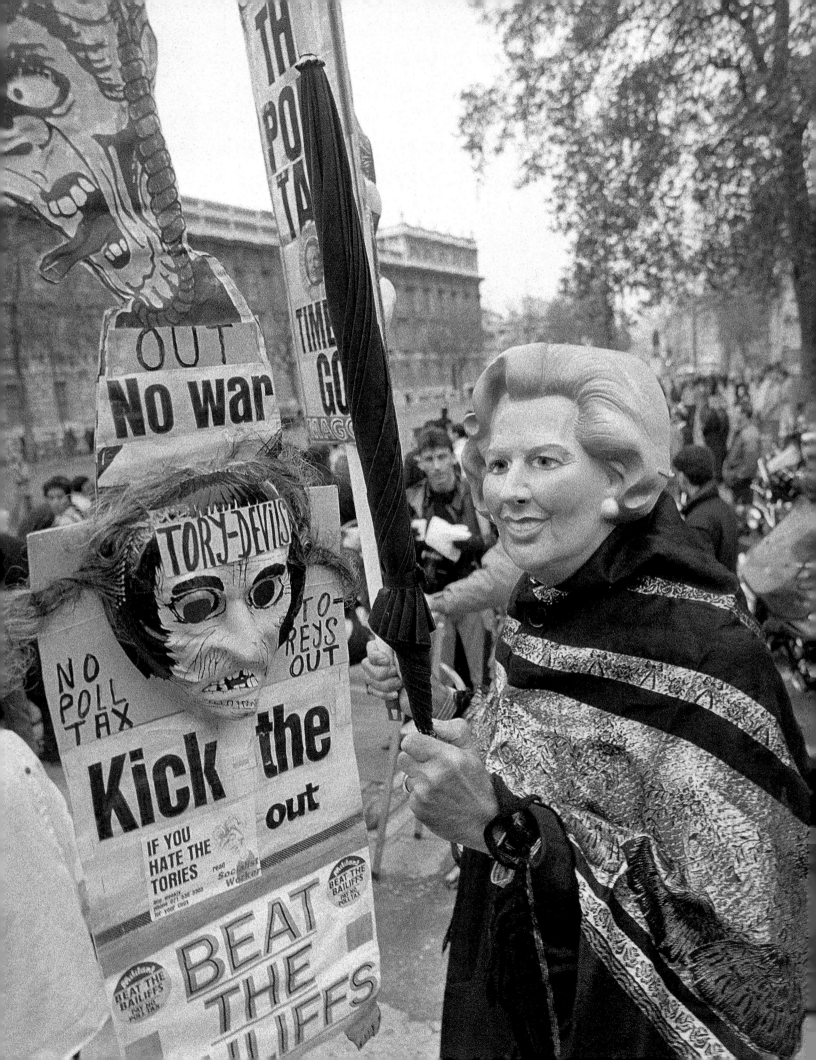

Mockery and anger end Thatcher's reign

Demonstrators mock the Prime Minister, Margaret Thatcher, as they protest against the deeply unpopular Poll Tax. Similar demonstrations in London were to erupt into riots.

Mrs Thatcher, nicknamed "The Iron Lady", gave her name to a political movement and ruled Britain as leader of the Conservative party for 11 years. Her government radically reduced trade union power, encouraged free enterprise and slowly privatised nationalised industries and services. Her victories over the Argentinians in 1982 and the miners in 1984 had persuaded many – possibly including herself – that she was unassailable. By November 1990, however, inflation was rising, the Poll Tax was proving as unsuccessful as it was unpopular and unease was stirring in the Conservative ranks.

On November 13, Sir Geoffrey Howe, the former Deputy Prime Minster, who had resigned over differences on European policy, made a speech openly attacking the Prime Minister. The next day, former Minister of Defence Michael Heseltine announced his decision to stand against her in a leadership contest. When Mrs Thatcher failed – by four votes – to secure an outright victory in the first leadership ballot on November 22, she resigned. She might not have been voted out of office, but it was clear support for her was waning fast. She made no secret of the fact that she felt she had been betrayed.

On November 28, Margaret Thatcher left 10 Downing Street as Prime Minister for the last time. John Major – who Mrs Thatcher described at the time as "pure gold" – was voted her successor by Conservative MPs. At 47, he was the youngest British Prime Minister this century.

Also this year...

Observer *journalist hanged in Iraq for spying*

Germany re-unified

Prisoners riot in Strangeways prison

John Gummer MP and his four-year-old daughter eat hamburgers to ally public fears about BSE

Ian Gow MP assassinated by IRA

Nintendo Game Boy launched

Nelson Mandela freed

Boris Yeltsin elected president of Russian federation

Lech Walesa president of Poland

Hubble Space telescope launched

Mary Robinson becomes first female president of Republic of Ireland

Britain joins the ERM

Paul Gascoigne cries as England lose World Cup semi-final to West Germany on penalties

Patricia Cahill and Karyn Smith arrested in Bangkok for drugs smuggling

Iraq, led by Saddam Hussein, invades Kuwait

Deaths: Ava Gardner, Aaron Copland, Laurence Durrell, Sir Len Hutton, A.J.P. Taylor, Greta Garbo, Max Wall, Sammy Davis Jr, Malcolm Muggeridge

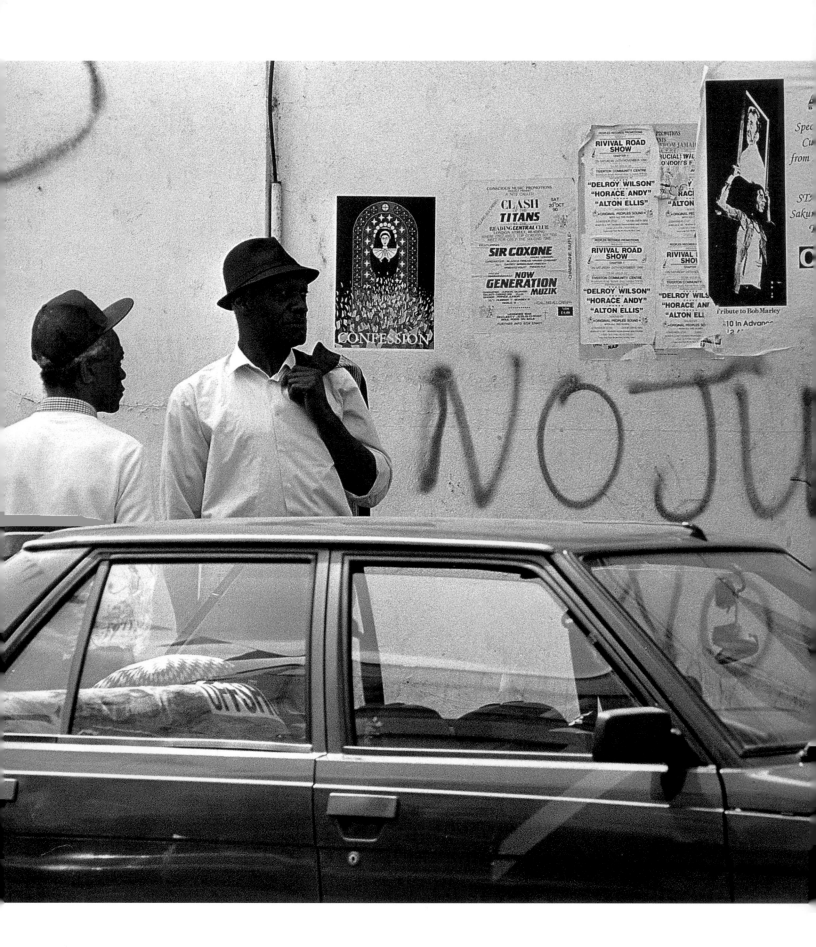

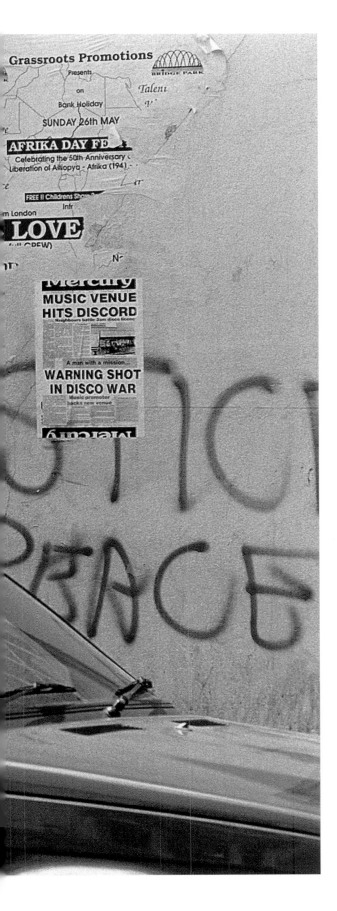

Operation Trident leads to urban chic

Two men look at a familiar sight: flyers and graffiti on the Portobello Road in west London's Notting Hill. The area had undergone some radical changes since it saw race riots in the fifties. A decade later, a large number of West Indian immigrants were well established in the area. The Notting Hill Carnival – which was to become a world-famous event attended by millions – was begun by locals, mainly of Trinidadian origin, in 1966. Throughout the sixties and seventies, the area's bohemian atmosphere attracted writers and artists.

Notting Hill had always had something of a split personality. While some areas were relentlessly chic – and correspondingly expensive – others remained stubbornly run-down. The All Saints Road was a particular black spot and by the mid-eighties it had become a no-go area, the target of frequent drugs raids by the police. Ian Hutcheson, deputy divisional commander of Notting Hill, remembered: "In 1987, we launched Operation Trident because there was an open street market in drugs and we had to … regain control of the streets."

The success of Operation Trident, despite claims of harassment by some young blacks, coincided with a dramatic shift in perceptions of the area generally. Within a decade, Notting Hill was to become one of the most sought-after addresses in London.

Also this year...

Allies launch operation "Desert Storm" on Iraq; Kuwait liberated; nine out of the 16 British soldiers killed were hit by "friendly fire"

IRA fire mortars at Downing Street

Hard-line coup in USSR fails; Gorbachev steps down in Yeltsin's favour; USSR dissolved, CIS formed

Bank of Credit and Commerce International (BCCI) collapses

Helen Sharman first Briton in space

Mike Powell long jumps 8.95 metres, breaking Bob Beamon's 22-year-old record

England wins Five Nations' Rugby Grand Slam for first time in 11 years

John McCarthy and Terry Waite, released by Islamic Jihad

Maastricht Treaty signed

Warsaw Pact dissolved

Yugoslav civil wars start as Slovenia and Croatia declare independence

Compulsory tests for seven-year-olds introduced in schools

President F.W. de Klerk announces end of South African apartheid

Miscarriage of justice upheld and "Birmingham six" freed after serving 16 years

Poll Tax abandoned

Bryan Adam's hit Everything I do, I do it for you *is number one for a record 16 weeks*

Deaths: Dame Margot Fonteyn, Graham Greene, Sir David Lean, Dame Peggy Ashcroft, Miles Davis, Rajiv Gandhi, Freddie Mercury, Robert Maxwell

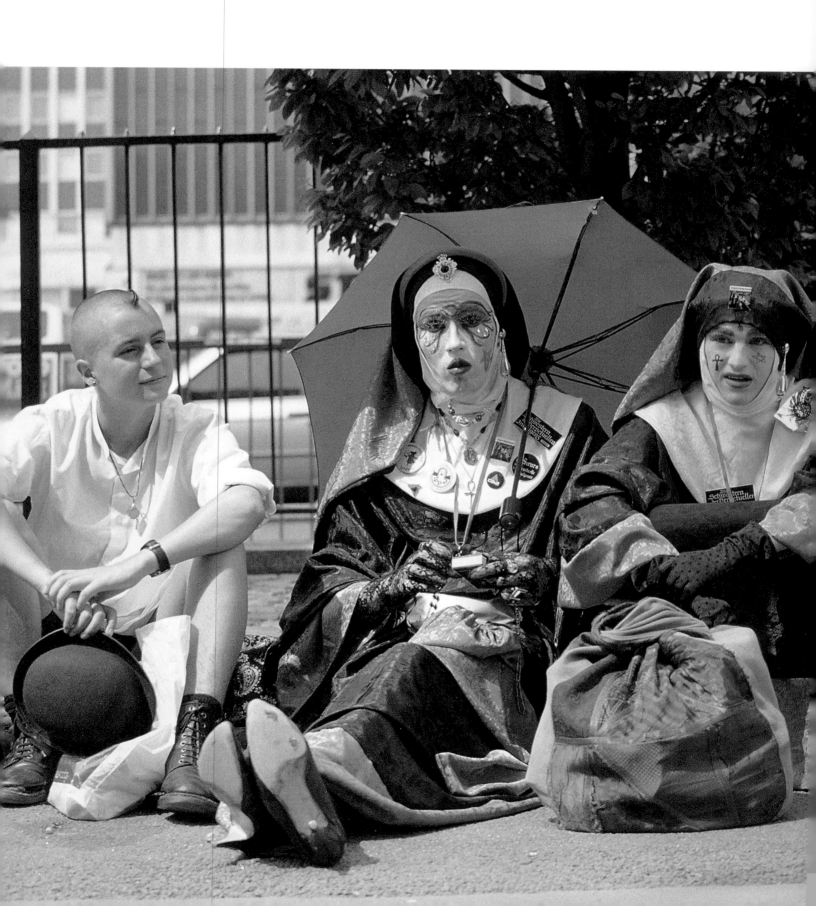

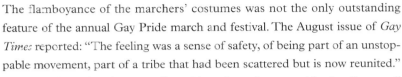

The tribe that marched with pride

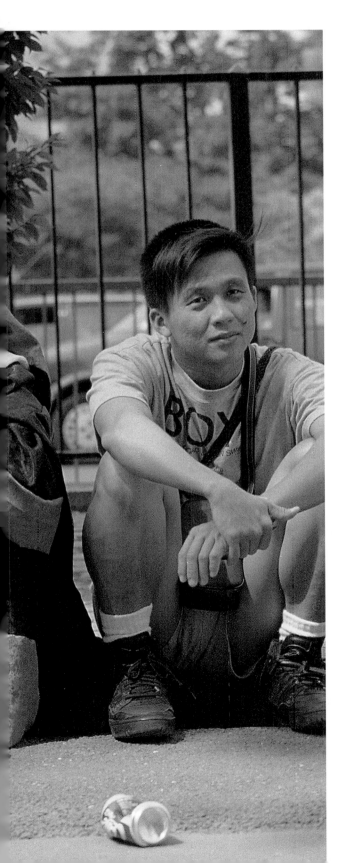

The flamboyance of the marchers' costumes was not the only outstanding feature of the annual Gay Pride march and festival. The August issue of *Gay Times* reported: "The feeling was a sense of safety, of being part of an unstoppable movement, part of a tribe that had been scattered but is now reunited."

Gay liberation is generally said to have begun with the Stonewall Rebellion in New York on the night of June 27, 1969 – which also happened to be the same day as gay icon Judy Garland's funeral. Riots started when police from the Public Morals Section of the First Division of the New York City Police Department used force to remove patrons from the Stonewall Inn, a gay bar in Greenwich Village. Gay liberation groups soon sprang up across the US and the following year across the world.

By the time the marchers pictured here took part in Pride '92, gay rights marches were well established in London. The Gay Liberation Front was the first to organise public protest marches in Britain – 80 protesters took part in a torchlit procession on Islington's Highbury Fields in November 1970. The first London march – known as Gay Pride – was held two years later, when an estimated 2,000 gays and lesbians marched to Hyde Park.

By 1992, thousands – gay and straight – had joined the march, which culminated in one of the largest free music festivals in the world, on Clapham Common. But the combined festival and march came to an end in 1998, when the festival collapsed due to lack of financial backing. The following year Gay Pride was replaced by the London Mardi Gras. The march became a "parade" and the festival moved to Finsbury Park.

Also this year...

Princess Anne divorces Captain Mark Phillips and marries Commander Tim Lawrence

Andrew Morton's Diana, Her True Story shocks Britain; Prince Charles and Princess Diana separate

Chris Patten becomes last governor of Hong Kong

Barcelona hosts Olympics

Civil war in Bosnia; Sarajevo besieged by Serb forces

Bill Clinton elected US president

John Major leads Conservatives to narrow election victory

John Smith becomes Labour leader

Lloyds of London reveals £2 billion loss

Polytechnics granted university status

Militant Hindus destroy Ayodhya mosque in India

Earth Summit held in Rio de Janeiro

Britain leaves ERM after pound collapses

Windsor Castle damaged by fire

Church of England votes for ordination for women

Deaths: Isaac Asimov, Menachem Begin, Willy Brandt, Leonard Cheshire, Alexander Dubcek, Benny Hill, Frankie Howerd, Francis Bacon, Marlene Dietrich

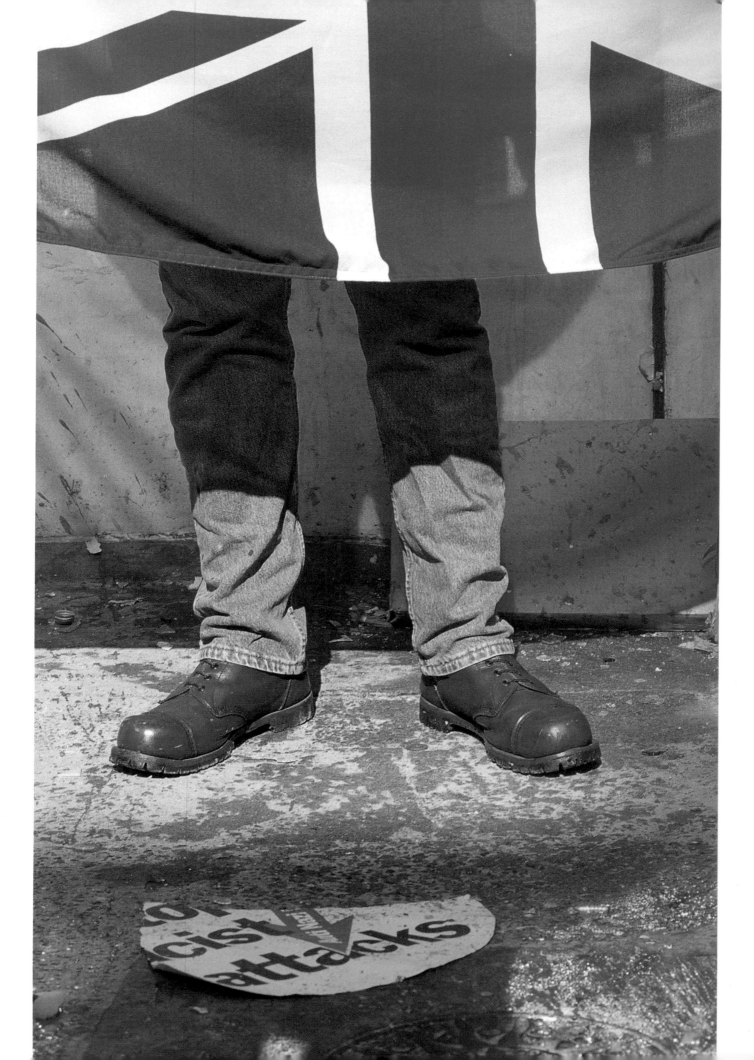

Fascism revisits the East End

The British National Party (BNP) demonstrate outside an Asian Halal shop in London's Brick Lane, on Sunday, September 19. The BNP, a small extremist right-wing party, believes, among other things, in ending immigration, introducing repatriation and reinstating the death penalty – shades of Oswald Mosley's Blackshirts who marched through the East End in the thirties.

Trouble was to break out when about 400 anti-Nazi protesters arrived and took over the market pitch that the BNP usually holds on Bethnal Green Road. Superintendent Nigel Wildman, one of around 200 police called to the skirmishes, said: "Normally, the two sides stand across the road shouting abuse at each other … Feelings were running high, but there were no serious injuries and the situation never got out of control."

Twenty-seven people were arrested, 23 of whom were anti-Nazi protesters. However, Richard Edmonds, deputy leader and national organiser of the BNP, and three others were later arrested for violent disorder after a black man, Steven Browne, was injured while walking past the Ship Pub in Bethnal Green with his white girlfriend. Edmonds was convicted of the attack in June the following year. Derek Beackon, who had recently been elected as BNP councillor for the Isle of Dogs, was present at the trial.

Earlier that year, on April 22, a black teenager, Stephen Lawrence, was stabbed to death by six white youths in Eltham, southeast London. Edmonds, acting as spokesman for the BNP, which denied connections with the murder, issued a statement claiming "We do not advocate violence to our members."

Also this year...

Oil slick near Shetlands from tanker Braer dispersed by wind and waves

Queen to pay income tax; Buckingham Palace opened to tourists

Single European Market in operation

Britain ratifies Maastricht Treaty

Czechoslovakia splits into Czech Republic and Slovakia

Jon Venables and Robert Thompson, both aged 10, charged with murder of two-year-old Jamie Bulger

Norman Lamont, Chancellor of Exchequer, dismissed

Boris Yeltsin suspends Russian parliament

Seven die in World Trade Centre bomb

Grand National abandoned after two false starts

Yassir Arafat, PLO leader, and Israeli Prime Minister Yitzhak Rabin sign Middle East peace deal

Fermat's Last Theorem solved

British and Irish Prime Ministers sign Northern Ireland peace deal

Deaths: Rudolf Nureyev, Audrey Hepburn, Arthur Ashe, Bobby Moore, Vincent Price, Les Dawson, Federico Fellini, Dizzy Gillespie, Jo Grimond, James Hunt, Sir William Golding, Anthony Burgess

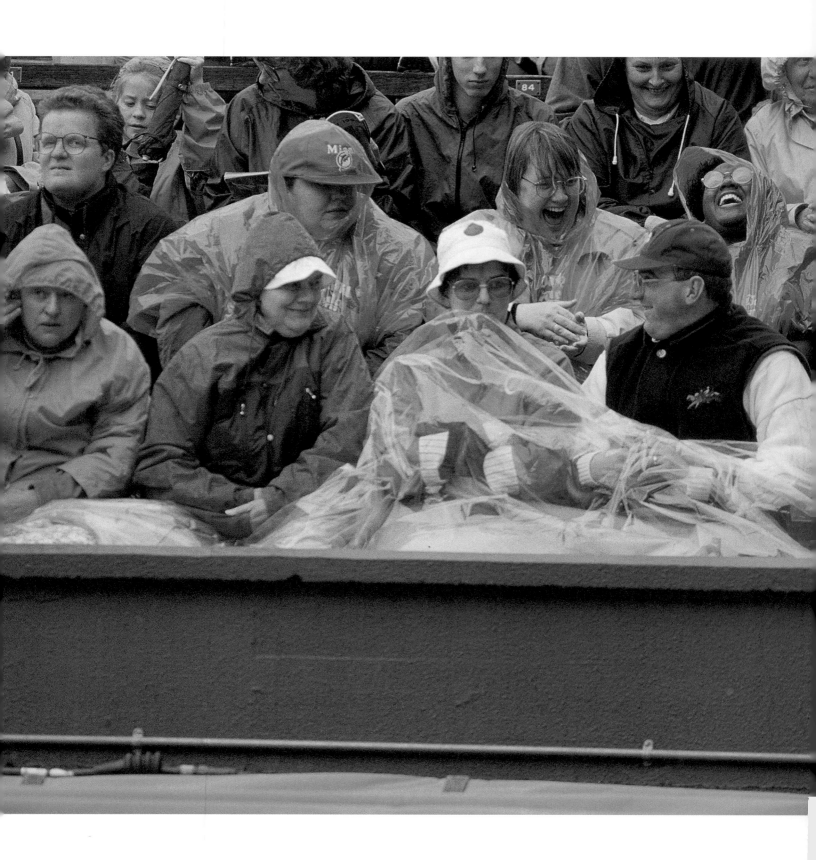

Strawberries and cream ... and rain

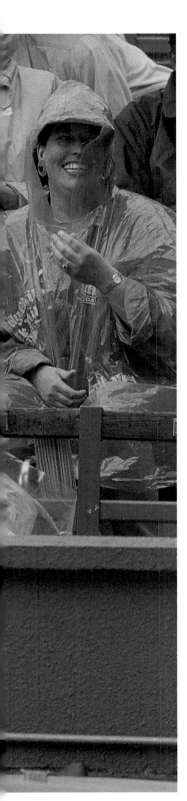

If anything captures the spirit of British life it is Wimbledon. For millions it has come to symbolise all that is best about sport, spiced with a dash of royalty and enjoyed with much jollity. That spirit has prevailed despite the coming of professionalism in 1968, the occasional tantrums by players on court – not least by the mercurial John McEnroe – and the growth of commercialisation through corporate entertaining.

The first Lawn Tennis Championships were held at The All England Croquet and Lawn Tennis Club in 1877. Originally an event for British amateurs, the Championships grew to attract international players, with the American May Sutton becoming the first non-British champion in 1905. Since then British players have not fared well: there have been two just native men's champions since 1907 (Arthur Gore in 1908-9 and Fred Perry in 1934-6). The women have done rather better.

In 1990, the Czech-born American Martina Navratilova became the first player to win the Ladies' Singles nine times. Navratilova is eloquent about her fondness for Wimbledon, in particular the crowds on Centre Court: "It goes beyond respect and the fact that they like the way I play. They've been with me for years and I feel like I'm playing in front of a whole bunch of friends."

Navratilova played her last Wimbledon in 1994. As she bowed out, the less charismatic American Pete Sampras beat Croatian Goran Ivanisevic to become Wimbledon men's champion for the second year running. Fred Perry, the last British singles champion, was not impressed. He remarked: "That must have been one of the most boring finals in history."

Also this year...

IRA declares ceasefire; Loyalists declare ceasefire seven weeks later

Lieutenant-General Sir Michael Rose appointed head of UN peace-keeping troops in Bosnia

South Africa re-joins Commonwealth

Tony Blair becomes Labour leader

John Major launches "Back to Basics" campaign

Homosexual age of consent lowered to 18

Fred West charged with 10 murders in Gloucester

Israel withdraws from Jericho and the Gaza Strip

Widespread killing of Tutsis in Rwanda

US troops invade Haiti

Brian Lara scores record 501 in a first-class cricket innings

NAFTA comes into effect

First Anglican women priests in Britain ordained

Channel Tunnel inaugurated

Sunday shop opening legalised

Deaths: Brian Johnston, Eugene Ionesco, Sir Matt Busby, Erich Honecker, Richard Nixon, John Osborne, Kurt Cobain, John Smith, Dennis Potter, Roy Castle, Sir Karl Popper, Burt Lancaster

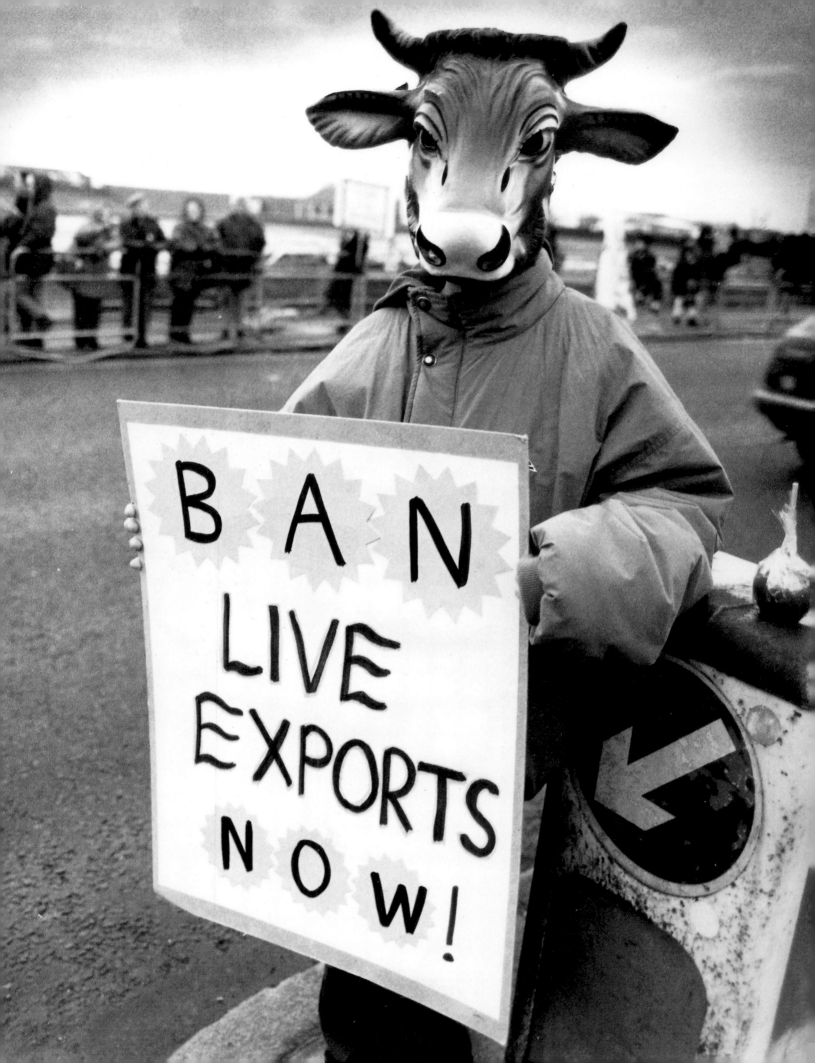

When Middle England rose in protest

A boy in a mask joins more than 250 protesters at Shoreham, West Sussex, to block the transportation of live animals across the Channel for slaughter. The protest erupted into violence the following day, January 3, when twice the number of activists attacked lorries and others threw themselves front of the vehicles. Jeremy Francis, a haulage contractor who was caught in the attack, complained to *The Times*: "I have a £120,000 vehicle which has been smashed to pieces. They have slashed air lines, smashed headlamps and thrown rocks and missiles through the windscreens." Compassion In World Farming, the largest group behind the protests, which was characterised by its support among the middle class and middle-aged, later claimed that the protest had been infiltrated by militant extremists.

The lucrative calf trade was a particular area of contention – hence the boy's mask. The majority of exported calves were transported to Holland and France where they were reared in crates to produce whiter meat for veal, a practice that had been banned in Britain on grounds of cruelty. In February, William Waldegrave, Minister of Agriculture, proposed a six-point action plan which included attempting to bring forward a European Commission review of veal crate-farming, looking into improving veal production in Britain and prosecuting those who failed Government livestock export standards.

The same day as the plan was announced, tragedy struck at Coventry Airport when Jill Phipps, 31, was killed at a protest against livestock flights when she threw herself at the cab of a slow-moving lorry.

Also this year...

Fred West hangs himself in custody

Footballer Eric Cantona attacks spectator

Austria, Sweden and Finland join EU

John Major and John Bruton present peace plan for Northern Ireland

Israeli Prime Minister Yitzhak Rabin assassinated

Clause IV of Labour's constitution replaced

David Trimble becomes Ulster Unionist leader

Barings Bank placed in administration after trader Nick Leeson accumulates massive losses

Aum Shinrikyo cult releases poison gas in Tokyo subway

Kobe earthquake kills 6,000

168 die in Oklahoma City bombing

Microsoft launches Windows 95

Third hottest July of the century

NATO launches air strikes against Serb forces in Bosnia; Dayton agreement produces peace plan for Bosnia

Princess Diana gives interview on Panorama about her marriage

Deaths: Peter Cook, Gerald Durrell, Fred Perry, James Herriot, Ronnie Kray, Ginger Rogers, Harold Wilson, Kingsley Amis, Alec Douglas-Home, Lana Turner, Harold Larwood

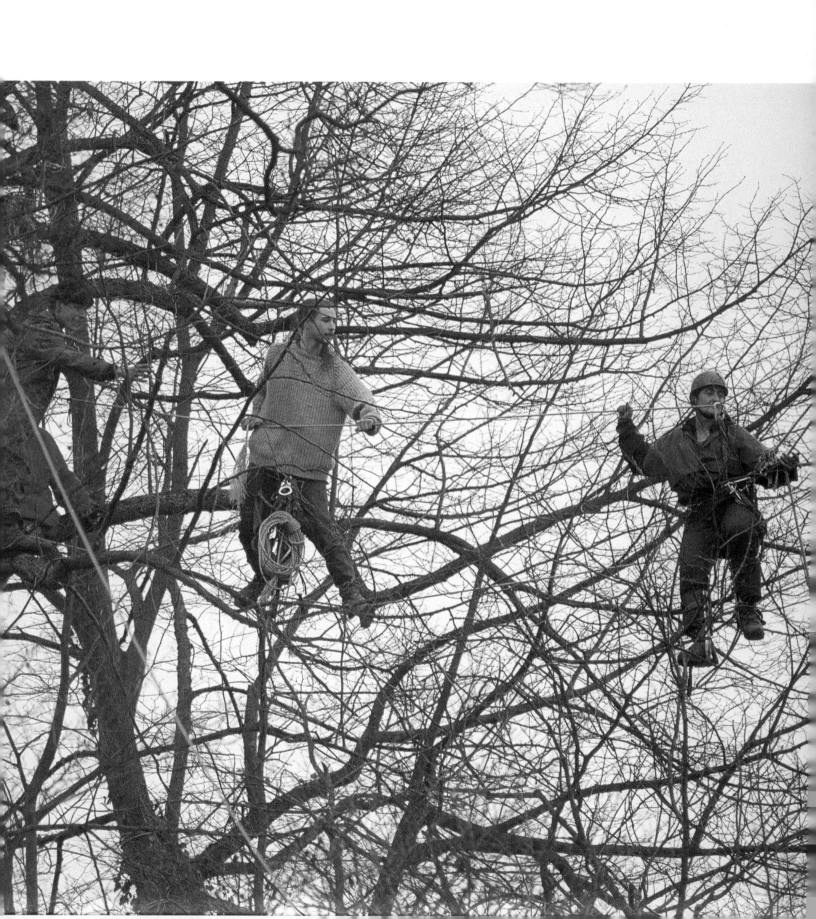

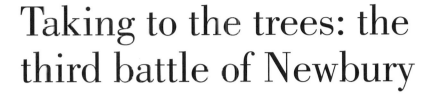

Taking to the trees: the third battle of Newbury

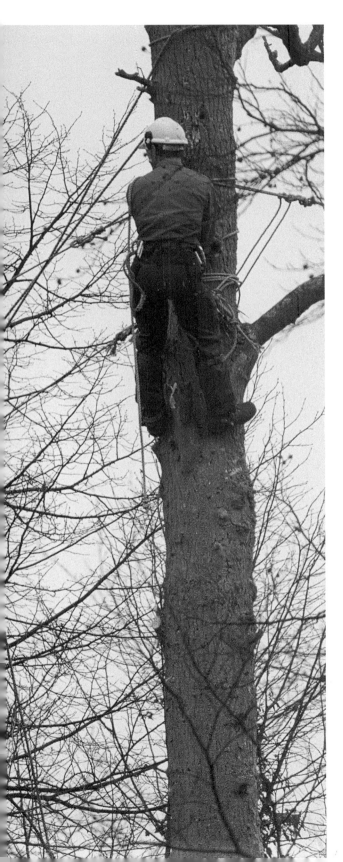

By the early nineties, Newbury, in Berkshire, suffered some of the worst traffic congestion in Europe with an estimated 50,600 vehicles passing through the town daily. Local shop owners believed commerce was adversely affected by the traffic; Newbury Racecourse goers were put off by the poor road access.

In July 1995, the Transport Secretary, Dr Brian Mawhinney, approved a nine-mile bypass, which was to cost £100 million. Protesters claimed the route of the road, to the west of the town, would damage the environment by crossing a protected Civil War battle site, one and a half acres of Snelsmore Common – home to a rare population of nightjars – and the Kennet and Lambourn rivers, where there was an endangered species of snail. It would also pass within 600 yards of Grade-I listed Donnington Castle.

Protesters hailed the dispute as The Third Battle of Newbury (the other two had been the Civil War encounters of 1643 and 1644). By January 1996, nine camps had been established along the route, each maintaining a 24-hour look-out. When the bulldozers came, the demonstrators – numbering 6,000 at the protest's height – planned to seek refuge either within an elaborate network of tunnels or in the trees. About 60 treehouses were constructed, linked with walkways and stocked with several weeks' supplies of food and water. A thousand people were arrested over nearly four months. One of the protesters, who styled himself "Swampy", earned public notoriety when he and other supporters burrowed away in underground tunnels to thwart bailiffs.

The Newbury bypass opened on Tuesday, November 17, 1998.

Also this year...

Prince and Princess of Wales divorce

Boris Yeltsin re-elected Russian president

Taliban capture Afghan capital Kabul

UN war crimes tribunal opens in The Hague

Restored Globe Theatre opens

Olympic Games held in Atlanta

First animal cloned, "Dolly" the sheep

Government admits a possible link between BSE and CJD; European Commission imposes a worldwide ban on British beef exports

IRA ceasefire ends as two are killed by Docklands bomb

Thomas Hamilton kills 16 children,

their teacher and himself in Dunblane

230 die when TWA flight 800 explodes between New York and Paris

England loses Euro 96 semi-final to Germany on penalties

Benjamin Netanyahu elected Israeli Prime Minister

Scott Report on arms sale to Iraq published

Deaths: Dr Timothy Leary, Ella Fitzgerald, Andreas Papandreou, Willie Rushton, Molly Keane, Jessica Mitford, Jean-Bédel Bokassa, Sir Frank Whittle, Beryl Reid, Terence Donovan, Marjorie Proops, François Mitterrand, Archbishop Derek Worlock, Gene Kelly

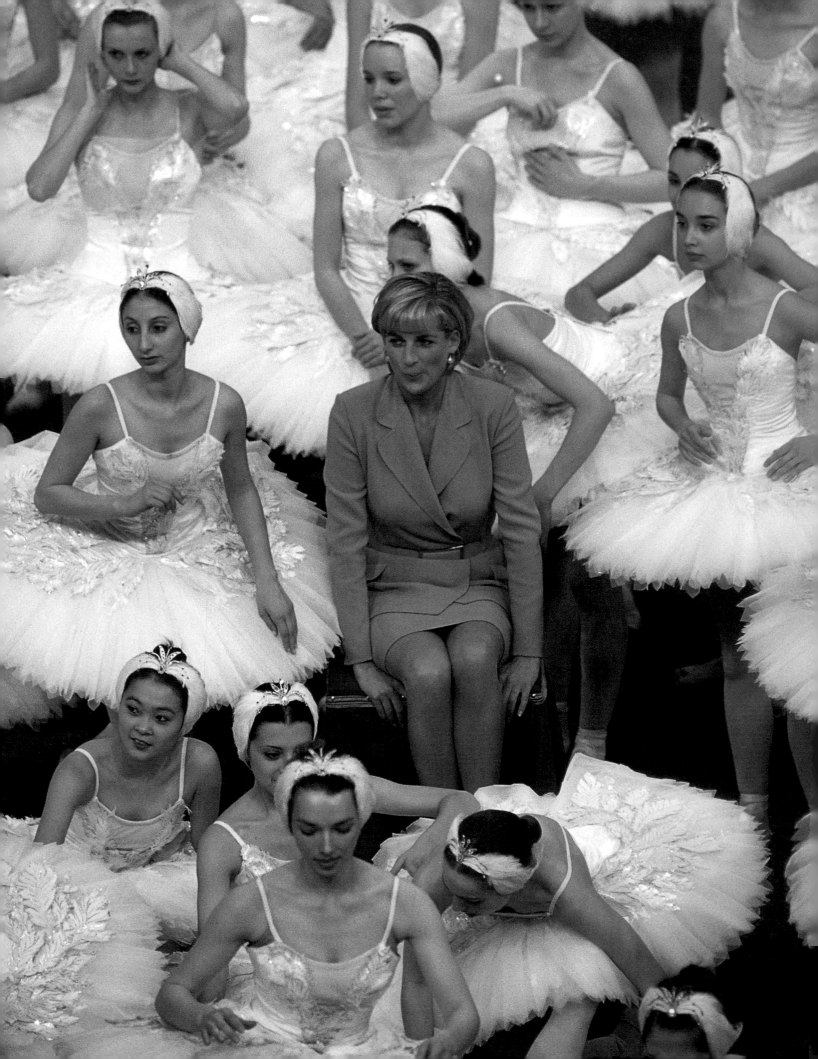

Dance for the muse of a time

Diana, Princess of Wales poses with members the English National Ballet at the Royal Albert Hall during rehearsals for a production of *Swan Lake*. The Princess was patron of the troupe for eight years and had, as a child, dreamt of dancing professionally herself.

Joanne Clarke, one of the ballerinas, remembered: "The princess would often arrive unannounced in the studios to watch a rehearsal or see a class … Once she even arrived with a huge birthday cake for us. She also showed a private interest in the welfare of individual members of the company." Diana's presence was enough to ensure that pictures of her with the dancers, taken to promote the ballet's production of *Swan Lake*, had an international appeal

The Princess remained the world media's favourite subject, despite her divorce from Prince Charles, and her own attempts to protect her privacy. Her relationship with Dodi Fayed caused a frenzy of media interest. When Diana and Dodi left the Ritz Hotel in Paris on August 31, they were pursued by the *paparazzi*. The chase culminated in tragedy in the underpass at the Pont d'Alema as their car crashed. Of the four passengers in the car, only Trevor Rees-Jones, a bodyguard, survived. It was later revealed that the driver, Henri Paul, was several times over the legal alcohol limit.

The Princess' death dominated the world's headlines and provoked an extraordinary surge of mourning across the world.

Also this year...

Tony Blair leads Labour Party to landslide general election victory

William Hague replaces John Major as Conservative Party leader

Hong Kong handed back to China

Kofi Annan becomes UN Secretary-General

Scottish and Welsh referendums vote for power shift from Westminster

Six British tourists die in Luxor massacre

British au pair Louise Woodward convicted of manslaughter in Massachusetts

Hungary, Czech Republic and Poland join NATO

Earthquake in Italy damages art treasures of Assisi

Comet Hale-Bopp visible across the world

Michael Stone charged with murder of Lin and Megan Russell

IRA restores its ceasefire; Mo Mowlam launches all-party Northern Ireland peace talks

Spice Girls take the pop world by storm

Deaths: Alan Ginsberg, Denis Compton, Laurie Lee, Jacques Cousteau, Deng Xiaoping, Gianni Versace, Hastings Banda, Robert Mitchum, Sir George Solti, Mother Theresa, Michael Hutchence, Sir Isaiah Berlin

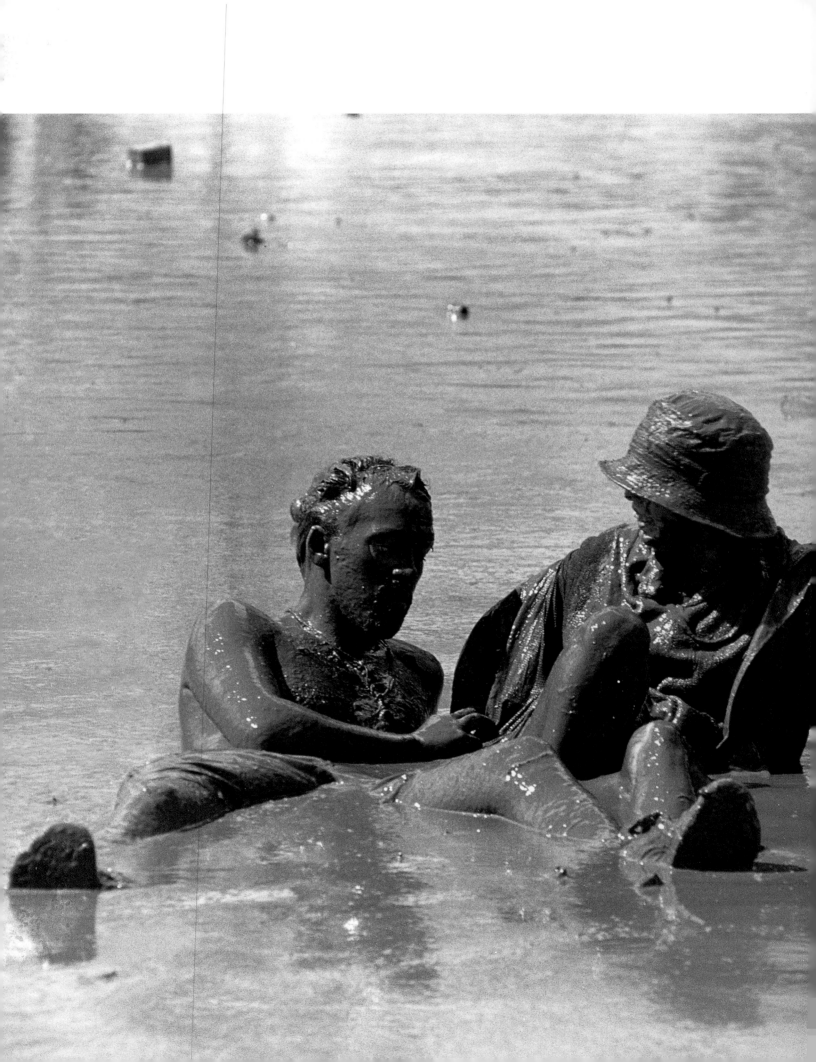

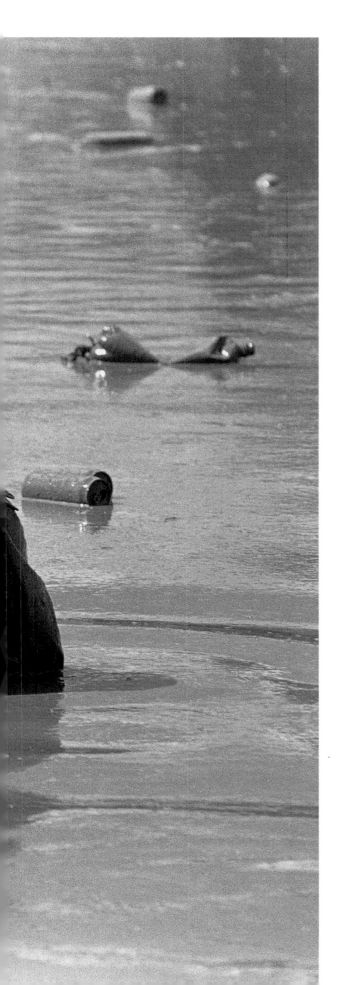

And the bands played on …

A pre-festival weather forecast on the web claimed that: "Reports from the site over the last few days say it is 'a little waterlogged', but as the weather is expected to improve the ground will dry out quite well – for farmland it drains VERY well."

Unfortunately for the 100,000 who attended the Glastonbury Festival in Somerset that year, the ground didn't drain as effectively as hoped. This was the second year running that Glastonbury had been almost swept away by bad weather. But attractions such as Pulp, Portishead, Catatonia and even Bob Dylan made sure it wasn't a complete wash-out.

But for many younger festival-goers, more distressing than the mud and wet was the increased percentage of a slightly maturer audience. Jason Holmes, spokesman for the festival, told *The Times*: "We've always had a wide cross-section of artists and fans here. We don't just want lots of indie kids, because it's for everyone. Think about it this way, if you came to the first festival aged 10, you'd be 40 now, and we have plenty of fans like that who come back and back."

Within the eight miles of the perimeter fence both young and old should have had room enough to do their own thing. For those bored with the bands, Glastonbury offered shops, food from around the world, alternative entertainment such as mime or cabaret and, this year, WaterAid's African-style "musical toe tapping toilets". The festival made donations to Greenpeace, Oxfam and WaterAid and a number of smaller organisations.

Also this year...

Japan offers official apology to Second World War PoWs

The Northern Ireland Peace Agreement is endorsed by referendum; David Trimble and John Hume awarded Nobel Peace Prize

President Clinton appeals for America's forgiveness over his relationship with Monica Lewinsky; he is impeached by the House of Representatives

Peter Mandelson resigns after scandal over home loan from Geoffrey Robinson

France wins World Cup on home soil

India and Pakistan carry out nuclear tests

Anthony Gormley's statue Angel of the North *erected overlooking Gateshead*

7,000 die as Hurricane Mitch strikes Central America

"Unabomber" Theodore Kaczynski sentenced to life imprisonment

12 Britons kidnapped in Yemen

Deaths: Frank Muir, Enoch Powell, Dr Spock, Sir Michael Tippett, Pol Pot, Linda McCartney, Frank Sinatra, Sir David English, Catherine Cookson, Maureen O'Sullivan, Lew Grade, Tammy Wynette, Lord Rothermere, Ted Hughes

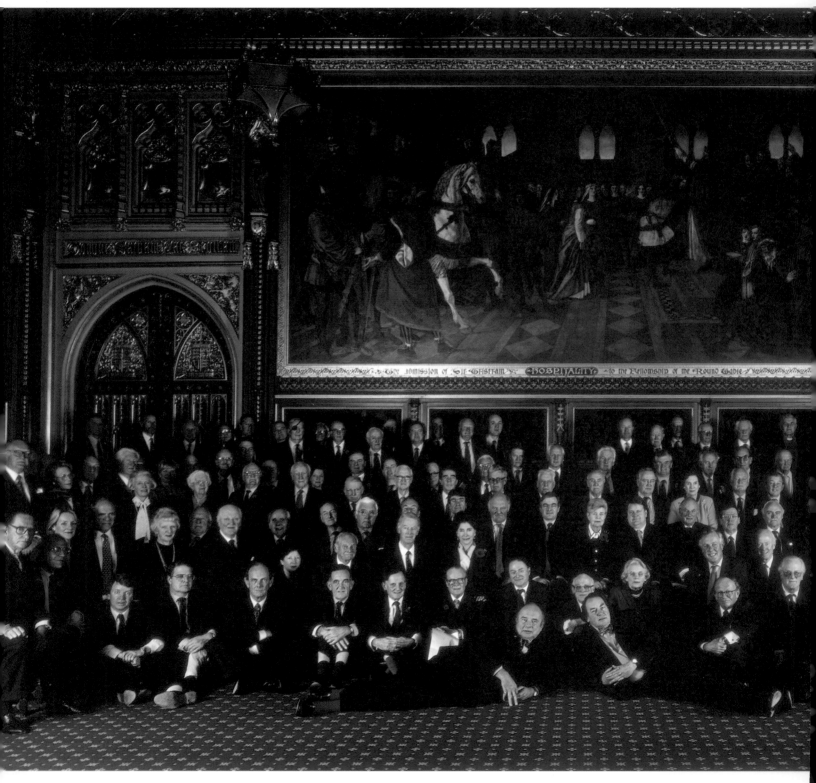

The end of the peer show

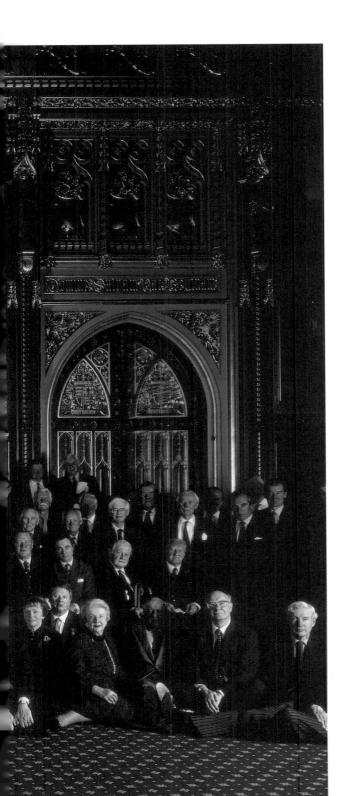

Eight hundred years of history, of power and privilege, came to an end when the House of Lords was prorogued at 5.18 pm on November 12 and scores of hereditary peers, many pictured here, lost their jobs. But not without a flutter of resistance. The hereditary peers accused the Prime Minister, Tony Blair, of trying to create an upper house filled with "Tony's cronies" and there were familiar objections that they were being ousted without a clear replacement. The Earl of Caithness complained that there would be almost a second hereditary system with a quarter of the members of a future house appointed by the Prime Minister. There was, however, no way of avoiding the inevitable. As the peers listened grim-faced, few grimmer than a funereally-dressed Baroness Thatcher, the Clerk of the Crown read out the words: "The House of Lords Act" and the Clerk of the Parliaments replied in the traditional Norman French: "La rayne le veult" With that – and one stifled boo – all but about 100 hereditary peers shuffled out of the chamber. Those who remained owed their place to a compromise measure which had allowed the hereditaries to elect 92 of their own number to remain in the Lords during a transitional period.

The departure of most hereditaries certainly changed the character of the house but had no immediate impact on its political balance. With 640 peers still *in situ* the Labour party were at first only able to muster about 180 supporters, though as many as 50 Labour peers were expected to be appointed to achieve parity with the Tories.

Earlier, 400 Tory peers had gathered for a last picture show in the sumptuous Robing Room, where the Queen puts on her ceremonial robes and crown before the State Opening of Parliament. The picture was taken by the Earl of Drogheda, better known under his professional name, the society photographer Derry Moore. It is a profession he can pursue with additional vigour. He was not re-elected.

Also this year...

NATO troops enter Kosovo after bombing campaign to halt ethnic cleansing of Kosovan Albanians

Scotland and Wales elect new devolved assemblies

Prince Edward marries Sophie Rhys-Jones

The Euro is launched

Nelson Mandela retires as South African president

British courts rule General Pinochet be extradited to Spain on torture charges

George Mallory's body found after 75 years on Everest

Total solar eclipse visible from Cornwall

TV presenter Jill Dando shot dead

30 killed in Paddington rail crash

Deaths: King Hussein of Jordan, Lord Denning, Stanley Kubrick, Yehudi Menuhin, Sir Alf Ramsey, Dirk Bogarde, Cardinal Basil Hume, Iris Murdoch, William Whitelaw, Ernie Wise, Screaming Lord Sutch, John F. Kennedy Jr, Alan Clark

Picture credits